Imaging in Management of Breast Diseases

Ekta Dhamija • S. V. S. Deo
Editors

Imaging in Management of Breast Diseases

Volume 2, Disease-based Approach

Springer

Editors
Ekta Dhamija
Department of Diagnostic and Interventional Onco-Radiology
Dr B.R.A.IRCH, All India Institute of Medical Sciences
New Delhi, Delhi, India

S. V. S. Deo
Department of Surgical Oncology
Indraprastha Apollo Hospital
New Delhi, Delhi, India

ISBN 978-981-96-4997-6 ISBN 978-981-96-4998-3 (eBook)
https://doi.org/10.1007/978-981-96-4998-3

This Springer imprint is published by the registered company Springer Nature Singapore Pte Ltd.
The registered company address is: 152 Beach Road, #21-01/04 Gateway East, Singapore 189721, Singapore

All India Institute of Medical Sciences, New Delhi
Our Land of Action
And
Our families who stayed with us during all ups and downs in the entire journey of this venture

Foreword

Imaging shapes a patient's entire treatment pathway; from the moment an abnormality is detected, it helps to determine the next steps, whether it's further investigation, surgical planning, or monitoring treatment response. This volume of the book is continuum of the previous efforts outlining the various facets involved in management of breast diseases. It includes disease-specific scenarios and surgical approaches to breast diseases, malignancies, and axillary nodes. What makes this book truly special is the collective expertise behind it. Radiologists, surgeons, oncologists, and pathologists have contributed their knowledge, ensuring a multidisciplinary perspective that reflects the realities of modern breast cancer care. This collaboration highlighted the role of different imaging modalities and multi-modality algorithmic approach with illustrative cases in specific scenarios, which would assist the readers in patient evaluation on routine basis.

The field of breast cancer diagnosis and treatment continues to evolve rapidly, and through shared knowledge and teamwork, we can make a meaningful impact in early detection, accurate diagnosis, and improved patient care. This volume has been complied to serve as a valuable resource for radiologists, breast surgeons, oncologists, and anyone involved in the care of patients with breast diseases. I hope this book becomes more than just a reference—it should feel like a guide, one that offers clarity when faced with complex cases.

New Delhi, India S. V. S. Deo

Preface

Breast imaging has become one of the most sought-after subspecialty among radiologists. One of the factor is the increasing incidence of breast cancer and the other is increasing awareness in the society. Investigation of any symptomatic female is like putting all the blocks of a puzzle together incorporating clinical inputs, radiology insights, and pathology results. At one end of the spectrum are the features that would indicate suspicion of breast cancer upfront, and on the other hand, there will be imaging features illustrating clear benign findings which would not need any further work-up. Radiologists are often on first line of detection and this makes their role deeply responsible. Therefore it becomes imperative to not only understand the basics of each imaging modality but also to be aware of when and how to utilize them appropriately

This book was thus planned in two volumes in order to do justice to this complex field where *Volume 1* was more like the groundwork elaborating on the various breast imaging techniques, exploring their clinical applications, and focused on the importance of a multidisciplinary approach in breast disease management. The bigger challenge in clinical practice is dealing with the patients in real-time and making the right decision even during uncertainty. That is what *Volume 2* aims to tackle. This volume consists of real-world, case-based learning because in day-to-day practice, no two patients present in the same way. The scenarios may vary from a teenager with hormonal breast changes to a woman with persistent nipple discharge, or an incidental calcification on a routine mammogram, each of these pose a different diagnostic challenge. The key isn't just recognizing the patterns but knowing what to do next. This book provides a step-by-step approach to evaluate different clinical presentations, incorporating multimodality imaging comparisons, algorithmic flowcharts, and case illustrations to help clinician in decision making. We have aimed to create content that is not just theoretical but practical, equipping clinicians with decision-making strategies that can be directly applied in their practice.

In addition, it also addresses the surgical approaches to breast cancer, axillary lymph node evaluation, and the growing role of personalized oncology. With advancements in molecular profiling and targeted therapies, imaging has evolved beyond detection. It has ability to assess treatment response, guide surgical management, and optimize patient care. We've included these aspects into this book to provide a multidisciplinary perspective on breast disease care.

Like the first volume, this book is a product of collaboration bringing together some of the most respected breast radiologists and clinicians of India, each of them contributing their expertise and real-world experience. Writing and compiling these volumes has been an incredible experience.

As we present *Volume 2* of *Imaging in Breast Diseases,* we hope that it serves as a go-to resource for radiology residents, practicing radiologists, breast surgeons, oncologists, and all those involved in breast cancer care. More than just a textbook, we hope this book becomes a trusted guide which will help in providing clarity in complex cases and confidence in clinical decisions.

New Delhi, India Ekta Dhamija

Acknowledgments

We would like to express our sincere gratitude to the entire team of authors and technicians involved in compilation of the chapters and illustrations.

We are sincerely thankful to Dr. Sushma Bhatnagar and Dr. Sanjay Thulkar for their continuous support.

We extend our appreciation to entire publishing team for their hard work and cooperation.

Last but not the least; we are grateful to the esteemed institute IRCH, AIIMS, where we could not only dream about this venture but could make it come true.

Contents

1 How to Approach Symptomatic Breast

Bhawna Satija, Ekta Dhamija, and Babul Bansal

Abstract

Breast symptoms are common in clinical practice with more than a quarter of females affected by breast disease once in their lifetime. Palpable breast mass, mastalgia and nipple discharge are the commonly encountered symptoms. The vast majority of patients presenting with breast symptoms are diagnosed with benign breast disease. A multidisciplinary team forms the basis of breast approach to management, and all patients with breast symptoms should undergo triple assessment. The aim of clinical and imaging evaluation of these patients is to institute appropriate treatment and exclude any underlying breast malignancy. The various imaging modalities available for evaluation of breast-related symptoms include mammography, breast ultrasound and breast Magnetic Resonance Imaging. It is essential to formulate an approach to investigate breast-related symptoms, which is simple to follow, avoids over-investigation in benign cases and prevents misdiagnosis in malignant lesions. This chapter outlines multimodality imaging assessment of the patients presenting with breast symptoms based on patient's demography and results of clinical breast examination. The results of imaging are communicated in terms of BI-RADS category which guides further management.

Keywords

Triple assessment · Breast lump · Mastalgia Mastitis · Nipple discharge · Digital mammography · Ultrasound · MRI · BI-RADS

B. Satija (✉)
Department of Radiodiagnosis, Lady Hardinge Medical College, New Delhi, India

E. Dhamija
Department of Diagnostic and Interventional Onco-Radiology, IRCH, AIIMS, New Delhi, India

B. Bansal
Department of Surgical Oncology, IRCH, AIIMS, New Delhi, India

1.1 Introduction

Breast cancer is common; nevertheless benign breast disease is commoner, and anxiety related with breast disease is very concerning. The vast majority of patients presenting with breast symptoms are diagnosed with benign disease or variations of normalcy. It is now universally accepted that a multidisciplinary team (MDT) forms the basis for the best approach to the management of patients with breast disease. Clinical and imaging evaluation of patients presenting with breast symptoms aim to achieve dual objective: firstly to

E. Dhamija, S. V. S. Deo (eds.), *Imaging in Management of Breast Diseases*,
https://doi.org/10.1007/978-981-96-4998-3_1

determine the cause of symptoms to institute appropriate management and secondly to exclude breast malignancy as the etiology responsible for the symptom.

1.2 Clinical Presentation

According to a study by Eberl et al., breast complaints were reported by female patients in about 3% of all visits to the family physicians [1]. In another study conducted over a 10-year period, 16% of women in the age group 40–69 years experienced breast symptoms, and 10% reported breast symptoms at the time of mammography [2]. The common complaints with which a female may present to the physician include palpable breast mass or lump, pain (mastalgia), and nipple discharge (Fig. 1.1).

The prevalence of breast cancer among women presenting with symptoms related to the breast is estimated to be less than 10%. There is an increased risk of malignancy in patients with breast lump as compared to patients with breast pain [3]. Although the cause of symptoms in majority of the patients is benign, the symptoms often cause significant anxiety to the patient, and ruling out underlying carcinoma is crucial. According to World Health Organization, breast cancer was the most common cancer in women in

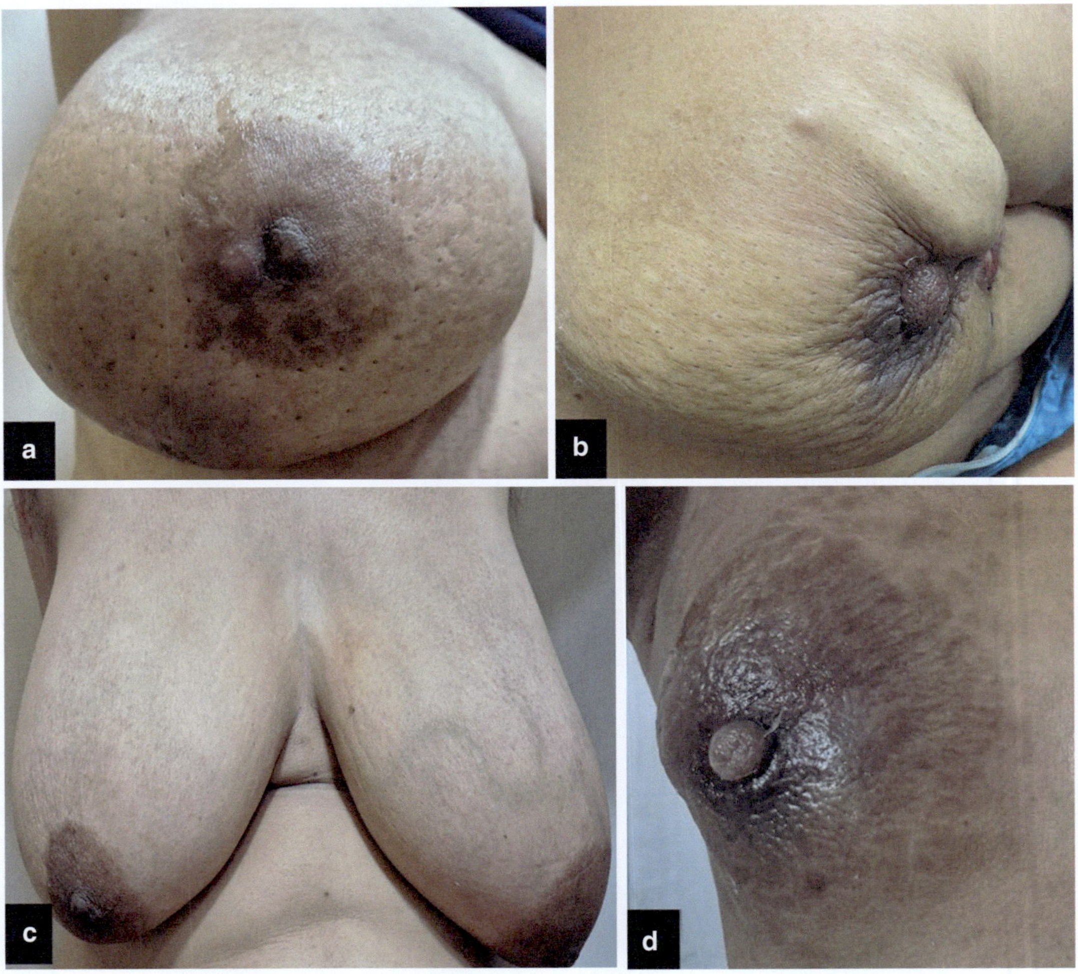

Fig. 1.1 Common breast-related symptoms. The patients may present with a lump (**a**, **b**), asymmetry in the size of the breast (**c**), skin (**d**) and nipple-areola complex changes (**b**, **d**) and nipple discharge

157 countries out of 185 and a cause of 670,000 deaths globally in 2022. Assessment and workup of a patient with breast symptoms are distinct from and do not substitute recommendations for breast cancer screening.

1.3 Triple Assessment

The diagnostic assessment of patients with breast complaints is based on triple assessment [4]. The investigations used in each case are guided by the patient's symptoms, clinical examination findings and age of the patient. Triple assessment includes three diagnostic components (Fig. 1.2).

- Medical history and clinical breast examination (CBE)
- Diagnostic imaging [Mammography and/or Ultrasound (US) (+/− Magnetic Resonance Imaging (MRI))]
- Non-excisional biopsy [fine needle aspiration cytology (FNAC) and core needle biopsy (CNB)]

The combination of these modalities, physical examination, imaging (mammogram and ultrasound) and biopsy, is more accurate than any modality alone [5]. The sensitivity of the triple test is more than either of the individual component and is recommended to achieve a maximum diagnostic accuracy while evaluating patients with breast symptoms. An appropriately employed triple test is accurate in detecting more than 99.6% of breast cancers. Any abnormal result achieved in any component of the triple assessment, which is either indeterminate, suspicious or malignant, requires referral to a specialist for further investigation and management. The probability of malignancy increases if more than one component is positive. Similarly, if the results are negative on all three components, further investigation is not warranted. A specialist intervention is recommended in case there are risk factors like positive family history or if the symptoms are persistent.

1.3.1 Medical History and Clinical Breast Examination

While addressing a breast complaint, an appropriate and detailed history taking is of paramount importance. Identification of known risk factors associated with breast diseases permits risk stratification of the patient. This includes a detailed family history of cancer with specific genetic mutations like BRCA1 and BRCA2, TP53, etc. Information regarding the patient's menstrual history (age of menarche and menopause), exogenous hormone administration (use of contraceptives, hormone replacement therapy or fertility

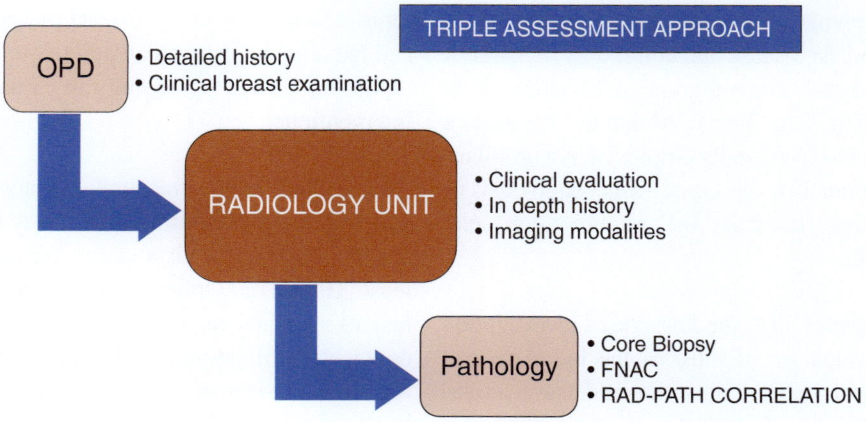

Fig. 1.2 Triple assessment approach to patients with breast symptoms

treatment), parity and lactational history and lifestyle risk factors such as smoking and alcohol consumption further add to the risk stratification process. The history of any previous breast pathology, breast surgery or radiation therapy is also significant.

A systematic physical examination of the breast is the next important step. The visual inspection is done in both upright and supine position. It is important to examine both breasts and observe the overall breast size, shape and symmetry. Some of the commonly adopted methods for clinical breast examination include the radial 'wagon wheel' method, the vertical strip method and the concentric circle method. The overall consistency of the breast is recorded as soft, firm or nodular. The position of any masses or focal tenderness is documented in terms of location in a conventional breast quadrant or clock face configuration and distance from the nipple mentioned. Eventually, the nipple-areola complex (NAC) should be carefully examined for morphology, skin changes and presence of nipple discharge, if any. Axillary and supraclavicular fossa examinations are an important part of any breast examination and should be examined for any palpable nodes.

1.3.2 Imaging

Radiological assessment of the breast is imperative for providing optimal breast health care to the patient. The choice of an appropriate diagnostic test is pivotal in establishing an accurate diagnosis of breast disease and commonly consists of ultrasound and mammogram, used alone or in combination. The breast Magnetic Resonance Imaging (MRI) is usually employed as a problem-solving modality in cases with equivocal or inconclusive findings on mammogram and ultrasound.

Mammography It is the first line of investigation for the evaluation of most of the breast-related symptoms. It helps in detection and characterization of lesions. Diagnostic mammograms are acquired to determine the cause of the symptom and essentially to exclude malignancy as the potential cause of symptoms.

Technique Digital mammography is preferred to film screen mammography, and the standard views include craniocaudal (CC) and mediolateral oblique (MLO) views. Even when symptoms are unilateral, bilateral mammograms should be performed to look for any asymmetry. Magnification and spot compression views can be obtained for further characterization if there is any suspicious abnormality on standard views. Supplementary views include lateral view, extended CC view, cleavage view, etc. for further characterization or detection of the abnormality. Digital breast tomosynthesis (DBT) is an advancement of digital mammography that creates volumetric reconstructions of the entire breast. It reduces the phenomena of summation and thereby reduces the masking effect of the overlapping normal breast tissue. This aids in better characterization of non-calcified lesions and avoids false-positive lesions. All the imaging modalities have been discussed in detail in the respective dedicated chapters.

Ultrasound It is an effective and well-established imaging modality for the evaluation of patients with breast symptoms. It is popular due to its wider availability and lack of radiation exposure. It is the first-line imaging modality of choice in women <30 years and a useful adjunct to mammography. The common indications for breast ultrasound include investigation of breast symptoms in female less than 30 years of age, pregnant and lactating women, as an adjunct to mammography or MRI, planning of image-guided interventions.

Technique Breast ultrasound is performed using real-time high-resolution linear array transducer (e.g. 6–12 MHz) with a centre frequency of at least 10 MHz. Optimal evaluation of breast lesions depends on technical factors like gain, depth, etc. Utilization of different settings including tissue harmonic imaging and compound imaging is beneficial. A thick layer of gel should be used for imaging superficial lesions and

NAC. The technique and lesion descriptors have been discussed in the dedicated chapter.

Magnetic Resonance Imaging MRI of the breast is an important addition to the diagnostic tools for the evaluation of the breast. It offers a very high sensitivity in the detection of breast cancer, although the specificity is low. Diagnostic breast MRI is used as a problem-solving tool in cases with equivocal or inconclusive findings on mammogram. In known cases of breast cancer, MRI is used for ascertaining the extent of disease, evaluating the response to chemotherapy and differentiating the scar from tumour recurrence.

Technique MRI of the breast involves utilization of at least 1.5 T magnet, dedicated breast surface coils and administration of gadolinium-based contrast media. A multiphasic dynamic contrast-enhanced study is imperative for both morphological and kinetic assessment of the lesion. MRI acquisition protocols may vary from centre to centre and can be individualized according to the indication. The findings seen on MRI should be described using the American College of Radiology (ACR)-breast imaging reporting and data system (BI-RADS) lexicon for the modality.

Ductography Historically, ductography (galactography) was the procedure of choice for the evaluation of intraductal lesions in patients with pathological nipple discharge. It involves mammographic examination after cannulation and injection of iodinated contrast into the lactiferous ducts with suspicious discharge. Ductography has higher sensitivity than mammography or US for the evaluation of intraductal pathology, but specificity is less. It also suffers from the disadvantage of being minimally invasive, uncomfortable to the patient and being time-consuming. The procedure is technically difficult, requires discharge to be present at the time of the examination to identify the suspicious duct and may lead to inadequate or incomplete results in up to 15% of the cases. It is contraindicated in lactating women and patients with acute mastitis. At present, the primary role of ductography is to localize intraductal lesions and assist in guiding surgical approach.

BI-RADS The BI-RADS is useful for interpretation and organization of imaging results (Table 1.1) [6]. It aims to standardize breast imaging terminology by utilizing a lexicon. It allows report organization and provides a structured reporting classification system for mammography, ultrasound and breast MRI. The BI-RADS reporting system enables communication of clear and consistent results by the radiologists to the treating physician, by providing a final assessment category with specific management recommendations.

1.3.3 Non-excisional Biopsy: FNAC and Core Biopsy

The gold standard for the final diagnosis of a breast abnormality is a core needle biopsy. Image-guided percutaneous biopsy helps obtain

Table 1.1 Breast imaging reporting and data system categories

Category	Assessment	Description	Recommendation
1	Normal/negative	Nothing more needed	Routine screening
2	Benign	Benign findings	Routine screening
3	Probably benign	Probability of being malignant <2%	Short interval follow-up
4	Suspicious finding	Not characteristic of cancer but probability >2% but <95%	Biopsy recommended
5	Highly suggestive of malignancy	High (≥95%) probability of being malignant	Biopsy recommended
6	Known malignancy	Known malignancy	Appropriate treatment

histopathological diagnosis and obviates the need of surgical excision in cases of benign diagnosis which are concordant with imaging findings. In cases of diagnosis of malignancy, immunohistochemistry can be performed to detect receptors on the surface of breast tumours. Also, preoperative histological diagnosis increases the possibility of obtaining clear histologic margins after surgery in cases of malignancy.

Image guidance should be used for biopsy even if the lesion is palpable- to target the most suspicious part of the lesion. The choice of imaging depends on which imaging modality the pathology is best depicted. Palpation guidance for biopsy is recommended only if the lesion is not visualized by any imaging modality.

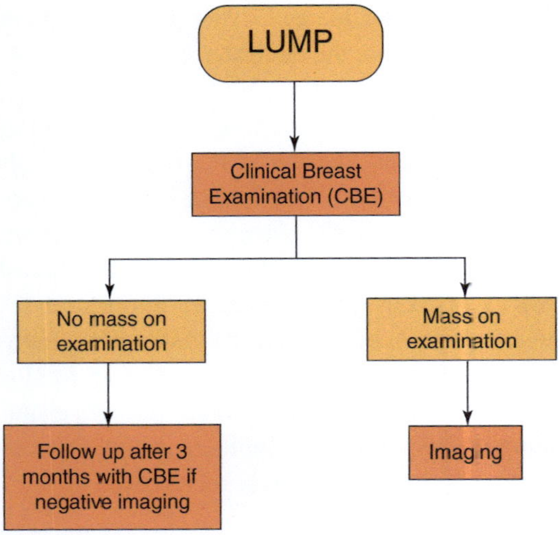

Fig. 1.3 Approach to a patient presenting with breast lump

1.4 Evaluation of Breast Lump

A palpable breast lump can either be detected by the patient or picked up at clinical breast examination. It is the most common presentation in patients with breast-related symptoms [7]. The cause of a palpable lump may either be a benign pathology, such as fibroadenoma, acute or chronic breast abscess, or it may be a manifestation of an ominous carcinoma breast. All patients who present with breast lump or swelling should be evaluated by triple assessment (Fig. 1.3).

Although physical examination may not reliably differentiate benign from malignant masses, benign masses are usually small, mobile, smooth and regular, whereas malignant masses are traditionally described as large, fixed, hard and heterogeneous in texture [8]. A palpable lump can cause significant anxiety to the patient resulting in repeated clinical examinations, imaging evaluation and biopsy. Therefore, it becomes imperative to define an unambiguous, systematic approach for the investigation of a palpable breast lump. This will avoid over-investigation in benign lesions and at the same time prevent the misdiagnosis of malignant breast lesions.

Breast Lump and Cancer There is an increased risk of breast cancer in patients presenting with breast mass [9]. Although majority of the breast lumps detected are benign, and breast cancer is diagnosed only in approximately 10% of the new breast lumps. The risk of a breast lump being diagnosed as a breast cancer increases with the increase in age of the patient, with 1/204 (0.49%) risk for a woman in her fourth decade, compared with 1/28 (3.54%) chance for a woman in the seventh decade of life [10]. The breast lumps in an adolescent are rarely malignant [11].

Imaging The aim of the imaging workup of a palpable breast lump is to accurately diagnose malignant lesions and avoid unnecessary interventions for a benign lesion. Imaging evaluation is indispensable to precisely characterize a palpable breast mass. There should be concordance between the results of clinical breast examination and diagnostic imaging evaluation [12]. The negative predictive value (NPV) of mammography with US in the evaluation of a palpable mass ranges from 97.4% to 100% [13–16]. Nevertheless, a biopsy should be performed even if imaging evaluation is negative, when a strongly suspicious finding is present on physical examination.

Ultrasound and mammography have a synergistic role in the evaluation of breast masses. Dynamic contrast-enhanced Magnetic Resonance

Imaging (CEMRI) may be considered when mammography and US are inconclusive. The mammography and ultrasound report for a breast mass should be described as per the ACR BI-RADS atlas lexicon and should include the size, shape, margin and density of the mass; its location and associated findings; and any change from previous examinations, if known. Finally, each report should be assigned an ACR BI-RAD final assessment category indicating the probability for cancer and further management recommendations. The following discussion includes patients presenting with breast lump in different case scenarios [17].

1.4.1 Age > 40 Years

Diagnostic mammography or DBT should be used for the initial imaging evaluation. A small radio-opaque marker may be placed on the skin over the palpable abnormality. Spot compression and magnification views and other supplementary views like cleavage view, lateral views, step-oblique views, etc. may be taken in addition to the standard craniocaudal and mediolateral oblique views. The sensitivity of mammography alone in patients with palpable breast mass is 86–91% and increases further in patients with entirely fatty breasts [18–21]. US may be considered as an initial imaging modality in patients with negative mammogram in previous 6–12 months. There is no role of MRI/core biopsy in initial evaluation of this subset [22–25].

Further management of patient depends on the results of initial imaging (Fig. 1.4).

Palpable breast mass with negative mammogram (BI-RADS I): If mammogram demonstrates negative results, ultrasound is considered as the next step in the evaluation of such cases. Addition of ultrasound to mammography increases the sensitivity to 93–100% [25]. If a suspicious finding is seen on US, US-guided core biopsy is recommended. However, even if the US is negative after a negative mammogram, palpation guided biopsy is recommended in cases with suspicious physical findings [26].

Palpable breast mass with benign findings on mammogram (BI-RADS II): Ultrasound is generally required when mammography findings do not correlate with the clinical findings. Definite benign masses on mammogram include lymph

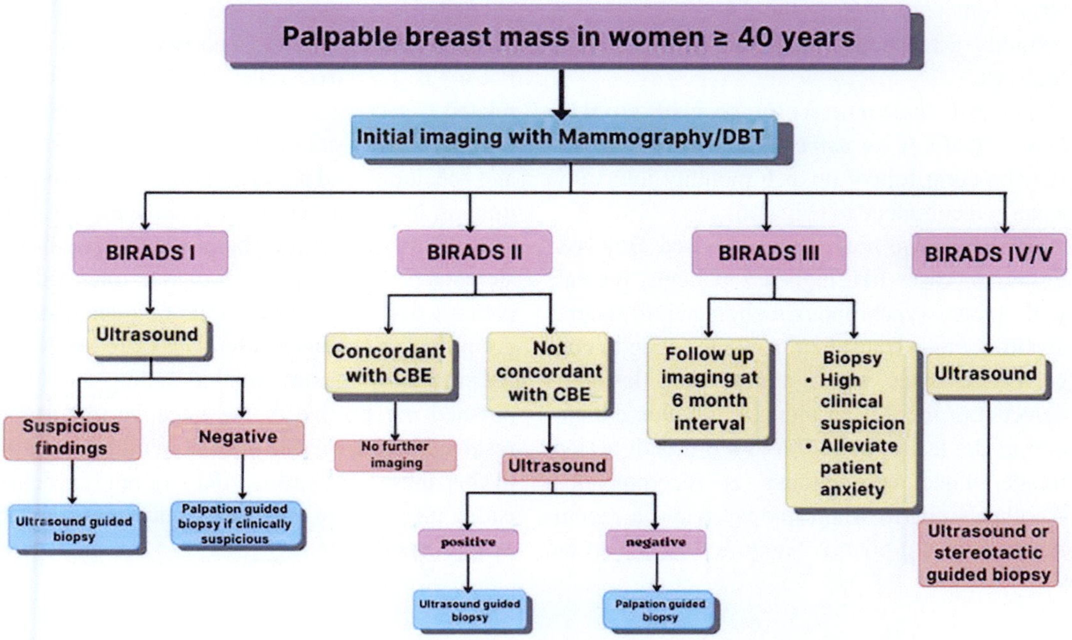

Fig. 1.4 Evaluation of palpable breast mass in women >40 years

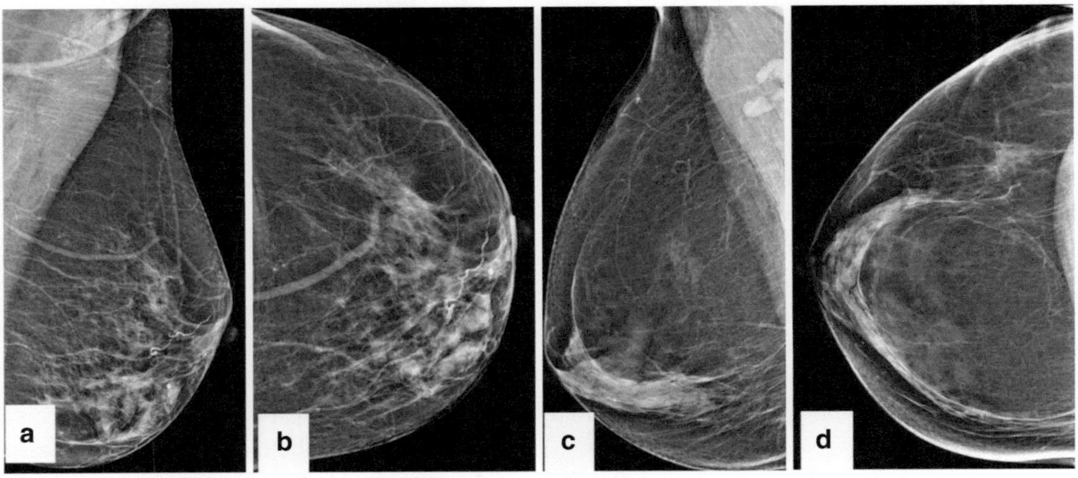

Fig. 1.5 BI-RADS II lesions on mammography: hamartoma (**a**, **b**) and lipoma (**c**, **d**) in the left and right breast in two different patients. No further imaging is required

nodes, hamartoma, fat-containing lesions, calcified involuting fibroadenoma, etc. which do not require further imaging if it correlates with the clinical findings (Fig. 1.5).

If both ultrasound and mammogram show negative or benign results, negative predictive value exceeds to 97%, and routine clinical follow-up is advised. MRI/core biopsy is not recommended. However, if there is any clinical suspicion, core biopsy should always be performed irrespective of benign imaging findings.

Palpable breast mass in case of probably benign findings on mammogram/US (BI-RADS III): Imaging follow-up at 6 monthly interval is usually recommended (Fig. 1.6).

Core biopsy is not routinely advised. However, in certain cases like high-risk patients, patients with known synchronous malignancies, patients awaiting organ transplant, patients trying to conceive and cases where a new mass lesion is detected or there is an increase in volume/diameter of the lesion by >20% in a 6-month period, image-guided core biopsy is recommended. Another scenario where biopsy may be recommended for a probably benign lesion is extreme patient anxiety [27, 28]. There is no role of MRI in evaluation of such patients.

Palpable breast mass with findings suspicious/highly suggestive of malignancy on mammogram (BI-RADS IV or V): Ultrasound is considered the next appropriate step in evaluation of such cases before any intervention is undertaken (Fig. 1.7).

Ultrasound has shown high sensitivity for characterizing mammographically detected suspicious findings [29]. Image-guided biopsy/FNAC is preferred after imaging as changes related to biopsy can result in altered interpretation of image. Core biopsy has higher sensitivity and specificity and provides accurate histological grading of breast masses as compared to FNAC [30]. Ultrasound-guided biopsy is preferred over stereotactic biopsy as it is better tolerated by patients due to lack of compression and can target posterior lesions easily [27]. Core biopsy of the suspicious mammographic finding should be pursued irrespective of the negative ultrasound results. There is no role of MRI in initial imaging in this subset. However, MRI can help in delineating the extent of the disease once confirmed to be malignant on biopsy [31].

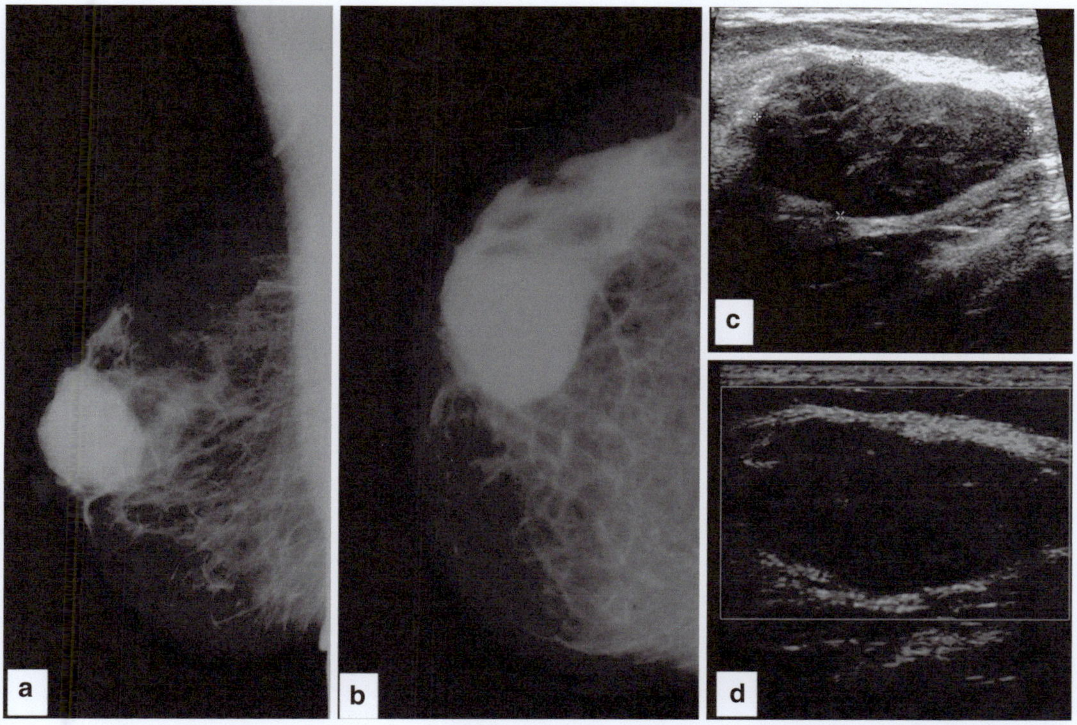

Fig. 1.6 BI-RADS III (probably benign) lesion in the right breast on mammogram (**a**, **b**) and ultrasound (**c**, **d**). Follow-up imaging at 6 months is recommended as there are no associated risk factors

1.4.2 Initial Imaging of Palpable Breast Mass in Women Aged 30–39 Years

DBT/diagnostic mammography or US has a complementary role in initial imaging evaluation of breast mass in women aged 30–39 years. Younger women have a higher density of the breast tissue, making mammography less sensitive in initial imaging workup. However, findings that are not well appreciated on ultrasound (microcalcifications or subtle architectural distortion) are readily detected on mammogram. DBT may also assess the extent of the disease in an ipsilateral breast more accurately and may identify lesions in a contralateral breast as well. A clinical correlation is important in this subset of patient before requesting a mammogram. US is reasonable for initial imaging, and mammography is used if the clinical examination is concerning or there are risk factors. If a suspicious mass is found on US, bilateral mammography is useful.

1.4.3 Age < 30 Years

Initial imaging recommendation is different in younger women owing to low incidence (less than 1%) of breast cancer in young women [32]. Younger women have a higher density of the breast tissue, making mammography less sensitive in initial imaging workup [33]. Thus, mammography is not useful as an initial imaging

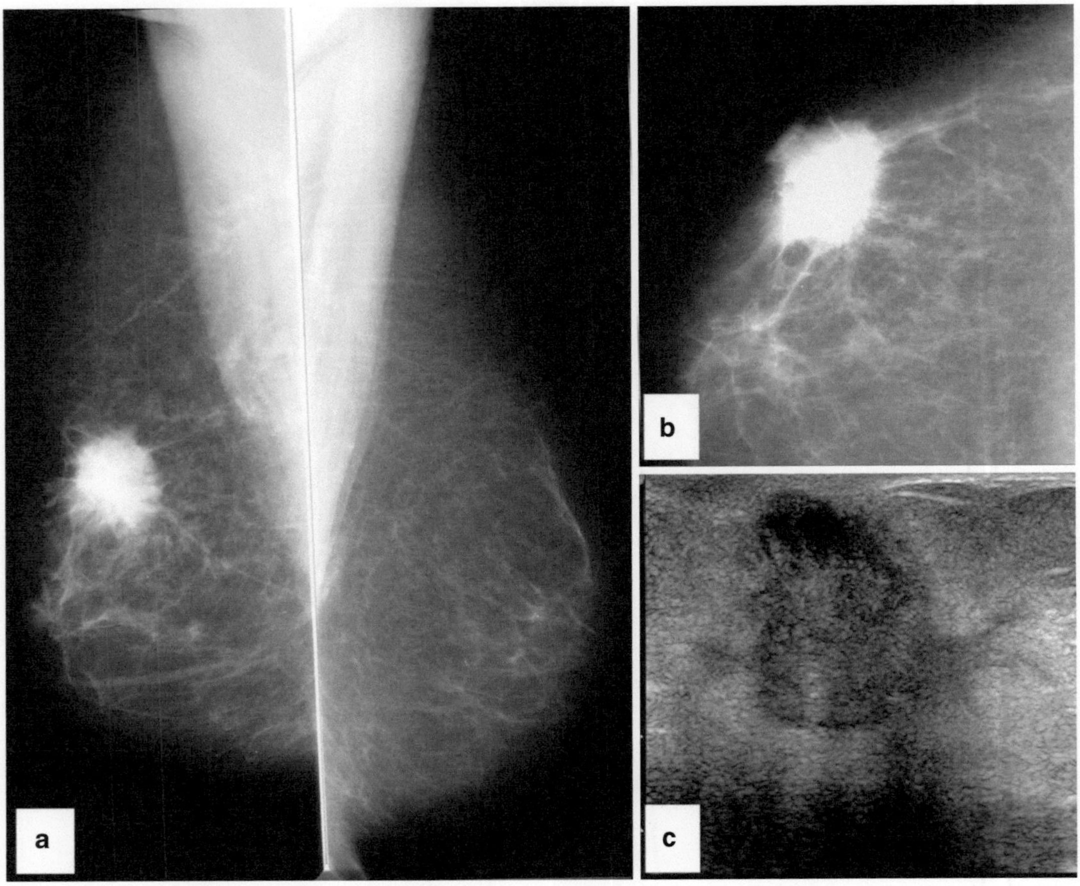

Fig. 1.7 MLO view of the bilateral breast (**a**) and CC view of the right breast (**b**) demonstrated an irregular high-density spiculated mass in the right upper and outer quadrant corresponding to a palpable lump on CBE. Ultrasound (**c**) showed an irregular, taller-than-wide, non-circumscribed, hypoechoic mass with spiculated margins and posterior acoustic shadowing. Further US-guided biopsy was performed, and histopathology confirmed invasive ductal carcinoma of the right breast

modality in women aged less than 30 years. Ultrasound is the most appropriate initial imaging modality to detect any abnormality, specifically targeting the palpable finding. There is no role of MRI/image-guided biopsy as initial imaging workup. Further management of patient depends on the results of initial imaging (Fig. 1.8).

Palpable lump with negative/normal ultrasound findings (BI-RADS I): No further imaging workup is recommended in this subset. Literature supports the role of diagnostic mammography only in cases with high clinical suspicion. Furthermore, stereotactic biopsy is recommended if mammography shows suspicious findings. Even if both DBT/mammography and US are negative, tissue sampling with core biopsy or surgical biopsy is warranted in a clinically suspicious palpable lump.

Palpable breast mass in case of benign findings on ultrasound (BI-RADS II): No further imaging workup is recommended in this subset. There is very less likelihood of a palpable breast mass that is benign on both clinical and ultrasound examination to be malignant (Fig. 1.9). Core biopsy is not required in this subset [34].

Palpable breast mass in case of probably benign findings on US (BI-RADS III): Ultrasound follow-up at 6 monthly interval is usually recom-

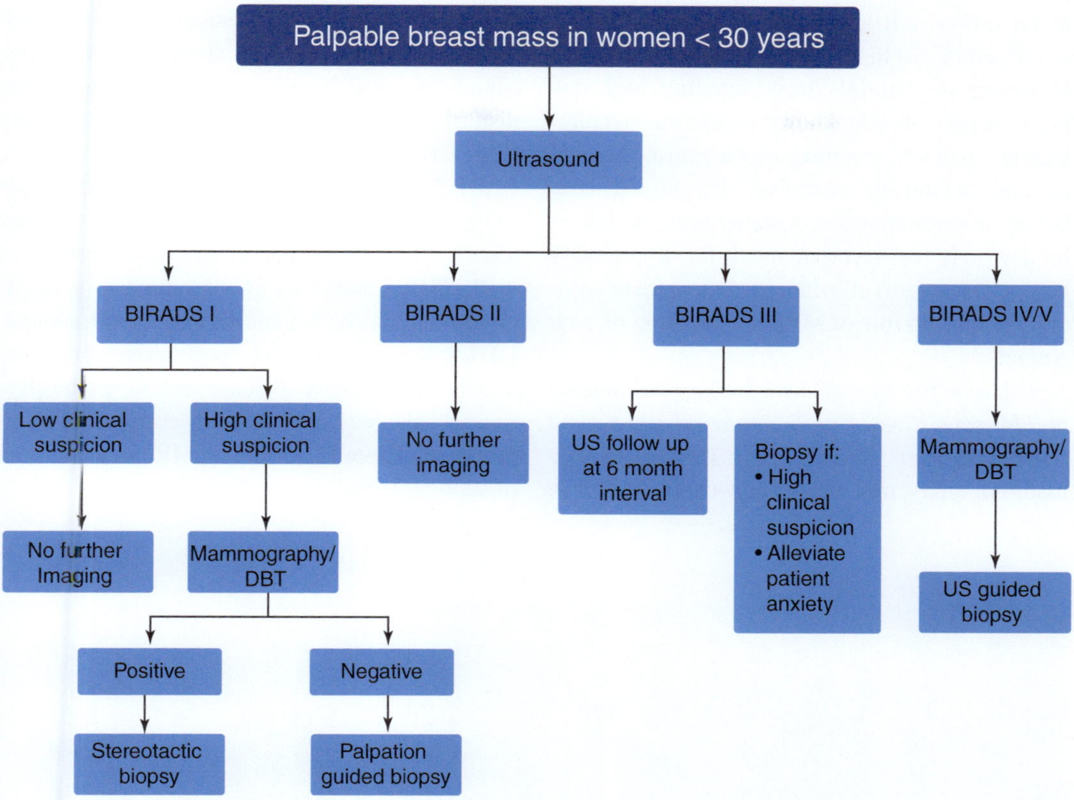

Fig. 1.8 Evaluation of palpable breast mass in women <30 years

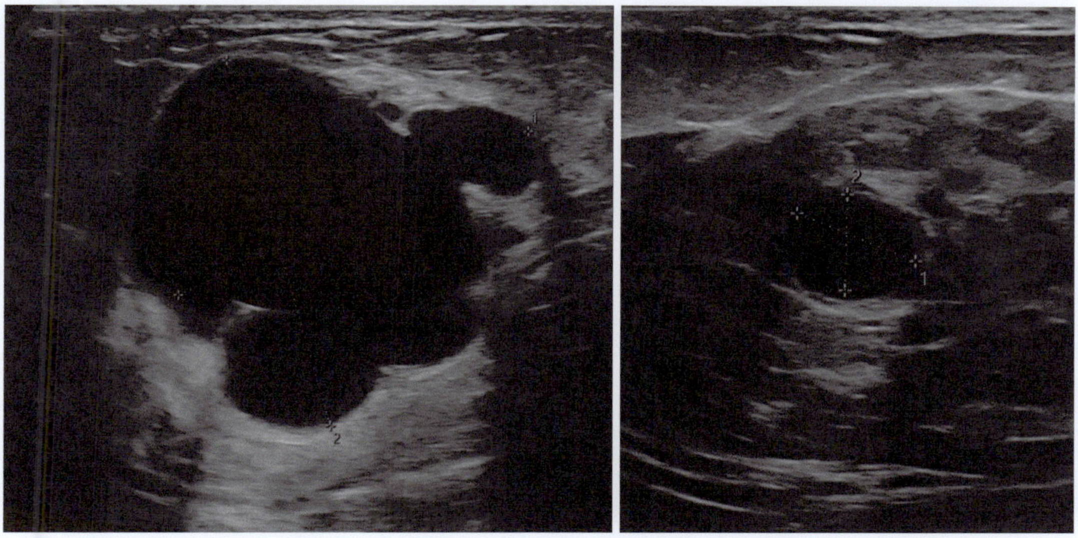

Fig. 1.9 BI-RADS II lesion on US in women aged <30 years. Simple cysts on ultrasound- do not require any further imaging workup

mended (Fig. 1.10), and there is no role of mammography. Core biopsy is not routinely advised. However, in certain cases including high-risk patients, patients with known synchronous malignancies, patients awaiting organ transplant, and patients trying to conceive, US-guided core biopsy is recommended. Another scenario where biopsy may be recommended for a probably benign lesion is to alleviate extreme patient anxiety. There is no role of MRI in evaluation of such patients.

Palpable breast mass with findings suspicious/highly suggestive of malignancy on ultrasound (BI-RADS IV or V, Fig. 1.11): DBT/diagnostic mammography has a role in women less than 30 years with suspicious sonographic findings. Findings that are not well appreciated on ultrasound (microcalcifications or subtle architectural distortion) are readily detected on mammogram (Fig. 1.12) [32].

DBT may also assess the extent of the disease in the ipsilateral breast more accurately and may identify lesions in the contralateral breast as well. Tissue sampling is warranted if a suspicious mass has been identified on the ultrasound. DBT/mammography is performed prior to biopsy to delineate disease extent as biopsy-related changes can alter or obscure image interpretation. There is no role of MRI in evaluation of such patients.

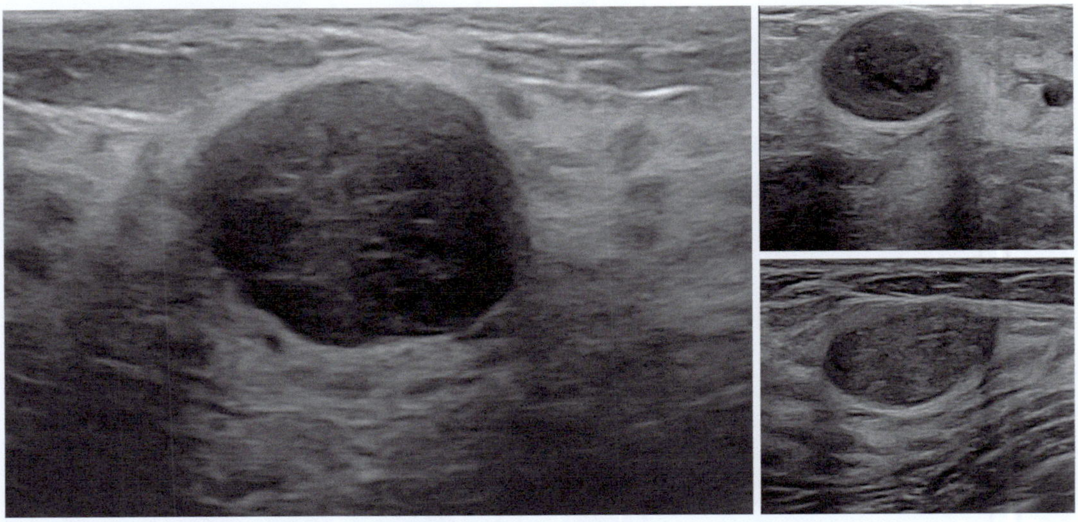

Fig. 1.10 BI-RADS III (probably benign) lesions on US in different patients aged <30 years with mobile lumps on CBE. Follow-up US at 6 months is recommended

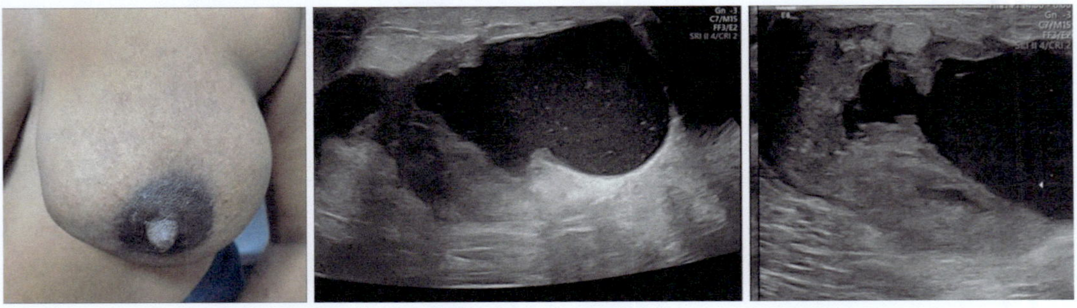

Fig. 1.11 Breast lump in the lower inner quadrant of the left breast in a 30-year-old woman. BI-RADS IV (probably malignant) complex cystic mass was seen on US. US-guided biopsy confirmed invasive ductal carcinoma

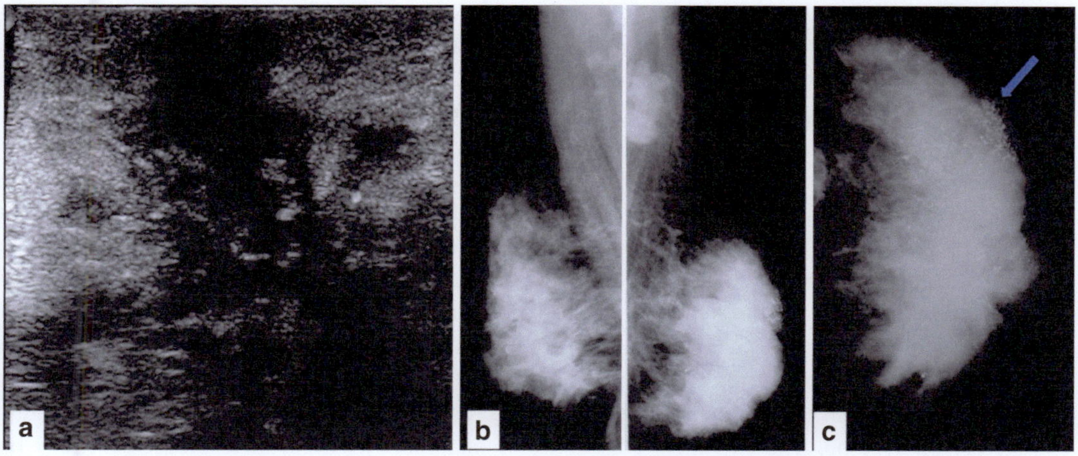

Fig. 1.12 BI-RADS IV (probably malignant) solid lesion on US (**a**). MLO views (**b**) of the bilateral breast and CC view of the left breast (**c**) show dense breasts with suspicious microcalcification (arrow)

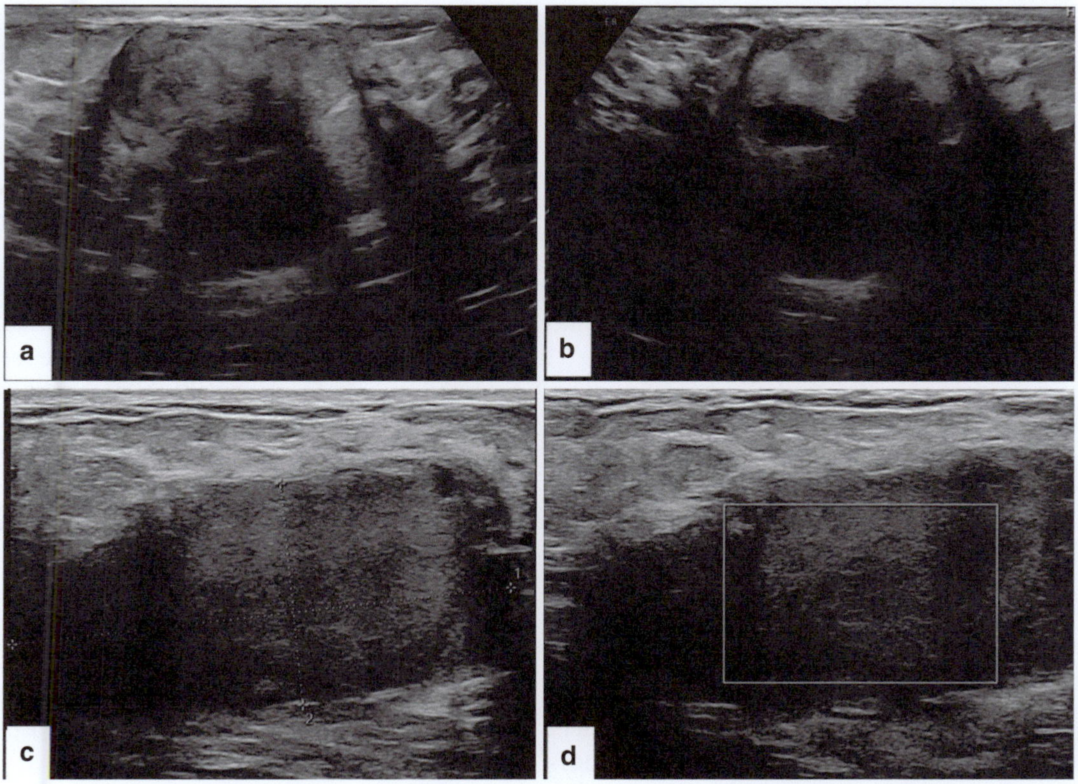

Fig. 1.13 US of breasts in lactating women presenting with pain and lump in the breast. A mixed solid cystic mass in the first patient (**a**, **b**) and cystic mass with echogenic contents in the second patient (**c**, **d**). No flow was demonstrated on colour Doppler (**d**). These masses in a lactating woman represent galactoceles

1.4.4 Breast Lump in Lactating or Pregnant Women

Ultrasound is the imaging modality of choice in this subset of patients at any age. The breasts are mammographically dense during this period. Any mass detected on US is further managed in accordance to the BI-RADS category (Fig. 1.13). Mammography may be considered in cases of equivocal or suspicious findings on US. It is better than US in delineation of calcifications and architectural distortion. CEMRI is not recommended during pregnancy but may be considered in lactation.

1.5 Breast Pain

Mastalgia or mastodynia is a common symptom reported by more than two thirds of the females at some time of their lives. It is the second most common breast symptom after breast lump. The etiology of breast pain is multifactorial and not completely understood. The two most common concerns for patients presenting with mastalgia are the risk of breast cancer associated with the symptom and the presence of severe pain itself which affects the quality of life [35].

Types of Breast Pain There are two main types of breast pain, cyclical and noncyclical, and need differentiation from pain of the non-mammary origin. The breast pain can further be categorized into diffuse, which involves more than 25% of the breast and axillary tissue or focal, which involves less than 25% of the breast and axillary tissue. The pain is called pinpoint if an area of the size of fingertip is involved [36, 37].

Cyclical Breast Pain This is the most common form of mastalgia which is usually diffuse and can be unilateral or bilateral. As the name suggests, the severity of the pain changes with the menstrual cycle and is most severe in the luteal phase, 1–2 weeks before the menstrual flow. This form of mastalgia is commonly seen in the age group 30–40 years. Resolution of the symptoms during pregnancy or menopause suggests a hormonal origin of the pain, although no consistent abnormality in the hormonal levels has been documented in patients with cyclical mastalgia. This suggests that there is an increased sensitivity of the breast to normal hormonal levels.

In the absence of other signs and symptoms, the likelihood of malignancy in a patient with cyclical mastalgia is extremely low. The majority of patients can be treated symptomatically and with reassurance. There may be spontaneous resolution of symptoms in up to 20% of patients.

Noncyclical breast pain This type of pain is usually unilateral and localized to a particular quadrant of the breast. The women presenting with this symptom are commonly in their fourth decade. This accounts for approximately one fourth of the cases of mastalgia and is usually inflammatory in origin. The etiology of noncyclical mastalgia may be benign, including cysts, mastitis, stretching of Cooper's ligaments, fat necrosis, Mondor's disease, diabetic mastopathy, or malignancy. Noncyclical breast pain may be experienced in pregnancy and lactation but is usually of short duration and often shows spontaneous resolution. Rarely, breast pain may be the first symptom of pregnancy. Noncyclical mastalgia is of shorter duration than cyclical breast pain and may resolve spontaneously in up to half of the patients. This type of breast pain requires further evaluation, irrespective of the presence or absence of additional signs and symptoms, to exclude an underlying benign or malignant breast lesion [38, 39].

Mastalgia MIMICS Ten to fifteen percent of cases of breast pain find their origin outside the breast tissue. The nerve supply to the breast is from intercostal nerves from T3 to T5, and irritation along its course anywhere can lead to breast or nipple pain. Common causes of the non-mammary origin of mastalgia include Tietze's disease, referred nerve root pain of cervical spondylitis, pectoral muscle strains, fibromyalgia, tuberculosis of chest wall, etc. Non-chest wall pain causing breast pain may arise from causes such as cardiac causes (ischemic heart disease), hepatobiliary causes (biliary pain), gastric (peptic ulcer) and herpes zoster.

Breast Pain and Cancer Although breast cancer does not commonly present with pain, mastalgia has been seen to be associated with increased breast cancer risk, especially in premenopausal women. The risk of malignancy in patients with breast pain has been described differently by different authors. Majority of the

Fig. 1.14 Types of breast pain

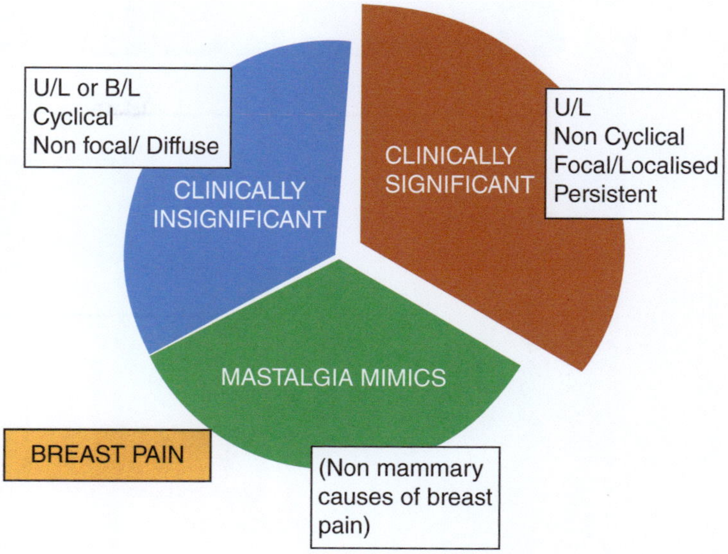

authors did not report any increased risk with some even reported reduced risk of breast cancer as compared to those without pain.

On the basis of the nature of breast pain, it is categorized into pain that is not suspicious for associated malignancy and pain that is clinically significant (Fig. 1.14).

Clinically insignificant pain is unilateral or bilateral, cyclical and diffuse. Clinically significant pain, though commonly associated with benign etiology, has shown association with malignancy. This type of pain is localized and persistent [40, 41].

Imaging The role of imaging in patients with mastalgia is to establish the cause in cases of benign etiology and rule out possibility of any associated malignancy. A negative imaging, though plays an important role in alleviating the patient's anxiety, can increase the odds of subsequent clinical visits. Mammography and ultrasound, alone or in combination, have been used to evaluate patients with mastalgia depending upon the nature of pain and age of the patient. The following discussion includes patients with breast pain without any other symptom (Fig. 1.15) [42].

When mastalgia is associated with any other symptom, e.g. lump or nipple discharge, it should be treated as a secondary symptom, and imaging workup should follow the other symptom. The following discussion includes patients presenting with breast pain in different case scenarios.

1.5.1 Woman with Clinically Insignificant Breast Pain: Non-focal, Diffuse or Cyclical

The literature evaluating the role of mammography and ultrasound in patients with cyclical and diffuse/ non-focal pain is limited. Nevertheless, limited studies done show no correlation between this type of breast pain and breast cancer. Considering this fact, the use of mammography beyond the usual screening is not recommended in this subset. Similarly, there is no role of DBT or MRI in the evaluation of these patients [43].

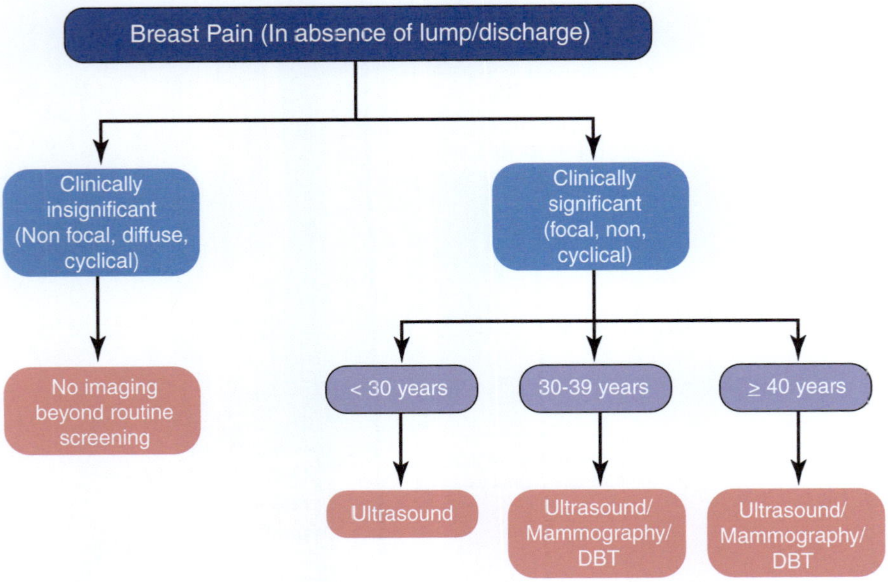

Fig. 1.15 Evaluation of patients with breast pain

1.5.2 Woman with Clinically Significant Breast Pain: Focal and Noncyclical

Age < 30 years: Mammography is considered less accurate in patients less than 30 years because of increased breast density and is not routinely recommended. Ultrasound has shown a high negative predictive value, sensitivity and specificity for evaluating patients with mastalgia for possible association of breast cancer [44, 45]. Moreover, ultrasound finds utility in identifying a benign, potentially treatable cause of breast pain (Fig. 1.16). So, ultrasound is considered appropriate in patients less than 30 years and with clinically significant breast pain. There is no role of DBT or MRI in evaluation of such patients.

Age 30–39 years: Despite a low incidence of cancer in patients with isolated breast pain, mammography finds its role in excluding malignancy in this subset of patients with a high sensitivity and negative predictive value [44]. Despite paucity of literature in evaluating the role of DBT, its superior lesion characterization as compared to conventional mammography offers its added role in evaluation of such patients [46].

There are very few studies evaluating the role of ultrasound as an independent imaging modality in evaluation of clinically significant breast pain in women aged 30–39 years old. Some authors did not find ultrasound useful in cases with a negative mammogram, especially in patients with nondense breasts. Nevertheless, it

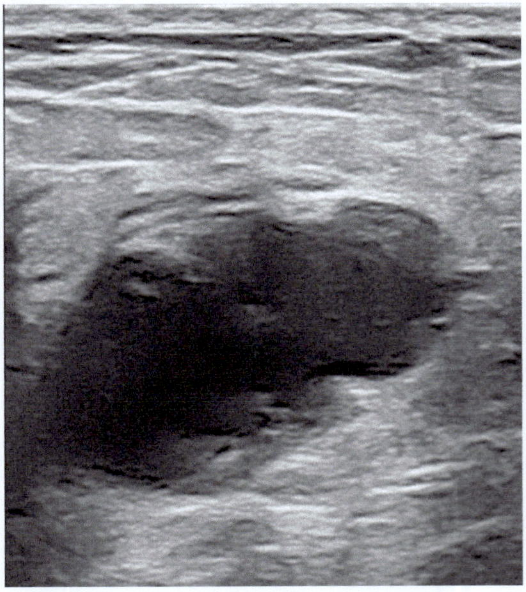

Fig. 1.16 A young 25-year-old woman with focal noncyclical breast pain. US evaluation shows a complicated cyst, a benign treatable cause of mastalgia.

has a definite utility in establishing a benign cause, including patients with negative mammogram. So, even with a low incidence of breast cancer in patients with clinically significant breast pain, ultrasound is useful in identifying a treatable benign cause [47]. Hence, mammography including DBT and ultrasound are considered as appropriate equivalent alternatives in patients aged 30–39 years with clinically significant breast pain. There is no role of MRI in evaluation of such patients.

Age ≥ 40 years: Similar to the women in age group 30–39 years, both mammography including DBT and ultrasound have a role in excluding malignancy in patients with breast pain. Ultrasound finds an additional benefit by establishing a treatable benign cause of mastalgia, especially in patients with nondense breasts. Thus, mammography and DBT are equivalent alternatives, and ultrasound is a complementary modality (Fig. 1.17). There is no role of MRI in evaluation of such patients [44, 47].

1.5.3 Imaging in Acute Mastitis

Mastitis refers to inflammation of the breast parenchyma and can be categorized into three groups: infectious mastitis, non-infectious mastitis and mastitis related to underlying malignancy [48]. Acute mastitis manifests as focal breast pain, induration, redness associated with fever and malaise. It can be puerperal, associated with lactation or non-puerperal. Mastitis is a clinical diagnosis and patients are managed conservatively. Imaging is recommended in patients who do not respond to conservative management or where the disease is progressive. Ultrasound is the modality of choice for evaluation of patients with acute painful breast as mammography requires compression and is technically not feasible. Ultrasound demonstrates heterogeneous echotexture with echogenic areas representing inflamed fat lobules and hypoechoic areas involving the glandular parenchyma, with associated mild skin thickening (Fig. 1.18).

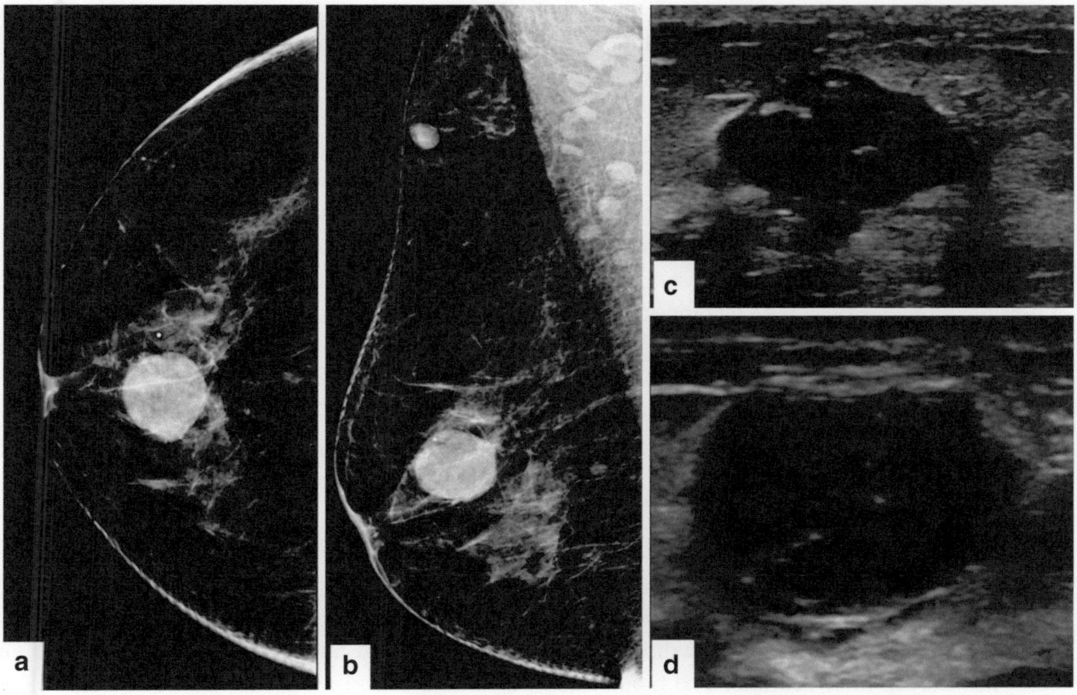

Fig. 1.17 Mammogram (**a**, **b**) and US (**c**, **d**) in a woman >40 years presenting with focal, noncyclical, persistent pain demonstrates a complex cyst in the right breast

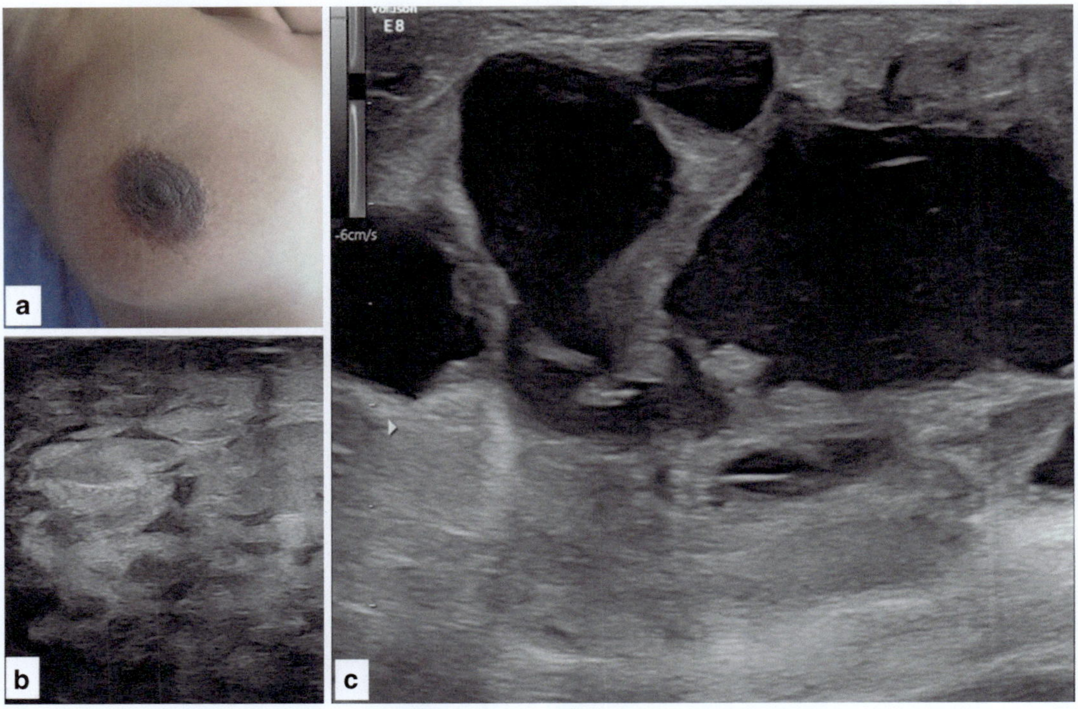

Fig. 1.18 Acute mastitis in a young female presenting with pain and redness of the skin of the right breast (**a**). (**b**) US evaluation shows hyperechogenicity with subcutaneous oedema suggestive of breast inflammation. US in another patient (**c**) with breast tenderness, lump and induration shows the presence of a breast abscess

There may be reactive enlargement of the axillary lymph nodes. Occasionally abscess formation may be visible. Surgical or ultrasound-guided drainage is recommended if mastitis has evolved into an abscess formation [49].

Follow-up mammography or sonography is recommended in non-puerperal mastitis after resolution of the acute symptoms. Any persistent or non-resolving lesion should be biopsied to rule out possibility of breast cancer [50].

1.6 Nipple Discharge

Nipple discharge is the third most common breast complaint after lump and pain and accounts for 2–5% of medical visits by women. Fifty to eighty percent of females in the reproductive age group experience nipple discharge at least once during their lifetime. The nipple discharge can be physiological or pathological (Fig. 1.19) [51].

Physiological Nipple Discharge This type of discharge is often provoked; may be yellow, green or white in colour; and is usually bilateral. It originates from multiple ducts and is not usually related to breast malignancy. Majority of the women in reproductive age group can express discharge. Galactorrhoea is milky discharge unrelated to normal milk production of lactation. In patients with galactorrhoea unrelated to pregnancy and lactation, the cause is usually an endocrinopathy with elevated prolactin levels. It may also manifest as a side effect of some commonly prescribed drugs like antidepressants and oral contraceptives.

Pathological Nipple Discharge It is spontaneous, unilateral, serous or blood-stained discharge which originates from a single duct. The causes of pathological nipple discharge may be benign or malignant. Intraductal papilloma and duct ectasia are the commonest benign causes (Figs. 1.20 and 1.21).

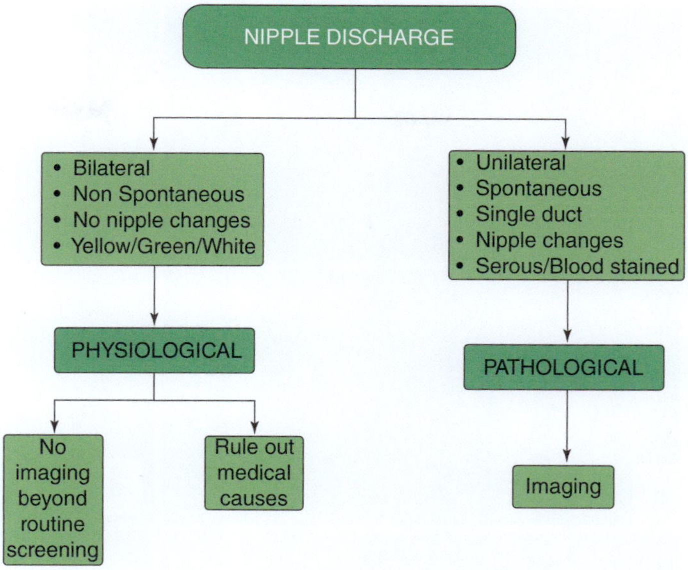

Fig. 1.19 Types of nipple discharge

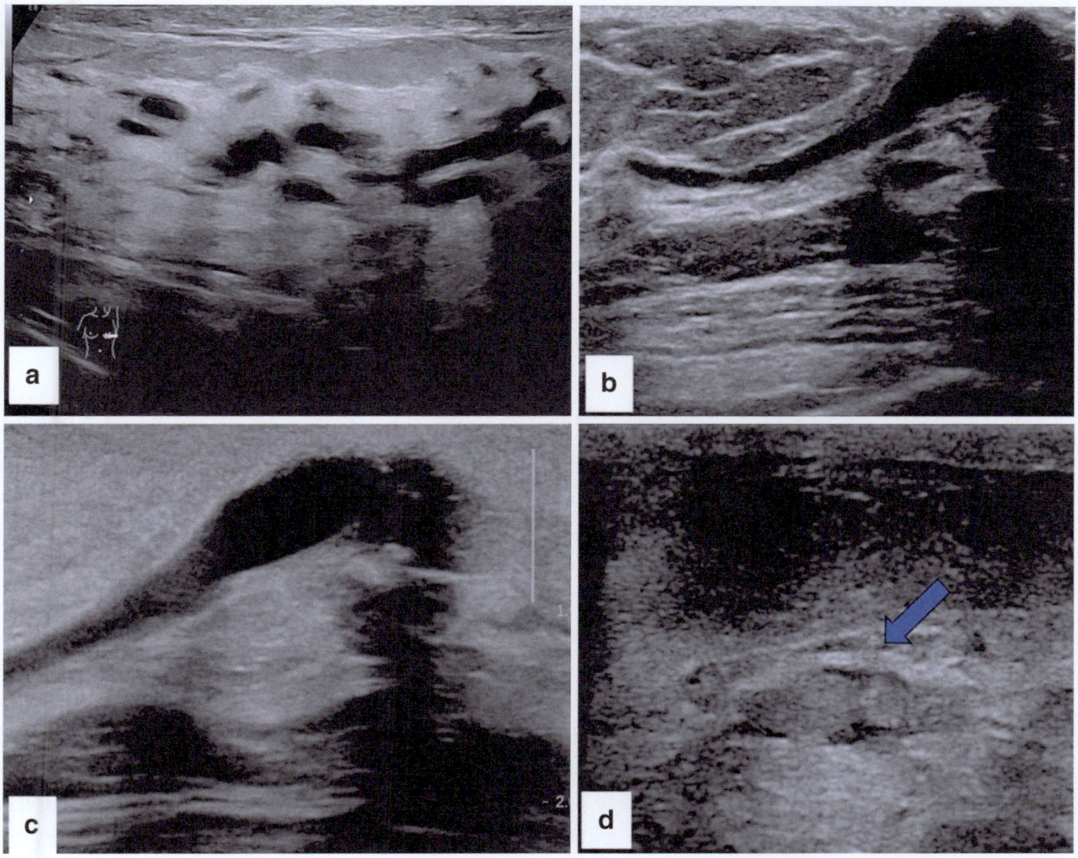

Fig. 1.20 Benign causes of nipple discharge. US evaluation of patients with nipple discharge showing multiple-dilated duct (**a**), single-dilated ducts (**b**) and single-dilated duct with intraductal papilloma (**c**, **d**)

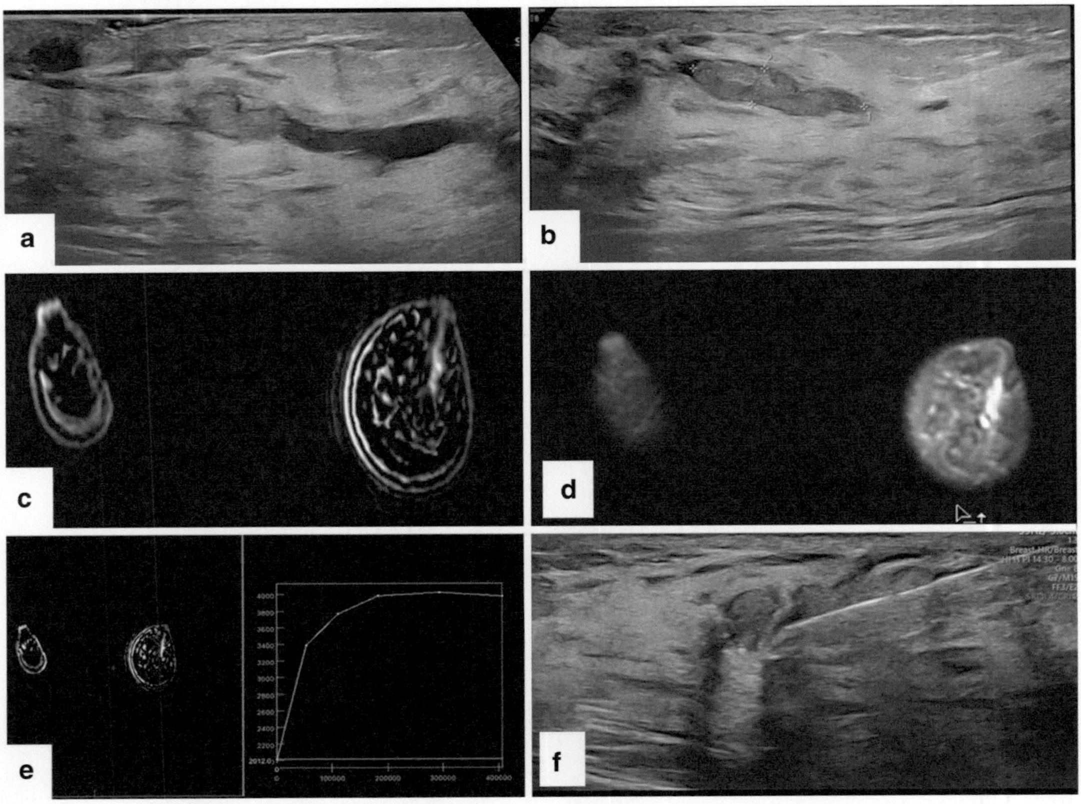

Fig. 1.21 Malignant cause of nipple discharge. A 30-year-old unmarried female presented with spontaneous serous unilateral nipple discharge from the left nipple. CBE was unremarkable. US evaluation of the breast (**a**, **b**) demonstrated single duct dilatation with an intraductal mass. Dynamic CEMRI was done for further evaluation. Coronal STIR image (**c**) and coronal dynamic post-contrast T1W subtracted image (**d**) demonstrated a solitary dilated duct in the left breast with linear non-mass enhancement (NME) showing type II Kuhl's kinetic curve (**e**). US-guided biopsy (**f**) confirmed malignancy

Nipple Discharge and Cancer Majority of the patients with nipple discharge do not have any underlying malignancy. In a study by Goksel et al. [52], only 0.3% of patients with non-spontaneous nipple discharge exhibited malignancy. Physiological nipple discharge is usually not associated with breast malignancy. The rate of malignancy in patients with pathological nipple discharge has been reported to be 11–16%. The patient demographics determines the risk of malignancy in patients with nipple discharge and increase in risk with increasing age. Any nipple discharge associated with a palpable mass or nipple inversions mandates a dedicated workup to rule out an underlying malignancy. Although uncommon but whenever present in men, nipple discharge is associated with malignancy in 23–57% of cases [53]. Nipple discharge cytology is neither sensitive nor specific and adds to the cost of the evaluation, hence not routinely recommended.

Imaging The standard evaluation of nipple discharge commences with detailed clinical assessment which comprises the patient's history and physical examination. This directs the requirement and type of diagnostic breast imaging. Mammography and breast ultrasound are the first step in evaluation. Historically ductography has been performed in patients with negative mammogram and sonogram. This has been replaced by breast MRI. It has a higher positive

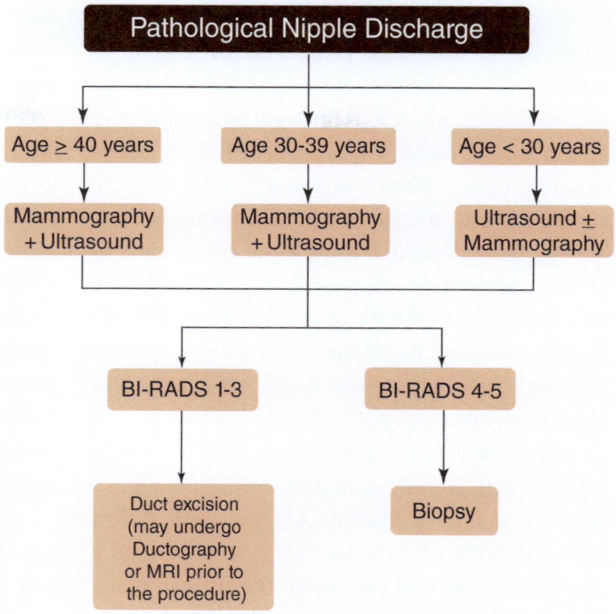

Fig. 1.22 Evaluation of women with pathological nipple discharge

and negative predictive value as compared to ductography in detecting malignancy in patients with pathological nipple discharge. The following discussion include patients presenting with nipple discharge in different case scenarios (Fig. 1.22) [54].

1.6.1 Adult Woman with Physiological Nipple Discharge

In a patient with nipple discharge, where medical history and clinical examination suggest physiological nature of the discharge, no radiological investigation is required beyond the routine screening mammography.

1.6.2 Adult Woman (≥40 Years) with Pathological Nipple Discharge

Mammography is the first-line imaging modality for evaluation of pathological nipple discharge in a patient in this age group. Since the lesions may be small, contain no calcification and may be intraductal in position, full-field mammography may fail to demonstrate such lesions. Additional mammographic views with spot compression and magnification may be useful to evaluate suspicious findings.

Mammography has a variable sensitivity (15–68%) and specificity (38–98%) for detection of malignancy (ductal carcinoma in situ (DCIS) and invasive cancer). The reported positive predictive value (PPV) is around 42%, and the NPV 90% [54]. The possible explanation for this variation in sensitivity includes variable breast density among different groups of patients and differences in imaging technology (digital versus film-screen mammography). Although there is no definite literature, early studies suggest a promising role of digital breast tomosynthesis in evaluation of patients with breast discharge.

Ultrasound has a role in detecting invasive cancer and assessing the extent of disease but has low sensitivity for detecting DCIS. In patients with pathologic nipple discharge, US can identify additional lesions in 63–69% of the cases with negative mammography [55]. It adds specificity for certain lesions by further characterizing the mammographic abnormality, for example, a simple cyst or duct dilatation. As compared to ductography, US can visualize and detect abnormalities in multiple rather than single duct and peripheral in addition to central ducts.

When used alone, US has a reported sensitivity of 56–80%, specificity of 61–75%, PPV of 9–39%, and NPV of 90–91% for the detection of underlying malignancy in patients with pathologic nipple discharge [56]. This difference in reported performance can be explained by variation in US technique. Although more sensitive than mammography, US is less specific in differentiating benign from malignant lesions. Volume averaging with the duct wall in a tortuous duct, fibrosis along the duct, intraductal blood clots or inspissated debris can lead to false-positive US. As mammography and US cannot reliably predict histology in patients with pathologic nipple discharge, histological diagnosis needs to be obtained by image-guided biopsy.

Ductography can detect high-risk lesions in patients with pathological nipple discharge and a negative mammogram and US, but with a low PPV and NPV of 19% and 63%, respectively. It can localize 76% of otherwise occult malignant/high-risk lesions and 91% of benign lesions. Even when mammography and US are positive, ductography may facilitate preoperative localization of the pathological lesion in 78% of cases [57].

Ductography is useful as it can demonstrate small lesions and localize the duct responsible for the nipple discharge. However, due to its minimally invasive nature, it is uncomfortable to the patient, and the procedure can be time-consuming. The procedure is technically limited and can be carried out only if there is active discharge on the day of ductography. Failure to cannulate the precise discharging duct may lead to a false-negative result. It is contraindicated in lactating women, patients with active mastitis and known hypersensitivity to iodinated contrast agents.

Ductography has higher sensitivity than mammography and US but is less specific than both modalities. A false-negative rate as high as 20–30% is reported, and a negative ductogram cannot reliably exclude an underlying cancer or high-risk lesion. At present, the primary role of ductography is localization of intraductal lesions to guide duct excision surgery.

Breast MRI has a high sensitivity for detecting invasive breast cancer, ranging from 93% to 100%, with a specificity of 37–97% [58]. Interpretation of MRI involves an analysis of a lesion's morphology and evaluation of enhancement kinetics to predict malignancy. Malignant lesions may appear as a mass or non-mass enhancement in a ductal or segmental distribution on MRI. Contrast-enhanced breast MRI has high sensitivity for detecting benign papillary lesions as well as in situ and invasive carcinoma. It also allows identification of pathological lesions located in peripheral ducts that are beyond the area normally encompassed by terminal duct excision, ductography, or targeted US. Index or synchronous lesions found only on MRI can be percutaneously biopsied with MRI guidance. This allows definitive surgical management in malignant cases and avoids unnecessary surgical excision for benign lesions.

MRI may be considered in cases of pathological nipple discharge with negative mammogram and sonogram and not as initial imaging in a patient with pathologic nipple discharge (Fig. 1.23).

Image-guided biopsy: Since mammography, US and ductography cannot predict histology in patients with pathologic nipple discharge, and histological diagnosis of lesions identified on imaging is imperative. The biopsy procedures may be guided by mammography (stereotactic), US or MRI, depending on the imaging modality that best depicts the lesion. CNB is preferred over FNA because it is more sensitive and specific and enables accurate histological grading of a lesion. A tissue marker may be placed at the end of the biopsy to allow needle localization and excision if the biopsied lesion yields malignant or high-risk histology. Vacuum-assisted biopsy is of great utility in assuring complete sampling of small intraductal papillary lesions. Although biopsy is a diagnostic procedure, there is near-complete removal of the intraductal soft tissue lesion during vacuum-assisted core biopsy. This procedure may result in eliminating nipple discharge in more than 90% of patients and thus provide therapeutic option.

According to the surgical literature, major duct excision continues to be the reference standard to exclude malignancy in patients with unremarkable imaging, as even a negative ductogram or MRI does not completely exclude an underlying cancer or high-risk lesion.

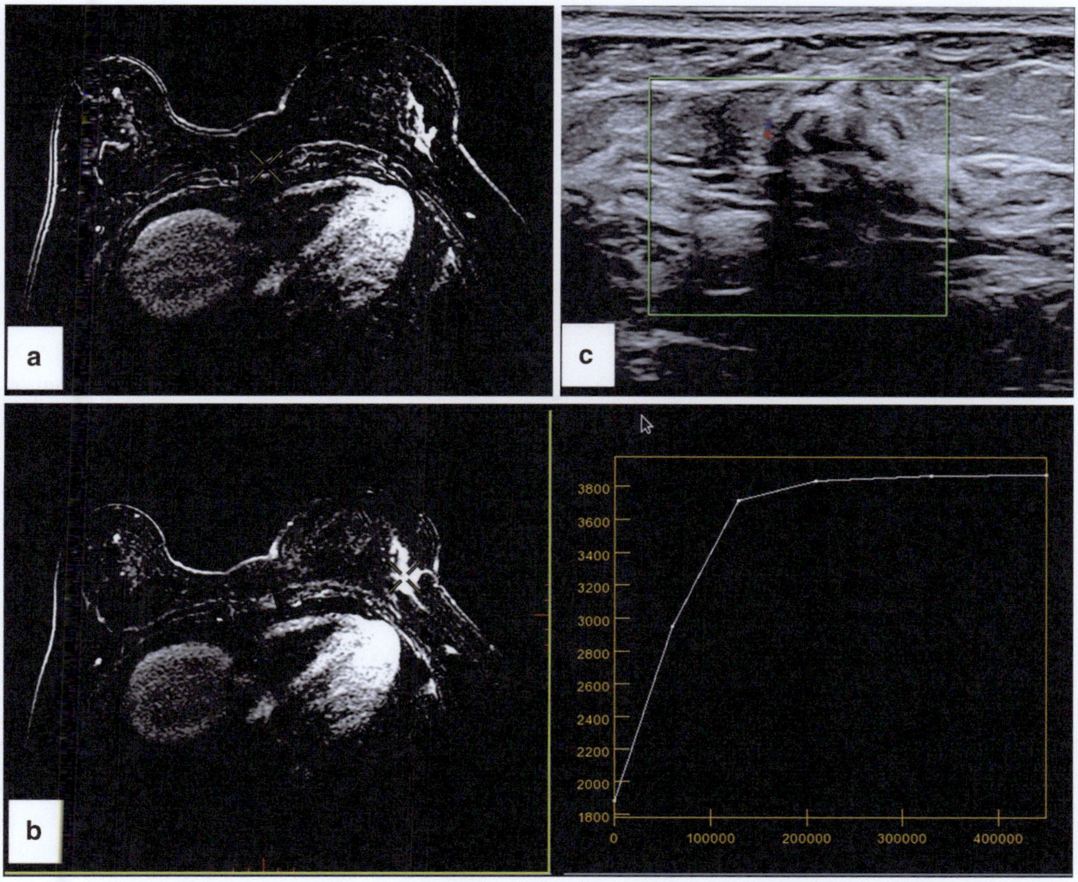

Fig. 1.23 A 43-year-old woman with pathological left nipple discharge and negative CBE. US and mammography were negative and did not demonstrate any pathology in either breast. Dynamic contrast-enhanced MRI (**a**) revealed heterogeneous NME in a segmental distribution in the outer and lower quadrant of the left breast, showing type II Kuhl's kinetic curve (**b**) suggesting a BI-RADS IV category. Subsequent targeted US (**c**) done showed some heterogeneity in the area. US-guided biopsy from the suspicious area confirmed invasive ductal carcinoma

To summarize, DBT or diagnostic mammography is usually recommended as equivalent alternatives in patients with pathologic nipple discharge and age more than or equal to 40 years for initial imaging evaluation. Breast US is complementary and may be performed in addition at the same time to better characterize the disease process. Ductography is limited due to its invasive nature and high false-negative results. CEMRI may be considered in patients with negative mammogram and sonogram.

1.6.3 Adult Woman (30–39 Years) with Pathological Nipple Discharge

The risk of breast cancer is relatively low in this age group. The sensitivity of ultrasound as compared to mammography is higher (95.7% vs 60.9%) in this age group [59]. However, suspicious microcalcifications are better depicted by mammography, and there is a high incidence of DCIS in patients presenting with nipple discharge. Either mammography or US can be used as an initial imaging modality based on institutional practice and case-by-case consideration.

Ductography has higher sensitivity than mammography and US but lower specificity than both modalities. It has a high false-negative rate and is not recommended for initial imaging. Ductography-guided localization of the lesion may help in surgical excision. CEMRI due to its very high sensitivity should be considered in patients with negative mammogram and sonogram.

1.6.4 Adult Woman (<30 Years) with Pathological Nipple Discharge

Breast cancer is extremely rare in women less than 30 years unless there is a risk factor including positive family history, history of irradiation to chest, etc. Ultrasound is most useful in initial imaging evaluation of these patients. Diagnostic mammography may be performed as an adjunct when some suspicious finding is picked up on US and MRI as problem-solving tool.

1.6.5 Nipple Discharge in a Male

Unilateral nipple discharge is rare in males but when present is more likely associated with malignancy. Imaging evaluation is required in all males with unilateral nipple discharge, irrespective of age [60]. DBT and mammography are appropriate for the initial imaging evaluation and are used as equivalent alternatives. Breast ultrasound has a role as a complementary modality and is used in addition to mammography for better characterization of the pathology. At present, there is no relevant literature to support the role of ductography or CEMRI in evaluation of nipple discharge in adult males.

1.7 Conclusion

Palpable breast mass, breast pain and nipple discharge are the common breast-related symptoms dealt by physicians in an outpatient department. All patients presenting with breast-related symptoms should undergo a triple assessment. MDT forms the basis for the best approach to management of patients with breast disease. The initial workup of patient begins with a detailed clinical history and physical examination. Further assessment by imaging is guided by the patient's demographics and results of clinical breast examination. Multimodality breast imaging is an integral part of comprehensive breast care. The results of imaging are communicated in terms of BI-RADS category which guides further management of the patients. The approach to symptomatic breast is continuously evolving with an ultimate goal of imaging being determination of cause of patient's symptoms and to rule out any underlying breast malignancy.

References

1. Eberl MM, Phillips RL, Lamberts H, Okkes I, Mahoney MC. Characterizing breast symptoms in family practice. Ann Fam Med. 2008;6(6):528–33.
2. Ryerson AB, Miller J, Eheman CR. Reported breast symptoms in the national breast and cervical cancer early detection program. Cancer Causes Control. 2015;26:733–40.
3. Barton MB, Elmore JG, Fletcher SW. Breast symptoms among women enrolled in a health maintenance organization: frequency, evaluation, and outcome. Ann Intern Med. 1999;130(8):651–7.
4. Karim MO, Khan KA, Khan AJ, Javed A, Fazid S, Aslam MI. Triple assessment of breast lump: should we perform core biopsy for every patient? Cureus. 2020;12(3):e7479.
5. Malherbe F, Nel D, Molabe H, Cairncross L, Roodt L. Palpable breast lumps: an age-based approach to evaluation and diagnosis. S Afr Fam Pract. 2022;64(1):5571.
6. Sickles EA. ACR BI-RADS® Atlas, Breast imaging reporting and data system. Reston: American College of Radiology; 2013. p. 39.
7. Salzman B, Collins E, Hersh L. Common breast problems. Am Fam Physician. 2019;99(8):505–14.
8. Boyd NF, Sutherland HJ, Fish EB, Hiraki GY, Lickley HL, Maurer VE. Prospective evaluation of physical examination of the breast. Am J Surg. 1981;142(3):331–4.
9. Aiello EJ, Buist DS, White E, Seger D, Taplin SH. Rate of breast cancer diagnoses among postmenopausal women with self-reported breast symptoms. J Am Board Fam Pract. 2004;17(6):408–15.
10. Lee H, Singh GK. Disparities in all-cancer and lung cancer survival by social, behavioral, and health status characteristics in the United States: a longitudinal fol-

low-up of the 1997–2015 National Health Interview Survey-National Death Index Record Linkage Study. J Cancer Prev. 2022;27(2):89.
11. Miller KD, Fidler-Benaoudia M, Keegan TH, Hipp HS, Jemal A, Siegel RL. Cancer statistics for adolescents and young adults, 2020. CA Cancer J Clin. 2020;70(6):443–59.
12. Lehman CD, Lee AY, Lee CI. Imaging management of palpable breast abnormalities. Am J Roentgenol. 2014;203(5):1142–53.
13. Dennis MA, Parker SH, Klaus AJ, Stavros AT, Kaske TI, Clark SB. Breast biopsy avoidance: the value of normal mammograms and normal sonograms in the setting of a palpable lump. Radiology. 2001;219(1):186–91.
14. Moy L, Slanetz PJ, Moore R, Satija S, Yeh ED, McCarthy KA, et al. Specificity of mammography and US in the evaluation of a palpable abnormality: retrospective review. Radiology. 2002;225(1):176–81.
15. Shetty MK, Shah YP. Prospective evaluation of the value of negative sonographic and mammographic findings in patients with palpable abnormalities of the breast. J Ultrasound Med. 2002;21(11):1211–20.
16. Chan CH, Coopey SB, Freer PE, Hughes KS. False-negative rate of combined mammography and ultrasound for women with palpable breast masses. Breast Cancer Res Treat. 2015;153:699–702.
17. Klein KA, Kocher M, Lourenco AP, Niell BL, Bennett DL, Chetlen A, et al. ACR appropriateness criteria® palpable breast masses: 2022 update. J Am Coll Radiol. 2023;20(5):S146–63.
18. Ciatto S, Houssami N. Breast imaging and needle biopsy in women with clinically evident breast cancer: does combined imaging change overall diagnostic sensitivity? Breast. 2007;16(4):382–6.
19. Murphy IG, Dillon MF, Doherty AO, McDermott EW, Kelly G, O'higgins N, et al. Analysis of patients with false negative mammography and symptomatic breast carcinoma. J Surg Oncol. 2007;96(6):457–63.
20. Shetty MK, Shah YP, Sharman RS. Prospective evaluation of the value of combined mammographic and sonographic assessment in patients with palpable abnormalities of the breast. J Ultrasound Med. 2003;22(3):263–8.
21. Linden OE, Hayward JH, Price ER, Kelil T, Joe BN, Lee AY. Utility of diagnostic mammography as the primary imaging modality for palpable lumps in women with almost entirely fatty breasts. Am J Roentgenol. 2020;214(4):938–44.
22. Amitai Y, Menes TS, Weinstein I, Filyavich A, Yakobson I, Golan O. What is the yield of breast MRI in the assessment of palpable breast findings? Clin Radiol. 2017;72(11):930–5.
23. Olsen ML, Morton MJ, Stan DL, Pruthi S. Is there a role for magnetic resonance imaging in diagnosing palpable breast masses when mammogram and ultrasound are negative? J Women's Health. 2012;21(11):1149–54.
24. Yau EJ, Gutierrez RL, DeMartini WB, Eby PR, Peacock S, Lehman CD. The utility of breast MRI as a problem-solving tool. Breast J. 2011;17(3):273–80.
25. Murphy IG, Dillon MF, Doherty AO, McDermott EW, Kelly G, O'higgins N, Hill AD. Analysis of patients with false negative mammography and symptomatic breast carcinoma. J Surg Oncol. 2007;96(6):457–63.
26. Gumus H, Gumus M, Mills P, Fish D, Devalia H, Jones SE, et al. Clinically palpable breast abnormalities with normal imaging: is clinically guided biopsy still required? Clin Radiol. 2012;67(5):437–40.
27. American College of Radiology. ACR practice parameter for the performance of ultrasound-guided percutaneous breast interventional procedures.
28. American College of Radiology. ACR practice parameter for the performance of stereotactic/tomosynthesis-guided breast interventional procedures.
29. Harvey JA. Sonography of palpable breast masses. In: Seminars in ultrasound, CT and MRI, vol. 27, No. 4. WB Saunders; 2006. p. 284–97.
30. Garg S, Mohan H, Bal A, Attri AK, Kochhar S. A comparative analysis of core needle biopsy and fine-needle aspiration cytology in the evaluation of palpable and mammographically detected suspicious breast lesions. Diagn Cytopathol. 2007;35(11):681–9.
31. American College of Radiology. ACR practice parameter for performing and interpreting magnetic resonance imaging (MRI).
32. Ciatto S, Bravetti P, Bonardi R, Rosselli del Turco M. The role of mammography in women under 30. Radiol Med. 1990;80(5):676–8.
33. Checka CM, Chun JE, Schnabel FR, Lee J, Toth H. The relationship of mammographic density and age: implications for breast cancer screening. Am J Roentgenol. 2012;198(3):W292–5.
34. Yue D, Swinson C, Ravichandran D. Triple assessment is not necessary in most young women referred with breast symptoms. Ann R Coll Surg Engl. 2015;97(6):466–8.
35. Holbrook AI. Breast pain, a common grievance: guidance to radiologists. Am J Roentgenol. 2020;214(2):259–64.
36. Scurr J, Hedger W, Morris P, Brown N. The prevalence, severity, and impact of breast pain in the general population. Breast J. 2014;20(5):508–13.
37. Groen JW, Grosfeld S, Bramer WM, Ernst MF, Mullender MM. Cyclic and non-cyclic breast-pain: a systematic review on pain reduction, side effects, and quality of life for various treatments. Eur J Obstet Gynecol Reprod Biol. 2017;219:74–93.
38. Kataria K, Dhar A, Srivastava A, Kumar S, Goyal A. A systematic review of current understanding and management of mastalgia. Indian J Surg. 2014;76:217–22.
39. Arslan M, Küçükerdem HS, Can H, Tarcan E. Retrospective analysis of women with only mastalgia. J Breast Health. 2016;12(4):151.

40. Khan SA, Apkarian AV. Mastalgia and breast cancer: a protective association? Cancer Detect Prev. 2002;26(3):192–6.
41. Fariselli G, Lepera P, Viganotti G, Martelli G, Bandieramonte G, Di Pietro S. Localized mastalgia as presenting symptom in breast cancer. Eur J Surg Oncol J Eur Soc Surg Oncol Br Assoc Surg Oncol. 1988;14(3):213–5.
42. Holbrook AI, Moy L, Akin EA, Baron P, Didwania AD, Heller SL, et al. ACR appropriateness criteria® breast pain. J Am Coll Radiol. 2018;15(11):S276–82.
43. Olawaiye A, Withiam-Leitch M, Danakas G, Kahn K. Mastalgia: a review of management. J Reprod Med. 2005;50(12):933–9.
44. Leddy R, Irshad A, Zerwas E, Mayes N, Armeson K, Abid M, et al. Role of breast ultrasound and mammography in evaluating patients presenting with focal breast pain in the absence of a palpable lump. Breast J. 2013;19(6):582–9.
45. Loving VA, DeMartini WB, Eby PR, Gutierrez RL, Peacock S, Lehman CD. Targeted ultrasound in women younger than 30 years with focal breast signs or symptoms: outcomes analyses and management implications. Am J Roentgenol. 2010;195(6):1472–7.
46. Hofvind S, Hovda T, Holen AS, Lee CI, Albertsen J, Bjorndal H, et al. Digital breast tomosynthesis and synthetic 2D mammography versus digital mammography: evaluation in a population-based screening program. Radiology. 2018;287(3):787–94.
47. Cho MW, Grimm LJ, Johnson KS. Focal breast pain: does breast density affect the need for ultrasound? Acad Radiol. 2017;24(1):53–9.
48. Tan H, Li R, Peng W, Liu H, Gu Y, Shen X. Radiological and clinical features of adult non-puerperal mastitis. Br J Radiol. 2013;86(1024):20120657.
49. Boakes E, Woods A, Johnson N, Kadoglou N. Breast infection: a review of diagnosis and management practices. Eur J Breast Health. 2018;14(3):136.
50. Yeh ED, Jacene HA, Bellon JR, Nakhlis F, Birdwell RL, Georgian-Smith D, et al. What radiologists need to know about diagnosis and treatment of inflammatory breast cancer: a multidisciplinary approach. Radiographics. 2013;33(7):2003–17.
51. Patel BK, Falcon S, Drukteinis J. Management of nipple discharge and the associated imaging findings. Am J Med. 2015;128(4):353–60.
52. Goksel HA, Yagmurdur MC, Demirhan B, Isıklar I, Karakayali H, Bilgin N, et al. Management strategies for patients with nipple discharge. Langenbeck's Arch Surg. 2005;390:52–8.
53. Carrasco RM, Benito MA, del Campo ER. Value of mammography and breast ultrasound in male patients with nipple discharge. Eur J Radiol. 2013;82(3):478–84.
54. Sanford MF, Slanetz PJ, Lewin AA, Baskies AM, Bozzuto L, Branton SA, et al. ACR appropriateness criteria® evaluation of nipple discharge: 2022 update. J Am Coll Radiol. 2022;19(11S):S304–18.
55. Morrogh M, Park A, Elkin EB, King TA. Lessons learned from 416 cases of nipple discharge of the breast. Am J Surg. 2010;200(1):73–80.
56. Bahl M, Baker JA, Greenup RA, Ghate SV. Diagnostic value of ultrasound in female patients with nipple discharge. Am J Roentgenol. 2015;205(1):203–8.
57. Morrogh M, Morris EA, Liberman L, Borgen PI, King TA. The predictive value of ductography and magnetic resonance imaging in the management of nipple discharge. Ann Surg Oncol. 2007;14:3369–77.
58. Comstock CE, Sung JS. Computer-aided detection for breast MRI. In: Molleran VM, Mahoney MC, editors. Breast MRI. Philadelphia: Elsevier Saunders; 2014.
59. Osako T, Iwase T, Takahashi K, Iijima K, Miyagi Y, Nishimura S, et al. Diagnostic mammography and ultrasonography for palpable and nonpalpable breast cancer in women aged 30 to 39 years. Breast Cancer. 2007;14:255–9.
60. Mainiero MB, Lourenco AP, Barke LD, Argus AD, Bailey L, Carkaci S, et al. ACR appropriateness criteria evaluation of the symptomatic male breast. J Am Coll Radiol. 2015;12(7):678–82.

Imaging in Adolescence, Pregnancy and Lactation

2

Sabita Desai, Saloni Desai, and Suchana Kushvaha

Abstract

The spectrum of breast disease in children differs from that in adults, and approach is usually conservative as breast malignancy in adolescents is very rare. Knowledge of normal physiological breast development is essential to distinguish from pathologies, and thus clinical examination is the most important step followed by ultrasound as the modality of choice. The purpose of this chapter is to elucidate imaging features of normal breast development, benign and rare malignant neoplasms, and metastatic conditions as a guidance for appropriate management options.

On the other hand, there is a wide spectrum of benign and malignant masses seen during pregnancy and lactation. The physiological changes that occur in the breast parenchyma during pregnancy and lactation are due to hormonal influences. This causes changes in the breast parenchyma and makes clinical examination and radiological imaging very challenging. It is important to have a good knowledge of the physiological changes that occur during this phase. A vast majority of the masses that are seen during pregnancy and lactation are benign; however, the possibility of pregnancy-associated breast cancer should be kept in mind as these cancers are detected late and are biologically aggressive. This chapter will include the common pathologies that are seen during pregnancy and lactation and their imaging features.

Keywords

Pregnancy · Lactation · Adolescence Mammography · Ultrasound · Pregnancy-associated breast cancer

2.1 Introduction

Breast complaints in children and adolescents are often a reason for anxiety for parents owing to the high incidence of breast malignancy in adults. However, the majority of conditions affecting this age group are benign, and only 0.1 in 100,000 females less than 20 years have been reported to have breast cancer [1]. However, the imaging features are overlapping which increases patient's, parent's and physician's anxiety. Hence, it is vital for the radiologist to know the spectrum of

S. Desai (✉)
Breach Candy Hospital Trust Mumbai, Mumbai, India

S. Desai
Sir H N Reliance Foundation Hospital, Mumbai, India

S. Kushvaha
Prajnam Breast Care, Gurugram, India

E. Dhamija, S. V. S. Deo (eds.), *Imaging in Management of Breast Diseases*,
https://doi.org/10.1007/978-981-96-4998-3_2

pathologies pertinent to children and adolescents to provide appropriate differential diagnoses and avoid unnecessary biopsies in the developing breast.

A thorough clinical examination is the most important step in addressing paediatric breast complaints as these are often developmental processes that do not need imaging. Owing to the lack of radiation hazard, ultrasound (US) forms the mainstay in assessment, while mammography (MG) is useful only in selected patients to look for microcalcifications. Computed tomography (CT) scan is generally not used due to radiation risk, while the role of MRI is limited to evaluate deep lesions for chest wall involvement, to delineate vascular anomalies and tumour extent, if present. Interventions in the paediatric breast including fine needle aspiration must be used extremely sparingly as they can lead to permanent breast bud arrest or disfigurement in later life. The exact reason is not known owing to the small number of cases that have been followed later in life. This might be due to the small size of breast bud, and hence even a small amount of trauma leads to breast tissue destruction [2, 3]. As used for adults, the American College of Radiology (ACR) Breast Imaging Reporting and Data System atlas is also used for reporting childhood pathologies.

2.2 Development of Breast and Expected Imaging Features

Breast development begins in utero in the 5th to 6th week of gestation when the epidermal cells invaginate into the deeper mesenchyme and form the primary mammary ridges or milk lines which extend symmetrically from the axillae to the groins. With time, the rest of these ridges involute, while the ones at the level of the fourth intercostal space develop into breast buds. Areolar development takes place in the 5th month of foetal life, and soon after birth, the nipple everts owing to mesodermal proliferation [4].

Breast development in both boys and girls is a result of the influence of placental oestrogen. The morphology is the same in both genders comprising of simple ducts and stroma. After birth, there is a rise in levels of gonadotropins and sex hormones and a drop in oestrogen levels [5]. A transient neonatal breast enlargement can be seen in the first few weeks of life in both genders that may be unilateral or bilateral. This is secondary to the maternal hormones crossing the placental barrier. This is seen in approximately 70% of term babies and is usually 1–2 cm in size. The falling blood levels of maternal hormones after birth lead to regression of the enlarged breasts, and this causes a rise in serum prolactin levels that may cause galactorrhoea [6, 7].

Galactorrhoea may be seen in normal newborns up to 2 months of age (also known as witch's milk) being more common in neonates with hypothyroidism and is associated with larger-than-average breast nodules [7, 8]. This breast nodule may show retroareolar density with simple branching ducts on US which needs to be differentiated from neonatal mastitis. The latter affects full-term infants at less than 5 weeks of age and is often unilateral. The most common pathogen found is *Staphylococcus aureus* followed by gram-negative bacteria presenting clinically with signs of local inflammation like breast tenderness, redness and swelling. If left untreated, it may progress to breast abscess which may need needle aspiration to prevent damage to the developing breast bud [9].

A period of mini-puberty in infancy caused by gonadotropin and sex steroid-level surge brings about varied changes in glandular development. Luteinizing hormone levels in boys peak at 1–3 months and return to prepubertal values by 4–6 months, while follicle-stimulating hormone levels peak in girls at 2–4 months and return to normal by 12–24 months. These can lead to changes in breasts, uterus and ovaries becoming a cause of parental concern [10, 11].

After the first in utero stage of breast development, the second stage in girls occurs at adolescence and is called thelarche, typically between 8 and 13 years of age. Under the influence of oestrogen, ductal growth gets stimulated, while progesterone leads to differentiation into the terminal duct lobular unit [12]. Normal pubertal breast development has been classified into five Tanner stages, and the US appearance of each stage has been well described (Table 2.1) [13]. Isolated premature thelarche prior to 2 years of age is likely to be non-progressive, and no further tests are usually required. However, if there are associated clinical features of sexual maturation, it should raise possibility of precocious puberty and warrants further investigations to look for the central (GnRH-dependent) or peripheral (GnRH-independent) causes of precocious puberty [14]. These may include biochemical tests, bone age estimation and abdominopelvic US for adrenal glands, uterus and ovaries to look for adrenal

Table 2.1 Tanner stages of breast development

Illustration	Tanner stages	Ultrasound (USG) appearances
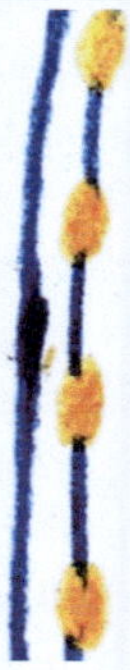	*Stage 1: Prepubertal* Nipple areola complex is present and is seen with the level of the skin of the adjoining chest wall. No glandular tissue present	
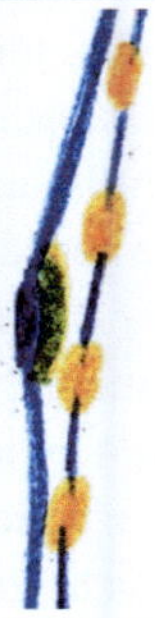	*Stage 2:* The breast bud develops beneath the areola such that NAC gets lifted up beyond the chest wall	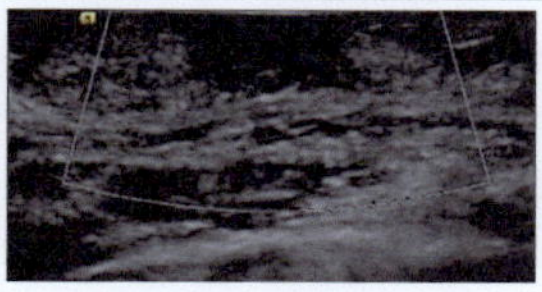
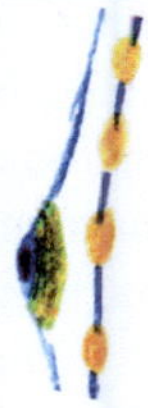	*Stage 3:* The developing breast bud enlarges and extends beyond the areolar margins. The NAC and the breast skin lie at one level	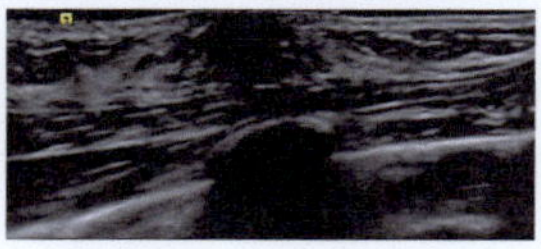
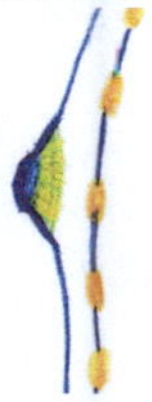	*Stage 4:* The areola becomes lifted up above the level of the breast skin (double scoop appearance)	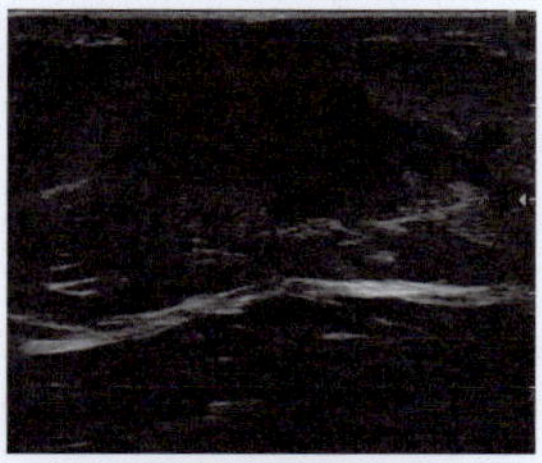
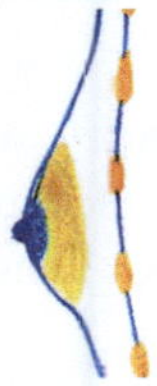	*Stage 5:* The areola becomes hyperpigmented, papillae develop, and the nipple protrudes out. The breast enlarges further	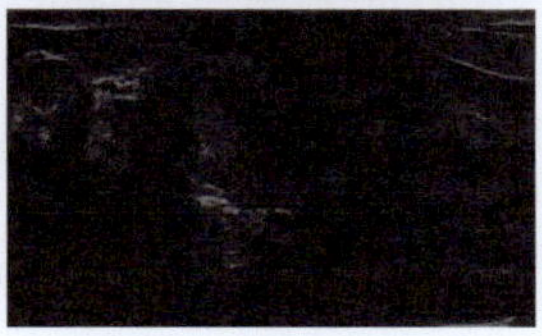

hyperplasia, gonadal sex cord stromal tumours like Sertoli/Leydig cell tumours and germ cell tumours like dysgerminomas, embryonal tumours and teratomas.

2.3 Congenital and Developmental Pathologies

The ectopic breast tissue may be seen due to incomplete regression of the mammary ridge anywhere from the axilla to the vulva but most commonly found in the axilla. Supernumerary nipples or polythelia can be found in 1–5% of the population, while the presence of supernumerary breasts or polymastia is less common, found in 0.4–0.6% of the population [15]. Asymmetry between the sizes of two breasts is a usual finding and a normal variant rather than a disease entity; however it may be disturbing cosmetically to the woman and affect her self-confidence. There are no objective criteria to define this asymmetry. The patient's decision for her image plays an important role for further counselling and surgical decision management. It is important for the treating team to understand the expectations of the patient well and also for the patient to understand that perfect symmetry may not be achieved before going ahead with any corrective surgery where the aim remains to bring down the difference in the two breasts to the minimum [16]. Usually, there is no identifiable cause; however, in some patients there may be an underlying reason like prior burns, trauma, radiation therapy or scoliosis.

The absence or hypoplasia of the breast can be seen in conditions like Poland syndrome. Poland syndrome is characterized by hypoplasia of the pectoralis major muscle. The underlying cause is not identifiable, and the most accepted theory says that there is ischemic injury that happens to the developing pectoral upper limb girdle that leads to non-development of the pectoralis major muscle, hypoplastic or absent breast bud. Clinically, there is asymmetrical chest wall development, and mammogram will show hypoplastic breast and non-visualization of the pectoral muscles. CT sections through the chest will reveal the absent pectoral muscle [17, 18].

Juvenile or virginal breast hypertrophy is uncontrolled breast development in adolescent girls without any underlying endocrine abnormality. It can affect one or both breasts. Sometimes the size may be huge enough to cause social embarrassment and health issues to the girl like chest wall pain and neck pain. The enlarged breast may present with pain, backache and social embarrassment, and treatment options would include anti-oestrogen medications and reduction mammoplasty after the cessation of breast development [17, 19].

Excessive breast development in neonates, adolescents and elderly males is termed as gynecomastia and is most commonly (60–75%) seen in adolescent boys [20]. Varying degrees of breast enlargement are seen frequently in boys which peak at 13–14 years of age and resolve within 2 years. Although mostly it is bilateral, it can be unilateral and familial and presents as firm, tender subareolar nodules. A decrease in testosterone and an increase in oestrogen levels are considered to be the triggering factor. The appearance of gynecomastia in prepubertal boys should warrant further tests to rule out endocrinopathy or tumours [14]. Tumours like testicular Leydig cell tumours and adrenal cortical tumours which produce oestrogen, and hepatoblastoma, choriocarcinoma and fibrolamellar hepatocellular carcinoma which secrete gonadotrophins, should be ruled out. Liver disease, Klinefelter syndrome, neurofibromatosis type 1, prolactinomas and drugs such as anabolic steroids, marijuana, tricyclic antidepressants, corticosteroids and herbal medications are other causes of breast development [21].

2.4 Benign Diseases at Puberty and in Young Females

2.4.1 Benign Cystic Masses

Retroareolar cysts or cysts of Montgomery are seen in adolescent girls due to blocked Montgomery glands at the areolar edge. These may be associated with pain or inflammation, and US may show thin-walled cysts which are usually less than 2 cm in diameter. These can be single or multiple and unilateral or bilateral and may contain debris. Management is generally conservative [15, 22].

Mammary duct ectasia is a rare condition seen in newborns and young children with the presentation of bloody nipple discharge or a palpable subareolar mass. The aetiology is unknown with infection or maternal hormones being considered as the contributing factors. On US, dilated ectatic retroareolar ducts are seen with or without debris within. The breast massage or nipple expression should be avoided, and the usual management is conservative and symptomatic. Their resolution post-cessation of breastfeeding corroborates the maternal hormones playing a role behind its occurrence [21, 23, 24].

Mastitis and breast abscesses can be seen in infants less than 2 months of age (mastitis neonatorum) and older children of 8–17 years' age group with clinical signs of inflammation like fever, erythema, tenderness and leucocytosis. *Staphylococcus aureus* is the most common causative organism followed by *Streptococcus* and *Enterococcus*. The abscess can be seen as a thick-walled collection with internal echoes on US which may need image-guided drainage (Fig. 2.1) [25].

Hematomas and fat necrosis usually result from an external injury, breast trauma or surgery; hence accurate history is essential for diagnosis. On US, the appearance of hematomas may be variable according to the stage of temporal evolution varying from echogenic irregular fluid collection to more organized and walled off heterogeneous area with internal echoes and septations. It can have associated overlying skin changes. In the appropriate clinical scenario, cold fomentation and adequate support to the breast should suffice, and a short-term interval follow-up is recommended to look for its resolution. Any increase in size over time must warrant a needle aspiration for further evaluation [23].

Galactoceles are cysts forming secondary to milk retention. These are seen predominantly in lactating women but have also been reported rarely in infants and adolescents. The three factors that are required for a galactocele to form are obstructed duct causing retention, prolactin stimulation and secretory breast epithelium. Usually there is no underlying endocrine disorder found [24]. The imaging features are similar in any age group, that is, unilateral or bilateral cysts with hypoechoic water component and hyperechoic fat component (fat-fluid level). Usually, these are self-limiting, and aspiration is reserved for symptomatic and atypical cases [23, 26].

2.4.2 Benign Solid Masses

The most common benign solid mass in paediatric or adolescent girls between 15 and 17 years is fibroadenoma [27]. The other reported benign masses include juvenile papillomatosis, pseudoangiomatous stromal hyperplasia (PASH) and vascular lesions like hemangiomas and vascular malformations. In cases with atypical imaging features or rapid increase in size, histopathological correlation should be considered.

Fibroadenomas are benign fibroepithelial lesions presenting clinically as a firm, non-tender,

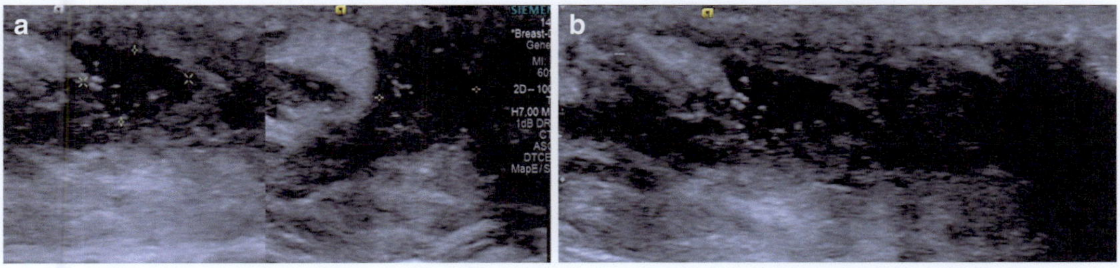

Fig. 2.1 Ultrasound of a 4-month-old baby shows hypoechoic collection with thick internal echoes in the retroareolar region with increased echogenicity of the surrounding fat (**a**, **b**—calipered area)

freely movable rubbery lump, arising as a result of the proliferation of connective tissue stroma around breast lobules. As these tumours are oestrogen sensitive, they can show rapid growth during puberty and pregnancy. Since male breasts do not have these lobules, fibroadenomas are not seen in the male breast, although a few rare case reports do exist with most of them reported in patients receiving oestrogen therapy as in transgender females or for prostate carcinomas [28]. A classical fibroadenoma (Fig. 2.2a) will be oval-shaped and hypoechoic with circumscribed or gently lobulated margins and parallel orientation on US, [20, 23, 29]. If the imaging features are characteristic, a conservative approach and a short-term interval follow-up should suffice. About 10% of these lesions are known to regress spontaneously [30]. A variant known as complex fibroadenoma (Fig. 2.2b) has been described on pathological evaluation where they can show foci of papillary apocrine metaplasia, sclerosing adenosis, cysts greater than 3 mm and calcifications on histology. These are usually seen in older children and are associated with a slightly higher risk of subsequently developing breast cancer [31].

Fibroadenomas larger than 5 cm in diameter are termed giant fibroadenomas. Juvenile or cellular fibroadenomas (Fig. 2.2c) are uncommon variants accounting for 7–8% of cases, common in African American girls and associated with rapid growth. Multiple and bilateral fibroadenomas can be seen in 10–25% of patients [32, 33]. US appearance of juvenile fibroadenomas overlaps with those of phyllodes tumour with the presence of cleft-like internal spaces, and hence surgical excision is usually advised [25].

PASH is benign breast stromal proliferation lined by myofibroblasts commonly seen in premenopausal women but reported in children and young adults as well. It is a close mimic of fibroadenoma clinically and radiologically, presenting as a firm, mobile rubbery mass which may show a rapid growth in adolescence. Associations with immunodeficiency conditions and neurofibromatosis type 1 have been reported [13, 23]. Sonographic features of PASH are similar to fibroadenoma, in the form of circumscribed oval hypoechoic lesion. Histologically, it can be confused with phyllodes or angiosarcoma due to the presence of anastomosing slit-like channels. Although these tumours are benign, a tendency of slow growth and recurrence after excision is known [34, 35].

Juvenile papillomatosis is a rare benign disorder of late adolescence seen at a mean age of 19 years that presents clinically as a firm mobile mass with no nipple discharge. It is also known as 'Swiss cheese' disease due to the presence of multiple cysts and dilated ducts separated by dense stroma [36]. Although clinical palpation mimics fibroadenoma, US reveals an ill-demarcated heterogeneously hypoechoic lesion with tiny cystic areas. It has been observed that 33–58% of patients with juvenile papillomatosis have a family history of breast cancer. Although juvenile papillomatosis is a benign entity, there is a chance of concurrent breast cancer in 5–15% patients; hence surgical excision is the treatment of choice [37]. In juvenile papillomatosis, there

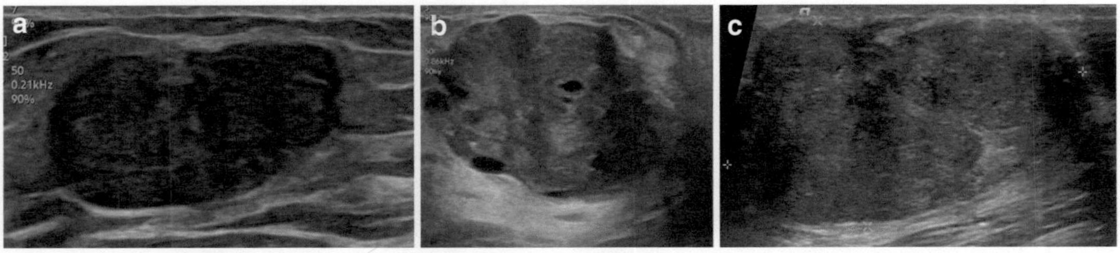

Fig. 2.2 *Imaging appearances of fibroadenoma:* (**a**) Classical fibroadenoma: oval-shaped parallel-oriented hypoechoic lesion with circumscribed margins in a 14-year-old female. (**b**) Complex fibroadenoma: oval-shaped heterogeneous lesion with circumscribed margins and internal cystic changes in a 22-year-old female. (**c**) Juvenile fibroadenoma: a rapidly increasing oval-shaped hypoechoic lesion with circumscribed margins and tiny internal cystic changes

are multiple cystic spaces representing focal dilated ducts, duct ectasia and papillary epithelial hyperplasia, ductal stasis, cysts with apocrine and non-apocrine epithelium, sclerosing adenosis, fibroadenomatoid hyperplasia and lobular hyperplasia. The papillary ductal hyperplasia is a different entity encompassing intraductal papillomas, intraductal papillomatosis and sclerosing papillomatosis [35].

Vascular tumours: The most common vascular lesion involving paediatric breast is haemangioma which may involve the chest wall as well as breast tissue. It can be capillary or infantile haemangioma which typically grows till the child is 11–12 months of age and subsequently involutes. Similar lesions can be seen elsewhere in the body as well. There would be skin changes that may appear as red or blue and often the history of their presence since birth is there. US with Doppler helps identify vascular channels within the lesion [38].

2.5 Malignant Masses at Puberty and Adolescence

Phyllodes is a rare fibroepithelial tumour comprising only 1% of paediatric breast lesions but is the most common primary breast malignancy in girls less than 20 years of age and more common in Asians. Histologically, these are categorized into low, intermediate and high grades, all of which have a propensity to recur and metastasize. Phyllode neoplasm was previously known as cystosarcoma phyllodes because just like sarcoma, it shows propensity for haematogenous spread to lungs as opposed to axillary lymph nodes [13]. Nonetheless, the majority of phyllodes seen in adolescence are benign in nature. Recurrence rates reported in benign and malignant phyllodes are 10–25% and 40%, respectively [39]. Juvenile fibroadenomas and phyllodes have similar clinical, US, and histopathological appearances, and hence biopsy is essential for further evaluation. Phyllodes vary in size from 1 to 20 cm, are generally heterogeneous with internal cleft-like spaces on US and can have circumscribed or lobulated margins. The presence of haemorrhagic infarction and necrosis raise the possibility of malignancy (Fig. 2.3) [40, 41]. If the tumour is larger than 5 cm, surgical excision with safe negative margins is recommended as on core biopsy it may not be possible to distinguish fibroadenoma from phyllodes [13, 23].

Metastatic breast disease is more common than primary breast malignancy in the paediatric age group and indicates a poor prognosis. Neuroblastoma, rhabdomyosarcoma, lymphoma and leukaemia have been reported to have dissemination to the breast. Malignant melanoma, renal cell carcinoma, Ewing sarcoma and primitive neuroectodermal tumours can also metastasize to the breast [27]. Metastases on US may appear as solid and hypoechoic circumscribed masses. In adolescents with known primary malignancy, one must be careful in interpreting breast masses because metastatic lesions have variable US appearances and may look like probably benign lesions (Fig. 2.4) [13].

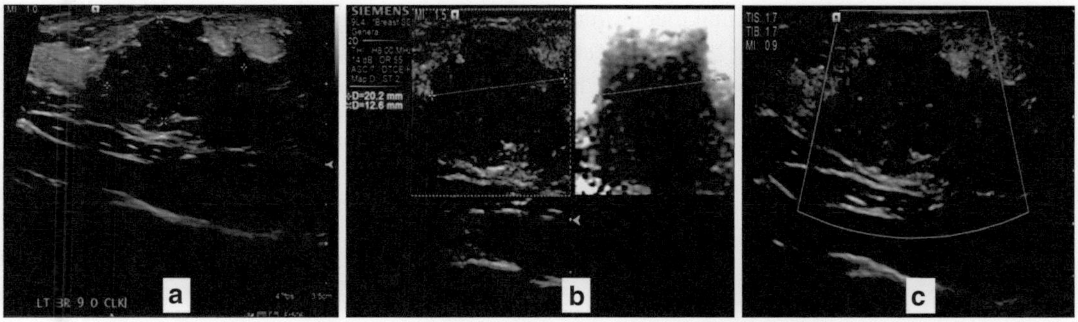

Fig. 2.3 Fibroepithelial tumour: USG reveals a hypoechoic irregular mass with angular margins in the left breast (**a**) which shows minimal vascularity on colour Doppler (**c**) and is hard on elastography (**b**)

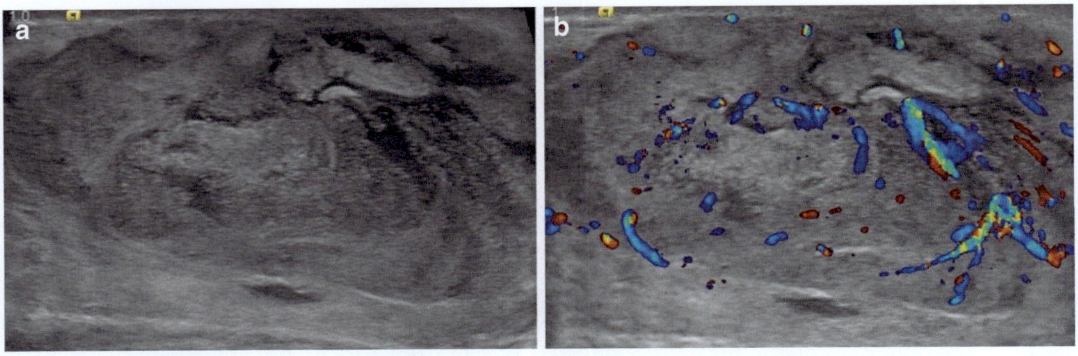

Fig. 2.4 *Lymphoma:* Grey-scale USG image (**a**) shows an irregular heterogeneous mass with indistinct margins and increased internal vascularity on colour Doppler (**b**) in a child with Burkitt's lymphoma

Primary breast carcinoma is exceedingly rare in children and adolescents with the reported incidence of 0.03 per 1,000,000 for females less than 20 years of age [42]. The most common subtype has been observed to be secretory (juvenile) carcinoma which has a favourable prognosis as compared to other less frequent subtypes like invasive ductal carcinoma, invasive lobular carcinoma and anaplastic, medullary and inflammatory carcinomas. Secretory carcinomas are usually painless circumscribed or microlobulated lesions, less than 3 cm in size and hypoechoic with internal heterogeneity on US. Patients treated with lumpectomy and radiation have shown a 5-year survival rate of 87.2% [43]. Children who have received mantle irradiation for Hodgkin's disease are found to be at increased risk of developing breast cancer (incidence of 12–20% by 40 years of age) [43]. Mantle radiation was a standard technique to treat Hodgkin's lymphoma from the 1970s till the 1990s. A large part of the neck, chest, armpits and mediastinum was included in the field to cover both the affected nodes and the normal lymph nodes. Now, it has been replaced by more focussed radiotherapy with lesser side effects. Thus, the American College of Radiology recommends annual screening with MRI in such patients starting after 25 years of age or for 8–10 years after treatment completion whichever is earlier [44].

2.6 Approach to Breast Lesions in Paediatrics and Adolescence

Most paediatric lesions are developmental or benign entities that require reassurance to the patient as well as caregiver. Short-interval follow-up US at 6 monthly interval for the first year is usually recommended and the next US at the end of the second year to monitor lesion size and growth. Biopsy should be done sparingly as it can cause permanent damage to the developing breast bud.

As the risk of breast malignancy in the paediatric age group is extremely low and harm to the developing breast bud should be avoided at all costs, a conservative approach to breast complaints has been suggested [2, 3]. Evaluation needs detailed history and clinical examination because the self-limiting conditions of newborns like nipple discharge and subareolar nodules would only need parental assurance.

Asymmetry of breast buds in the prepubertal age group is common, and US may be used for confirmation. Physiologic gynecomastia is frequently seen in neonates and adolescent boys, while gynecomastia in prepubertal boys requires further investigations to rule out tumours and endocrinopathies. Small palpable masses in young girls are likely to be fibroadenomas which would need US for confirmation of characteristic features with subsequent follow-up US. Lumps larger than 5 cm and rapidly growing lesions may need a biopsy to rule out other worrisome pathologies. High-risk conditions in children and adolescents would include the presence of extramammary malignancy, prior chest irradiation and genetic mutations. Any breast mass seen in the high-risk group should be viewed with suspicion. Management of breast masses in children differs from that in adults, and knowledge of the spectrum of conditions affecting the paediatric age group helps in guiding appropriate treatment.

2.7 Physiological Changes During Pregnancy and Lactation

There is a spectrum of benign and malignant diseases that are seen during pregnancy and lactation. It is important to know the appearance of the breast parenchyma in both conditions as imaging in pregnancy and lactation can be very challenging due to physiological changes that take place in the breasts causing an alteration in the echogenicity of the breast parenchyma. The choices of imaging modalities during pregnancy and lactation are US, MG and MRI where every imaging modality has its own benefits and risks.

During pregnancy, the breast undergoes numerous changes in preparation for lactation. These changes occur in response to an increase in circulating hormones, i.e. oestrogen, progesterone and prolactin, which begin early in the 2nd month of the first trimester of pregnancy [45]. Oestrogen causes marked ductular sprouting with some branching and discrete lobular growth, simultaneous involution of the fibrofatty stroma and an increase in glandular vascularity, often accompanied by infiltration by mononuclear cells [45].

During the first, second and third trimesters of pregnancy, the echogenicity of glandular elements relative to fat varies slightly. The glandular tissues are isoechoic during the early pregnancy but become slightly hypoechoic as lactational change fills the intralobular acini with secretions. The breast is diffusely hypoechoic during pregnancy, due to the increase in glandular tissue (Fig. 2.5) [46].

During lactation, the fall in the oestrogen and progesterone levels and rise in prolactin and oxytocin levels cause the breast tissue to secrete milk. This change from the proliferative to the secretory phase in the breast at delivery is called lactogenesis. This is seen on ultrasound as diffusely increased echogenicity of glandular parenchyma with dilated ducts containing milk (Fig. 2.6) [46].

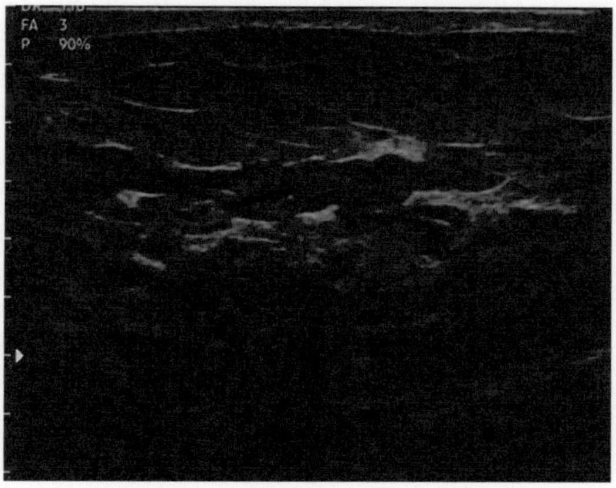

Fig. 2.5 USG image shows a hypoechoic glandular parenchyma in a pregnant patient

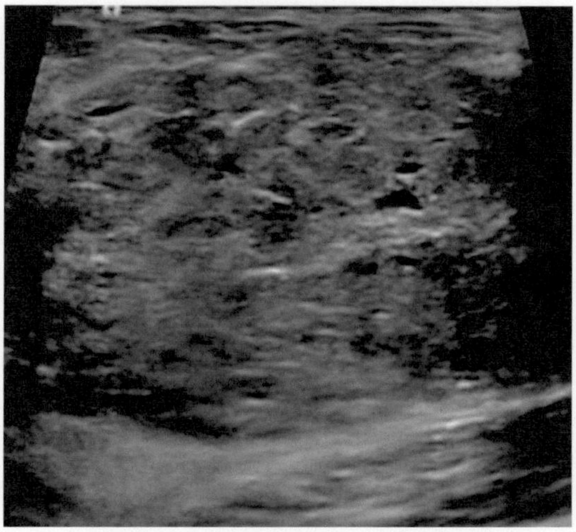

Fig. 2.6 USG image shows a diffuse increase in the echogenicity of glandular parenchyma during lactation owing to secretory changes in the breast

2.8 Imaging Modalities During Pregnancy and Lactation

Imaging of the breasts during pregnancy and lactation is extremely challenging due to the various physiological and structural changes owing to the variation of related hormones. US is the modality of choice for evaluation of the breast in pregnancy and lactation as it is radiation-free and comfortable for the females with a sensitivity of 86.7% and 100%, respectively [47]. Also, the breasts become denser limiting the mammogram quality; however, the quality is not compromised to such an extent that one should not utilize it when clinically indicated [48]. It should be avoided in the first trimester owing to the theoretical risk of malformations in the foetus, though the exposure is minimal to cause any detrimental effects [46].

The breast parenchyma shows diffuse hypoechogenicity due to the proliferative phase in pregnancy and is diffusely hyperechoic with prominent ductal dilatation and increased vascularity in lactating phase [49]. The sensitivity and negative predictive value for detection of pregnancy-associated breast cancer (PABC) is up to 100% with US [49]. Thus, MG of the breasts is not the initial imaging modality of choice in pregnant women; however, if the US reveals any suspicious masses, then a bilateral mammogram can be done to look for calcifications. In such circumstances, an abdominal shield using a lead apron should be used which can decrease the dose to the uterus by up to 50% [49]. The radiation dose to the breast is 3 mGy which is roughly equivalent to 7 weeks of background radiation, and the radiation dose to foetus is <0.03 microGy which is a fraction of the total 50 microGy threshold causing teratogenic effects in the foetus [49].

MRI does not play a role in the diagnostic workup of the breast during pregnancy. This is due to foetal safety concerns which are associated with gadolinium-based contrast agents as they are known to cross the placenta [50]. However, gadolinium-based contrast is considered safe for administration during lactation. Although the ACR Manual on Contrast Media notes that breastfeeding after the IV administration of gadolinium is safe [51], a mother can always choose to pump and discard milk for 24 hours following gadolinium administration.

The preferred intervention for breast masses during pregnancy and lactation is an US-guided core needle biopsy. The patient should be informed of the complications while taking consent for the procedure. The common complication of a core needle biopsy in these patients is bleeding, infection, bloody nipple discharge and milk fistula formation owing to increased parenchymal vascularity and milk-filled ducts acting as culture medium for bacterial growth. Bloody nipple discharge can occur post-biopsy and resolves spontaneously. These risks can be minimized by cessation of breastfeeding before core biopsy, practising strict asepsis during the procedure and adequate manual compression or ice pack post-procedure. The patient can resume breastfeeding post-biopsy and should continue an adequate support to the breast [52].

2.9 Benign Diseases Related to Physiological Changes of Pregnancy and Lactation (Table 2.2)

Rusty pipe syndrome is a self-limiting condition that can be seen during pregnancy but is more common in early lactation. The name has been acquired due to the presence of blood in the breastmilk which renders a rusty or brownish colour to it. It occurs because of the increased vascularization of rapidly developing alveoli which have delicate networks of capillaries, and these capillaries get traumatized easily and result in bleeding from nipples. However, if it is spontaneous, involves single duct and is unilateral, then it has to be evaluated further to rule out malignancy [51]. Ultrasound is often asked for nonresolving cases or for psychological reasons of the mother and is usually normal. One may see an intraductal lesion in cases with pathological discharge.

Galactocele is the most common benign physiologic change that is seen in lactating women which is caused by an obstruction in the lactiferous duct or terminal ductal lobular units with resultant formation of a milk-filled retention cyst [51]. They can also be seen in the third trimester of pregnancy, and clinically they can present as single or multiple palpable masses. The US appearance is variable and depends on the proportion of fat and protein content in the milk. Commonly it is seen as a cystic mass with a layering of the fat and fluid content, and this is the typical appearance of a galactocele with the fat layering above and the fluid below. Sometimes, the high viscosity or low-fat content of the breast milk may not allow separation of the fat and water contents, and then a galactocele can resemble a hamartoma or also known as a pseudo-hamartoma. It can also be seen as a simple or a complicated cyst. Infection is a common complication of a galactocele which can be treated with an US-guided aspiration, and the fluid should be sent for culture and sensitivity. On MG they are seen as fat-containing masses; however, MG is not the imaging modality of choice (Fig. 2.7).

Table 2.2 Breast disorders in pregnancy and lactating females

Physiologic changes
Gestational and secretory hyperplasia
Galactocele
Gigantomastia
Inflammatory and infectious diseases
Puerperal mastitis
Granulomatous mastitis
Mastopathy
Juvenile papillomatosis
Benign tumours
Lactating adenoma
Changes in fibroadenoma: growth/infarction
Malignant tumours
Pregnancy-associated breast cancer
Pregnancy-related Burkitt's lymphoma

Gigantomastia is a very rare condition that complicates about 1 of every 100,000 pregnancies. It is characterized by massive enlargement of the breasts, resulting in tissue necrosis, ulceration, infection and haemorrhage. Although its cause remains unknown, gigantomastia is believed to represent an abnormal response to hormonal stimulation during pregnancy [45].

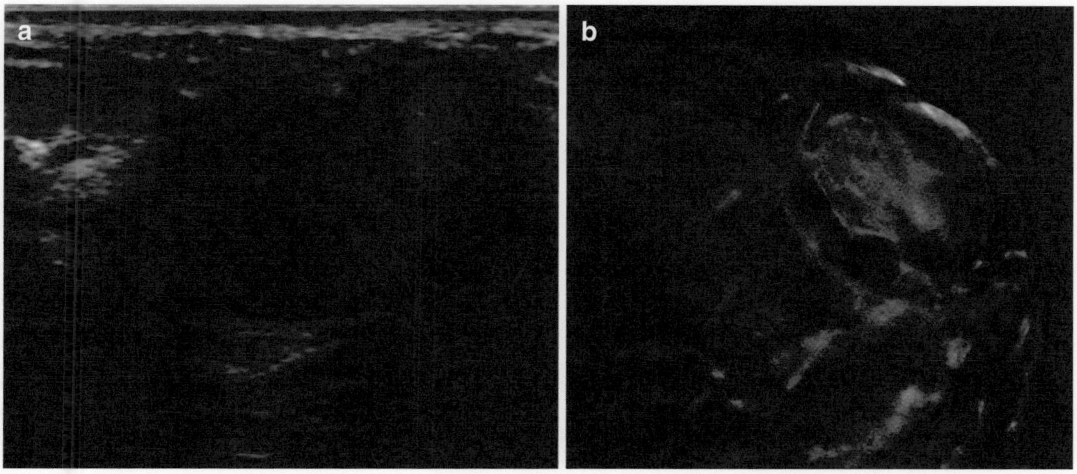

Fig. 2.7 *Galactocele:* (**a**) USG image showing an oval lesion circumscribed margins and with echogenic and cystic components within. (**b**) Limited mammography of the left breast in the CC view reveals a fat containing area within the equal density lesion with circumscribed margins

2.10 Inflammatory and Infectious Diseases

Mastitis is commonly seen during lactation and rarely during pregnancy. The organisms that commonly cause infection are *Staphylococcus aureus* and *Streptococcus*. These organisms are present in the nasopharynx and throat of the nursing infant which can enter the ductal system through disrupted epithelial surface in a cracked nipple or skin abrasion. The stasis of milk is a good culture medium for the bacteria to thrive [45]. Abscesses tend to occur more frequently with *Staphylococcus aureus*, whereas *Streptococcus* infection causes diffuse mastitis (Fig. 2.8). The imaging modality of choice is US to diagnose and treat with guided aspiration of the abscess. On US, abscesses are seen as a cystic collection with thick walls and thick internal echoes or debris within (Fig. 2.9). Colour Doppler reveals the presence of peripheral vascularity. There is a thickening of the overlying skin and increased echogenicity of the surrounding fat lobules. MG is done only if the abscess does not resolve with antibiotics and a malignancy is suspected. If it is suspicious for malignancy, then a core biopsy should be done from the wall of the abscess.

Granulomatous mastitis is an inflammatory disease of unknown aetiology. It is seen in women with a history of pregnancy in the past 5 years [2]. The organism *Corynebacterium* as a causative organism of granulomatous mastitis has been reported in literature supported by the fact of its isolation and growth from the pus samples [53]. The diagnosis of granulomatous mastitis is based on exclusion since it depends on the demonstration of a particular histologic pattern: a noncaseating, nonvasculitic granulomatous inflammatory reaction centred on lobules [45]. On US, the masses are heterogeneous in echotexture with indistinct/angular margins. The linear fluid-tracking pattern in the subcutaneous tissue is typical of granulomatous mastitis. On MG, they are seen as high-density irregular masses with indistinct margins and mimic malignancy. A core needle biopsy clinches the diagnosis (Fig. 2.10).

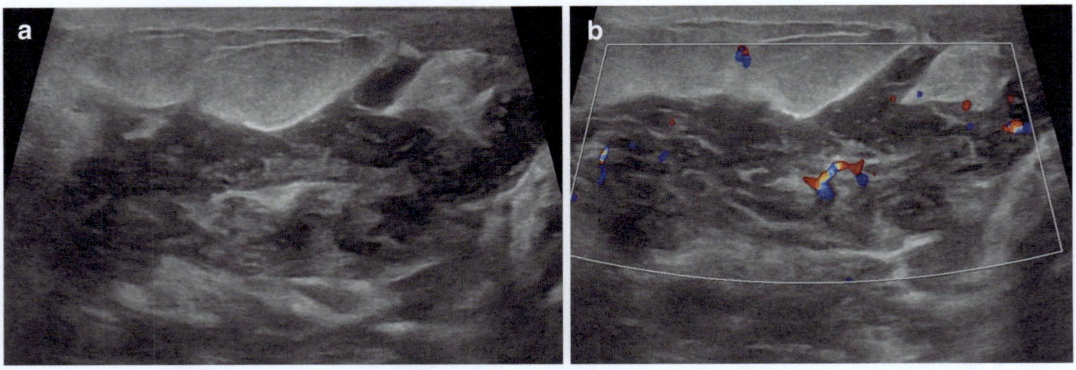

Fig. 2.8 *Mastitis:* There is a heterogeneous area in the breast with a tract towards the skin with increased echogenicity of the surrounding fat. (**a**) There is increased vascularity on color doppler (**b**)

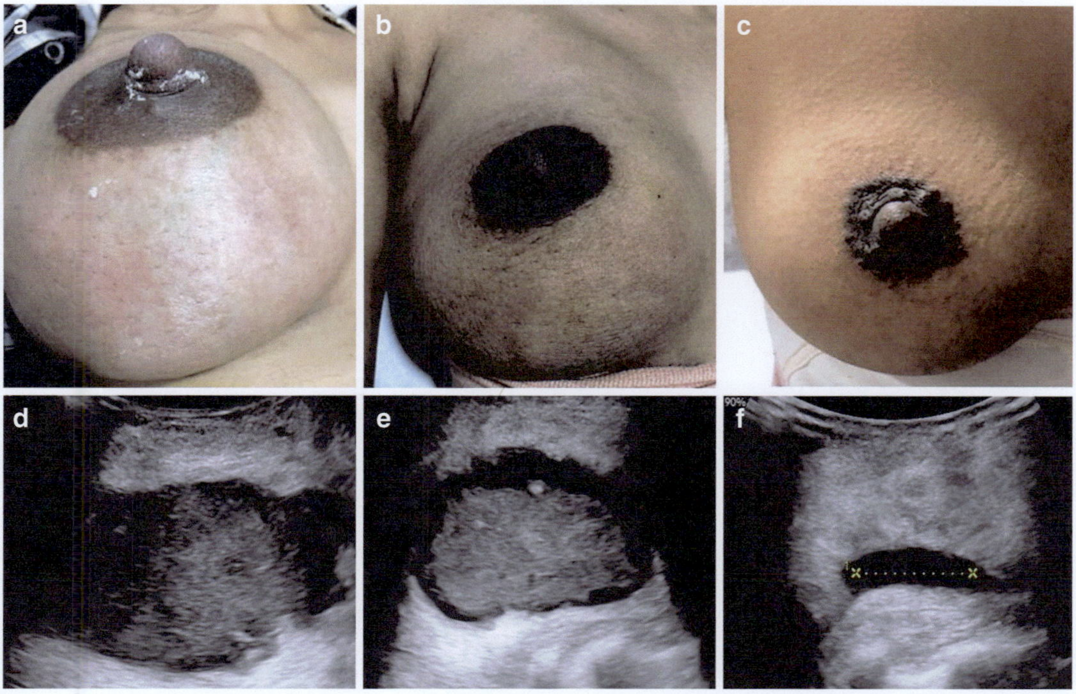

Fig. 2.9 *Abscess:* (**a–c**) Clinical pictures of the right breast of a lactating mother on serial visits showing resolution post-needle aspiration and course of antibiotics. (**d–f**) Correlative grey-scale USG of the right breast shows a reducing abscess size on serial visits post-needle aspiration and course of antibiotics

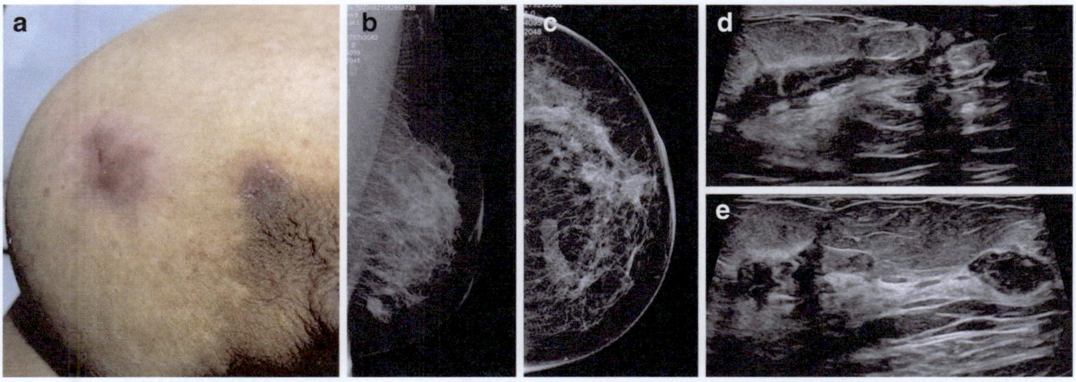

Fig. 2.10 *Granulomatous mastitis:* (**a**) Clinical image of the left breast showing on and off discharging skin sinuses. (**b**, **c**) Left breast MLO and CC view there is an equal density area with circumscribed margins in the lower and inner quadrant. (**d**, **e**) US images demonstrating fluid-filled tracking channels within the parenchyma

2.11 Benign Tumours Closely Related to Pregnancy and Lactation

Fibroadenoma is a common benign tumour seen in pregnant and lactating patients. They are hormone sensitive, and due to the increased hormone levels during this period, they undergo morphologic and physiologic changes and hence can grow in size. This also accounts for the pre-existing or unknown fibroadenomas which are discovered during pregnancy [45]. Fibroadenomas

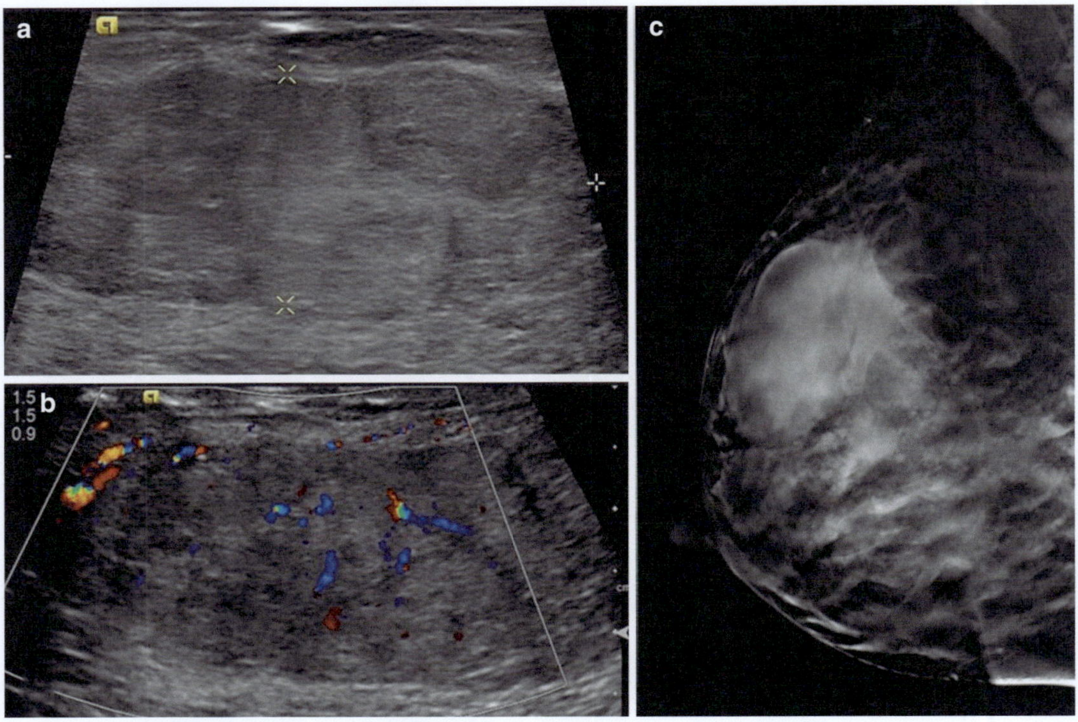

Fig. 2.11 *Lactating adenoma:* (**a**) USG of the right breast shows an oval iso to hypoechoic lesion with circumscribed margins in the right breast. (**b**) Colour Doppler image shows both peripheral and internal vascularity. (**c**) Limited mammography of the right breast in the MLO view reveals a high density oval mass, margins of which are partially circumscribed amd partially obscured by overlying fibroglandular parenchyma

can undergo an increase in size and infarction or can have secretory hyperplasia or lactational changes. Due to these changes, fibroadenomas can have varied imaging appearances. On US, fibroadenomas are seen as oval hypoechoic masses with circumscribed margins and minimal vascularity. During pregnancy and lactation, the echotexture may be heterogeneous with cystic areas within representing a complex fibroadenoma. In view of this, a core biopsy should be done to confirm the diagnosis.

Lactating adenoma is a benign breast lesion that is thought to occur in response to the physiologic changes that characterize pregnancy and lactation [45]. Lactating adenoma has been suggested to be a variant of fibroadenoma, tubular adenoma or lobular hyperplasia, and it can spontaneously regress after pregnancy and lactation [49]. On imaging they are seen as equal-density masses with circumscribed margins; however, the imaging modality of choice is US. On US, they are seen as hypoechoic or isoechoic masses, which are homogeneous and oval and with circumscribed margins. Increased vascularity is seen on the colour Doppler (Fig. 2.11). If these masses show any atypical appearance like indistinct margins or irregular shape, then a core biopsy of the mass is recommended.

2.12 Pregnancy-Associated Breast Cancer

PABC is defined as breast cancer that occurs during pregnancy and/or the first year of postpartum [54]. According to a study done by Chunchun Shao et al. in 2020, the definition of the duration of the postpartum period has been controversial, and this may lead to diverse results regarding prognosis [54]. PABC occurs in 1 out of every 3000–10,000 pregnancies and represents up to 3% of all breast malignancies [55]. PABC mani-

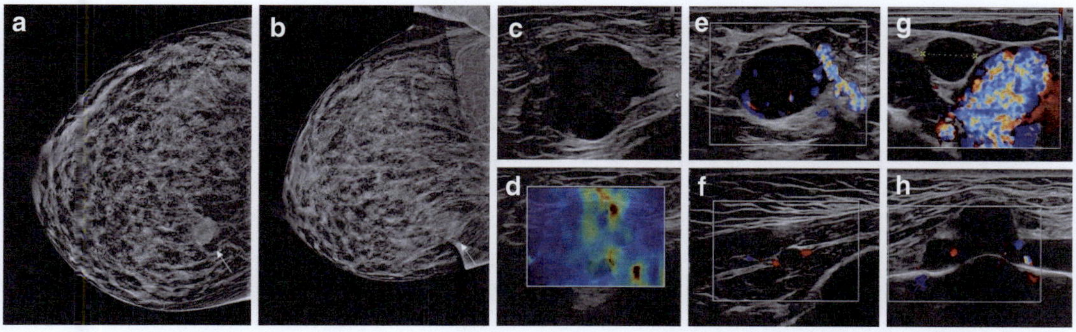

Fig. 2.12 *Pregnancy associated breast cancer:* (**a**, **b**) Right breast CC and MLO view showing an isodense mass with obscured margins in the posterior third of lower inner quadrant (arrow). (**c**, **d**) Correlative grey-scale USG and elastography show a solid hypoechoic mass with angular margins, hard on elastography. Suspicious lymph nodes at level I (**e**), level II (**f**), supraclavicular (**g**) and internal mammary (**h**) region

fests as a painless palpable mass, and there may be a delay in the diagnosis due to the hormonal changes that take place in the breast making clinical breast examination very challenging. Patients with PABC tend to have larger, more advanced neoplasms at diagnosis and a poorer outcome than other women of the same age with breast cancer [54]. More than 50% of patients present with high-grade tumours along with high rates of inflammatory tumours [54]. There is a high prevalence of hormone receptor-negative and *HER2/neu* tumours that support their aggressive biological growth pattern [54]. Clinically, patients with PABC present with a painless lump in the breast. They can also uncommonly present with redness and diffuse enlargement of the breast. Ultrasonography of the breasts is done to evaluate and characterize the mass and also to evaluate the axilla. It is also useful in monitoring the response to neoadjuvant chemotherapy. MG of the breasts is done if there is a suspicion of malignancy on US to visualize if there are any suspicious calcifications and also to determine whether it is multifocal, multicentric or bilateral. On imaging, PABC is seen as hypoechoic/heterogeneous masses with angular/indistinct margins. Enlarged axillary lymph nodes with hypoechoic/thickened cortex may be seen (Fig. 2.12). The treatment of PABC depends on which trimester it is diagnosed. In the first trimester of pregnancy, unless it is a precious pregnancy, the patient should be offered a medical termination of pregnancy. In the second trimester, either a mastectomy or breast conservation surgery can be done. Some chemotherapeutic agents are considered safe. In the third trimester, early induction of labour is done with surgery and chemotherapy after delivery [56]. BRCA1 and BRCA2 mutation carriers constitute a specific group of women who are at risk for breast cancer [45]. This makes strict surveillance mandatory. Pregnant patients with mutation must be strictly assessed before pregnancy and after delivery, and a complete clinical and radiological assessment is necessary [45].

2.13 ACR Appropriateness Criteria During Pregnancy and Lactation for Screening and Diagnostic Imaging [56]

The breast imaging in pregnant and lactating females is challenging due to the increased breast volume, increased mammographic density and increased echogenicity secondary to the development of lobules, stroma, increased vascularity, water retention, secretions and milk [56]. Nevertheless, it is indicated for screening of breast cancer and for diagnostic evaluation in this group of patients.

Mammography exposes the foetus to negligible radiation dose (<0.03 mGy for four-view mammogram) and hence can be performed safely with a lead apron over the abdomen [57, 58]. DBT has been found useful in this set of patients as the increased breast density may mask smaller lesions. In lactating females, it is advisable that the lady breastfeeds and empties her breasts prior to undergoing a mammogram [56].

Ultrasound is the safest option available as it is devoid of any radiation or contrast. However, it is not recommended as for screening purposes as the sole modality but may be done to compliment the MG/DBT.

For diagnostic evaluation of pregnant or lactating patients, this is the most appropriate first modality of choice. Depending upon the findings of USG, one may do a mammogram [56].

MRI is used for screening of breast cancer in high-risk group of patients less than 40 years of age. It utilizes dynamic post-contrast enhancement sequences to detect the cancers early. Gadolinium-based contrasts are not recommended for use in pregnancy patients due to the possible toxic effects of free gadolinium ions that can cross the placental barrier on developing foetus. So, contrast-enhanced MRI (CEMRI) should not be done in pregnant patients for the purpose of screening or diagnosis. It may be used only in evaluation and staging of already diagnosed cases of breast cancer in whom the pregnancy would be aborted like the ones diagnosed in first trimester [56]. CEMRI can be used safely for screening or diagnostic purposes in lactating females. The female does not need to stop breastfeeding before or after the MRI [50].

The ACR-appropriate criteria have been summarized in Tables 2.3 and 2.4.

Table 2.3 ACR recommendations for breast imaging in pregnant women

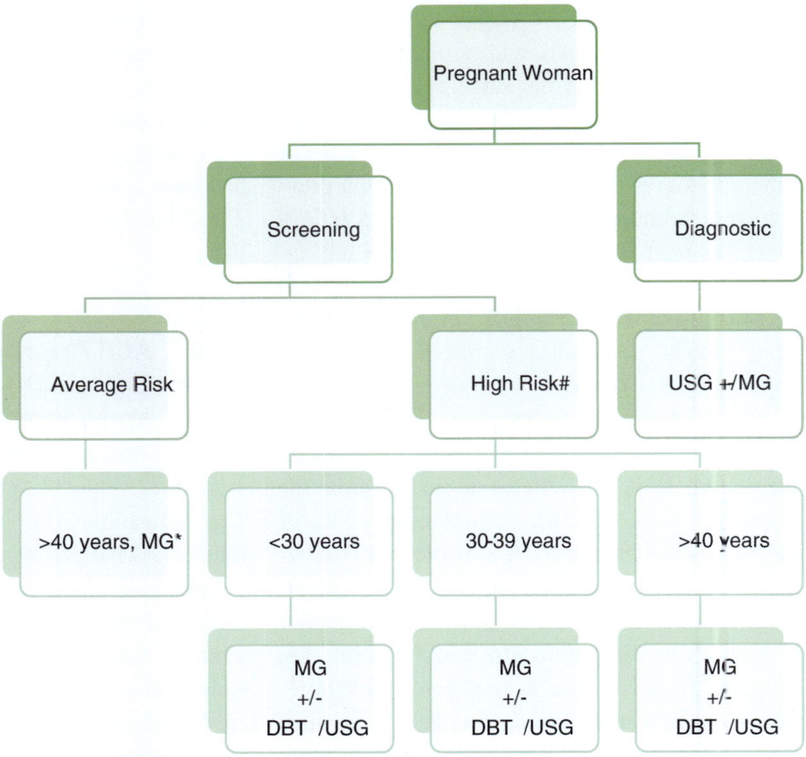

Table 2.4 ACR recommendations for breast imaging in lactating women

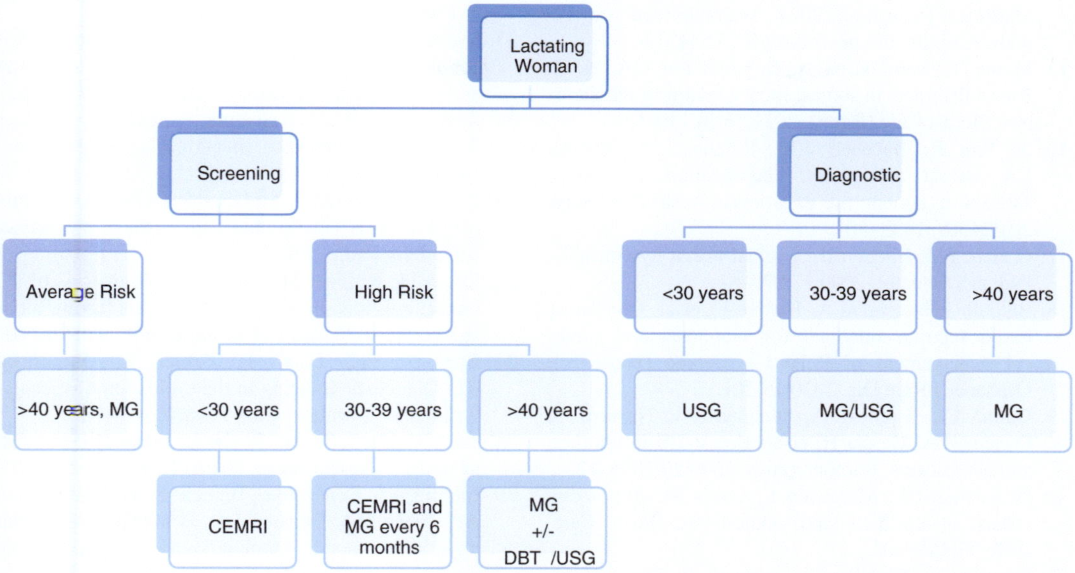

2.14 Conclusion

Clinical examination and imaging during pregnancy and lactation can be very challenging due to the physiological changes that occur in the breast due to hormonal changes. The majority of the masses in the breasts are benign; however the possibility of PABC should be kept in mind as this can cause the disease to be detected in the advanced stage.

References

1. Chang DS, McGrath MH. Management of benign tumors of the adolescent breast. Plast Reconstr Surg. 2007;120:13e–9e.
2. Howard BA, Gusterson BA. Human breast development. J Mammary Gland Biol Neoplasia. 2000;5:119–37.
3. Rudoy RC, Nelson JD. Breast abscess during the neonatal period. A review. Am J Dis Child. 1975;129(9):1031–4.
4. Lanciotti L, Cofini M, Leonardi A, et al. Up-to-date review about mini puberty and overview on hypothalamic-pituitary-gonadal axis activation in fetal and neonatal life. Front Endocrinol (Lausanne). 2018;9:410.
5. Amer A, Fischer H. Images in clinical medicine. Neonatal breast enlargement. N Engl J Med. 2009;360:1445.
6. Madlon-Kay DJ. 'Witch's milk': galactorrhea in the newborn. Am J Dis Child. 1986;140:252–3.
7. Wroblewska-Seniuk K, Jarząbek-Bielecka G, Kędzia W. Gynecological problems in newborns and infants. J Clin Med. 2021;10(5):1071.
8. Jawahar A, Vade A. Sonographic features of physiologic neonatal breast enlargement. J Clin Neonatol. 2014;3:106–8.
9. McHoney M, Munro F, Mackinlay G. Mammary duct ectasia in children: report of a short series and review of the literature. Early Hum Dev. 2011;87:527–53.
10. Amer A. Fischer H Images in clinical medicine. Neonatal breast enlargement. N Engl J Med. 2009;360:1445.
11. Bock K, Duda VF, Hadji P, et al. Pathologic breast conditions in childhood and adolescence: evaluation by sonographic diagnosis. J Ultrasound Med. 2005;24:1347–54.
12. Chung EM, Cube R, Hall GJ, González C, Stocker JT, Glassman LM. From the archives of the AFIP: breast masses in children and adolescents: radiologic-pathologic correlation. Radiographics. 2009;29(3):907–31.
13. Dixon JM, Mansel RE. ABC of breast diseases. Congenital problems and aberrations of normal breast development and involution. BMJ. 1994;309(6957):797–800.

14. Kota AS, Ejaz S. Precocious puberty. [Updated 2023 Jul 4]. In: StatPearls [Internet]. Treasure Island: StatPearls Publishing; 2024. Available from: https://www.ncbi.nlm.nih.gov/books/NBK544313/.
15. Mareti E, Vatopoulou A, Spyropoulou GA, et al. Breast disorders in adolescence: a review of the literature. Breast Care (Basel). 2021;16(2):149–55.
16. de Vita R, Buccheri EM, Villanucci A, Ragusa LA. Breast asymmetry, classification, and algorithm of treatment: our experience. Aesth Plast Surg. 2019;43(6):1439–50.
17. O'Hare PM, Frieden IJ. Virginal breast hypertrophy. Pediatr Dermatol. 2000;17:277–81.
18. Baldelli I, Baccarani A, Barone C, et al. Consensus based recommendations for diagnosis and medical management of Poland syndrome (sequence). Orphanet J Rare Dis. 2020;15:201.
19. García CJ, Espinoza A, Dinamarca V, Navarro O, Daneman A, García H, et al. Breast US in children and adolescents. Radiographics. 2000;20:1605–12.
20. Greydanus DE, Matytsina L, Gains M. Breast disorders in children and adolescents. Prim Care. 2006;33:455–502.
21. Huneeus A, Schilling A, Horvath E, Pinochet M, Carrasco O. Retroareolar cysts in the adolescent. J Pediatr Adolesc Gynecol. 2003;16:45–9.
22. Valeur NS, Rahbar H, Chapman T. Ultrasound of pediatric breast masses: what to do with lumps and bumps. Pediatr Radiol. 2015;45:1584–99.
23. Faden H. Mastitis in children from birth to 17 years. Pediatr Infect Dis J. 2005;24(12):1113.
24. Welch ST, Babcock DS, Ballard ET. Sonography of pediatric male breast masses: gynecomastia and beyond. Pediatr Radiol. 2004;34(12):952–7.
25. Kaneda HJ, Mack J, Kasales CJ, Schetter S. Pediatric and adolescent breast masses: a review of pathophysiology, imaging, diagnosis, and treatment. AJR Am J Roentgenol. 2013;200:W204–12.
26. Coffin CM. The breast. In: Stocker JT, Dehner LP, editors. Paediatric pathology. 2nd ed. Philadelphia: Lippincott Williams & Wilkins; 2002. p. 993–1015.
27. Simmons PS. Diagnostic considerations in breast disorders of children and adolescents. Obstet Gynecol Clin N Am. 1992;19(1):91–102.
28. Morikawa H, Nobuoka M, Amitani M, et al. Fibroadenoma in a young male breast: a case report and review of the literature. Clin Case Rep. 2021;9(11):e05114.
29. West KW, Rescoria FJ, Scherer LR III, Grosfeld JL. Diagnosis and treatment of symptomatic breast masses in the pediatric population. J Pediatr Surg. 1995;30:182–6; discussion, 186–7
30. Sanchez R, Ladino-Torres MF, Bernat JA, Joe A, DiPietro MA. Breast fibroadenomas in the pediatric population: common and uncommon sonographic findings. Pediatr Radiol. 2010;40:1681–9.
31. Dehner LP, Hill DA, Deschryver K. Pathology of the breast in children, adolescents, and young adults. Semin Diagn Pathol. 1999;16:235–47.
32. Breast RJ. In: Rosai J, editor. Rosai and Ackerman's surgical pathology. 9th ed. St Louis: Mosby; 2004. p. 1769–73.
33. Kronemer KA, Rhee K, Siegel MJ, Sievert L, Hildebolt CF. Gray scale sonography of breast masses in adolescent girls. J Ultrasound Med. 2001;20:491–6.
34. Ibrahim RE, Sciotto CG, Weidner N. Pseudoangiomatous hyperplasia of mammary stroma. Cancer. 1989;63:1154–11.
35. Rosen PP, Cantrell B, Mullen DL, DePalo A. Juvenile papillomatosis (Swiss cheese disease) of the breast. Am J Surg Pathol. 1980;4:3–12.
36. Rosen PP, Kimmel M. Juvenile papillomatosis of the breast: a follow-up study of 41 patients having biopsies before 1979. Am J Clin Pathol. 1990;93:599–603.
37. Burrows PE, Laor T, Paltiel H, Robertson RL. Diagnostic imaging in the evaluation of vascular birthmarks. Dermatol Clin. 1998;16:455–88.
38. Tse GM, Niu Y, Shi HJ. Phyllodes tumor of the breast: an update. Breast Cancer. 2010;17:29–34.
39. Liberman L, Bonaccio E, Hamele-Bena D, Abramson AF, Cohen MA, Dershaw DD. Benign and malignant phyllodes tumors: mammographic and sonographic findings. Radiology. 1996;198:121–4.
40. Yabuuchi H, Soeda H, Matsuo Y, et al. Phyllodes tumor of the breast: correlation between MR findings and histologic grade. Radiology. 2006;241:702–9.
41. Gutierrez JC, Housri N, Koniaris LG, Fischer AC, Sola JE. Malignant breast cancer in children: a review of 75 patients. J Surg Res. 2008;147:182–8.
42. Horowitz DP, Sharma CS, Connolly E, GideaAddeo D, Deutsch I. Secretory carcinoma of the breast: results from the survival, epidemiology and end results database. Breast. 2012;21:350–3.
43. Freitas V, Scaranelo A, Menezes R, Kulkarni S, Hodgson D, Crystal P. Added cancer yield of breast magnetic resonance imaging screening in women with a prior history of chest radiation therapy. Cancer. 2013;119(3):495–503.
44. Apostolou P, Fostira F. Hereditary breast cancer: the era of new susceptibility genes. Biomed Res Int. 2013;2013:747318.
45. de Holanda AA, Gonçalves AK, de Medeiros RD. Ultrasound findings of the physiological changes and most common breast diseases during pregnancy and lactation. Radiol Bras. 2016;49(6):389–96.
46. Canoy JM, Mitchell GS, Unold D, et al. A radiologic review of common breast disorders in pregnancy and the perinatal period. Semin Ultrasound CT MR. 2012;33:78–85.
47. Joshi S, Dialani V, Marotti J, et al. Breast disease in the pregnant and lactating patient: radiological-pathological correlation. Insights Imaging. 2013;4:527–38.
48. Swinford AE, Adler DD, Garver KA. Mammographic appearance of the breasts during pregnancy and lactation: false assumptions. Acad Radiol. 1998;5:467–72.
49. Vashi R, Hooley R, Butler R, Geisel J, Philpotts L. Breast imaging of the pregnant and lactating patient:

imaging modalities and pregnancy-associated breast cancer. AJR Am J Roentgenol. 2013;200(2):321–8.
50. American College of Radiology. Manual on contrast media. Available at: https://www.acr.org/Clinical-Resources/Contrast-Manual. Accessed 18 Apr 2024.
51. Lee SE, Bae YK. Breast lesions during pregnancy and lactation: a pictorial essay. Ultrasonography. 2020;39(3):298–310.
52. Sabate JM, Clotet M, Torrubia S, et al. Radiologic evaluation of breast disorders related to pregnancy and lactation. Radiographics. 2007;27(Suppl 1):S101–24.
53. Taylor GB, Paviour SD, Musaad S, Jones WO, Holland DJ. A clinicopathological review of 34 cases of inflammatory breast disease showing an association between corynebacteria infection and granulomatous mastitis. Pathology. 2003;35:109–19.
54. Shao C, Yu Z, Xiao J, et al. Prognosis of pregnancy-associated breast cancer: a meta-analysis. BMC Cancer. 2020;20:746.
55. Keyser EA, Staat BC, Fausett MB, Shields AD. Pregnancy-associated breast cancer. Rev Obstet Gynecol. 2012;5(2):94–9.
56. Expert Panel on Breast Imaging, diFlorio-Alexander RM, Slanetz PJ, Moy L, Baron P, Didwania AD, Heller SL, Holbrook AI, Lewin AA, Lourenco AP, Mehta TS, Niell BL, Stuckey AR, Tuscano DS, Vincoff NS, Weinstein SP, Newell MS. ACR appropriateness criteria® breast imaging of pregnant and lactating women. J Am Coll Radiol. 2018;15(11S):S263–75. PABC in BRCA Germline Mutation Carrier
57. Tremblay E, Therasse E, Thomassin-Naggara I, Trop I. Quality initiatives: guidelines for use of medical imaging during pregnancy and lactation. Radiographics. 2012;32:897–911.
58. NCCN Clinical Practice Guidelines in Oncology. Breast cancer screening and diagnosis. Version 3.2023. 31 Oct 2023.

3 Imaging Approach in Breast Masses

Rupa Renganathan and Prema Subramaniam

Abstract

Breast masses are one of the common symptoms across all ages. Although the majority of breast masses are benign, palpable breast lump is the most common presenting symptom for breast cancer. Evaluation with imaging is indicated in all palpable masses irrespective of the age of presentation. The choice of imaging is primarily based on the age of patient. On both mammography and ultrasound, margin is one of the most important characteristics in assessing if the mass is benign or suspicious. Both contrast-enhanced mammography and MRI provide the functional aspects of the mass through enhancement parameters. Advanced imaging techniques like elastography and diffusion-weighted MRI add as supplementary techniques in further characterising the masses.

The majority of the breast masses can be categorised as benign and suspicious based on the imaging findings. Biopsy can be safely avoided for the masses which have typical benign features. Biopsy of the mass is performed to evaluate the masses which are indeterminate on imaging or to confirm the malignancy in case the mass is suspicious. In this chapter we will discuss characterisation of breast masses using basic and advanced imaging techniques and illustrate the imaging approach to breast masses.

Keywords

Breast mass · Mammography · Ultrasound breast · Elastography · Diffusion-weighted image

3.1 Introduction

A mass is defined as a three-dimensional space-occupying lesion with convex outer margins [1]. Although the majority of breast masses are benign, palpable breast lump is the most common presenting symptom for breast cancer [2]. Evaluation with imaging is indicated in all palpable masses irrespective of the age of presentation. The primary aim of imaging is to characterise the masses using the American College of Radiology-Breast Imaging Reporting and Data System (ACR-BIRADS) [1]. The majority of the breast masses can be categorised as benign and suspicious based on the imaging findings. Biopsy can be safely avoided for the masses which have typical benign features. Biopsy of the mass is

R. Renganathan (✉) · P. Subramaniam
Division of Breast and Women's Imaging, Department of Diagnostic and Interventional Radiology, Kovai Medical Centre and Hospitals, Coimbatore, Tamil Nadu, India

E. Dhamija, S. V. S. Deo (eds.), *Imaging in Management of Breast Diseases*,
https://doi.org/10.1007/978-981-96-4998-3_3

performed only to evaluate the masses which are indeterminate on imaging or to confirm the malignancy in case the mass is suspicious. In this chapter we will review breast mass characterisation using basic and advanced imaging techniques and discuss the imaging approach to breast masses.

3.2 Clinical and Radiological Assessment

Due to variable combinations of the fibroglandular tissue and fat in the breast, it is often difficult to determine if the mass is benign or malignant only with clinical examination. True masses are asymmetrical in relation to the other breast, distinct from surrounding tissues and three-dimensional. Palpable breast thickening, defined as increased firmness of one area of the breast compared to other breast or other quadrants of the ipsilateral breast, can also be a presenting symptom of cancer in approximately 5% of cases [3]. Benign masses typically are mobile with a soft or rubbery texture, whereas malignant masses are hard and fixed on clinical examination.

Cysts and solid breast masses cannot be reliably distinguished only by palpation. In a study, out of 66 palpable cysts, only 58% were correctly characterised by physical examination [4]. The other associated features of malignant masses that can be present include dimpling or retraction of the skin, nipple retraction, fixation to deep structures, skin oedema and axillary adenopathy. Distinguishing benign and malignant masses with clinical examination is not reliable [5]. This highlights the importance of imaging evaluation of all palpable breast abnormalities.

The first and foremost step in imaging the breast mass is to choose the right modality. This is primarily based on the age of presentation, pregnant and lactational status.

3.2.1 Choice of Modality

Women who present with palpable lump and are less than 30 years of age, or pregnant, or lactating should undergo ultrasonography (USG) as the initial investigation [6]. Digital mammography (MG) with or without digital breast tomosynthesis (DBT) is indicated only if US or clinical findings are suspicious or when the mass is already proven to be malignant.

For women who are above 40 years of age, MG with or without DBT is the initial investigation of choice along with USG targeted to the clinical abnormality and clinical evaluation by interpreting radiologist.

For women between 30 and 40 years, the initial imaging modality can be either USG or MG ± DBT.

The radiologist must be able to establish the clinical imaging concordance for all palpable breast lumps [7]. The negative predictive value of MG combined with USG ranges from 97.4% to 100% [8, 9]. It is important to highlight that negative imaging should never overrule a finding that is strongly suspicious on physical examination or vice versa. Any highly suspicious finding on imaging or clinical examination should undergo biopsy unless contraindicated.

There is little role for other advanced imaging modalities like breast MRI, positron emission tomography-computed tomography or molecular breast imaging in the initial evaluation of palpable breast masses.

Mammography and Digital Breast Tomosynthesis In several studies on evaluation of palpable breast lumps, the sensitivity of MG alone ranges from 86% to 91% [10, 11]. The sensitivity of MG significantly reduces with increasing density of the breast tissue, i.e. increasing fibroglandular tissue and lesser fatty tissue. This has been shown to bring down the sensitivity to about 57% in women with dense breasts as compared to 93% in women with high breast adiposity [12, 13]. If a clearly benign lesion corresponding to the palpable abnormality can be identified on MG, no further imaging evaluation or biopsy is required [6]. If no imaging correlate is identified on MG or the correlate identified is not clearly benign, targeted USG for the palpable abnormality is indicated for further evaluation [6].

To further evaluate the findings on MG, additional views such as spot compression view for architectural distortion and magnification view for microcalcifications can be performed. The use of DBT can address some of the limitations of standard MG and may avoid additional views. With DBT, lesion masking by the overlapping normal tissue can be reduced leading to better characterisation of non-calcified lesions and margin evaluation in the diagnostic setting [14].

Several studies have demonstrated that the diagnostic accuracy of one-view tomosynthesis to be equivalent or better than supplemental mammographic views in screening recalls and diagnostic workup [15, 16]. The disadvantages of DBT include increased interpretation time and increased radiation dose, if standard two-dimensional (2D) images are obtained in addition to DBT images [17]. However current data suggest that synthesised reconstructed 2D images from DBT perform as good as standard full-field digital images and may replace them [15]. Implementation of direct tomosynthesis with synthesised 2D views can reduce additional radiation, avoid additional radiation from supplemental views used and can be used in better characterisation of breast masses [18].

Ultrasound (USG) USG is the first-line imaging modality in women with palpable breast masses who are <30 years of age [6]. It is also the essential next step in the evaluation of women above 30 years of age who had mammograms as an initial imaging with no definite clearly benign lesion (fat density mass or calcified fibroadenoma) corresponding to the palpable abnormality [6].

USG may be definitely able to characterise certain indeterminate mammographic findings and may identify certain mammographically occult findings [19]. If a palpable breast can be definitively characterised as benign lesion on USG, further sampling is usually not indicated.

USG is the best imaging modality to differentiate cystic and solid masses and also to further characterise both solid and cystic masses [20].

Any suspicious finding on MG or USG should be followed by tissue sampling unless contraindicated. Image-guided sampling is preferred especially if the mass is vaguely palpable, deep or small or if there are multiple lesions and if the mass is a complex solid cystic mass [21]. Even if the lesion is well palpable clinically, image guidance will have advantages such as confirmation of accurate targeting and placement of marker clip after the biopsy.

The choice of the modality depends on the modality in which the lesion is best seen. If the mass is seen equally well on MG and USG, USG is the preferred modality because of many advantages such as patient comfort, lack of radiation, cost-effectiveness and real-time needle visualisation [22]. Core biopsy is proven to be superior to fine needle aspiration in terms of sensitivity, specificity and histopathological grading of tumours [23].

MRI Though MRI is highly sensitive in detecting invasive breast cancer, it is not used as the initial imaging modality [24]. In the setting of palpable breast lumps, it is cost-effective to use MG and USG as the initial imaging modalities. MRI is proven to be highly sensitive but less specific in patients with palpable breast lumps with negative or equivocal conventional imaging findings [25].

3.2.2 Advanced Imaging Techniques

Contrast-Enhanced Ultrasound Contrast-enhanced ultrasonography (CEUS) aims to improve the Doppler sensitivity to blood flow particularly in small vessels measuring <100um. CEUS can differentiate benign and malignant lesions by analysing the acquired images both qualitatively and quantitatively [26, 27]. The sensitivity and specificity of this method for diagnosis of breast lesions are 100% and 87.5%, respectively [28]. Benign characteristics on CEUS include well-defined margins with no enhancement or homogeneous centrifugal enhancement pattern and numerous dendritic branching vessels. Malignant characteristics include ill-defined lesion margins, heterogeneous centripetal enhancement, filling defects and distorted vessels, early uptake, peritumoral enhancement and significantly shorter time to peak, high peak intensity and increased wash-in slopes.

Ultrasound Elastography of the Breast Elastography has the potentiality to quantify tissue stiffness which was judged subjectively on palpation [29, 30]. This has become an excellent technique for characterising breast lesions as benign and malignant [31]. Elastography can be strain or shear types. Strain elastography assesses the relative strain between a lesion and the encompassing tissue [32]. Shear wave elastography measures tissue stiffness and the speed and propagation pattern of shear waves in target tissue [33]. Lower speed indicates a softer tissue, and higher speed means a hard tissue.

Contrast-Enhanced Mammography Contrast-enhanced MG (CEM) is a newer emerging modality combining the digital MG with injection of iodinated contrast material providing structural as well as functional information like MRI [1, 34]. The sensitivity of CEM ranges between 93 and 100%, and specificity is 63% [35]. CEM involves acquisition of low and high energy images, leading to mild increased radiation dose compared to standard digital MG, but the total dose is well within the accepted range [36]. Both low and high energy images are interpreted together and given as a single report based on MG and CEM lexicon by ACR and assessed with appropriate BIRADS category [1, 34, 36].

Diffusion-Weighted MRI of the Breast Diffusion-weighted imaging of the breast is a newer imaging technique used for the differentiation of benign and malignant breast lesions. It can be incorporated into the routine dynamic contrast-enhanced MRI protocols for characterisation of masses, and it may potentially reduce unnecessary biopsies [37].

The apparent diffusion coefficient (ADC) value for the malignant masses ranges from ≤ 0.9 to 1.3×10^{-3} mm^2/s, and the ADC value for benign masses ranges from 1.7 to $\geq 2.1 \times 10^{-3}$ mm^2/s. The ADC value between 1.3 and 1.7×10^{-3} mm^2/s is of intermediate concern [37].

3.3 Imaging Features of Breast Masses

Breast masses in mammogram, USG, MRI and contrast-enhanced MG are described using the ACR-BIRADS [1]. In each modality, there are specific descriptors to characterise breast masses as shown in Table 3.1.

The breast is an organ without specific anatomical landmarks. Also, the positioning of the breast is different in MG, USG and MRI leading to difficulties in triangulation. To overcome these limitations, the location of the mass should be described in terms of side, quadrant, clock-face location, depth of the lesion and distance from the nipple, and it should be consistent across the modalities [1].

Based on the descriptors and associated findings which include calcification or architectural distortion and skin changes, the mass can be assigned under appropriate BIRADS category and as BIRADS 1 if the palpable mass represents a normal breast tissue.

Across all modalities, the shape descriptors used for masses are as follows: round, oval and irregular [1]. Irregular shape is defined as a shape that is neither round nor oval and also includes mass with >3 lobulations. Irregular masses are suspicious findings and need histopathological evaluation.

Fat density masses on MG are almost always benign, and no further evaluation is necessary (Fig. 3.1). Examples of masses with fat density include lipoma, galactocele, hamartoma, oil cyst, intramammary lymph node and fat necrosis. Masses with circumscribed margins with coarse or popcorn calcifications within represent calcified fibroadenomas, and they are also benign [BIRADS 2] (Fig. 3.1). Multiple bilateral circumscribed masses (at least three in both breasts and at least one in each breast] on MG are also assessed as benign findings [38].

Table 3.1 Descriptors for breast masses in MG, USG, MRI and CEM

Modality	MG	USG	MRI	CEM
Mass descriptors	Size Location Shape Margins Density	Size Location Shape Margins Echo pattern Orientation Posterior features	Size Location Shape Margins Enhancement pattern Kinetics	Size Location Shape Margins Conspicuity Enhancement pattern

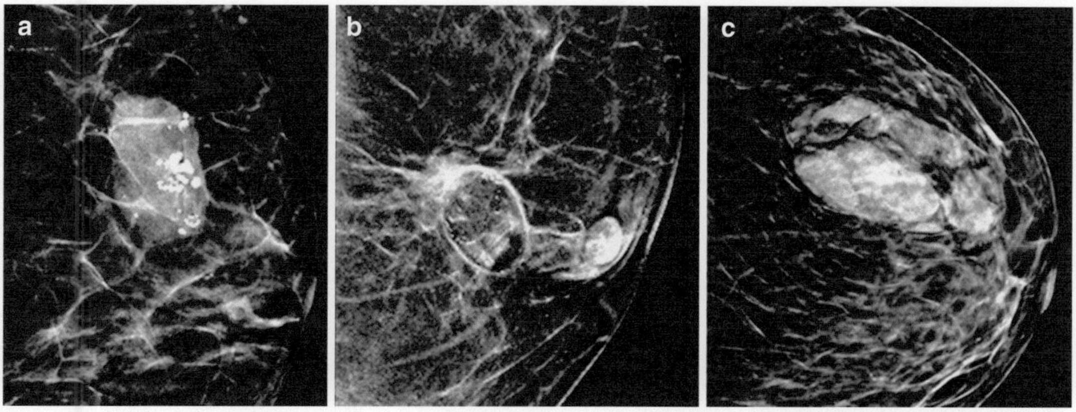

Fig. 3.1 Benign (BIRADS 2) lesions on mammography. (**a**) Calcified fibroadenoma, (**b**) oil cyst, and (**c**) hamartoma

High-density masses on mammograms are suspicious findings and have a high probability of malignancy.

In USG, anechoic masses represent simple cysts, and they are benign. Echogenicity of most of the benign and malignant masses is hypoechoic, and it is a less specific feature in differentiating benign and malignant lesions [1].

Parallel orientation of the mass indicates benign pathology, whereas nonparallel orientation is a suspicious feature [1].

Among the posterior features, shadowing represents fibrosis, and the differentials include post-surgical scar, fibrous mastopathy and breast cancer with a desmoplastic reaction. Posterior enhancement is seen in cysts and homogeneous solid lesions including high-grade cancers [1].

Among all the descriptors, margin of the mass is the most corroborative feature in characterising the mass as benign or malignant. In MG, margins should be assessed in both craniocaudal (CC) and mediolateral oblique (MLO) views and tomosynthesis views whenever available [39]. Tangential views or tomosynthesis confirms the skin lesions. If there are calcifications, a magnification view is indicated. Even if a small proportion of the mass is not circumscribed, it should be considered suspicious, as the worst margin features should guide further management.

Circumscribed Margins Majority of the masses with circumscribed margins seen on MG are benign. Only 1.4% of masses with circumscribed margins seen on screening MG turn out to be malignant, and 9% of circumscribed masses undergoing biopsy can be malignant [40]. The examples of benign circumscribed masses include simple and complicated cysts, fibroadenomas, benign phyllodes tumours, hamartoma, lipoma, galactocele, intramammary lymph node and benign papilloma.

Ultrasound can reliably categorise a circumscribed mass detected on mammogram as solid or cystic and can also further categorise cystic masses (Fig. 3.2, Table 3.2). When circumscribed masses are seen in both breasts and are multiple (at least three), they can be dismissed as benign.

When circumscribed masses are seen in both breasts and are not multiple or when such masses are unilateral, a BIRADS 3 category is assigned, and a follow-up is advised as per the ACR guidelines.

Cystic lesions with circumscribed margins: USG is the best modality to diagnose and characterise cystic breast masses. Based on the morphological criteria on USG, complex cystic and solid masses are classified into four types [39]: type 1 when there is a thick wall or thick internal septations (>5 mm); type 2 masses have nodular peripheral intracystic masses; type 3 masses have mixed cystic and solid parts and are at least 50% cystic; and type 4 masses are at least 50% solid [41] (Fig. 3.3).

Colour Doppler can be used to differentiate solid masses from complicated cysts with inter-

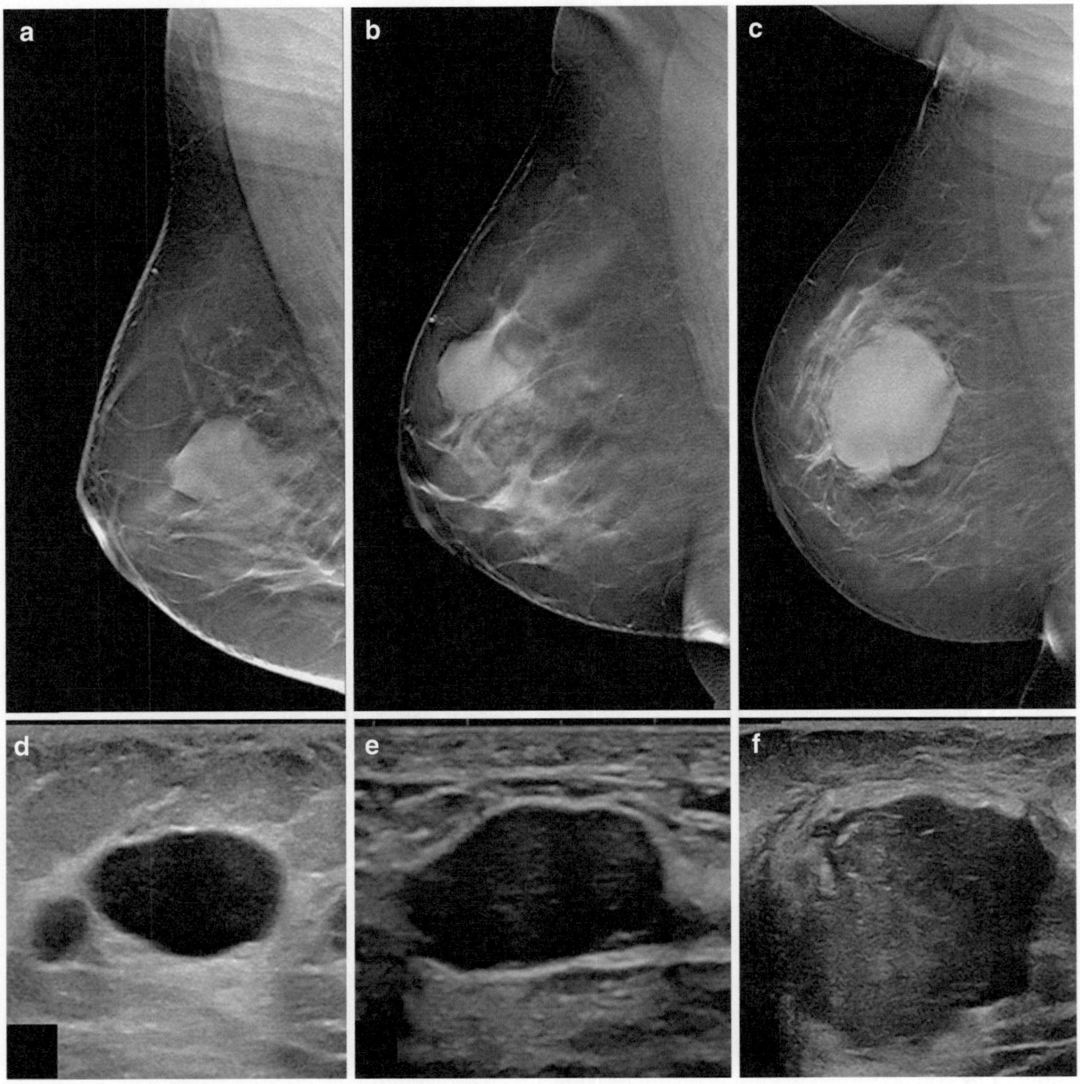

Fig. 3.2 Masses with circumscribed margins seen on mammogram need supplementary USG for further characterisation. (**a**, **d**) A mass with circumscribed margins on mammogram (**a**) corresponds to simple cyst on USG (**d**) (BIRADS 2 finding). (b and e) A mass with circumscribed margins on mammogram (**b**) corresponds to an oval hypoechoic parallel mass with circumscribed margins on USG (**e**) (BIRADS 3 finding). (**c**, **f**) A mass with circumscribed margins on mammogram (**c**) corresponds to a round isoechoic nonparallel mass with focal indistinct margins on USG (**f**) (BIRADS 4 finding)

Table 3.2 BIRADS categorisation of cysts and their management recommendation

Type of cyst	BIRADS category	Recommendation
Simple cyst	BIRADS 2	Annual screening
Clustered microcysts	BIRADS 2 If new or concerning in a post-menopausal women (BIRADS 3)	Annual screening Short interval follow-up after 6 months
Asymptomatic complicated cysts with multiple simple cysts	BIRADS 2	Annual screening
Isolated asymptomatic complicated cyst with moving internal echoes/ fluid debris levels	BIRADS 2	Annual screening
Incidental isolated round or oval mass with circumscribed margins (difficulty in differentiating solid mass and complicated cyst with homogeneous echoes)	BIRADS 3	Short interval follow-up after 6 months
Palpable complicated cyst with multiple simple cysts	BIRADS 3	Aspiration may be considered for symptomatic relief
Isolated palpable complicated cyst seen as mass with obscured margins on mammogram	BIRADS 4a	Aspiration is indicated

nal echoes and to identify solid components in a complex solid cystic lesion.

Solid mass with circumscribed margins: Among the solid masses with circumscribed margins, incident masses and masses that are presenting as palpable lumps in a young patient (<30 years) are assigned a BIRADS category 3, and short interval follow-up after 6 months is indicated. Any new, concerning or dominant mass with circumscribed margins especially in females above 30 years needs decision-making on a case-by-case basis with histopathological confirmation in the presence of any suspicious features.

Irregular masses (presence of >3 lobulations) with circumscribed margins are BIRADS category 4a lesions with low suspicion (>2% to ≤10%) for malignancy. Biopsy is indicated for those lesions.

On MRI, T2 hyperintensity generally indicates a benign pathology such as cysts and fibroadenomas. Exceptions include metastatic lymph nodes, mucinous carcinomas, papillary carcinomas and high-grade infiltrating ductal carcinomas with necrosis [42]. Lesions with dark internal septations on post-contrast images represent fibroadenomas. Masses which show progressive kinetics on MRI are benign and which show rapid washout are suspicious.

Malignancies that present as masses with circumscribed margins include triple-negative breast cancer, mucinous carcinoma, medullary carcinoma, papillary carcinoma, malignant phyllodes tumour and high-grade infiltrating ductal carcinomas [43]. They should be considered as differentials, and biopsy is warranted if the mass shows a significant increase in size, has associated suspicious features or is newly palpable in an elderly patient.

Obscured Margins This terminology should only be used in MG if more than 75% of margins are circumscribed and the rest of the margins are obscured [1]. It should not be used in USG or MRI as in both these modalities, three-dimensional visualisation is possible. DBT or spot compression views can help in better margin visualisation in case of obscured margins on 2D [15].

All the masses with obscured margins on MG need further evaluation with USG to determine the margins. After full diagnostic workup, the most suspicious margin of the mass should be used for assigning the BIRADS category (Fig. 3.4) [1].

Microlobulated Margins (Fig. 3.5) Microlobulated margins are defined as small undulations or lobu-

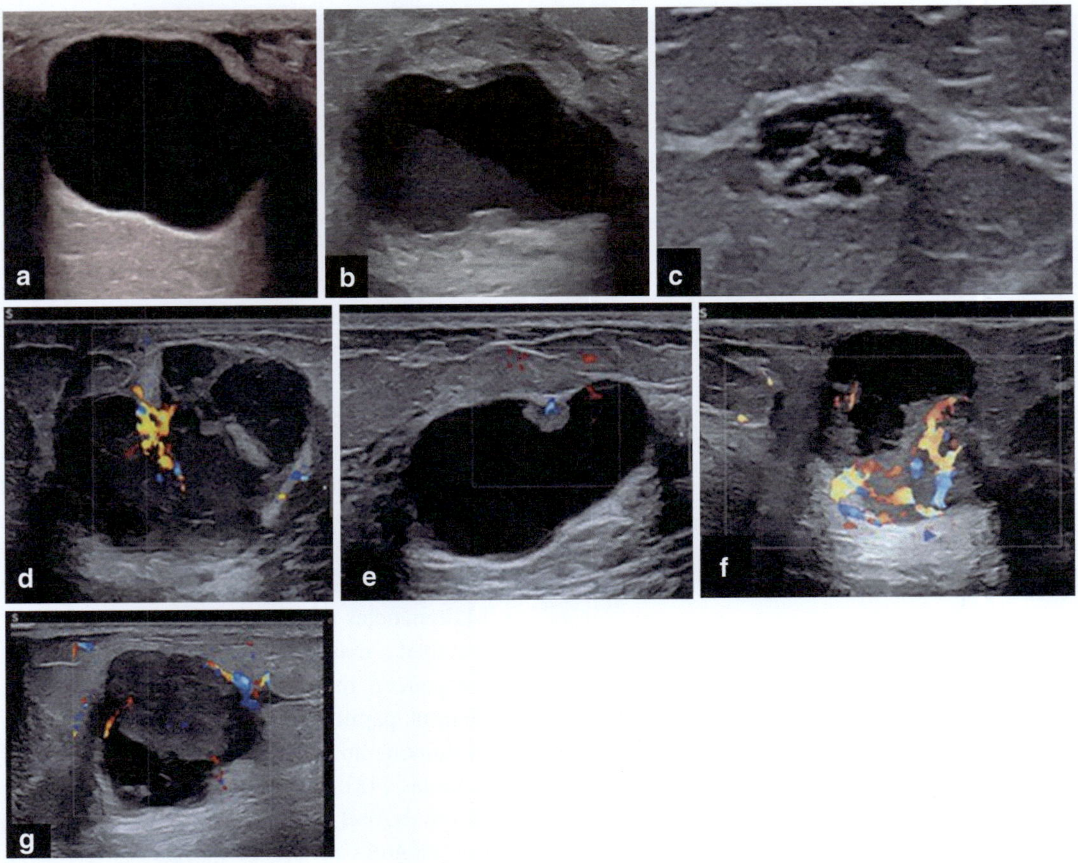

Fig. 3.3 Types of cysts. (**a**) Simple cyst, (**b**) complicated cyst with thick walls and fluid debris levels, (**c**) and clustered microcysts. (**d–g**) Types of complex solid cystic masses. (**d**) Type 1 with thick septations and septal vascularity, (**e**) type 2 showing a mural solid nodule, (**f**) type 3 with at least 50% cystic component and (**g**) type 4 with >50% solid component

lations on the surface of mass. It generally indicates a suspicious finding on mammogram, and targeted USG is indicated. On USG, a small proportion of these masses could represent clustered microcysts. If they are without solid components or thick septations, they are generally considered benign and assigned a BIRADS 2 or 3 based on the diagnostic confidence [44].

All the solid and complex cystic and solid masses with microlobulated margins are assessed as suspicious findings, and biopsy is recommended [1]. Other differentials for masses with microlobulated margins include fibroadenomas, phyllodes tumours, lactating adenomas, invasive ductal carcinomas, ductal carcinoma in situ and lobular carcinoma in situ [40].

Indistinct Margins Margins are indistinct when there is no clear demarcation between the mass and the surrounding tissue. Spot compression views or DBT helps differentiate focal asymmetry from masses with indistinct margins. In USG, the presence of thick echogenic irregular rim suggests malignancy. In MRI, the margins may appear circumscribed in early post-contrast images because of blooming. To avoid that artefact, the masses should be seen in delayed images after the contrast washes out [45].

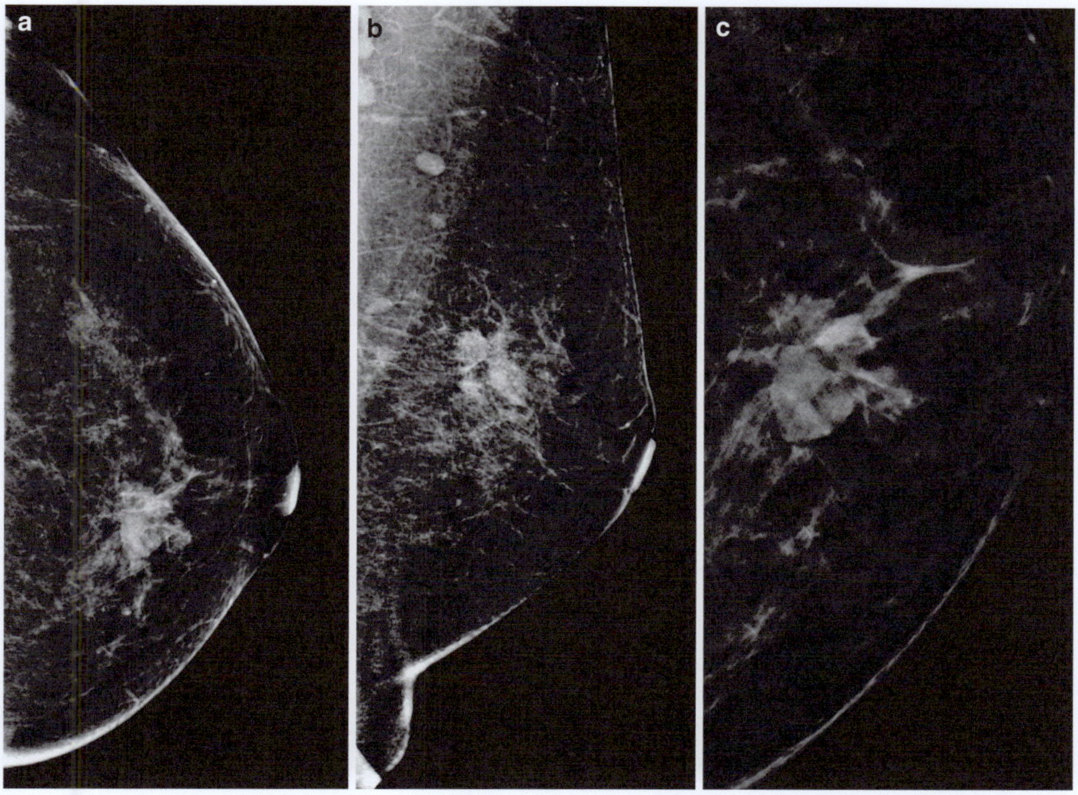

Fig. 3.4 CC and MLO images and CC tomosynthesis (**a**–**c**, respectively) of the left breast show an irregular mass in the upper inner quadrant. On tomosynthesis images (**c**), the margins are circumscribed in the medial aspect, whereas the lateral and anterior margins have a wide zone of transition with indistinct margins. The lesion is categorised as having indistinct margins which is the most suspicious feature. Biopsy was suggestive of invasive ductal carcinoma, not otherwise specified

Masses with indistinct margins are commonly malignant. Some of the high risk and locally aggressive lesions such as lobular carcinoma in situ, atypical papilloma, fibromatosis and borderline/ malignant phyllodes can also have indistinct margins (Fig. 3.6). Benign causes of indistinct margins include fat necrosis, ruptured cyst and abscess. Indistinct masses are assigned BIRADS category 4, and biopsy is recommended [46].

Spiculated Margins Spiculated margins are defined as sharp lines radiating from a mass. Spiculations are best seen on DBT or spot compression DBT. On USG, spiculations are best seen on 3D imaging, and they often show a stiff rim on elastography. It should be distinguished from architectural distortion which is an associated finding.

The common differential diagnosis for masses with spiculated margins include malignancies such as infiltrating ductal carcinomas, tubular carcinomas and invasive lobular carcinomas, radial scars, post-surgical scars, fat necrosis, granular cell tumours, fibromatosis and plasma cell mastitis (Fig. 3.7) [47]. Masses with spiculated margins have the highest probability of malignancy with a positive predictive value of 81–91%. Seventy-one percent of spiculated malignancies are luminal A group. Spiculated high-density masses with associated suspicious calcifications are categorised as BIRADS 5 lesions [1].

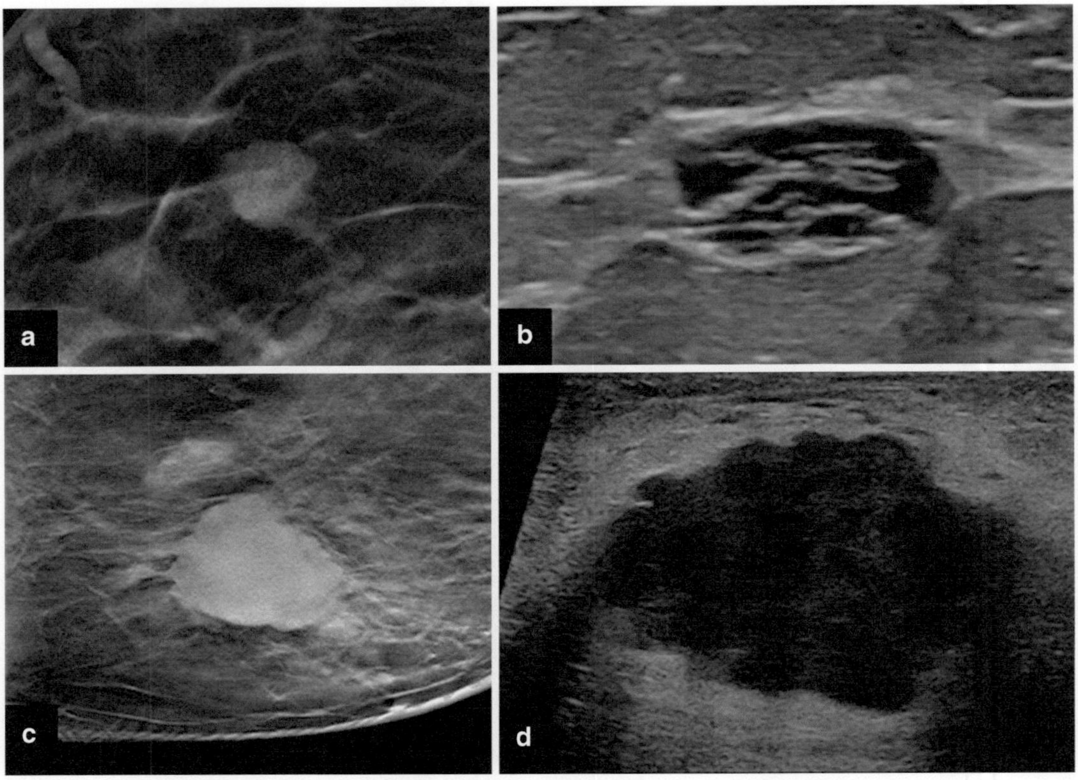

Fig. 3.5 Masses with microlobulated margins. (**a**, **b**) A mass with microlobulated margins on mammogram (**a**) corresponds to clustered microcysts on USG (**b**). (**c**, **d**) A mass with microlobulated margins on mammogram (**c**) corresponds to a solid hypoechoic mass with microlobulated margins on USG (**d**) which is a biopsy-proven malignancy

Enhancement Characteristics Apart from morphological features, contrast enhancement patterns and kinetics are obtained from MRI and CEM. The masses showing homogeneous enhancement and dark internal septations are more likely to be benign. Heterogeneous enhancement is a suspicious finding. Rim enhancement is seen in complicated cysts, abscesses and high-grade carcinomas with central necrosis. Complicated cysts have smooth inner walls, whereas malignancies show thick, nodular and irregular walls (Fig. 3.8) [1].

Breast MRI and CEM use the principle of neoangiogenesis in detecting breast cancers. In addition to morphological assessment as in MG and USG, functional information in the form of enhancement characteristics is possible with MRI. As breast malignancies have leaky capillaries, they show early intense enhancement and rapid washout in post-contrast dynamic images [48]. In contrast, benign lesions show minimal enhancement in the early phase with a progressive increase in enhancement in the delayed phase.

There are three types of time intensity curves based on the enhancement pattern in dynamic post-contrast images [1].

Type 1: Persistent—slow rise in the initial phase (<50% of peak enhancement in first 2 minutes) with >10% increase in signal intensity after 2 minutes.

Type 2: Plateau—medium rise in the initial phase (50–100% of peak enhancement in first 2 minutes) with <10% change in signal intensity at 2–5 minutes.

Type 3: Washout—rapid rise (100% of peak enhancement within first 2 minutes) with

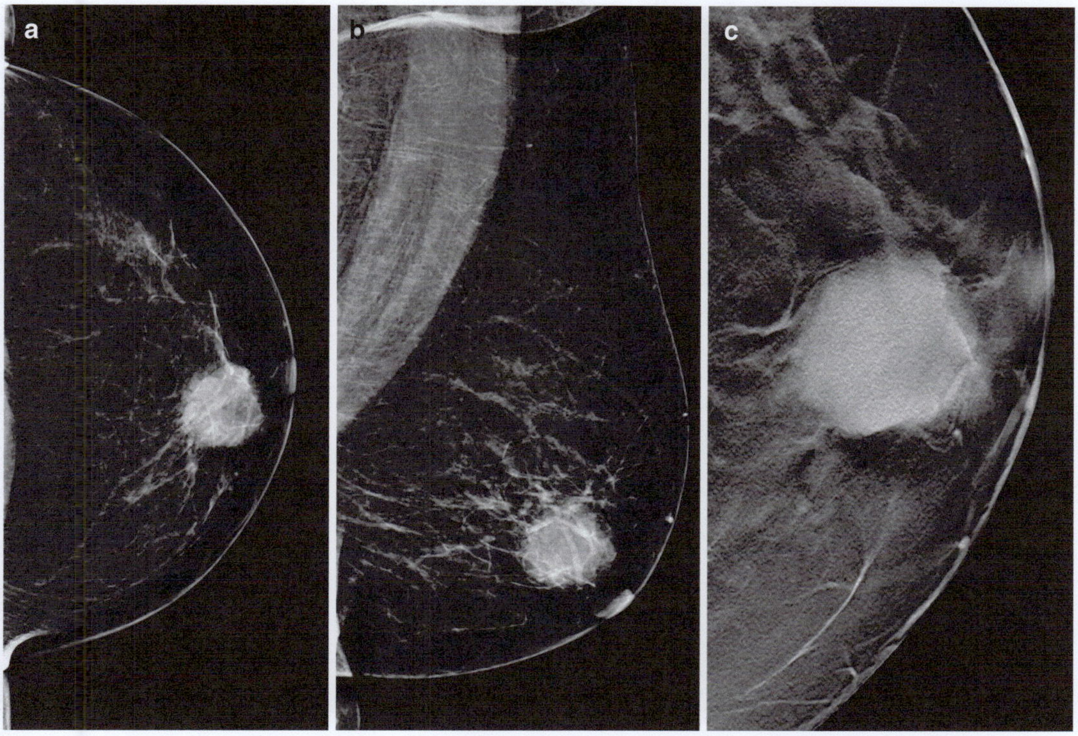

Fig. 3.6 CC and MLO image and CC tomosynthesis (**a**–**c**, respectively) of the left breast shows an irregular mass in the retroareolar region. The margins are indistinct with a wide zone of transition. Biopsy was suggestive of solid papillary carcinoma

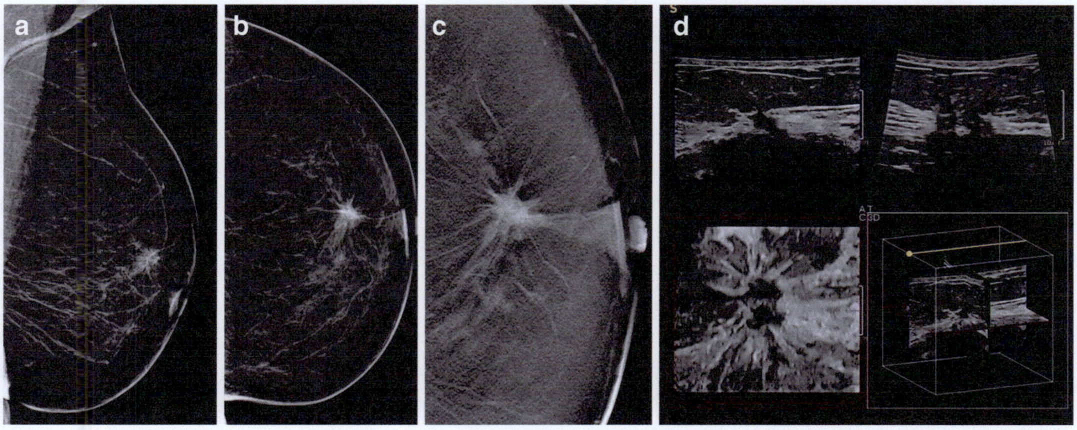

Fig. 3.7 MLO, CC and CC tomosynthesis (**a**–**c**, respectively) of the left breast shows an irregular mass in the upper central quadrant. The margins show radiating spicules all around suggestive of spiculated margins. (**d**) An USG image showing an irregular hypoechoic mass with spiculated margins with surrounding architectural distortion. The findings are well depicted in the coronal plane. Biopsy was suggestive of invasive ductal carcinoma, not otherwise specified

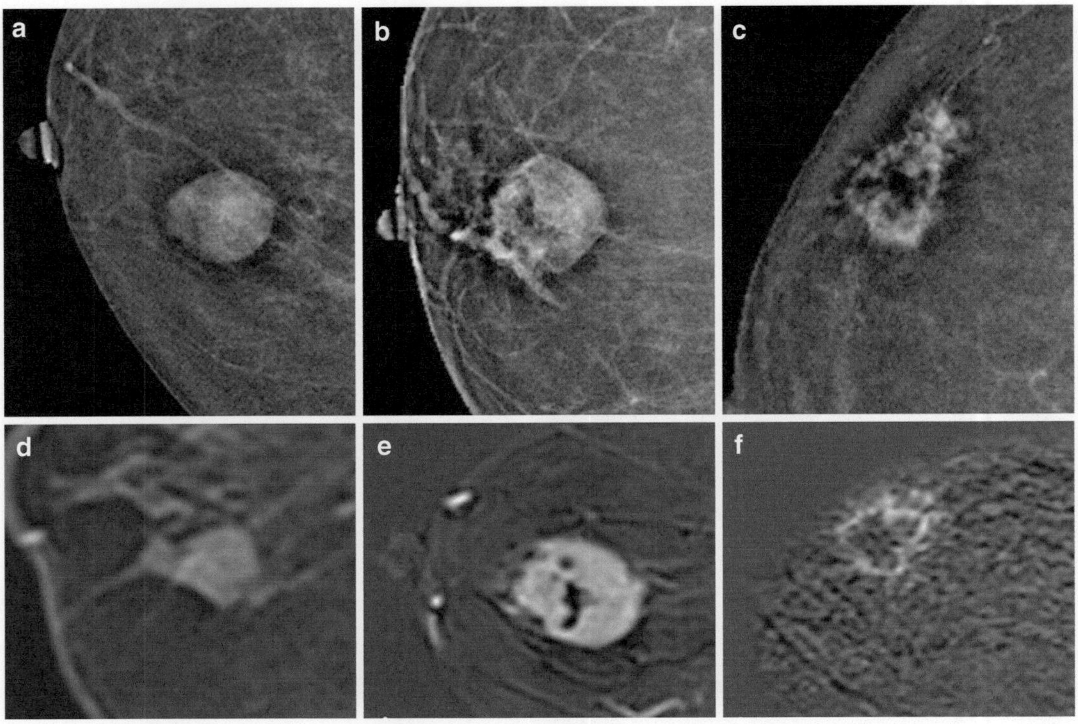

Fig. 3.8 CEM-recombined images (**a**–**c**) and MRI breast post-contrast subtraction images (**d**–**f**) demonstrating homogeneous (**a**, **d**), heterogeneous (**b**, **e**) and rim (**c**, **f**) enhancement

>10% reduction in signal intensity between 2 and 5 minutes.

Type 1 kinetics generally indicates a benign pathology, type 3 kinetics indicates a malignant pathology and type 2 kinetics is indeterminate.

In CEM, though kinetic assessment is currently not standardised, there are studies on assessment of kinetics in CEM, and CEM kinetics has comparable accuracy to MRI kinetics in differentiating benign and malignant masses [49].

Morphological and kinetic information of masses are evaluated together; even if anyone feature is suspicious, the mass should be categorised as suspicious, and biopsy should be recommended [1].

Imaging features of benign and malignant masses in each modality are shown in Table 3.3 and Figs. 3.9 and 3.10 [1, 49].

BIRADS Assessment and Management Recommendations When the mass is benign on imaging, BIRADS 2 assessment is given, and annual screening mammogram is recommended. If the mass has suspicious imaging features, it is assessed as BIRADS 4 or BIRADS 5 depending on the level of suspicion, and biopsy is recommended.

Masses with >0% to ≤2% malignancy are assessed as BIRADS 3 lesions, and short interval follow-up is recommended. The diagnostic approach to breast masses has been illustrated in Fig. 3.11.

Table 3.3 Imaging features of benign and malignant breast masses

	Mammogram	USG	CEM/CE-MRI
Benign features (Fig. 3.9)	Fat density Coarse or popcorn calcifications Oval shape Circumscribed margins	Oval shape Circumscribed margins Parallel orientation Thin pseudocapsule Soft on elastography	Oval shape Circumscribed margins No diffusion restriction Homogeneous enhancement Dark internal septations Type I kinetics
Malignant features (Fig. 3.10)	High density Irregular shape Noncircumscribed margins Associated features: Architectural distortion Skin or nipple retraction Skin invasion and thickening Microcalcifications Axillary lymphadenopathy	Irregular shape Noncircumscribed margins Nonparallel orientation Shadowing Ductal extensions Calcifications Hard on elastography	Irregular shape Noncircumscribed margins Restricted diffusion Heterogeneous or rim enhancement Type II or III kinetics

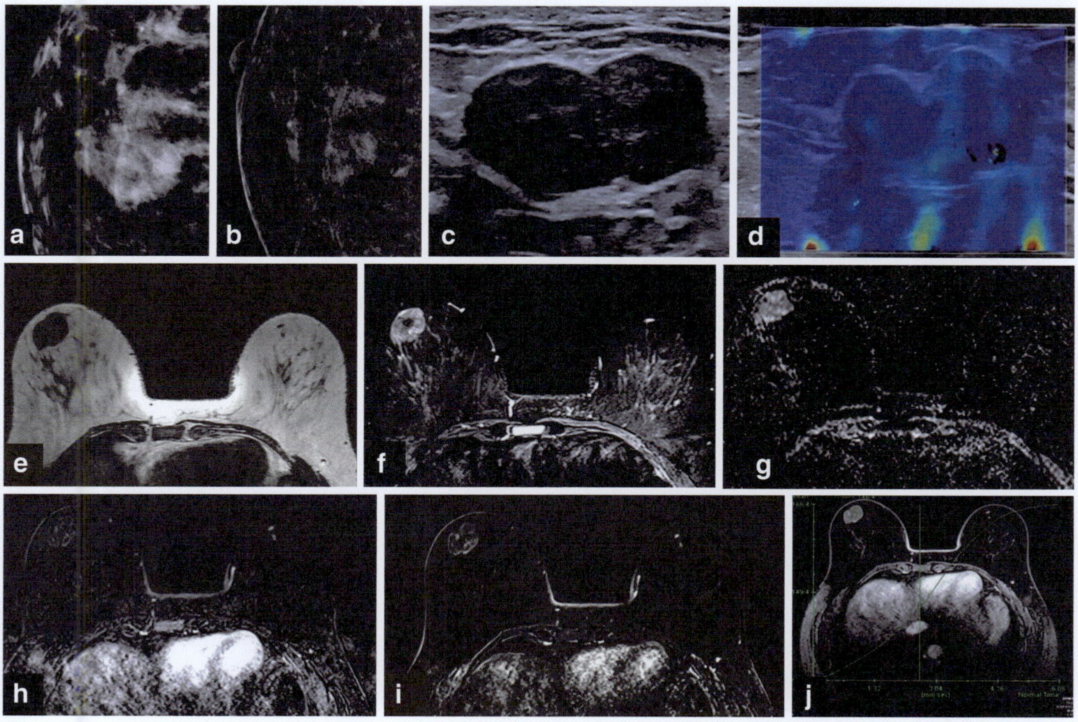

Fig. 3.9 Imaging characteristics of a benign breast mass. (**a**) Mammogram showing an oval mass with partly circumscribed and partly obscured margins. (**b**) CEM shows complete enhancement of low conspicuity. (**c**) Circumscribed margins on US with thin echogenic pseudocapsule. The mass was soft on elastography (**d**). On MRI the mass shows an oval shape and circumscribed margins and is isointense on T1 (**e**), hyperintense on IR (**f**), shows no diffusion restriction (**g**—ADC image) and heterogeneous enhancement with persistent (type 1) kinetics (**h**–**j**)

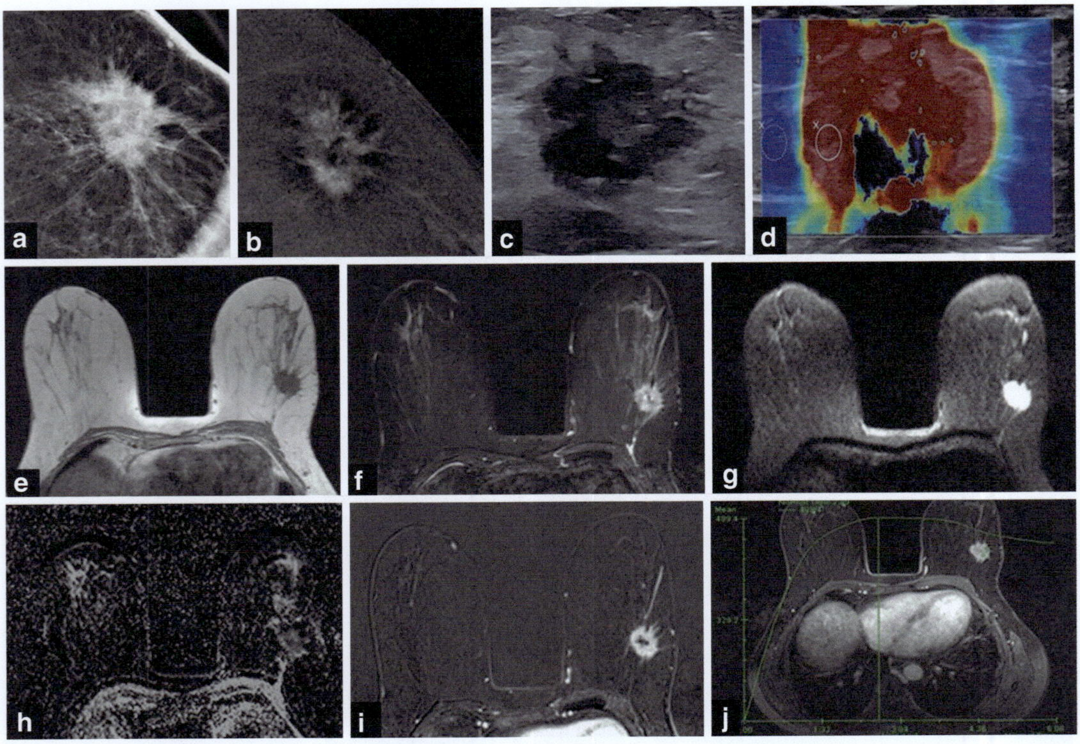

Fig. 3.10 Imaging characteristics of a malignant breast mass. (**a**) Mammogram showing an irregular high-density mass with spiculated margins. (**b**) On contrast-enhanced mammogram, the mass shows heterogeneous enhancement of moderate conspicuity. (**c**) USG showing an irregular hypoechoic nonparallel mass with spiculated margins which is hard on elastography (**d**). On MRI the mass shows irregular shape and spiculated margins and is isointense on T1 and IR (**e**, **f**), shows diffusion restriction (**g**, **h**) and heterogeneous enhancement with washout (type 3) kinetics (**i**, **j**)

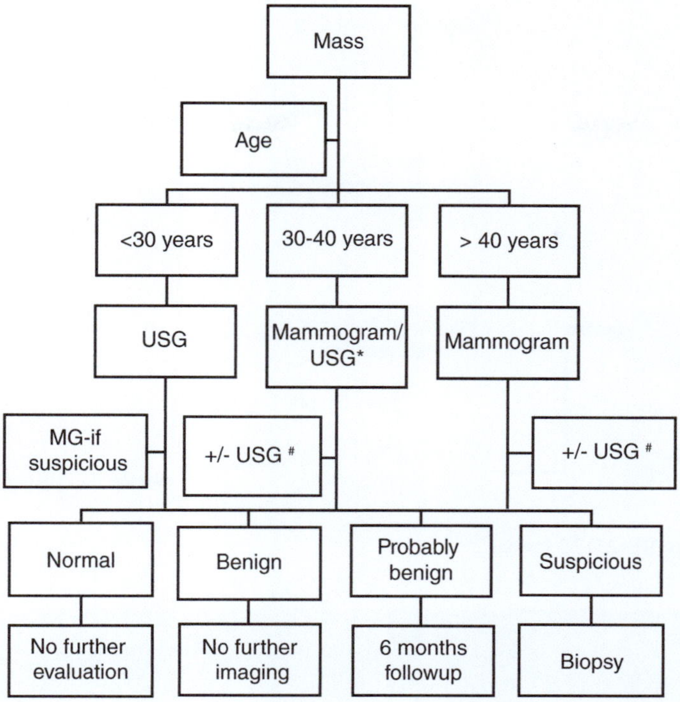

Fig. 3.11 Algorithmic approach to breast masses. USG, ultrasonography; MG, mammogram. *For patients who are 30–40 years presenting with palpable breast masses, the initial investigation can be mammogram or USG depending on the clinical scenario and level of suspicion. #When a mammogram is the primary investigation for a palpable abnormality, supplementary USG is indicated if the mammogram is negative or the findings are indeterminate or suspicious

3.4 BIRADS 3 Masses

Probably benign category (BIRADS 3) is given for specific imaging findings known to have a greater than 0% but ≤2% likelihood of representing malignancy [1].

BIRADS 3 in MG and USG: Among all the breast masses, BIRADS 3 is assigned only to a non-calcified well-circumscribed mass after full diagnostic workup and found to be iso- or hypoechoic on USG.

Diagnostic workup with USG helps identify characteristically benign findings (BIRADS 2) such as simple cysts and intramammary lymph nodes and also helps identify malignancies with circumscribed margins at an early stage. The use of BIRADS 3 in screening MG is discouraged [50].

BIRADS 3 is the most difficult category to assign and proven to have considerable interobserver variability especially in MG and MRI [51].

These imaging features are compatible with fibroadenoma or complicated cyst with internal debris. BIRADS 3 masses require an initial short interval follow-up at 6 months followed by 12 and 24 months to establish stability. During the follow-up period, if the lesion decreases in size, it can be downgraded to BIRADS 2. If it shows a significant increase in size (generally accepted as more than 20% in 6 months), it is upgraded as a suspicious abnormality, and biopsy is recommended [52]. If the lesion is stable at 24 months follow-up, BIRADS 2 category is assigned, and the patient returns to routine screening. Follow-up protocol for BIRADS 3 lesions has been highlighted in Figs. 3.12 and 3.13.

BIRADS 3 in MRI: In MRI, typically BIRADS 3 is assigned to a round or oval mass with well-circumscribed margins and persistent or plateau kinetic curve [53]. Other typical features of BIRADS 3 lesions include T2 hyperintensity and

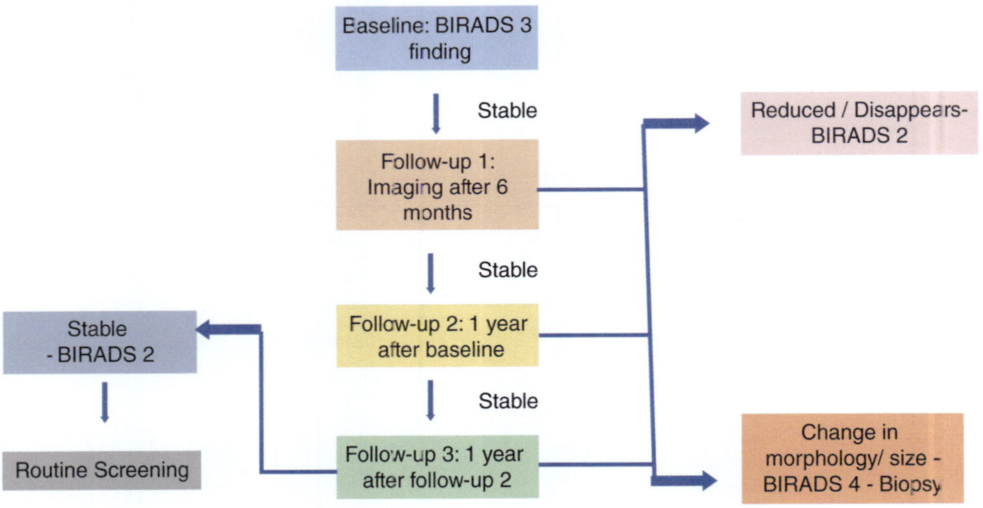

Fig. 3.12 Protocol for BIRADS 3 lesions

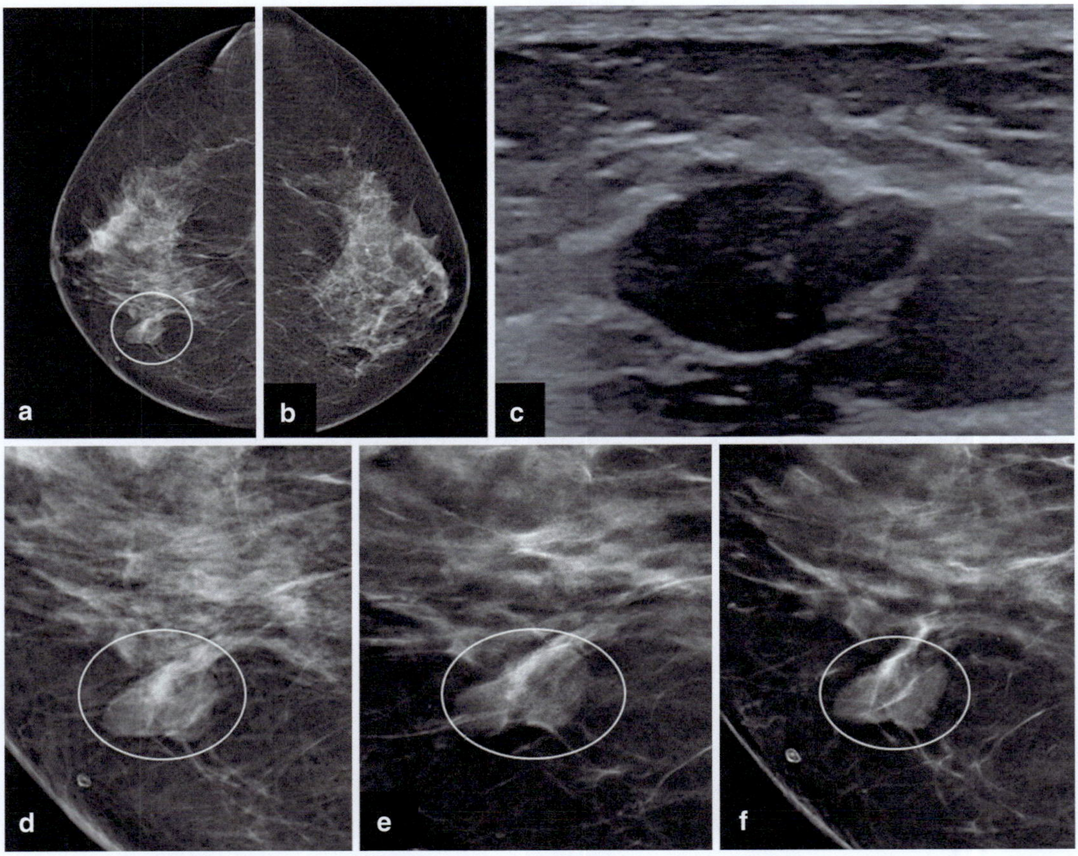

Fig. 3.13 CC images of right and left breasts (**a**, **b**) show an oval mass with circumscribed margins in the inner quadrant of the right breast (marked by white circle). An USG image (**c**) shows an oval hypoechoic parallel mass with circumscribed margins in the right breast corresponding to the mammographic abnormality. BIRADS 3 assessment (probably benign) was given, and short interval follow-up was suggested. Follow-up at 6 months, 1 year and 2 years (**d–f**, respectively) demonstrated an interval stability of the lesion, and it was downgraded to BIRADS 2 category (benign finding)

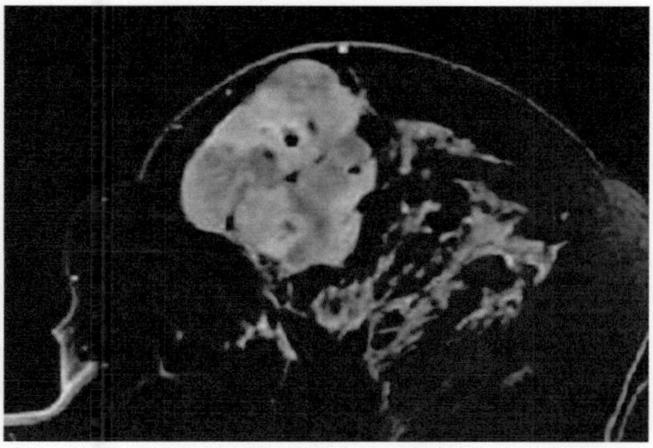

Fig. 3.14 A post-contrast T1 FS image shows a homogeneously enhancing mass with circumscribed margins and non-enhancing septations referred as dark internal septations. Biopsy from the mass revealed fibroadenoma

the presence of dark internal septations in post-contrast images (Fig. 3.14).

3.5 Conclusion

Breast masses are one of the common symptoms across all ages, and imaging plays a crucial role in evaluation. The choice of imaging is based primarily on the age at presentation. On both MG and USG, margin is one of the most important characteristics in assessing if the mass is benign or suspicious. Typically, a benign mass on MG or USG needs no further evaluation, and negative MG and USG on a clinically palpable mass have close to 100% negative predictive value. Both CEM and CE-MRI provide the functional aspects of the mass through enhancement parameters. Advanced imaging techniques like USG elastography and diffusion-weighted MRI add as supplementary techniques in further characterising the masses.

References

1. D'Orsi CJ, Sickles EA, Mendelson EB, Morris EA, et al. ACR BI-RADS® atlas, breast imaging reporting and data system. Reston: American College of Radiology; 2013.
2. Ma I, Dueck A, Gray R, et al. Clinical and self breast examination remain important in the era of modern screening. Ann Surg Oncol. 2012;19:1484–90.
3. Kaiser JS, Helvie MA, Blacklaw RL, Roubidoux MA. Palpable breast thickening: role of mammography and US in cancer detection. Radiology. 2002;223:839–44.
4. Rosner D, Blaird D. What ultrasonography can tell in breast masses that mammography and physical examination cannot. J Surg Oncol. 1985;28:308–13.
5. Boyd NF, Sutherland HJ, Fish EB, Hiraki GY, Lickley HL, Maurer VE. Prospective evaluation of physical examination of the breast. Am J Surg. 1981;142:331–4.
6. Expert Panel on Breast Imaging, Moy L, Heller SL, Bailey L, D'Orsi C, DiFlorio RM, Green ED, Holbrook AI, Lee SJ, Lourenco AP, Mainiero MB, Sepulveda KA, Slanetz PJ, Trikha S, Yepes MM, Newell MS. ACR appropriateness criteria® palpable breast masses. J Am Coll Radiol. 2017;14(5S):S203–24. https://doi.org/10.1016/j.jacr.2017.02.033. PMID: 28473077
7. Lehman CD, Lee AY, Lee CI. Imaging management of palpable breast abnormalities. AJR Am J Roentgenol. 2014;203:1142–53.
8. Shetty MK, Shah YP. Prospective evaluation of the value of negative sonographic and mammographic findings in patients with palpable abnormalities of the breast. J Ultrasound Med. 2002;21:1211–6.
9. Soo MS, Rosen EL, Baker JA, Vo TT, Boyd BA. Negative predictive value of sonography with mammography in patients with palpable breast lesions. AJR Am J Roentgenol. 2001;177:1167–70.
10. Ciatto S, Houssami N. Breast imaging and needle biopsy in women with clinically evident breast cancer: does combined imaging change overall diagnostic sensitivity? Breast. 2007;16:382–6.
11. Joshi P, Singh N, Raj G, et al. Performance evaluation of digital mammography, digital breast tomosynthesis and ultrasound in the detection of breast cancer using pathology as gold standard: an institutional experience. Egypt J Radiol Nucl Med. 2022;53:1. https://doi.org/10.1186/s43055-021-00675-y.
12. Greenwood HI, Dodelzon K, Katzen JT. Impact of advancing technology on diagnosis and treatment of breast cancer. Surg Clin. 2018;98(4):703–24.
13. Friedewald SM. Breast cancer screening: the debate that never ends. In: Gradishar W, editor. Optimizing breast cancer management. Cancer treatment and research, vol. 173. Cham: Springer; 2018.
14. Dhamija E, Gulati M, Deo SV, Gogia A, Hari S. Digital breast tomosynthesis: an overview. Indian J Surg Oncol. 2021;12(2):315–29.
15. Zuley ML, Guo B, Catullo VJ, et al. Comparison of two-dimensional synthesized mammograms versus original digital mammograms alone and in combination with tomosynthesis images. Radiology. 2014;271:664–71.
16. Waldherr C, Cerny P, Altermatt HJ, et al. Value of one-view breast tomosynthesis versus two-view mammography in diagnostic workup of women with clini-

cal signs and symptoms and in women recalled from screening. AJR Am J Roentgenol. 2013;200:226–31.
17. Dang PA, Freer PE, Humphrey KL, Halpern EF, Rafferty EA. Addition of tomosynthesis to conventional digital mammography: effect on image interpretation time of screening examinations. Radiology. 2014;270:49–56.
18. Zuckerman SP, Maidment ADA, Weinstein SP, McDonald ES, Conant EF. Imaging with synthesized 2D mammography: differences, advantages, and pitfalls compared with digital mammography. AJR Am J Roentgenol. 2017;209(1):222–9. https://doi.org/10.2214/AJR.16.17476.
19. Durfee SM, Selland DL, Smith DN, Lester SC, Kaelin CM, Meyer JE. Sonographic evaluation of clinically palpable breast cancers invisible on mammography. Breast J. 2000;6:247–51.
20. Hooley RJ, Scoutt LM, Philpotts LE. Breast ultrasonography: state of the art. Radiology. 2013;268(3):642–59. https://doi.org/10.1148/radiol.13121606.
21. Liberman L, Ernberg LA, Heerdt A, et al. Palpable breast masses: is there a role for percutaneous imaging-guided core biopsy? AJR Am J Roentgenol. 2000;175:779–87.
22. American College of Radiology. ACR practice parameter for the performance of stereotactic-guided breast interventional procedures. Available at: http://www.acr.org/w/media/ACR/Documents/PGTS/guidelines/Stereotactically_Guided_Breast.pdf.
23. Garg S, Mohan H, Bal A, Attri AK, Kochhar S. A comparative analysis of core needle biopsy and fine-needle aspiration cytology in the evaluation of palpable and mammographically detected suspicious breast lesions. Diagn Cytopathol. 2007;35:681–9.
24. Berg WA, Gutierrez L, NessAiver MS, et al. Diagnostic accuracy of mammography, clinical examination, US, and MR imaging in pre-operative assessment of breast cancer. Radiology. 2004;233:830–49.
25. Spick C, Szolar DH, Preidler KW, Tillich M, Reittner P, Baltzer PA. Breast MRI used as a problem-solving tool reliably excludes malignancy. Eur J Radiol. 2015;84:61–4.
26. Vraka I, Panourgias E, Sifakis E, Koureas A, Galanis P, Dellaportas D, Gouliamos A, Antoniou A. Correlation between contrast-enhanced ultrasound characteristics (qualitative and quantitative) and pathological prognostic factors in breast cancer. In Vivo. 2018;32:945–54. https://doi.org/10.21873/invivo.11333.
27. Li C, Gong H, Ling L, Du L, Su T, Wang S, Wang J. Diagnostic performance of contrast-enhanced ultrasound and enhanced magnetic resonance for breast nodules. J Biomed Res. 2018;32:198–207. https://doi.org/10.7555/JBR.32.20180015.
28. Iranmakani S, Mortezazadeh T, Sajadian F, et al. A review of various modalities in breast imaging: technical aspects and clinical outcomes. Egypt J Radiol Nucl Med. 2020;51:57. https://doi.org/10.1186/s43055-020-00175-5.
29. Eisenbrey JR, Dave JK, Forsberg F. Recent technological advancements in breast ultrasound. Ultrasonics. 2016;70:183–90. https://doi.org/10.1016/j.ultras.2016.04.021.
30. Mesurolle B, El Khoury M, Chammings F, Zhang M, Sun S. Breast sonoelastography: now and in the future. Diagn Interv Imaging. 2019;100(10):567–77. https://doi.org/10.1016/j.diii.2019.03.009.
31. Hari S, Paul SB, Vidyasagar R, Dhamija E, Adarsh AD, Thulkar S, Mathur S, Sreenivas V, Sharma S, Srivastava A, Seenu V. Breast mass characterization using shear wave elastography and ultrasound. Diagn Interv Imaging. 2018;99(11):699–707.
32. Shahzad R, Fatima I, Anjum T, Shahid A. Diagnostic value of strain elastography and shear wave elastography in differentiating benign and malignant breast lesions. Ann Saudi Med. 2022;42(5):319–25. https://doi.org/10.5144/0256-4947.2022.319. Epub 2022 Oct 6. PMID: 36252146; PMCID: PMC9557788
33. Youk JH, Gweon HM, Eun Ju Son D. Shear-wave elastography in breast ultrasonography: the state of the art. Ultrasonography. 2017;36:300–9.
34. Subramaniam P, Renganathan R, Rajalakshmi PR, Thakur V. Contrast enhanced mammography descriptors using breast imaging and reporting and data system. Indographics. 2022;2022(1):161–70.
35. Lalji UC, Houben IP, Prevos R, Gommers S, van Goethem M, Vanwetswinkel S, et al. Contrast-enhanced spectral mammography in recalls from the Dutch breast cancer screening program: validation of results in a large multireader, multicase study. Eur Radiol. 2016;26(12):4371–9.
36. Polat DS, Evans WP, Dogan BE. Contrast-enhanced digital mammography: technique, clinical applications, and pitfalls. AJR Am J Roentgenol. 2020;215(5):1267–78. https://doi.org/10.2214/AJR.19.22412. Epub 2020 Sep 2. PMID: 32877247
37. Baltzer P, Mann RM, Iima M, et al. Diffusion-weighted imaging of the breast—a consensus and mission statement from the EUSOBI International Breast Diffusion-Weighted Imaging working group. Eur Radiol. 2020;30:1436–50. https://doi.org/10.1007/s00330-019-06510-3.
38. Cohen EO, Tso HH, Leung JWT. Multiple bilateral circumscribed breast masses detected at imaging: review of evidence for management recommendations. AJR Am J Roentgenol. 2020;214(2):276–81. https://doi.org/10.2214/AJR.19.22061.
39. Nakashima K, et al. Comparison of visibility of circumscribed masses on digital breast tomosynthesis (DBT) and 2D mammography: are circumscribed masses better visualized and assured of being benign on DBT? Eur Radiol. 2017;27(2):570–7.
40. Berg WA, Leung JWT. Diagnostic imaging: breast. 3rd ed. Philadelphia: Elsevier; 2019. p. 246–8.
41. Chotai NC, Yim H, Fok ECM, Loke SC, Lim HMY. Complex cystic breast masses: an ultrasound imaging review. Adv Breast Cancer Res. 2022;11:31–49. https://doi.org/10.4236/abcr.2022.111002.

42. Gibson AL, et al. Shedding light on T2 bright masses on breast MRI: Benign and malignant causes. J Breast Imaging. 2022;4(4):430–40. https://doi.org/10.1093/jbi/wbac030.
43. Bernent H, Becette V, Mohallem M, Ferreira F, Chérel P. Masses in mammography: what are the underlying anatomopathological lesions? Diagn Interv Imaging. 2014;95(2):124–33. https://doi.org/10.1016/j.diii.2013.12.010.
44. Goldbach AR, Tuite CM, Ross E. Clustered microcysts at breast US: Outcomes and updates for appropriate management recommendations. Radiology. 2020;295(1):44–51. https://doi.org/10.1148/radiol.2020191505.
45. Malich A, Fischer DR, Wurdinger S, Boettcher J, Marx C, Facius M, Kaiser WA. Potential MRI interpretation model: differentiation of benign from malignant breast masses. AJR Am J Roentgenol. 2005;185(4):964–70. https://doi.org/10.2214/AJR.04.1073.
46. Salkowski LR. Mass with indistinct margins. In: Lee CI, Lehman CD, Bassett LW, editors. Breast imaging, Rotations in radiology. online ed. New York: Oxford Academic; 2018. https://doi.org/10.1093/med/9780190270261.003.0024.
47. Andrejeva L, Geisel JL, Harigopal M. Spiculated masses. In: Lee CI, Lehman CD, Bassett LW, editors. Breast imaging, Rotations in radiology. online ed. New York: Oxford Academic; 2018. https://doi.org/10.1093/med/9780190270261.003.0025.
48. Xiao J, Rahbar H, Hippe DS, Rendi MH, Parker EU, Shekar N, Hirano M, Cheung KJ, Partridge SC. Dynamic contrast-enhanced breast MRI features correlate with invasive breast cancer angiogenesis. NPJ Breast Cancer. 2021;7(1):42. https://doi.org/10.1038/s41523-021-00247-3. PMID: 33863924; PMCID: PMC8052427
49. Subramaniam P, Renganathan R, Suganya P, et al. Diagnostic accuracy of subjective kinetic assessment of masses in contrast-enhanced mammography in comparison with contrast-enhanced magnetic resonance imaging. Egypt J Radiol Nucl Med. 2023;54:89. https://doi.org/10.1186/s43055-023-01039-4.
50. Stavros AT, Thickman D, Rapp CL, Dennis MA, Parker SH, Sisney GA. Solid breast nodules: use of sonography to distinguish between benign and malignant lesions. Radiology. 1995;196(1):123–34.
51. Michaels AY, Chung CSW, Frost EP, Birdwell RL, Giess CS. Interobserver variability in upgraded and non-upgraded BI-RADS 3 lesions. Clin Radiol. 2017;72(8):694.e1–6.
52. Gordon PB, Gagnon FA, Lanzkowsky L. Solid breast masses diagnosed as fibroadenoma at fine-needle aspiration biopsy: acceptable rates of growth at long-term follow-up. Radiology. 2003;229(1):233–8.
53. Spick C, Szolar DH, Baltzer PA, Tillich M, Reittner P, Preidler KW, et al. Rate of malignancy in MRI-detected probably benign (BI-RADS 3) lesions. AJR. 2014;202(3):684–9.

Approach to Calcifications

4

Suma Chakrabarthi and Sugat Sanyal

Abstract

Calcifications in the breast are often benign but may also indicate malignant change in the breast. Identifying and characterizing calcifications is an important art and science of breast imaging. In this chapter we discuss the clinical impact of breast calcifications, pathophysiology of benign and malignant calcifications and assessment of calcifications on various imaging modalities. As calcifications are best demonstrated on mammography, we will discuss in detail the appearances on mammography including the typically benign features of some calcifications and also delve into assessment of suspicious calcifications. Classifying suspicious calcifications into various BI-RADS assessment categories to enable appropriate management of calcifications has also been discussed. Biopsy and localization of calcifications and the importance of radiology-pathology correlation have also been addressed. Artefacts mimicking calcifications, disappearing calcifications and prognosis prediction using calcifications have also been touched upon. With scientific progress and successful experiments using the concept of Raman spectroscopy, there are interesting future possibilities of detection and investigation of calcifications in the breast, which we discuss briefly. This chapter provides an overall understanding of breast calcifications with an emphasis on radiological assessment and management of these very important indicators of breast disease.

Keywords

Breast calcifications · Breast microcalcifications · Suspicious calcifications · Benign calcifications · Calcification BI-RADS Radiology-pathology correlation

4.1 Introduction

Calcification on mammography (MG) is often an indicator of the changes occurring in the breast parenchyma at the cellular level, sometimes the tip of the iceberg that unravels the elusive diagnosis. The job of reassuring the patient that the calcification is benign is as important as the skill to identify malignant calcifications. Hence it is imperative that a good breast radiologist should be able to identify and characterize calcifications optimally. In this chapter we aim to give you an overall understanding of breast calcifications with an emphasis on radiological assessment and

S. Chakrabarthi (✉)
Department of Radiology, Peerless Hospitex Hospital, Kolkata, India

S. Sanyal
Department of Histopathology, Peerless Hospitex Hospital, Kolkata, India

E. Dhamija, S. V. S. Deo (eds.), *Imaging in Management of Breast Diseases*,
https://doi.org/10.1007/978-981-96-4998-3_4

management of these very important markers of breast disease. We discuss the pathophysiology of benign as well as malignant calcifications. Biopsy and preoperative localization of calcifications as well as the importance of radiology-pathology correlation (RPC) have been discussed. Most importantly we hope that you will be equipped with the knowledge to interpret calcifications effectively and make a positive contribution to patient care.

4.2 Clinical Impact of Calcifications

Calcifications are seen in the breast tissue either as a result of physiological or pathological change either in the past or at present. We would not be writing or reading an entire chapter on calcifications if finding and characterizing them did not have an impact on the clinical care of the patient! Especially to the radiologist, they are of immense value as subtle calcifications can lead the radiologist to deadly disease in the breast. Similarly benign calcifications can be used to characterize breast disease and reassure the patient. Seventy-five percent of breast carcinomas have histologically detectable microcalcifications, whereas only 35–40% breast carcinomas have radiologically detectable microcalcifications [1]. This means that we only appreciate about 50% of the microcalcifications on mammography! It is therefore important that we assess these vital informers of malignant change and make a difference to our patients.

Calcifications on MG are very common and are actually seen in 80% of the mammograms, and they are mostly benign in nature [2]. However, they have a big role in early detection of malignant change in the breast. Fifty-five percent of nonpalpable malignant lesions in the breast demonstrate mammographically visible microcalcifications. Eighty-five to ninety-five percent of cases of ductal carcinoma in situ (DCIS) in screening MG are detected due to microcalcifications [3]. Forty-two to seventy-two percent of DCIS have calcifications. Calcifications are more common in DCIS with high-grade neoplastic change and in younger women [4]. Up to 50% of high-grade carcinoma in situ (CIS) and high-grade in situ component of invasive cancers contain calcifications. Low-grade CIS calcifies in approximately 25% of cases [5].

In the screening population, the recall rate for calcifications ranges from 0.4 to 2% of the women screened. Mammographic calcifications investigated as a result of screening MG yield a diagnosis of malignancy in 0.3% women screened [6]. The extent of suspicious calcifications helps decide surgical options such as mastectomy, wide local excision and oncoplastic reconstruction, as calcifications extending beyond the palpable and/or sonographic mass may only be visualized on MG. Morphology of some calcifications may indicate the genetic and molecular features of the neoplasm and also provide prognostic information.

Male breast mammogram also demonstrates microcalcifications, although they are less frequent than in females and are reported in 13 to 30% of male breast cancers. Microcalcifications are most likely seen in DCIS component of the masses, which are not frequently present in male breast cancer. They tend to be coarser and less likely to be linear when compared to female breast cancer. Benign breast calcifications can also be seen on male mammography, although less common than on female mammography [7, 8].

4.3 Pathophysiology and Biochemical Composition of Calcifications

Mammary calcification can be an active pathological mineralization process as well as a passive process, such as degeneration or necrosis. Pathophysiology of calcification in breast lesions involves a complex interplay of cellular processes, hormonal influences, inflammation and microenvironmental factors. Microcalcifications are associated with benign, premalignant and malignant breast lesions. Distinguishing between benign and malignant calcifications is critical for appropriate patient care. Core biopsy and pathological examination remain essential in confirming the benign nature of lesions, ensuring that patients are spared unnecessary anxiety and aggressive treatments [9, 10]. The primary calcification types are composed of calcium oxalate (CO) and calcium phosphate, usually in the form of hydroxyapatite (HA).

4.3.1 Biochemistry of Calcifications

At the biochemical level, microcalcifications have been categorized into the following: type I, composed of CO, and type II, composed of HA. CO is usually associated with benign conditions, while the others remain primarily associated with malignancy. Table 4.1 summarizes the biochemistry of microcalcifications.

4.3.2 Cellular Dynamics and Molecular Alterations in Benign Lesions

Cellular Mechanism A multitude of cellular mechanisms are responsible for calcification. The most predominant factor is the turnover of epithelial cells within the mammary parenchyma. Apoptotic cell debris from normal cellular turnover serves as nucleation sites for calcium phosphate deposition, initiating the formation of calcifications. In addition, the presence of myoepithelial cells, responsible for regulating tissue integrity, plays a role in the calcification process. Dysfunctions in these cellular processes contribute to the formation of benign calcifications [13, 14].

Hormonal Influences The hormonal balance at the cellular level of the breast parenchyma potentially impacts the pathophysiology of calcification. Oestrogen and progesterone, which are key hormones in breast development and function, influence cellular activities. Hormonal fluctuations during menstrual cycles and changes occurring after hormone replacement therapy significantly affect the proliferation and differentiation of mammary epithelial cells, leading to the formation of microcalcifications [15, 16].

Inflammatory Processes Chronic inflammation causes the release of cytokines and growth factors modulating cellular behaviour and tissue remodelling. Macrophages, the key components of the immune response, release matrix vesicles that serve as initiation sites for calcium phosphate deposition, contributing to the formation of microcalcifications [17].

Extracellular Matrix Remodelling Changes in the composition of the extracellular matrix (ECM) contribute to calcification in benign breast lesions. Fibroblasts and myoepithelial cells regulate ECM remodelling, and alterations in their function greatly influence the mineralization process at the tissue level. Dysregulation of these cellular components results in changes in composition of the ECM causing deposition of calcium in the ECM, leading to calcifications [18, 19].

Microenvironmental Factors Factors such as tissue acidity, oxygen levels and the presence of growth factors influence the mineralization process. Understanding how these microenvironmental factors interact with cellular processes provides insights into the diverse patterns of calcification observed in benign lesions [20].

Table 4.1 Features of and differences between type I, type II and Mg-HA calcifications [2, 11, 12]

Features of MC	Type 1	Type 2	Mg-HA
Biochemistry	CO (CaC2O42H2O)	Calcium HA [Ca10(PO4)6(OH)2]	Mg-HA [Mg10(PO4)6(OH)2]
Pathology	Benign	Benign and malignant	Mostly malignant
Optical microscopy	Amber or transparent	Opaque, grey/white	Opaque, grey/white
Birefringence	Birefringent	Non-birefringent	Non-birefringent

MC microcalcifications, *CO* calcium oxalate, *HA* hydroxyapatite, *Mg-HA* magnesium-substituted HA

4.3.3 Cellular Dynamics and Molecular Alterations in Malignant Lesions

Dysregulated Cellular Processes Dysregulated cellular process is the starting point. Tumour cells develop aberrant proliferation, survival and death, causing the release of cellular debris. Apoptotic bodies and necrotic tissue fragments form nucleation sites for calcium phosphate deposition, initiating microcalcification formation [21].

Angiogenesis and Vascular Calcification Complex interplay between angiogenesis and vascular wall calcification play a dominant role. Pro-angiogenic factors, including vascular endothelial growth factor, induce the formation of leaky vascular channels. Microcalcifications develop within the wall of vasculature due to the abundance of calcium ions and create a distinctive mammographic pattern [22, 23].

Genetic Alterations and Molecular Pathways Genetic mutations like BRCA1 and BRCA2 disrupt cell cycle control, DNA repair mechanisms and apoptosis, promoting the process of microcalcification formation. Dysregulation in the control pathway of matrix metalloproteinases and tissue inhibitors of metalloproteinases impacts the extracellular matrix microenvironment, leading to calcification [24, 25].

Microenvironmental Factors Interactions between cancer cells and stromal components, inflammatory responses and alterations in the extracellular matrix composition contribute to a favourable microenvironment crucial for microcalcification and are also responsible for the heterogeneity of calcification patterns [26, 27].

4.3.4 Histomorphological Hallmarks

While type I calcifications are usually associated with cysts or fat necrosis (dystrophic calcification), type II calcifications are associated with abnormal epithelial cells. Histologically, microcalcifications are calcium-related deposits in the breast duct lobular units associated with an epithelial component or are entrapped within the mesenchymal component, either in the stroma or within a fibrotic healing process. It is of utmost importance to identify microcalcifications and mention their presence in the pathology report, as it confirms that the biopsied area is the actual target of the examination. It is important to ascertain, if possible whether microcalcifications are irregular or birefringent. When the fragments labelled as 'with microcalcifications' are microscopically analysed, it may not be easily identifiable, as they may lie deeper in the paraffin block, or they may be lost during sample processing [2, 28].

Insights into the pathogenesis and pathophysiology of microcalcification lead to the concept of targeted therapeutic interventions. Modulating calcium signalling pathways and angiogenic factors need to be explored. Therapies targeting genetic mutations associated with breast cancer can alter the process of microcalcifications [29, 30].

4.4 Assessment of Calcifications with Imaging Modalities

Mammography is the best tool for identification and assessment of calcifications. Full-field digital mammography has established itself as better than film-screen mammography in detection of microcalcifications [31, 32]. Suspicious calcifications seen on the standard mediolateral oblique (MLO) and craniocaudal (CC) views need to be assessed further with additional views. A lateral view helps assess the true position of the calcifications in the superoinferior plane and is most useful with calcifications at the level of the nipple on MLO, to decide if they are actually above or below the nipple. CC or lateral spot magnification views aid better characterization of the morphology and extent of calcifications which in turn help in the assessment of the probability of malignancy [33]. Digital breast tomosynthesis (DBT) has a high sensitivity for detection of malignant calcifications, but some calcifications may not be detected on DBT-only screening. However, it may demonstrate associated masses and architectural distortions better as it reduces tissue overlap and increases image contrast [34].

Improvement in technology has made some calcifications visible on ultrasound. It is a good modality to look for the associated soft tissue suggestive of invasion and also to assess axillary lymph nodes [6]. Hence a breast ultrasound is to be done prior to biopsy of the calcifications. The low sensitivity and specificity of breast MRI for calcifications not associated with masses makes this a suboptimal tool for assessment of mammographically detected microcalcifications [35]. Diffusion-weighted imaging and radiomics assessment of DCIS with MRI are active areas of research [36].

4.5 Artefacts Mimicking Calcifications

Artefacts resulting from dust on compression paddles and detectors can mimic calcifications. These artefacts usually occur on images of multiple patients and at the same site on the image. Also one must check for artefacts if calcifications are seen on only one view. A coarse flaky skin due to fungal infections may mimic soft calcifications [37]. Metallic particles in certain ointments, deodorants, powders, creams and antiperspirants can mimic calcifications. Hence patients should be advised not to apply anything over the breasts and underarms prior to MG. Although artefacts seem to be a straightforward thing to deal with, there are times when even the experienced breast radiologist may be duped by these, so beware of them! Always think of artefacts if things don't add up between the different views of the same breast (Fig. 4.1).

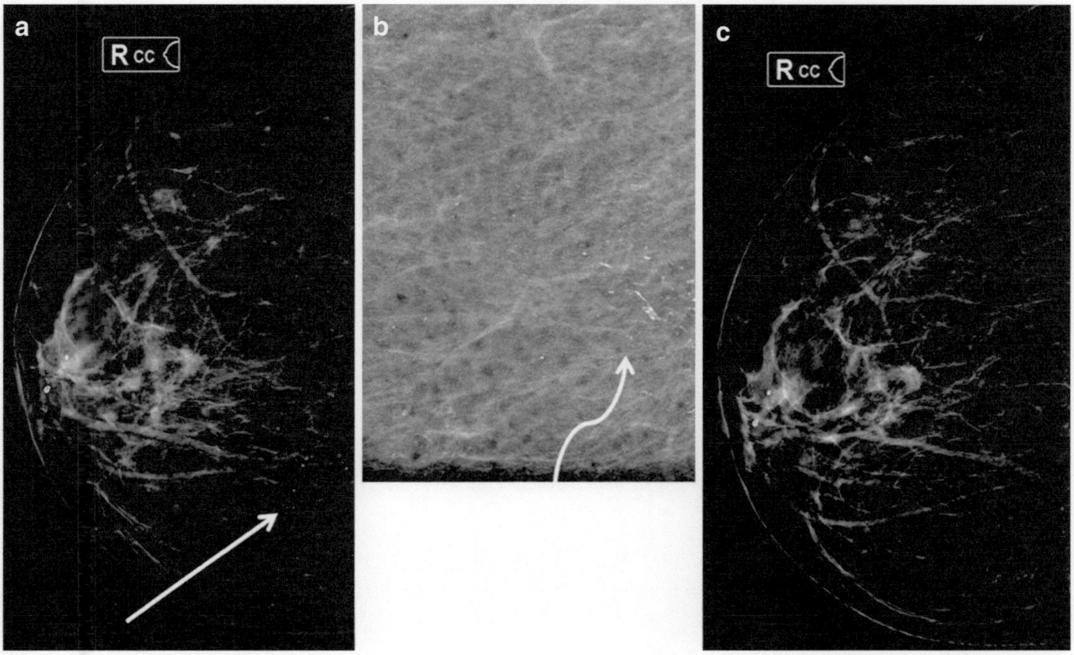

Fig. 4.1 (**a**) Artefact (arrow) mimicking calcifications in the posterior medial breast due to ointment applied for rashes. (**b**) Magnified view of the same (curved arrow). (**c**) Artefact no longer seen on the CC view repeated after cleaning the area

4.6 Typically Benign Calcifications

Some calcifications are characteristically benign and need no further mammography views, correlating ultrasound or biopsy to confirm their nature. Benign calcifications tend to be larger in size and are termed macrocalcifications when they are >2 mm calcium deposits in the breast tissue. However size alone cannot be used to confirm benignity. Morphology and distribution of calcifications are very important determinants of benign etiology. Calcifications that are diffusely scattered involving all quadrants of the breasts, often bilateral, tend to be benign, as these are due to generalized breast changes such as fibrocystic disease [33]. Morphology is mostly decided by the structure within which the calcification arises. For example, morphological appearance of the calcifications can help deduce if they originate in the walls of cysts or within the arterial wall. Benign calcifications tend to be very dense, and individual particles are well defined and of typical shapes that indicate the structure they arise in and are less likely to be segmental [5]. Some of the typically benign calcifications are discussed below (Fig. 4.2).

(a) Vascular calcifications: These calcifications involve the middle layer of arteries and are called Mönckeberg calcifications. They are due to medial calcific sclerosis as opposed to calcifications seen in the intimal layer in atherosclerotic arteries elsewhere in the body. They tend to be diffusely distributed, are thin and mostly involve the entire circumference of the arteries. Parallel linear calcifications along the course of a vessel visualized on at least one mammographic view are benign vascular calcifications, and these have a distinct tram-track or railroad track configuration. Although linear, they have a serpentine course in contrast to the branching or casting linear ductal calcifications which follow the pattern of ductal distribution. However early vascular calcifications deposited on only one

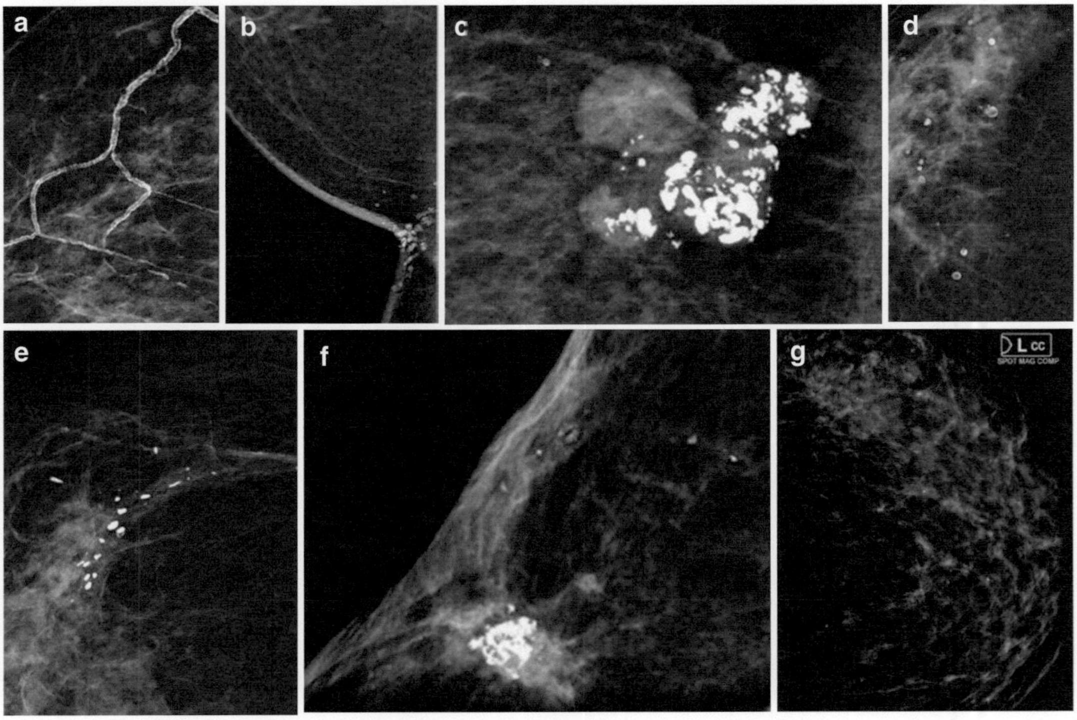

Fig. 4.2 Benign calcifications: vascular (**a**), skin calcifications in the medial breast (**b**), coarse or popcorn-like (**c**), rim (**d**), large rod-like (**e**), dystrophic (**f**) and round diffuse (**g**)

side of a vessel may appear intraductal, but often careful examination demonstrates an associated smooth tubular vessel [38, 39].

(b) Skin calcifications: These are most commonly located in the inframammary fold, parasternal region, axilla and around the areola. They are easily identified on DBT by their location as they are seen on the first and last three images of the DBT sequence when the skin touches either the compression paddle or the detector. However if the skin with calcifications is not touching one of these, the calcifications will appear on the deeper images [34]. They are also well identified on digital mammography and are often polygonal or round, grouped, with central lucency, as they are mostly calcified skin cysts [40]. They may be seen within the skin in one of the views. The tangential view may be used to confirm a cutaneous location in some cases [33]. Calcifications that maintain a fixed relationship to each other on different views suggest skin calcification, also known as the tattoo sign [41] (Fig. 4.3).

(c) Coarse or 'popcorn-like': This is typically seen in postmenopausal women when fibroadenomas regress and become hyalinized with calcification [4]. They may be seen as small calcifications at the periphery of a circumscribed low-density mass to start with, which over time become larger than 2–3 mm and coarse, to finally coalesce and form the typically benign popcorn calcification. In small involuting fibroadenomas which calcify, only calcification may be visible with no appreciable soft tissue component of the mass [8].

(d) Large rod-like: These are large thick smooth linear calcifications within the ducts due to benign intraductal or periductal pathology such as duct ectasia or plasma cell mastitis. Hence they are in ductal distribution radiating towards the nipple and may occasionally branch. They are also called 'secretory' calcifications. They are seen in 3% of the mammograms. They do not have central lucencies if they are intraductal. Periductal calcification however will have central lucency. They are usually greater than 0.5 mm in diameter and bilateral [42].

(e) Rim calcification: These are <1 mm thin calcifications on the surface of a spherical structure such as an oil cyst. These are also referred to as eggshell or ring calcifications. The centre is of low or fat density. They can be of varying sizes and may sometimes present with a history of trauma [4, 42].

(f) Milk of calcium calcifications: Small saccular dilatations of the terminal duct lobular units (TDLU) forming micro or macrocysts containing calcium oxalate within them look amorphous on the CC view but are seen to be

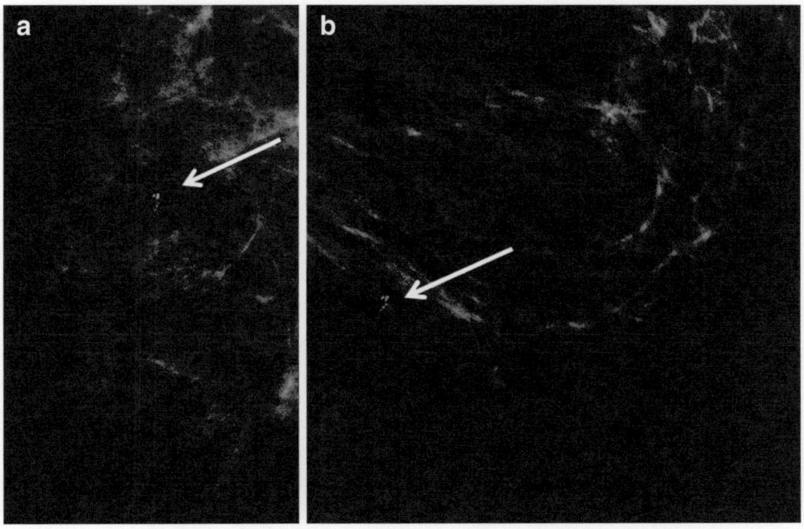

Fig. 4.3 Small grouped calcifications are noted in the left lower central breast. Calcifications (arrow) maintain a fixed relationship to each other on both CC (**a**) and MLO (**b**) views suggesting skin calcifications, also known as the tattoo sign

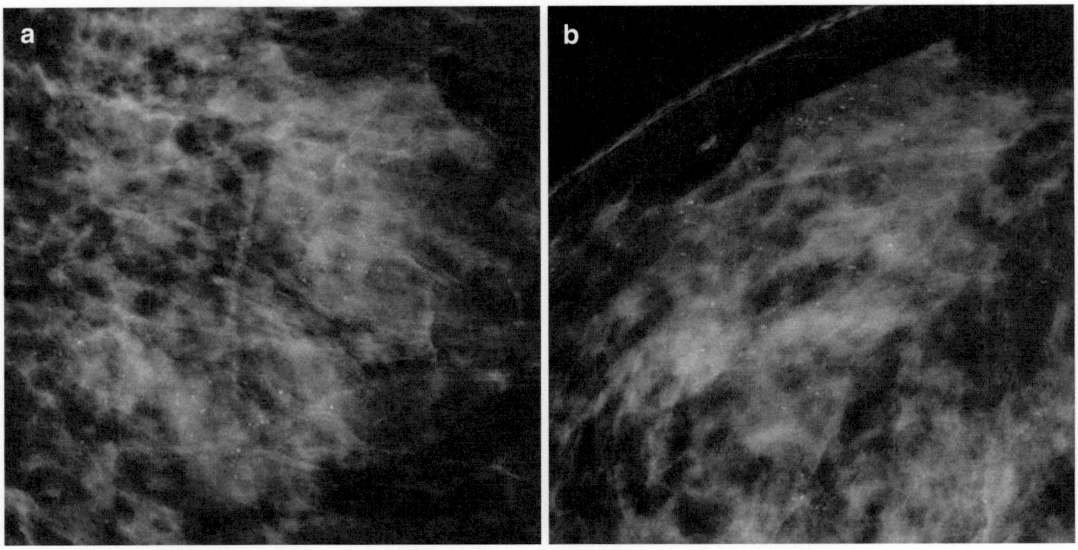

Fig. 4.4 Milk of calcium calcifications: The CC view shows amorphous and punctuate calcifications (**a**). The lateral view shows many calcifications layering, some are horizontal and some have crescent shapes (**b**)

dependent and layering on the lateral view, creating a crescent with upper concavity or linear-shaped calcifications. The best visualization of these 'teacup' calcifications is on the lateral view, preferably with the patient seated for about 2 to 5 minutes before the image, to allow for the calcium to sediment (Fig. 4.4). These calcifications are most common in perimenopausal and postmenopausal women [42, 43]. Sometimes correlating cysts with dependent echogenic material can be seen on ultrasound.

(g) Dystrophic calcifications: These are seen after surgery, radiotherapy or trauma to the breast. They are usually greater than 1 mm, have irregular shapes and can coalesce to sometimes form large palpable chunks of calcification with bizarre shapes. The fat density area within or around it to support fat necrosis is helpful to make a diagnosis of benign calcification. Dystrophic breast calcifications can also be caused by systemic diseases such as hyperparathyroidism and collagen diseases [44, 45].

(h) Suture calcifications: These are typically benign with linear, arc or knot-shaped calcification overlying the surgical sutures.

(i) Round calcifications: These are round or spherical in shape, are variable in size and are called 'punctate' if smaller than 0.5 mm [46]. These calcifications are mostly formed in the acini of the lobules. These are considered benign when they are diffuse or regional, <1 mm and small [46]. However follow-up or biopsy may be warranted in some distribution patterns and will be discussed in the section on suspicious calcifications.

4.7 Suspicious Calcifications

Sometimes early benign calcification may cause confusion. Early calcification within a fibroadenoma, early unilateral secretory calcification or early dystrophic calcification at the site of the scar post-surgery may give rise to diagnostic dilemmas. Unless the morphology and distribution are typically benign, it is best to manage these calcifications with guarded suspicion.

Suspicious calcifications need to be assessed based on both their morphology and distribution. Both of these aspects of the calcifications are indicators of the site of origin of the disease, the pathological change and the extent of disease, which in turn help us decide what the diagnosis may be and if the calcifications need to biopsied. In general multiple bilateral diffuse calcifications are likely to be benign. There are various terminologies used over the years to describe the morphology and distribution patterns of suspicious calcifications. We are going to use the terminologies based on the American College of Radiology (ACR) Breast Imaging Reporting and Data System (BI-RADS) as these are the most used in the literature at present and will make it a lot easier for the readers to correlate with most of the recent publications [46]. We will look at the five morphology and five distribution patterns that are used to describe suspicious calcifications.

Calcifications with a diameter less than 1 mm are referred to as microcalcifications [47]. It is well known that microcalcifications can be malignant. However not all microcalcifications are malignant. For example, punctate calcifications usually arising from the lumen of lobular acini may indicate a benign disease as well as DCIS. Similarly not all calcifications >1 mm are benign. For example, coarse heterogeneous or dystrophic calcifications >1 mm in size may be seen in malignant lesions. Hence size is not the only criterion to confirm or refute malignant etiology. Also the stability of probably benign calcifications such as grouped punctuate microcalcifications over a period of time may indicate a benign disease; hence follow-up mammography plays a role in the management of this subgroup of calcifications. However the stability of suspicious microcalcifications, for example, in segmental distribution is not to be considered reassuring as these should always be deemed suspicious. Hence follow-up is not an option when calcification is of suspicious category. Morphology, distribution, size and stability of calcifications are all taken into consideration to make a decision about biopsy and treatment of calcifications [47].

4.7.1 Morphology Subtypes

The five morphology subtypes have been discussed below (Figs. 4.5, 4.6, 4.7, 4.8, and 4.9):

(a) Round/punctate calcifications: Although this is considered a benign morphology in general, certain distribution patterns such as linear and segmental dictate biopsy. Grouped punctate calcifications on baseline MG are probably benign, and follow-up of these is appropriate. However if the group is new or increasing, biopsy is recommended. Also grouped punctate calcifications adjacent to a known cancer needs biopsy [46]. (We are often judged by the close friends we make!) Follow-up or biopsy of grouped punctate calcifications is advisable as 15% of DCIS calcification clusters have predominantly punctuate calcifications [48, 49].

(b) Amorphous calcifications: These are indistinct calcifications that are too hazy and/or too small for their margin or shape to be clearly defined. Amorphous calcifications are mostly found in benign conditions such as fibrocystic changes, fibrosis and sclerosing adenosis. They are also found in high-risk lesions such as atypical ductal hyperplasia, atypical lobular hyperplasia and lobular carcinoma in situ. About 20% of amorphous calcifications are malignant, most of which are DCIS. Grouped, linear, segmental amorphous calcifications should be biopsied. Bilateral diffuse amorphous calcifications can be deemed benign and do not warrant biopsy. However magnification views to evaluate the calcifications optimally if seen on baseline mammography is useful to characterize the calcifications [46, 50].

(c) Coarse heterogeneous calcifications: These are conspicuous, have irregular shape and may be found in benign lesions such as fibroadenomas and fibrosis. These are generally 0.5 to 1 mm in size. Early dystrophic calcifications can be coarse heterogeneous, but as they coalesce and become larger, they show the typical characteristics of benign dystrophic calcifications. Hence coarse heterogeneous calcifications can be seen after trauma, surgery or hematoma. In general, coarse heterogeneous calcifications are benign, and the likelihood of malignancy is around 13%, most of which are DCIS [3, 51]. If there are

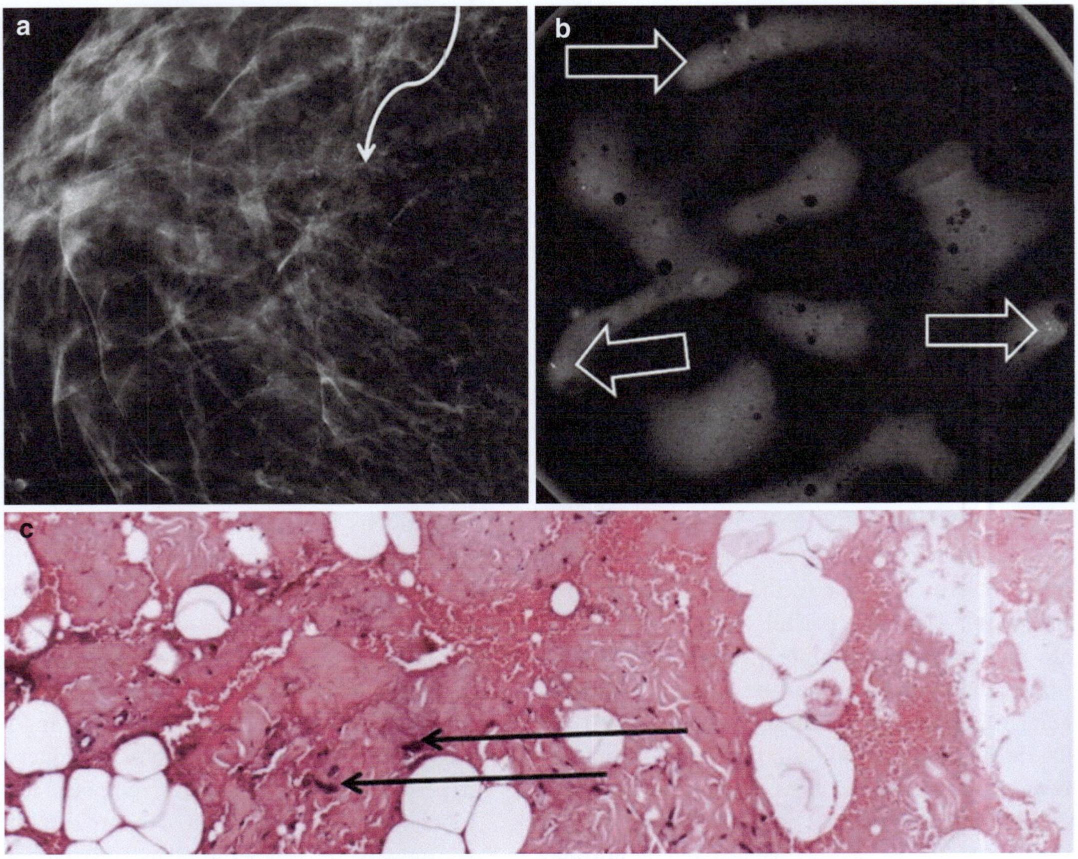

Fig. 4.5 (**a**) Regional punctate calcifications on mammography (curved arrow). (**b**) A specimen radiography from stereotactic biopsy shows calcifications in cores (thick arrows). (**c**) Calcifications (straight arrow) seen within benign sclerotic stroma on histology

numerous bilateral grouped coarse heterogeneous calcifications, they are likely to be benign. However magnification views on baseline mammography is useful [46].

(d) Fine pleomorphic calcifications: These are small <0.5 mm calcifications which have varying shapes and sizes. They do not have fuzzy margins like amorphous calcifications and do not have fine linear calcifications. They have a positive predictive value of 29% for malignant etiology, which is higher than the amorphous and coarse heterogeneous groups [3, 46, 51].

(e) Fine linear and fine-linear branching: This is the most suspicious of all morphologies with the highest positive predictive value of 70%. These are thin linear calcifications <0.5 mm in calibre. The calcifications are irregular,

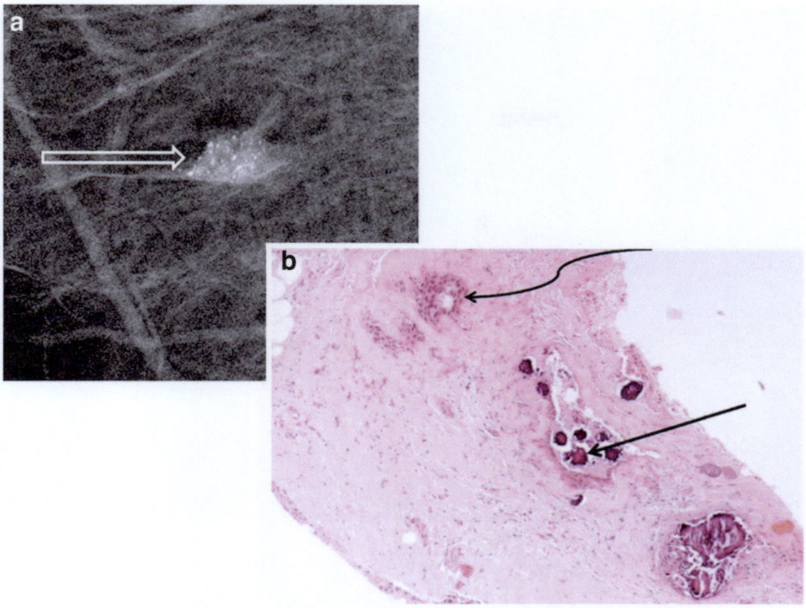

Fig. 4.6 (**a**) Grouped amorphous calcifications on mammography (thick arrow). (**b**) Calcifications seen within an area of comedonecrosis on histology (straight arrow). A small focus of DCIS (curved arrow) is also seen in the same image

and some branching calcifications may be seen suggesting intraductal calcifications involved by breast cancer [3, 10, 51]. These differ from benign linear calcifications such as seen in plasma cell mastitis which are regular with well-defined margin, may have lucent centres and are usually thicker. Intraductal calcifications are due to calcification of cellular debris or secretions within the distal TDLU. Sometimes these intraductal calcifications may form casts of the entire involved ductal system which may be fragmented. These casting-type calcifications are highly suspicious for malignant etiology and indicate segmental or lobar patterns of malignant change in a sick lobe. Casting-type calcifications are also associated with neoductgenesis, but in this case, they are not distributed in a segmental fashion delineating the usual ductal branching pattern of a segment or lobe [5, 33].

4.7.2 Distribution Subtypes

The five distribution subtypes have been discussed below (Fig. 4.10):

(a) Diffuse: This refers to calcifications scattered throughout the breast and tend to be benign especially if they are bilateral punctate or amorphous calcifications. Diffuse randomly scattered calcifications such as skin calcifications and lobular calcifications in the acini such as seen in fibrocystic disease are benign [46, 52]. There are many studies that have shown that none of the diffuse calcifications were malignant [3,

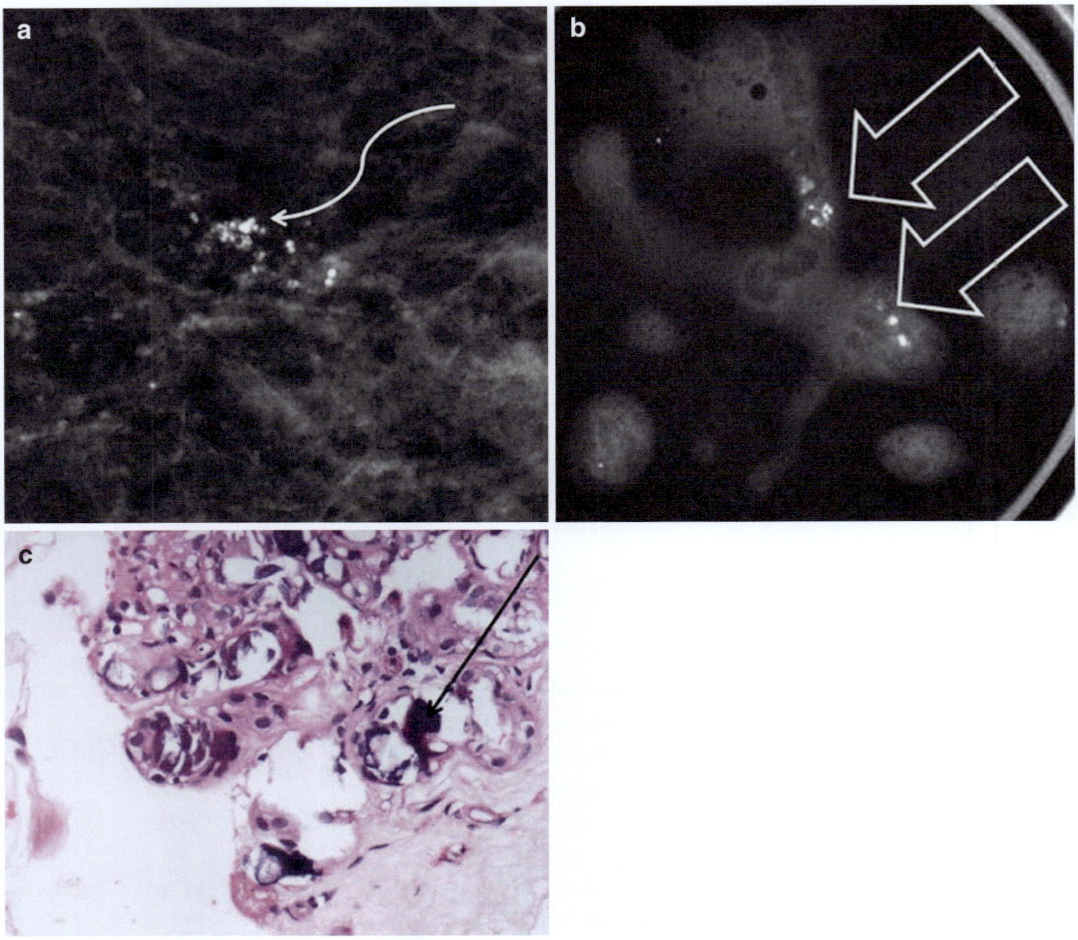

Fig. 4.7 (**a**) Grouped coarse heterogeneous calcifications on mammography (curved arrow). (**b**) A specimen radiography from stereotactic biopsy shows calcifications in cores (thick arrows). (**c**) Multiple coarse calcifications (straight arrow) seen on histology demonstrating fibrocystic mastopathy with sclerosing adenosis as the dominant component

10, 51]. However morphology must be checked, and biopsy should be performed if any of the calcifications show a suspicious morphology.

(b) Regional: Numerous calcifications in a large area of the breast which is more than 2 cm in greatest dimension, but not conforming to a duct distribution, are deemed to be regional in distribution. This may involve a large area, even more than a quadrant. While some studies reported no malignancy in calcifications of regional distribution, a study has demonstrated malignant regional calcifications of fine pleomorphic and amorphous morphology. Overall the positive predictive value for this distribution pattern is 26% [46].

(c) Grouped: Calcifications clustered together into small groups are termed grouped calcifications. At least five calcifications within 1 cm of each other are required to be termed as grouped calcifications. A larger number of calcifications grouped within a distance of up to 2 cm of each other can be accepted as grouped calcifications. If the area of calcifications is more than 2 cm, it should be termed regional calcification. Thirty percent of grouped calcifications may demonstrate malignant histology upon biopsy [46].

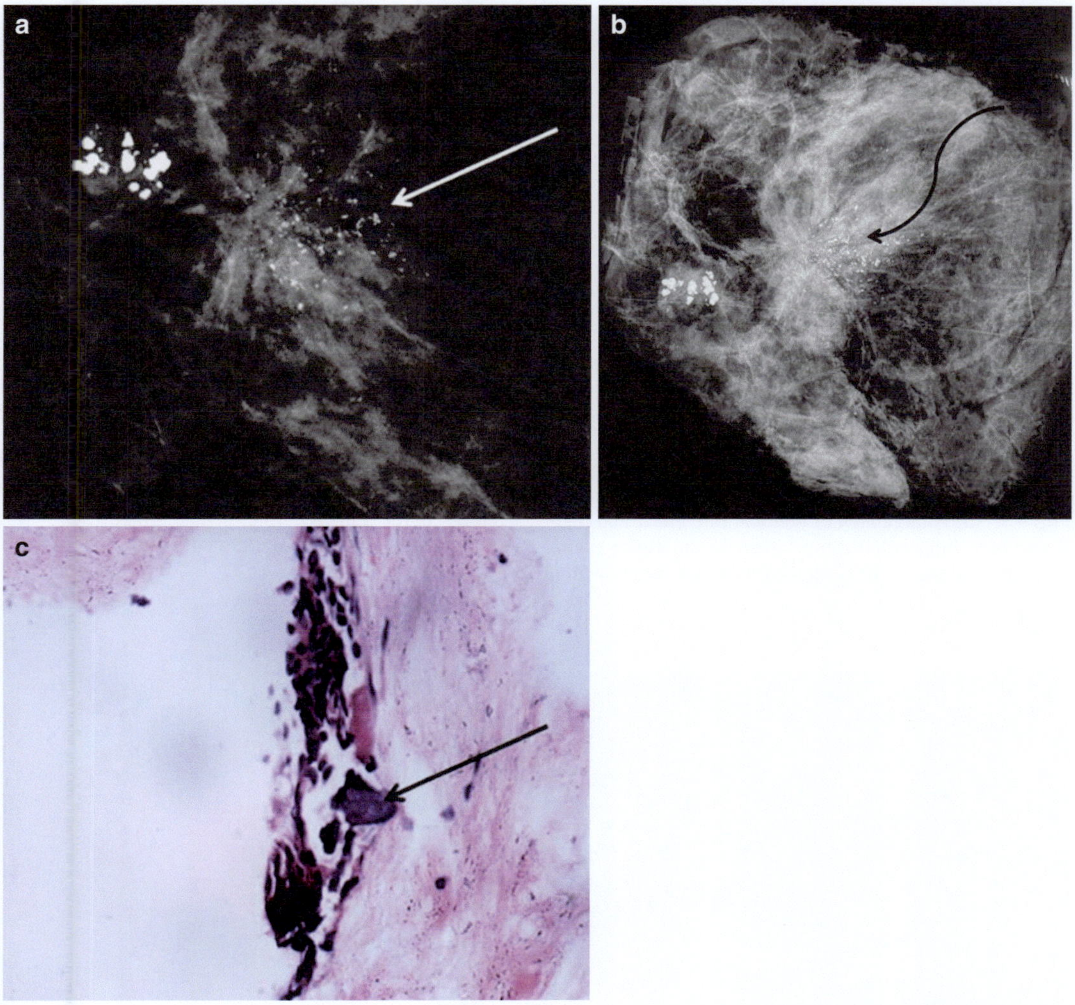

Fig. 4.8 (**a**) Regional fine pleomorphic calcifications with associated architectural distortion on mammography (white arrow). (**b**) A specimen radiography after surgical excision demonstrates the calcifications in the excised tissue (curved arrow). (**c**) Histology: chronic lymphocytic lobulitis. Calcification seen within sheets of lymphocytes (straight black arrow). Note: The low-density circumscribed mass with benign coarse calcifications close to the above-mentioned abnormality was confirmed to be a fibroadenoma on histology

(d) Linear: Calcifications arranged in a line are called linear. This is different to the term linear used in morphology where the individual particles are linear. Deposits of calcium within a duct are likely to have a linear distribution, and hence this distribution pattern is regarded suspicious with a positive predictive value of 60%. Linear distribution of typically benign vascular calcifications and thick rod-like secretory calcifications is not worrying, and these are considered in the benign calcification section [3, 10, 46, 51].

(e) Segmental: With 62% positive predictive value, calcifications delineating a segment are the most suspicious distribution pattern as they may indicate multifocal neoplastic change within a lobe or segment of the breast. These calcifications outline abnormal ductal systems with calcifications deposited within them, sometimes giving casting calci-

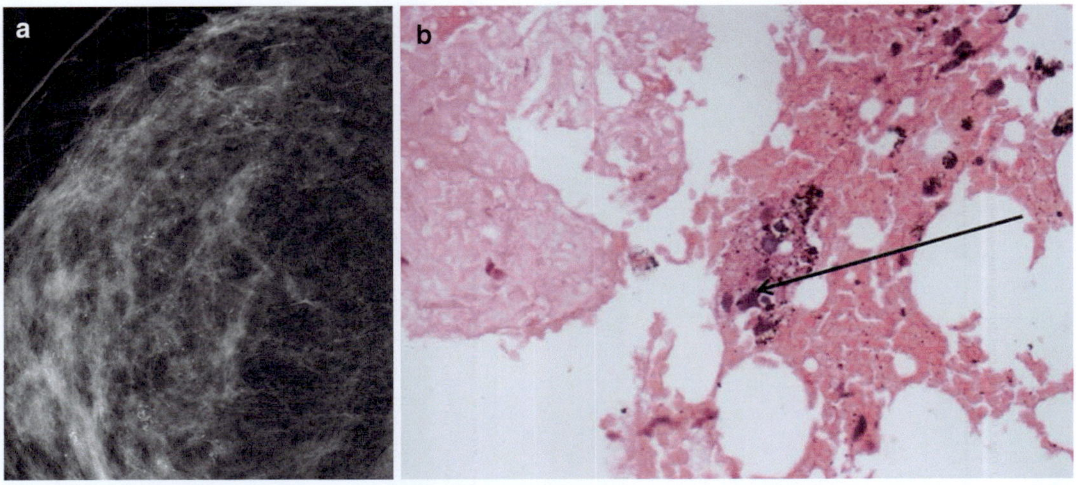

Fig. 4.9 (**a**) A large area of regional fine linear and fine-linear branching calcifications seen in the entire mammography image. (**b**) Calcifications are seen within necrotic tissue (arrow). Intermediate-grade DCIS was seen on histology (not demonstrated on this image)

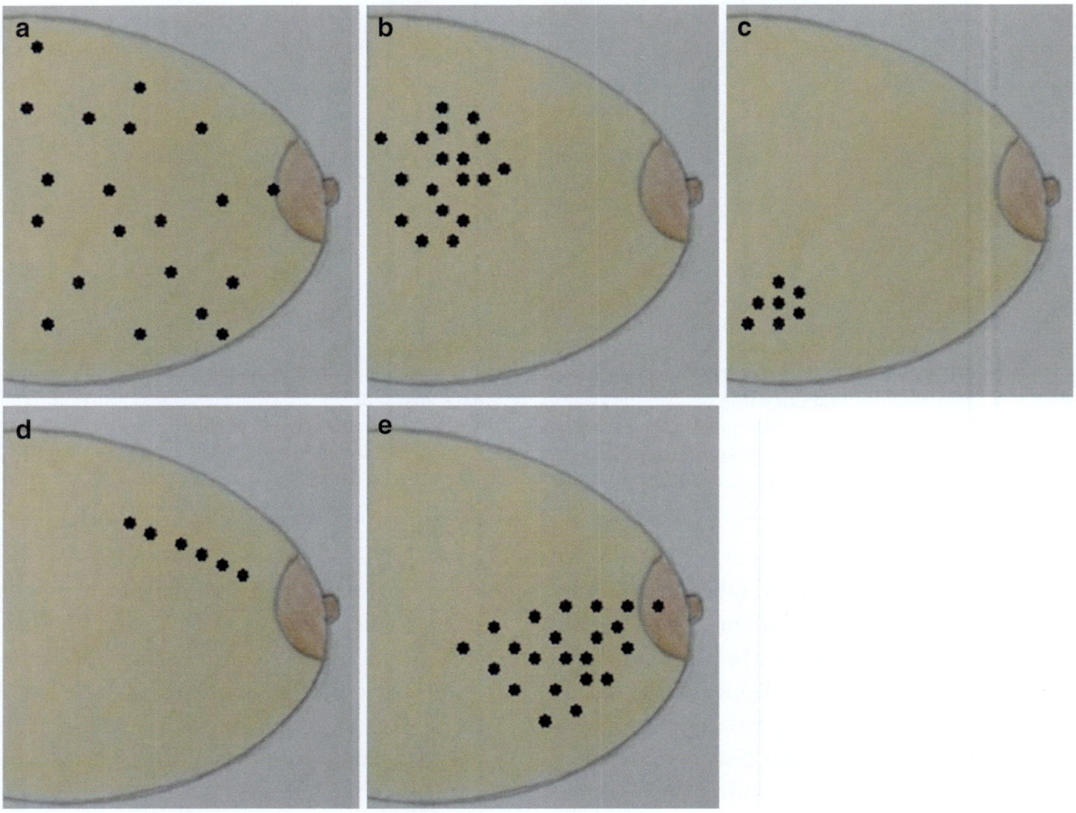

Fig. 4.10 Distribution patterns of breast calcifications: Diffuse (**a**), regional (**b**), grouped (**c**), linear (**d**), and segmental (**e**)

fications within the ducts. Even the less suspicious punctuate morphology calcifications warrant a biopsy if they are found in segmental distribution.

4.8 Reporting and BI-RADS® Assessment Categories

Morphology, distribution and location of calcifications along with any significant associated feature such as adjacent skin change or abnormal axillary lymph nodes should be mentioned in the mammography report. Comparison with available previous mammography images and comment on stability of calcifications should be made. An assessment category as per ACR BI-RADS should be awarded to the calcifications and specific management recommendations made as part of the report [46].

Typically benign calcifications are categorized as BI-RADS assessment category 2 and do not warrant a follow-up or biopsy. The only calcifications that can be put into BI-RADS assessment category 3 are the grouped punctate calcifications on baseline mammography as these are probably benign with a $\leq$ 2% chance of malignancy. Follow-up of these at 6 months, 1 year and 2 years (and 3 years if required) is appropriate. However, biopsy can be considered if the patient chooses biopsy or if there is an overriding clinical concern.

All other suspicious calcifications need to be biopsied. They are BI-RADS assessment category 4 (including 4A, 4B and 4C) if there is >2% and < 95% chance of malignancy. 4A, 4B and 4C categories indicate that the range of likelihood of malignancy is >2% to $\leq$10%, >10% to $\leq$50% and >50% to <95%, respectively. 4A, 4B and 4C categories indicate low, moderate and high suspicion of malignancy, respectively. New or increasing grouped punctate calcifications are of BI-RADS 4 assessment category. Calcifications are BI-RADS assessment category 5 if there is a $\geq$ 95% chance of malignancy, i.e. if they are highly suggestive of malignancy. No single feature can attribute a BI-RADS 5 categorization. However multiple suspicious features such as a segmental distribution pattern with fine-linear branching morphology can put calcifications in BI-RADS 5 category. Biopsy is advised for calcifications of BI-RADS 4 and BI-RADS 5 categories. An algorithm for determination of assessment categories of calcifications has been given [46] (Algorithm 4.1).

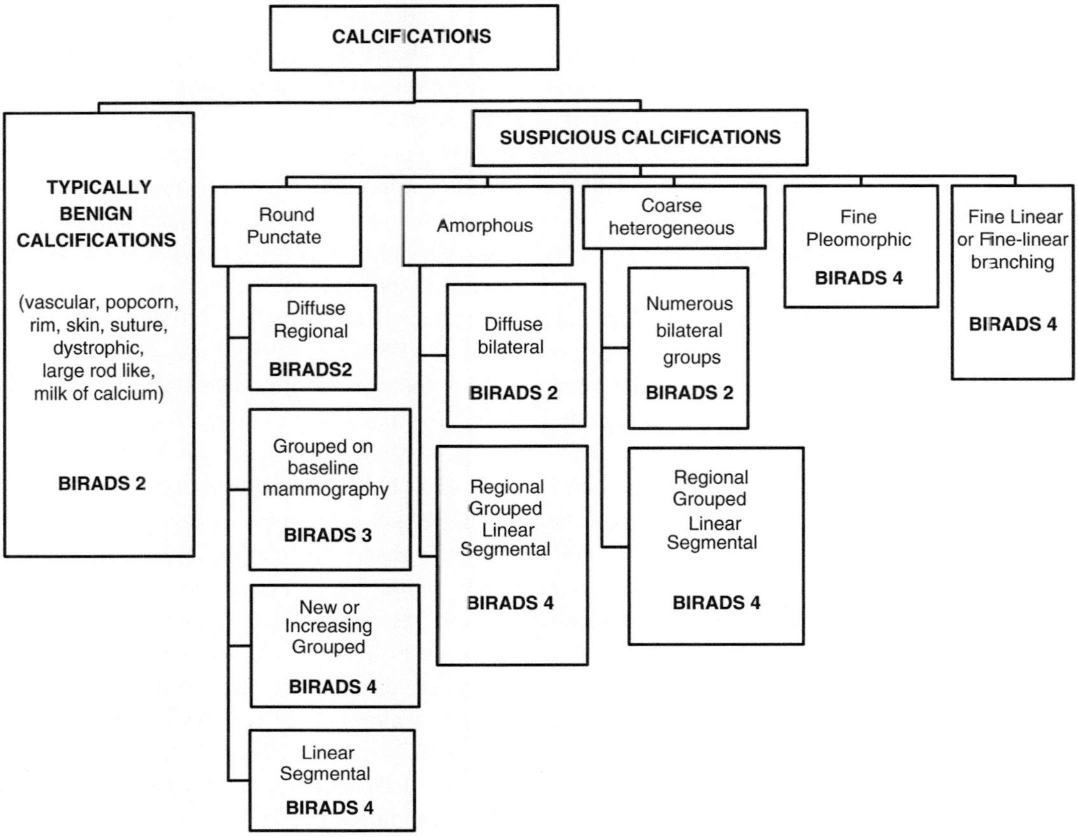

Algorithm 4.1 BI-RADS assessment categories of calcifications in the breast [46]

4.9 Biopsy and Localization of Suspicious Calcifications

Stereotactic biopsy under MG guidance is the method of choice as calcifications in general are better demonstrated on mammography. However, when calcifications are visualized with confidence on ultrasound, ultrasound-guided biopsy can be performed and is quicker and more comfortable for the patient [53]. It is important to be certain that the quadrant, o'clock position and distance from skin and nipple all correlate with the mammographic abnormality when biopsying calcifications under ultrasound guidance. Immediate specimen radiography of the cores acquired is required to confirm that the calcifications have indeed been sampled, both for stereotactic and ultrasound-guided biopsies. Calcifications should preferably be present in more than one core, depending on the extent of calcifications. A minimum of five flecks of calcifications or calcifications in at least three separate cores should be demonstrated to ensure optimum sampling [6]. In my practice for ultrasound-guided biopsies, I do not radiograph the cores if the calcification is undoubtedly part of a suspicious mass as the mass is my main target. I radiograph all cores of calcifications that are not within a mass as I cannot be otherwise certain if I have definitely biopsied the calcification under ultrasound guidance, as hyperechoic speckles seen on ultrasound are not always calcifications.

Core biopsy with 14-gauge fully automated biopsy gun and vacuum-assisted biopsy (VAB) are both options to biopsy calcifications. Stereotactic biopsy of microcalcifications is most effectively performed using VAB devices of 11 gauge or larger [6]. If representative calcification is not seen on specimen radiograph and the histology demonstrates a benign disease, a repeat biopsy, preferably VAB, is advised to confirm that a malignant lesion is not missed. The type of biopsy device used is dictated by the availability of equipment and expertise of the operator. If the lesion being biopsied is small and may be removed at biopsy or may not be easily identified for excision at a later date, a metal marker should be placed at the site of the lesion at the time of biopsy. Multiple different-shaped markers may be placed to differentiate the biopsy sites if multiple abnormalities are biopsied [54].

Currently hookwire-guided localization is the most common technique used for preoperative localization of nonpalpable breast lesions. The calcifications themselves are the markers for localization, unless all or most of the calcifications were excised during biopsy, in which case the radio-opaque marker placed at the time of biopsy is used for localization. Either an alphanumeric paddle or stereotactic equipment can be used for hookwire localization of the suspicious calcifications, as most calcifications would need mammography-guided preoperative localization. Ultrasound guidance can be used for those few cases where suspicious calcifications can be well visualized on ultrasound. After surgery, the excised tissue must be radiographed to confirm the presence of the suspicious calcifications (or the radio-opaque marker if calcifications have been fully removed at biopsy) and the localizing device in the specimen [55].

4.10 Radiology-Pathology Correlation for Suspicious Calcifications

The best forum to perform RPC is breast multidisciplinary meeting (MDM). RPC is vital preoperatively to confirm that the abnormal calcification has been adequately sampled and that there is concordance between the mammographic appearance and the pathological diagnosis. Postoperatively it is vital to correlate with the preoperative imaging findings, the specimen radiographs of the excised tissue and the final histological diagnosis. This gives feedback to the radiologist about the initial mammographic assessment and adequacy of biopsy samples, to the surgeon about adequacy of the performed surgery and to the pathologist about whether pathology findings correspond to the radiological findings or if the specimen was undersampled [5]. If concordance has not been established, repeat biopsy or follow up, as deemed appropriate by the MDM, must be performed. An algorithm for management of suspicious calcifications has been provided [46, 54] (Algorithm 4.2).

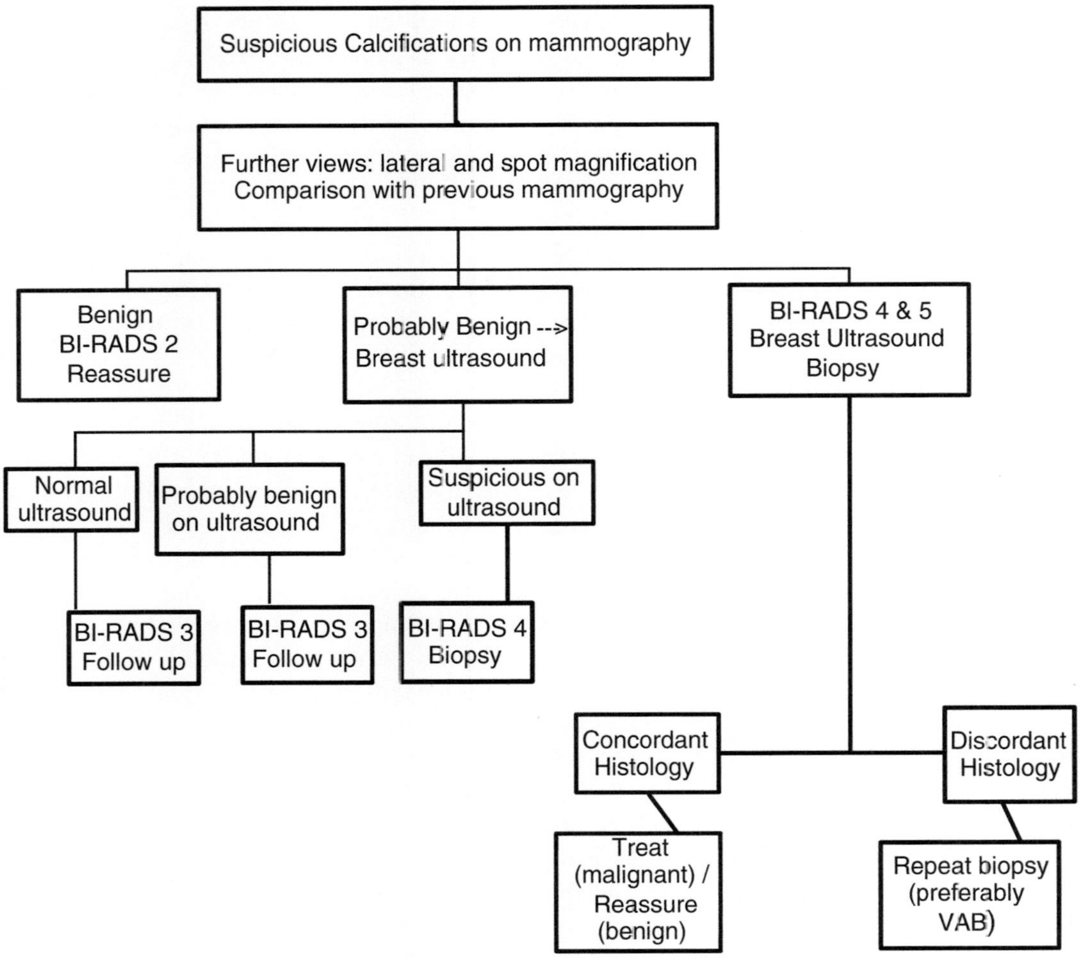

Algorithm 4.2 Management of suspicious breast calcifications [46, 54]

4.11 Disappearing Calcifications

Benign calcifications are more likely to disappear than malignant calcifications. Local Ph, calcium and phosphate ion concentrations may contribute to this phenomenon. If the initial calcification was of suspicious category, its disappearance should be taken seriously, and breast ultrasound and biopsy (if needed) should be performed. This is an obvious decision sometimes when the calcification gets replaced by a mass, focal asymmetry or architectural distortion which are suspicious for invasive disease [56, 57]. In my practice I perform an ultrasound for disappearing suspicious calcifications even if there is no abnormality demonstrated on mammography.

4.12 Microcalcifications as Prognosis Predictors

The tumour size refers to the largest dimension of the largest invasive focus of the cancer. Most malignant microcalcifications are seen in DCIS, and hence microcalcifications are less likely to influence the tumour size. The extent of the disease or whole tumour measurement refers to the entire volume of the breast tissue with malignant change which the surgeon needs to excise with clear margins and hence includes the entire invasive and DCIS disease [5]. This is a very important prognostic indicator, and studies have shown that the disease extent of $\geq$4 cm is an independent marker of local recurrence, with a cumulative 10-year relapse rate more than three times of the risk for the rest of the patients [58]. Casting microcalcifications are considered an independent negative prognostic marker [5]. DCIS of a high histology grade is a negative prognostic marker, being associated with extensive disease and hence higher mastectomy rates. Local recurrence is more frequent with a shorter time to relapse. Higher grades have a higher mortality rate [5]. Up to 50% of high-grade CIS and high-grade in situ component of invasive cancers contain calcifications. However low-grade CIS calcifies in approximately 25% of cases. Low-grade CIS is similar to the normal epithelium and hence is more likely to express oestrogen and progesterone receptors and almost never over-expresses human epidermal growth factor receptor 2 (HER2). High-grade CIS, on the other hand, expresses hormone receptors less often and is much more likely to be HER2-positive [5].

4.13 Breast Calcifications and Non-breast Disease Associations

Benign vascular calcifications are regarded as a biomarker for cardiovascular disease, and multiple studies indicate that they may improve cardiovascular risk stratification in women. Associations have also been shown between vascular calcifications and hypertension, diabetes, renal disease, hypervitaminosis, hyperparathyroidism and autonomic neuropathy in some studies [38, 39].

4.14 Further Developments: Things to Watch Out For!

Raman spectroscopy (RS) is an optical spectroscopic technique that produces a Raman spectrum or a specific spectral fingerprint which contains numerous bands of various frequencies that are unique to a particular molecule based on the structural features and functional groups of that molecule. Unlike mammography which relies on the visual information such as morphology and distribution, RS relies on the chemical composition of calcifications to characterize them. As calcium oxalate and calcium hydroxyapatite have different spectral signatures, RS can differentiate between type 1 and type 2 microcalcifications. As malignant ducts contain lower levels of carbonate and higher amounts of protein, RS can further differentiate between benign and malignant type 2 calcifications [59, 60].

RS can be performed with fibre-optic probes compatible with VAB needles. This can be utilized for detecting microcalcifications during stereotactic biopsies [59]. Attempts are being made to detect and evaluate microcalcifications in the clinic. But the main hurdle at present is the weakening of the Raman signal as the tissue sampling depth increases. If this could be overcome, a day may arrive when we assess microcalcifications by putting in probes into the areas of calcifications rather than biopsy or excise calcifications! Even more exciting is the research that is exploring RS techniques to analyse serum to help diagnose breast cancer [60].

References

1. Gershon-Cohen J, Berger SM, Curcio BM. Breast cancer with microcalcifications: diagnostic difficulties. Radiology. 1966;87(4):613–22.
2. Logullo AF, Prigenzi KCK, Nimir CCBA, Franco AFV, Campos MSDA. Breast microcalcifications: past, present and future (Review). Mol Clin Oncol. 2022;16(4):81.
3. Bent CK, Bassett LW, D'Orsi CJ, Sayre JW. The positive predictive value of BI-RADS microcalcification descriptors and final assessment categories. Am J Roentgenol. 2010;194(5):1378–83.
4. Tse GM, Tan PH, Pang ALM, Tang APY, Cheung HS. Calcification in breast lesions: pathologists' perspective. J Clin Pathol. 2007;61(2):145–51.
5. Tot T, Gere M, Hofmeyer S, Bauer A, Pellas U. The clinical value of detecting microcalcifications on a mammogram. Semin Cancer Biol. 2021;72:165–74.
6. Wilkinson L, Thomas V, Sharma N. Microcalcification on mammography: approaches to interpretation and biopsy. Br J Radiol. 2016;90(1069):20160594.
7. Chen L, Chantra PK, Larsen LH, Barton P, Rohitopakarn M, Zhu EQ, et al. Imaging characteristics of malignant lesions of the male breast. Radiographics. 2006;26(4):993–1006.
8. Shi AA, Georgian-Smith D, Cornell LD, Rafferty EA, Staffa M, Hughes K, et al. Radiological rea-

soning: male breast mass with calcifications. Am J Roentgenol. 2005;185(6_supplement):S205–10.
9. Berg WA, Zhang Z, Lehrer D, Jong RA, Pisano ED, Barr RG, et al. Detection of breast cancer with addition of annual screening ultrasound or a single screening MRI to mammography in women with elevated breast cancer risk. JAMA J Am Med Assoc. 2012;307(13):1394–404.
10. Liberman L, Abramson AF, Squires FB, Glassman JR, Morris EA, Dershaw DD. The breast imaging reporting and data system: positive predictive value of mammographic features and final assessment categories. Am J Roentgenol. 1998;171(1):35–40.
11. Haka AS, Shafer-Peltier KE, Fitzmaurice M, Crowe J, Dasari RR, Feld MS. Identifying microcalcifications in benign and malignant breast lesions by probing differences in their chemical composition using Raman spectroscopy. Cancer Res. 2002;62(18):5375–80.
12. Frappart L, Boudeulle M, Boumendil J, Lin HC, Martinon I, Palayer C, et al. Structure and composition of microcalcifications in benign and malignant lesions of the breast: Study by light microscopy, transmission and scanning electron microscopy, microprobe analysis, and X-ray diffraction. Hum Pathol. 1984;15(9):880–9.
13. Davies JD. Diagnostic histopathology of the breast. O. L. Page and T. J. Anderson, with several contributors. Churchill Livingstone, Edinburgh, 1987. No. of pages: 362. Price: £65.00. ISBN: 0 443 02240 2. J Pathol. 1988;156(3):271–2.
14. Schnitt SJ, Collins LC. Biopsy interpretation of the breast. 3rd ed. Philadelphia: Wolters Kluwer; 2017.
15. Russo J, Russo IH. Development of the human breast. Maturitas. 2004;49(1):2–15.
16. Pike MC, Spicer DV, Dahmoush L, Press MF. Estrogens, progestogens, normal breast cell proliferation, and breast cancer risk. Epidemiol Rev. 1993;15(1):17–35.
17. Shacter E, Weitzman SA. Chronic inflammation and cancer. Oncology (Williston Park). 2002;16(2):217–26, 229; discussion 230–2.
18. Paszek MJ, Zahir N, Johnson KR, Lakins JN, Rozenberg GI, Gefen A, et al. Tensional homeostasis and the malignant phenotype. Cancer Cell. 2005;8(3):241–54.
19. Provenzano PP, Inman DR, Eliceiri KW, Knittel JG, Yan L, Rueden CT, et al. Collagen density promotes mammary tumor initiation and progression. BMC Med. 2008;6(1):11.
20. Hu M, Yao J, Carroll DK, Weremowicz S, Chen H, Carrasco D, et al. Regulation of in situ to invasive breast carcinoma transition. Cancer Cell. 2008;13(5):394–406.
21. Lakhani SR, Ellis IO, Schnitt SJ, Tan PH, van de Vijver MJ. WHO classification of tumours of the breast. 4th ed. Lyon: International Agency for Research on Cancer (IARC); 2012.
22. Folkman J. Angiogenesis: an organizing principle for drug discovery? Nat Rev Drug Discov. 2007;6(4):273–86.
23. New SEP, Aikawa E. Role of extracellular vesicles in De Novo mineralization. Arterioscler Thromb Vasc Biol. 2013;33(8):1753–8.
24. Miki Y, Swensen J, Shattuck-Eidens D, Futreal PA, Harshman K, Tavtigian S, et al. A strong candidate for the breast and ovarian cancer susceptibility gene BRCA1. Science. 1994;266(5182):66–71.
25. Nagase H, Visse R. Matrix metalloproteinases and tissue inhibitors of metalloproteinases: Structure, function, and biochemistry. Circ Res. 2006;79(6):525–35.
26. Bonnans C, Chou J, Werb Z. Remodelling the extracellular matrix in development and disease. Nat Rev Mol Cell Biol. 2014;15(12):786–801.
27. Bissell MJ, Hines WC. Why don't we get more cancer? A proposed role of the microenvironment in restraining cancer progression. Nat Med. 2011;17(3):320–9.
28. Morgan MP, Cooke MM, McCarthy GM. Microcalcifications associated with breast cancer: an epiphenomenon or biologically significant feature of selected tumors? J Mammary Gland Biol Neoplasia. 2005;10(2):181–7.
29. Clapham DE. Calcium signaling. Cell. 2007;131(6):1047–58.
30. Miller KD, Nogueira L, Mariotto AB, Rowland JH, Yabroff KR, Alfano CM, et al. Cancer treatment and survivorship statistics. CA Cancer J Clin. 2019;69(5):363–85.
31. Skaane P, Hofvind S, Skjennald A. Randomized trial of screen-film versus full-field digital mammography with soft-copy reading in population-based screening program: follow-up and final results of Oslo II study 1. Radiology. 2007;244:708–17.
32. Hambly NM, McNicholas MM, Phelan N, Hargaden GC, O'Doherty A, Flanagan FL. Comparison of digital mammography and screen-film mammography in breast cancer screening: a review in the Irish breast screening program. Am J Roentgenol. 2009;193(4):1010–8.
33. Demetri-Lewis A, Slanetz PJ, Eisenberg RL. Breast calcifications: the focal group. Am J Roentgenol. 2012;198(4):W325–43.
34. Horvat JV, Keating DM, Rodrigues-Duarte H, Morris EA, Mango VL. Calcifications at digital breast tomosynthesis: imaging features and biopsy techniques. Radiographics. 2019;39(2):307–18.
35. Bazzocchi M, Zuiani C, Panizza P, Del Frate C, Soldano F, Isola M, et al. Contrast-enhanced breast MRI in patients with suspicious microcalcifications on mammography: results of a multicenter trial. Am J Roentgenol. 2006;186(6):1723–32.
36. Grimm LJ, Rahbar H, Abdelmalak M, Hall AH, Ryser MD. Ductal carcinoma in Situ: state-of-the-art review. Radiology. 2022;302(2):246–55.
37. Geiser WR, Haygood TM, Santiago L, Stephens T, Thames D, Whitman GJ. Challenges in mammography: part 1, artifacts in digital mammography. Am J Roentgenol. 2011;197(6):W1023–30.
38. Oliveira ELC, Freitas-Junior R, Afiune-Neto A, Murta EFC, Ferro JE, Melo AFB. Vascular calcifications seen on mammography: an independent factor indi-

cating coronary artery disease. Clin Sao Paulo Braz. 2009;64(8):763–7.
39. Lai KC, Slanetz PJ, Eisenberg RL. Linear breast calcifications. Am J Roentgenol. 2012;199(2):W151–7.
40. Giess CS, Raza S, Birdwell RL. Distinguishing breast skin lesions from superficial breast parenchymal lesions: diagnostic criteria, imaging characteristics, and pitfalls. Radiographics. 2011;31(7):1959–72.
41. Homer MJ, D'Orsi CJ, Sitzman SB. Dermal calcifications in fixed orientation: the tattoo sign. Radiology. 1994;192(1):161–3.
42. Arancibia Hernández PL, Taub Estrada T, López Pizarro A, Díaz Cisternas ML, Sáez TC. Calcificaciones mamarias: descripción y clasificación según la 5.a edición BI-RADS. Rev Chil Radiol. 2016;22(2):80–91.
43. Guth TA, Bhatt AA. The "teacup sign": significance in breast imaging. Clin Imaging. 2023;104:110009. Available from: https://www.clinicalimaging.org/article/S0899-7071(23)00229-2/abstract.
44. Kim SM, Park JM, Moon WK. Dystrophic breast calcifications in patients with collagen diseases. Clin Imaging. 2004;28(1):6–9.
45. Lee KM, Lee JE, Cha ES, Chung J, Kim JH, Moon BI. Dystrophic calcifications in the breast from secondary hyperparathyroidism. Breast Care. 2018;13(1):44–6.
46. Sickles EA, D'Orsi CJ, Bassett LW, et al. ACR BI-RADS® mammography. In: ACR BI-RADS® atlas, breast imaging reporting and data system. Reston: American College of Radiology; 2013.
47. Henrot P, Leroux A, Barlier C, Génin P. Breast microcalcifications: the lesions in anatomical pathology. Diagn Interv Imaging. 2014;95(2):141–52.
48. Dinkel HP, Gassel AM, Tschammler A. Is the appearance of microcalcifications on mammography useful in predicting histological grade of malignancy in ductal cancer in situ? Br J Radiol. 2000;73(873):938–44.
49. Evans A. The diagnosis and management of preinvasive breast disease: radiological diagnosis. Breast Cancer Res. 2003;5(5):250.
50. Berg WA, Arnoldus CL, Teferra E, Bhargavan M. Biopsy of amorphous breast calcifications: pathologic outcome and yield at stereotactic biopsy. Radiology. 2001;221(2):495–503.
51. Burnside ES, Ochsner JE, Fowler KJ, Fine JP, Salkowski LR, Rubin DL, et al. Use of microcalcification descriptors in BI-RADS 4th edition to stratify risk of malignancy. Radiology. 2007;242(2):388–95.
52. Dev B, Vakamudi U, Thambidurai L, Joseph LD, Srinivasan JP. Imaging and pathological correlation in spectrum of fibrocystic breast disease and its Mimics – our experience. Arch Breast Cancer. 2022;9:465–73.
53. Moy L, Giess CS, Aminololama-Shakeri S, Appleton CA, Destounis SV, Gupta D, et al. ACR practice parameter for the performance of ultrasound-guided percutaneous breast interventional procedures. Revised 2021 (Resolution 31)*. Reston: American College of Radiology; 2021. Available from: https://www.acr.org/-/media/ACR/Files/Practice-Parameters/US-GuidedBreast.pdf.
54. Borrelli C, Cohen S, Duncan A, Given-Wilson R, Jenkins J, Kearins O, et al. Clinical guidance for breast cancer screening assessment. NHSBSP publication number 49. 4th ed. London: Public Health England; 2016. Available from: https://associationofbreastsurgery.org.uk/media/1414/nhs-bsp-clinical-guidance-for-breast-cancer-screening-assessment.pdf.
55. Sarkar DK. Breast diseases: guidelines for management. Routledge & CRC Press; 2024.
56. Parker MD, Clark RL, McLelland R, Daughtery K. Disappearing breast calcifications. Radiology. 1989;172(3):677–80.
57. Nguyen QD, Nguyen NT, Dixon L, Posleman Monetto FE, Robinson AS. Spontaneously disappearing calcifications in the breast: a rare instance where a decrease in size on mammogram is not good. Cureus. 2020;12(6):e8753.
58. Lindquist D, Hellberg D, Tot T. Disease extent ≥4 cm is a prognostic marker of local recurrence in T1-2 breast cancer. Pathol Res Int. 2011;10(2011):e860584.
59. Barman I, Dingari NC, Saha A, McGee S, Galindo LH, Liu W, et al. Application of Raman spectroscopy to identify microcalcifications and underlying breast lesions at stereotactic core needle biopsy. Cancer Res. 2013;73(11):3206–15.
60. Hanna K, Krzoska E, Shaaban AM, Muirhead D, Abu-Eid R, Speirs V. Raman spectroscopy: current applications in breast cancer diagnosis, challenges and future prospects. Br J Cancer. 2022;126(8):1125–39.

Asymmetries and Architectural Distortion

5

Smriti Hari, Pratyaksha Rana, and Ekta Dhamija

Abstract

Asymmetries and architectural distortion are some of the frequent imaging findings of early breast cancer. They can be difficult to identify due to subtle and variable appearances. Both represent common findings in retrospective assessment of false-negative mammograms. Apart from malignancy, various benign breast entities can also manifest with these non-mass findings. Knowledge about the normal breast architecture and pattern is important to recognize the abnormal findings. Breast imaging ACR BI-RADS atlas (fifth edition) recognizes four types of asymmetries with variable management and presentation. Architectural distortion can arise secondary to surgery or trauma and also due to various benign and malignant breast pathologies, with clinical correlation being crucial for avoiding unnecessary interventions. Targeted ultrasound, additional mammographic views, and further imaging with magnetic resonance imaging or contrast-enhanced mammogram play a crucial role in the workup of asymmetries and architectural distortion.

Keywords

Architectural distortion · Asymmetry · Focal asymmetry · Developing asymmetry · Mammogram · Ultrasound · Breast cancer

5.1 Introduction

Timely detection of invasive breast cancer has an important implication on the prognosis and overall survival of patients [1]. Imaging reveals diverse manifestations of breast cancer, including masses, calcifications, asymmetries, and architectural distortion, with masses and calcifications being more easily identifiable [2, 3]. In the early stages, breast cancers may present as nonspecific findings including focal asymmetry or subtle architectural distortion before they develop into recognizable masses [4]. Detecting asymmetry and architectural distortion can be challenging as they may be subtle and exhibit variable appear-

S. Hari (✉)
Radiodiagnosis & Interventional Radiology, AIIMS, New Delhi, India

P. Rana
Department of Radiology, UN Mehta Institute of Cardiology and Research Center, Ahmedabad, India

E. Dhamija
Department of Diagnostic and Interventional Onco-Radiology, IRCH, AIIMS, New Delhi, India

E. Dhamija, S. V. S. Deo (eds.), *Imaging in Management of Breast Diseases*,
https://doi.org/10.1007/978-981-96-4998-3_5

ances. That is why these findings are commonly encountered in retrospective assessments of false-negative mammograms [5–7]. Identifying these non-mass findings requires a deep understanding of normal breast anatomy and the architectural pattern of normal breast parenchyma as seen on mammograms [8, 9]. This chapter aims to highlight the various causes, imaging findings, challenges, and an algorithm for the workup and management of asymmetries and architectural distortion.

5.2 Normal Mammographic Appearance

Identification of asymmetries and architectural distortion necessitates a fundamental understanding of normal breast anatomy and the appearance of normal breast parenchyma on various imaging modalities like mammogram (MG) and ultrasound (US). A variable amount of fat and fibroglandular tissue constitutes the mammogram of a normal breast, depending on the natural history of development and involution of the breast tissue.

Young women usually have a highly glandular, dense breast tissue, which appears white on a normal mammogram. With advancing age, the glandular tissue involutes to fat, with asymmetric distribution of the glandular tissue and fat within the breast. The upper outer portion of the breast has more of the dense glandular tissue, while the medial and the lower part of the breast is composed more of the fatty tissue. In some women, the breast is predominantly composed of fat. Posterior to the glandular tissue is a retroglandular fat, described by Dr. Laszlo Tabar as "no man's land" in which no glandular tissue should be seen. Normally, the edge of the fibroglandular tissue is scalloped gently anteriorly as well as posteriorly. The fibroglandular tissue pattern is fairly symmetrical or mirror image from side to side. The mammograms of both the breasts must be viewed back to back, to be able to identify asymmetries easily. Usually, a normal mammogram does not change over years, after taking into account the normal involution of the glandular tissue over time. It is important to compare old studies with current examinations to evaluate for new or developing changes (Fig. 5.1).

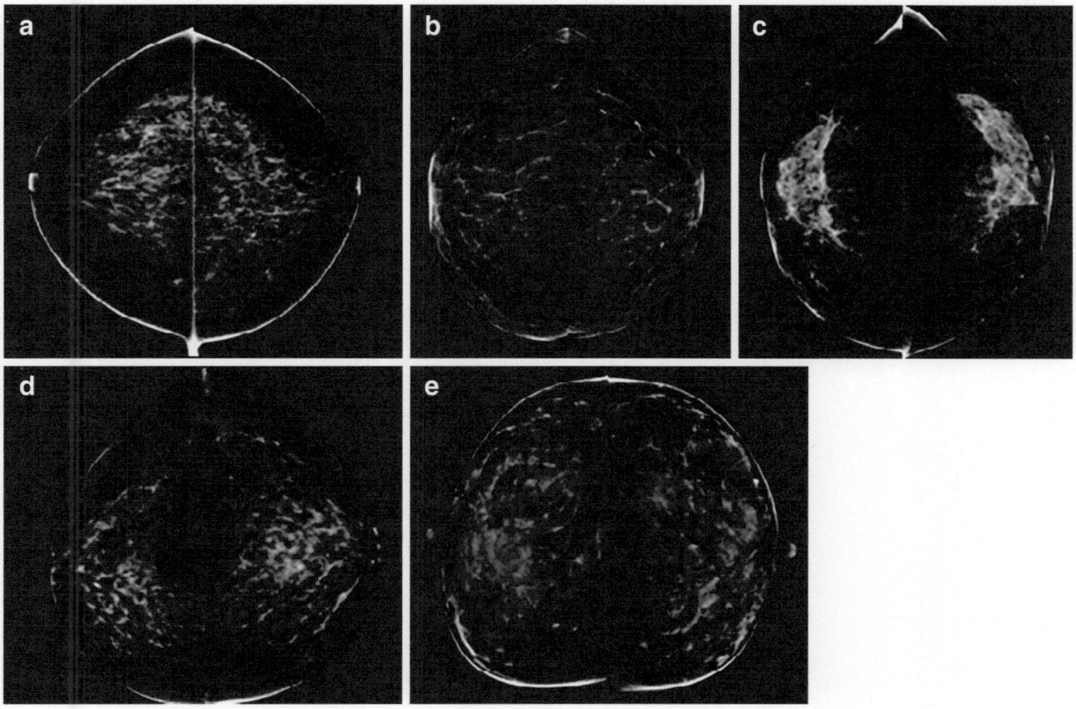

Fig. 5.1 A craniocaudal (CC) view of a standard mammogram depicting normal Tabar's mammographic patterns. Type 1 pattern (**a**) represents a balanced proportion of all components of the breast tissue, pattern II (**b**) shows predominance of the fat tissue, and pattern III (**c**) represents predominance of the fat tissue with retroareolar residual fibrous tissue. Pattern IV (**d**) and pattern V (**e**) are high-risk patterns characterized by predominantly nodular densities and fibrous tissue, respectively. Note the fairly symmetrical pattern side to side

5.3 Types and Classification of Asymmetry

Asymmetries constitute a range of mammographic imaging findings that indicate the presence of unilateral deposits of the fibroglandular tissue, without a corresponding mirror-image correlate in the opposite breast [10]. The ACR-Breast Imaging Reporting and Data System (BI-RADS) (fifth edition) atlas defines four types of asymmetries, namely, asymmetry, global asymmetry, focal asymmetry, and developing asymmetry, each with varying management approaches and recommendations (Table 5.1 and Fig. 5.2) [10].

Asymmetry is visible only on a single mammographic projection, while the other asymmetries can be seen on both craniocaudal and mediolateral views. Asymmetries are planar with concave-outward borders and are often interspersed with fat. In contrast, a mass is characterized by convex-outward borders, either partially or completely, and appears denser in the center compared to the periphery [10]. Various factors can contribute to the presence of asymmetries including normal overlapping tissue, asymmetric breast tissue, and a multitude of benign and malignant breast lesions [11]. Identification and further diagnostic evaluation of asymmetries is particularly challenging, as they often appear similar to the normal fibroglandular tissue at mammogram. Additional mammographic views like spot compression views with or without magnification, rolled/angled views, and lateral views are often required for precise triangulation of the asymmetry to demonstrate its true nature [12–14].

There is a growing role of digital breast tomosynthesis (DBT) as a valuable tool for assessing

Table 5.1 Definition of various types of asymmetries

Type of asymmetry	BIRADS category (after excluding worrisome features)	Definition (BIRADS-5th edition, atlas)
Asymmetry	I	***Discrete asymmetric area of fibro glandular-density tissue that is visible on only one mammographic projection***
Global asymmetry	II	***Two-view mammographic finding characterized by large amount of asymmetric fibro glandular breast tissue occupying at least one quadrant ,judged relative to corresponding area in the contralateral breast***
Focal asymmetry	III	***Two-view mammographic finding representing a relatively small amount of fibro glandular -density tissue over less than one quadrant ,judged relative to the corresponding location in the contralateral breast.***
Developing asymmetry	IV	***Focal asymmetry that is new, larger, or more conspicuous than on a previous examination***

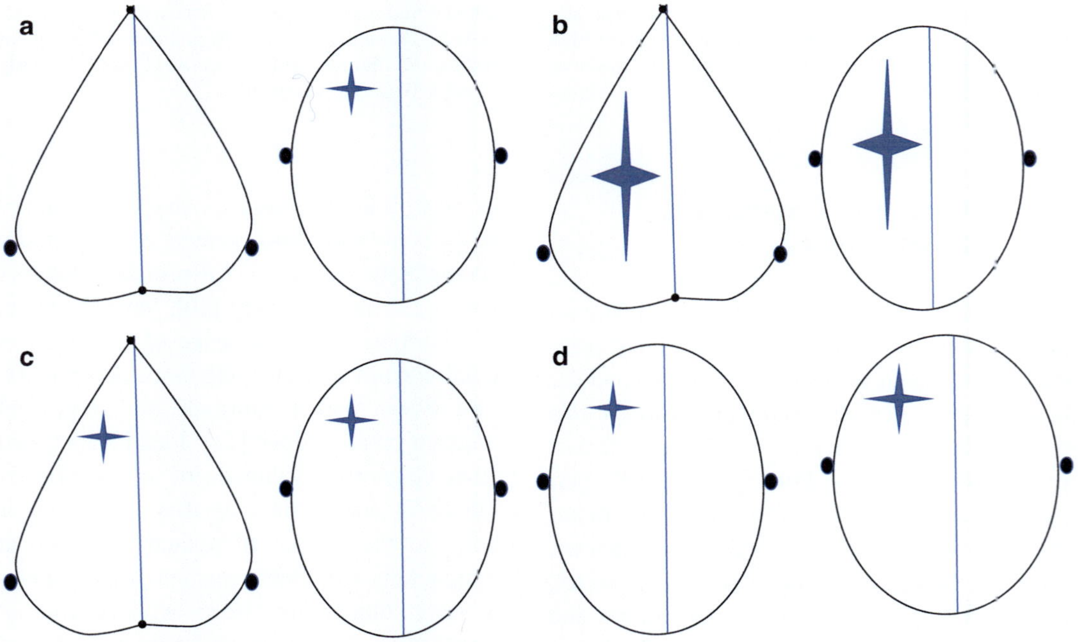

Fig. 5.2 Pictorial representations of the type of asymmetries. (**a**) is suggestive of asymmetry, single-view finding on CC projection of the right breast. (**b** and **c**) represent global and focal asymmetry, respectively, which are two view findings occupying more than (global asymmetry) and less than one quadrant (focal asymmetry) of the right breast in comparison to the left breast. (**d**) represents developing asymmetry with an increase in size and conspicuity of asymmetry in the recent CC view (right image) as compared to the previous mammogram (left image). CC, craniocaudal

asymmetries [15, 16]. By diminishing the impact of overlapping breast tissue and summation artifacts, DBT enhances the visibility of asymmetries and associated features. It aids in accurate localization and characterization, particularly for focal and developing asymmetries [17, 18].

All true asymmetries should be assessed with targeted US, and patient can be reassured if the US reveals a normal breast tissue that correlates with the asymmetric finding on the MG [19]. Magnetic resonance imaging (MRI) and contrast-enhanced mammograms (CEM) are problem-solving tools for further characterization and have shown promising results [20–24].

5.3.1 Asymmetry

Asymmetry refers to a discrete area of the asymmetric fibroglandular-density tissue that is seen only on one mammographic projection. Asymmetries are typically detected during screening MG, and more than 80% of these screen-detected asymmetries are actually summation artifacts, resulting from the superimposition of normal breast structures [25]. In rare cases, persistent asymmetries may turn out to be malignant, with invasive lobular carcinoma (ILC) being the common cause [26].

5.3.2 Global Asymmetry

Global asymmetry is a two-view mammographic finding, observed in approximately 3% of screening MG [12]. It is characterized by a significant amount of the asymmetric fibroglandular breast tissue occupying at least one quadrant, without any associated mass, suspicious calcifications, or architectural distortion [10]. Any form of asymmetry should be assessed in relation to the corresponding area in the opposite breast. In most cases, global asymmetry occurs due to either a developmental variant or as a result of different responses to the hormonal stimuli within the breast. One should not see the appearance of the global asymmetry in a previously normal tissue volume. However, there are several benign factors which may cause its appearance. These include distinctive imaging techniques and positioning, weight changes, hormone replacement therapy, or surgical/interventional procedures. Occasionally, an underlying breast cancer can manifest as a global asymmetry, especially if it is associated with palpable abnormality. On the other hand, long-term stability in comparison to previous imaging confirms its benign nature, resulting in BI-RADS 2 categorization (Fig. 5.3) [10]. Generally additional US evaluation is not necessary for global asymmetry, unless there is a specific concern regarding its pathological nature.

5.3.3 Focal Asymmetry

Focal asymmetry is a confined asymmetry with a similar shape on two views but does not fit the criteria of a mass: that is, it lacks convex outer borders and conspicuity. In contrast to global asymmetry, it occupies a relatively smaller volume of less than one quadrant of the breast. Although the area of involvement is smaller compared to global asymmetry, focal asymmetry is a more worrisome finding, particularly when it measures less than 1 cm [10]. It is worth noting that many cases initially described as focal asymmetry during screening MG are later identified as ill-defined masses upon further evaluation. The use of "focal asymmetry" as descriptor reduces when DBT is performed, as underlying mass margins may be better delineated with this technology.

(i) *Focal asymmetry with a palpable or sonographic correlate and/or other associated features*

A focal asymmetry that has a clinically palpable correlate requires careful evaluation. When an US correlate is present, the management and recommendation are based on the degree of suspicion indicated by the US features [19, 27]. For instance, if a focal asymmetry corresponds to a simple cyst on US, no further evaluation is needed, and it can be assigned a BI-RADS 2 category. However, if an irregular mass on US or

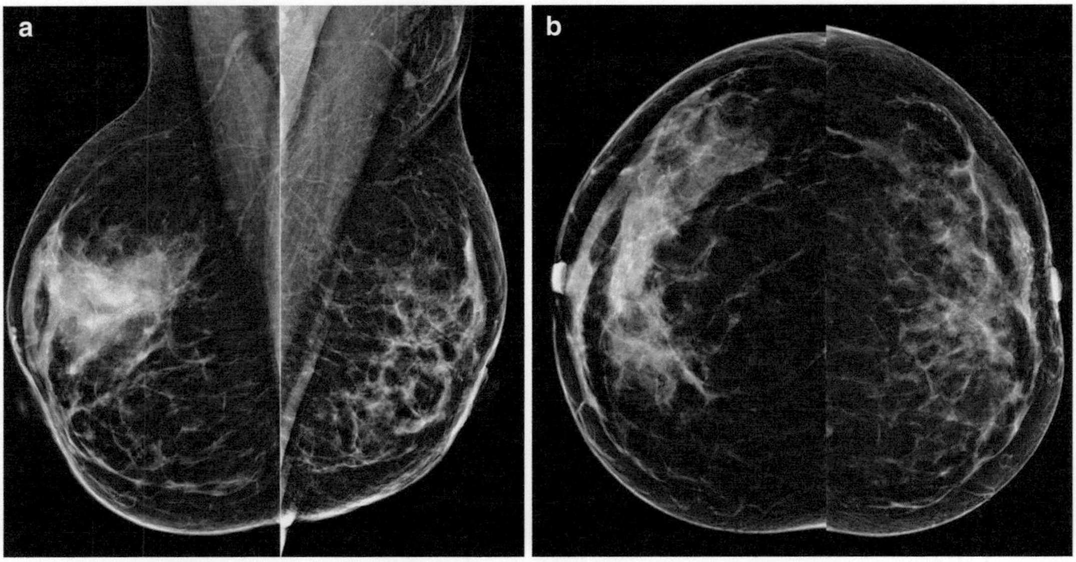

Fig. 5.3 A screening mammogram of a 52-year-old, (mediolateral oblique (MLO, left) and cranio-caudal (CC, right) views) shows an asymmetric fibroglandular breast tissue occupying more than one quadrant of the right breast in relation to the corresponding area in the left breast suggestive of global asymmetry. No other suspicious features or palpable correlate was seen, and findings were stable as compared to the previous mammogram. Overall assessment is BI-RADS 2 category

suspicious features such as architectural distortion or microcalcifications are observed on MG, a higher BI-RADS category is assigned, prompting biopsy for diagnosis and further management (Fig. 5.4 and Table 5.2).

(ii) *Isolated focal asymmetry with no palpable or sonographic correlate*

When a focal asymmetry is identified on MG without any associated mass, calcifications, or architectural distortion, and there is no palpable or sonographic correlate to the finding, the assessment category and further management recommendation differ based on the accessibility of prior mammograms for comparison. If the prior mammograms are not available, focal asymmetry is assigned a probably benign (BI-RADS category 3) assessment, with a recommendation for short-interval follow-up. In this scenario the chance of malignancy is approximately 0.5–1%, according to published literature [10, 28, 29]. If the focal asymmetry demonstrates stability over a 2–3-year surveillance period or in comparison with previous mammograms, it can be assigned a benign (BI-RADS category 2). However, it is important to note that the lesion morphology takes precedence over stability. If a focal asymmetry exhibit features suspicious for malignancy, further assessment is warranted regardless of apparent stability because it may correspond to a slow-growing cancer.

5.3.4 Developing Asymmetry

A developing asymmetry is defined as a focal asymmetry that is new, larger, or denser compared to a previous mammogram [10]. Developing asymmetry manifesting as an area of increasing density may not be apparent over a shorter follow-up period. Hence it is crucial to compare the current study with the previous studies performed at least 2 years earlier. A developing asymmetry that cannot be accounted for by differences in imaging technique and positioning, due to various other factors like hormone replacement therapy, surgery, trauma, or infection at the site,

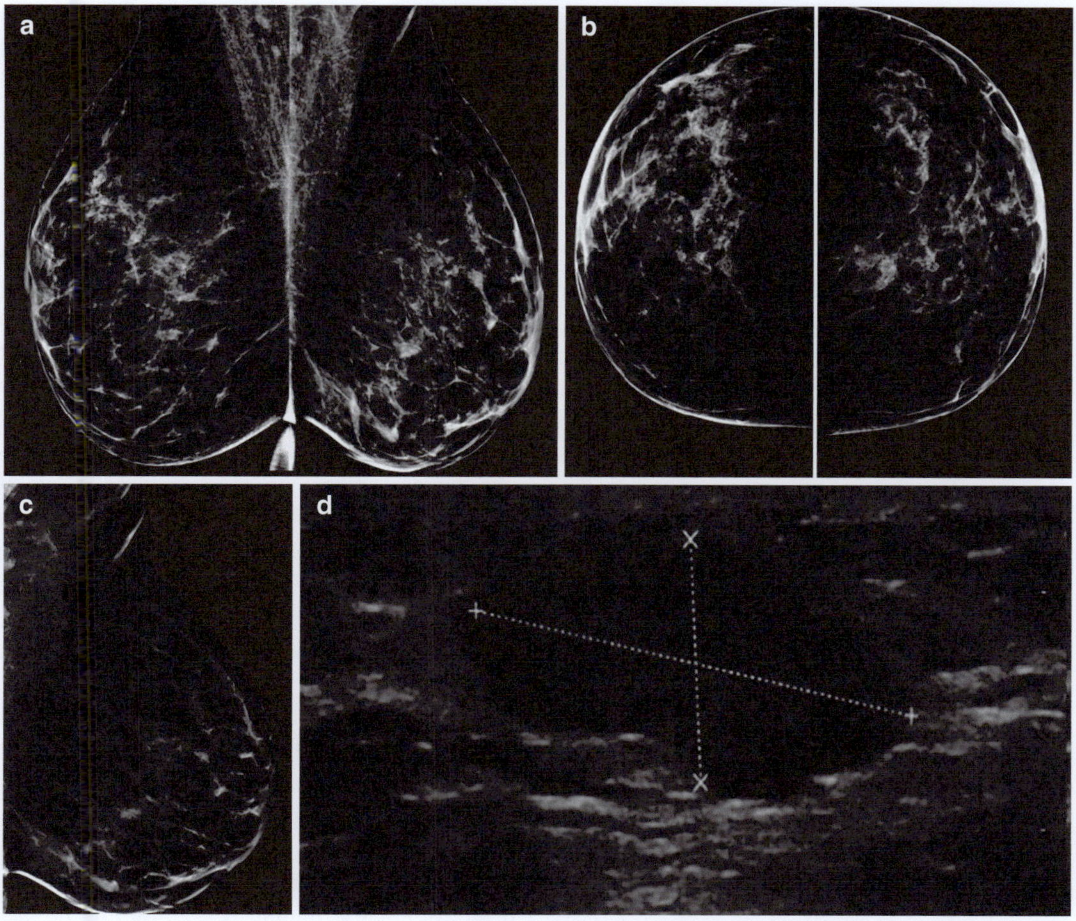

Fig. 5.4 A 42-year-old with complaints of a lump in the left breast. MLO and CC views (**a** and **b**) of diagnostic mammogram show focal asymmetry in the lower inner quadrant of the left breast which was confirmed to be a mass on a DBT image (**c**). Target US (**d**) shows an irregular parallel-oriented hypoechoic microlobulated mass corresponding to the site of focal asymmetry

Table 5.2 Benign and malignant causes of focal and developing asymmetry

Benign	Malignant
Benign breast tissue	Invasive carcinomas: ductal, lobular, tubular, mucinous types
Breast cysts	High risk lesions: DCIS, LCIS, ADH
Fibroepithelial lesions	Primary lymphoma
Fibrocystic change	
Fat necrosis	
Scar	
Infective and noninfective mastitis	
Radial scar/complex sclerosing lesions	
Papillomas	

should raise suspicion. While this is a rare finding, there is a substantial likelihood of malignancy, with approximately 15% of developing asymmetries turning out to be malignant [21]. Even in the absence of a sonographic correlate, a suspicious assessment for developing asymmetry is reasonable (BI-RADS 4 category), and tissue diagnosis should be obtained [10, 30]. Other associated suspicious findings and clinically palpable correlate increase the likelihood of malignancy. In a clinical setting of recent breast trauma, infection, or breast interventions and surgeries, a short-term interval follow-up at 1 month can be done, with biopsy of the lesion in case of persistence of the findings [10].

5.3.5 Imaging Evaluation and Management of Asymmetric Finding

The first step in evaluating an asymmetric finding is to identify whether it is a true finding or a projection artifact arising due to overlapping of the normal fibroglandular tissue. One of the methods to confirm its real three-dimensionality is by comparing projections at MG. To differentiate asymmetry (single-view finding) from a focal asymmetry (two-view finding), one can determine the location of the asymmetry on the projection in which it is visible and then evaluate the corresponding tissue on the other projection. The arc method uses the distance from the nipple to the lesion as the radius of an arc with the nipple as its center (Fig. 5.5). The lesion should lie on the arc at the same distance from the nipple on both projections. If a corresponding asymmetric finding is not visible on the other projection, it is regarded as an "asymmetry."

When assessing a potential asymmetry, it is prudent to check if the asymmetry is one view only because on the other view it can be obscured by the dense tissue, located outside the field of view (difficult anatomic locations like the axillary tail, inframammary fold, or posterior breast), or the positioning is poor during mammographic examination [31]. In case of any doubt, repeat imaging or appropriate additional views should be performed.

The other method for determining whether the asymmetric finding is real is to slightly alter the projection in which it is seen. A true finding will not change its appearance on alteration of the angle of projection, in contrast to the overlapping breast tissue [13]. For an asymmetry seen only on a mediolateral oblique (MLO) view, a straight lateral view should be obtained, while for an asymmetry seen only on a CC view, a rolled view should be obtained. If one is confident of not seeing the asymmetry on the additional view, it likely represents a summation shadow, and a BI-RADS category 1 can be assigned. After confirming the finding to be real, further workup warrants triangulating the three-dimensional location precisely on the orthogonal mammographic views.

In DBT, the localization bar can be helpful in defining the potential location of the lesion on the other view. Triangulation allows accurate positioning of the spot compression paddle for additional standard or magnification views and enables a more specific targeted US examination. If an asymmetric finding is seen on two projec-

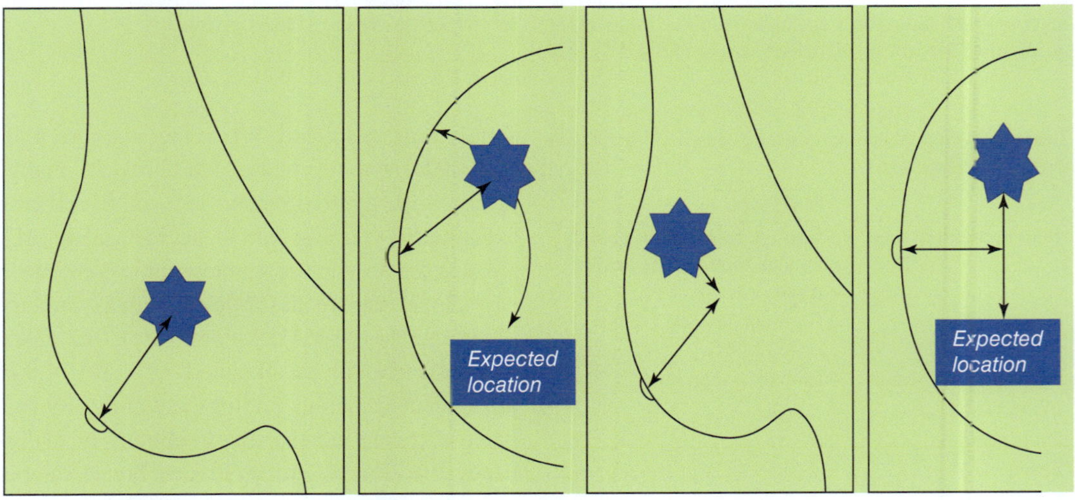

Fig. 5.5 Triangulation methods on 2D mammogram for exact lesion localization. The arc method uses the distance from the nipple to the lesion as the radius of an arc with the nipple as its center. The straight-line method measures the distance straight back from the nipple to a point where it is perpendicular to a line from the lesion that is parallel to the chest wall. The lesion should fall on an arc or line at the same distance from the nipple on both projections

tions, it is important to identify the cause of the focal asymmetry, that is, whether it represents a true lesion or an island of the normal breast tissue. An island of the normal breast tissue constitutes a vast majority of the focal asymmetries encountered in a day-to-day practice. This normal tissue is usually apparent on a closer look, representing superimposed structures with interspersed fat within (Fig. 5.6). However one must ensure the absence of an associated mass, architectural distortion, or suspicious calcifications in cases of focal asymmetry corresponding to an island of the breast tissue. The lack of specific benign characteristics, denser center, focused rather than a diffuse asymmetry should be viewed with suspicion and warrants further evaluation, especially in the presence of a palpable correlate. Spot compression views, rolled views, or different angles of the x-ray beam may help spread or reorient tissue structures to help define and characterize an underlying lesion more clearly.

The further step in evaluation of the focal asymmetry includes targeted US, which helps in further characterization of the abnormality. Targeted US should be done in the region of the breast where the palpable asymmetric finding is correlated or where the anatomic location of a focal abnormality is determined on the MG (Fig. 5.4). In cases where the exact location of the focal radiological abnormality cannot be determined, US may be applied to a larger area in searching for the presumed lesion. Although this approach is useful in certain cases, it is not very reliable as direct correlate of the mammographic finding cannot be firmly established. To overcome this challenge, one can place a needle in the abnormality seen on US and repeat the MG for establishing the concordance. Skin markers can also be useful. When no logical inference as to the location of the density can be established mammographically or clinically, US is unreliable in evaluating the asymmetric finding.

A algorithm that can be used for evaluation of asymmetric breast findings is summarized in Fig. 5.7.

5.3.6 Role of MRI and CEM

MRI is now an indispensable tool in breast imaging, pertaining to its high sensitivity and high negative predictive value (NPV). It may be sparingly utilized in cases where thorough diagnostic MG and targeted US fail to confirm the finding or when attempts to sample the lesion are unsuccessful, but there is still suspicion of a

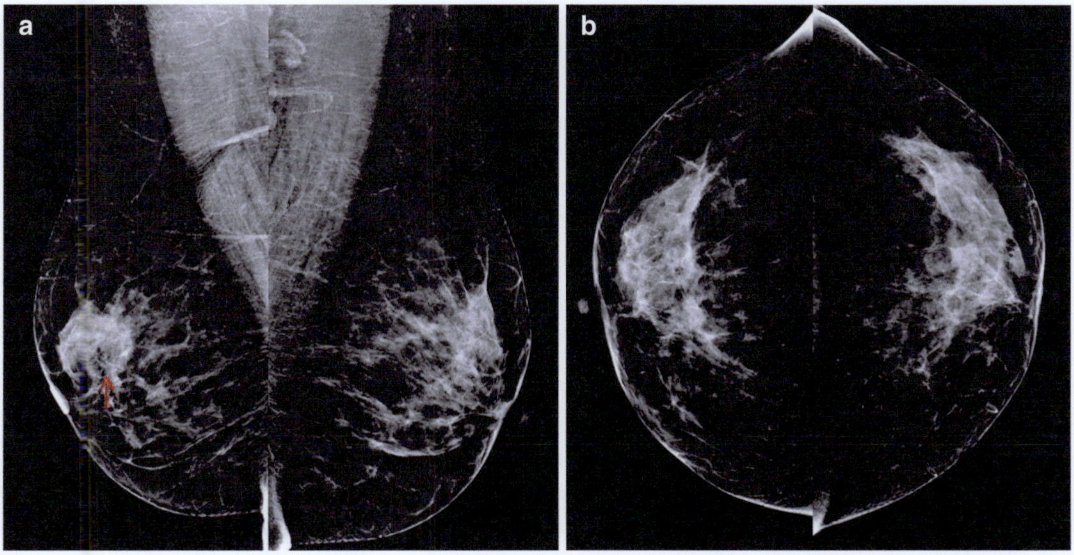

Fig. 5.6 A screening mammogram of a 62-year-old lady. MLO (**a**) and CC (**b**) views show an asymmetry in the upper quadrant of the right breast, with no correlate on the CC view. Note the interspersed fat within (red arrow)

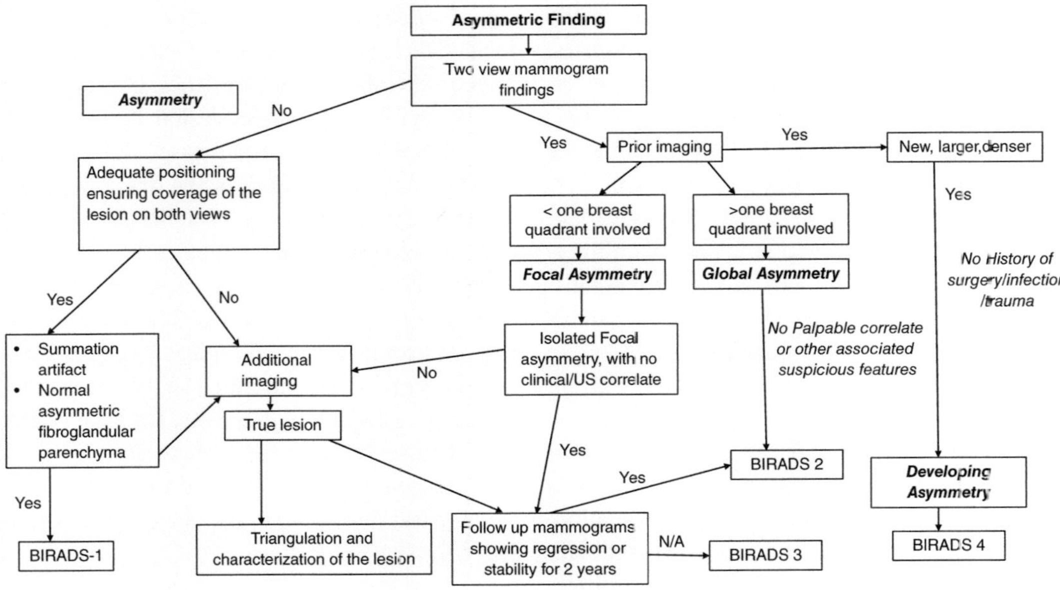

Fig. 5.7 Workup algorithm for the asymmetric breast findings. *HRT* hormonal replacement therapy, *Hx* history, *N/A* not available, *Wt* weight

lesion [13, 17]. If the asymmetric finding is clearly visible at MR imaging and is without associated architectural distortion or contrast enhancement, its likelihood of being a cancer is low, and it can be assigned a benign or probably benign category [20, 22].

Similar to MRI, CEM offers both functional and morphological information about breast lesions. It can be utilized to characterize breast asymmetries as physiological, benign or malignant and is particularly useful for identifying lesions in dense breasts [20–24]. The term "enhancing asymmetry" refers to the enhancement observed within the asymmetry, on recombined images. In some cases, the asymmetry may only be identified on recombined images without a correlate on the low energy images. The enhancement pattern of the asymmetry can be either homogenous with uniform enhancement or heterogeneous with non-uniform enhancement in a random pattern, with normal parenchyma or fat separating the areas of enhancement. While the presence of enhancement can aid in perceiving and characterizing the asymmetry, it does not significantly alter the management approach [32].

5.3.7 Percutaneous Biopsy

When a focal or developing asymmetry has been categorized as suspicious with the presence of US correlate, US-guided percutaneous biopsy can be executed, and a localization clip should be placed following tissue sampling. In cases where the sonographic correlate is absent or uncertain, a stereotactic biopsy may be considered. Identifying the asymmetry on scout images can be challenging, especially when it is subtle. In such cases, reviewing the diagnostic mammogram images or obtaining a mammogram with alphanumeric grid to place a skin marker can be helpful. Similar to US, it is crucial to deploy a post-biopsy clip for accurate targeting and to aid in subsequent imaging evaluations and pathological correlation. Radiological-pathological correlation is of utmost importance, as it guides further management decisions.

5.4 Architectural Distortion

Architectural distortion is defined in the fifth edition of ACR-BI-RADS atlas as the distortion of the normal architecture of breast parenchyma without any discernible mass [10]. This includes the presence of spicules radiating from a point, focal retraction, and straightening or distortion at the edge of the parenchyma (Fig. 5.8). Architectural distortion is the third most common manifestation of non-palpable breast cancer, accounting for 6% of detected abnormalities on screening mammograms [33]. It is also a frequent imaging finding in post-procedural or postoperative surveillance mammograms. Most patients with architectural distortion are clinically asymptomatic, although some patients may experience palpable thickening, skin or nipple retraction, or a lump [34]. Sometimes an apparent or pseudo-architectural distortion may appear on imaging due to summation artifact, which can be resolved with careful examination, additional mammographic view, or DBT.

5.4.1 Imaging Findings of Architectural Distortion

Architectural distortion manifests as spiculations or thin, straight lines extending from a central point on MG. It can also manifest as localized retraction, straightening, or distortion at the front or back boundary of the fibroglandular tissue. Women with a dense breast tissue often exhibit an outwardly curved contour of the breast parenchyma. However, in cases of cancer, the normal outward margin may exhibit distortion, reminiscent of the action of a crochet hook pulling the tissue toward the cancer (Fig. 5.9). Consequently, the subcutaneous fat is pulled into this region, resulting in the formation of straight lines (referred to as architectural distortion) with an angular fat density invaginating within the underlying breast parenchyma. This is very important to recognize, as it can be the only sign of a hidden non-palpable cancer within the dense breast tissue. The term "tent sign" has been used to describe architectural distortion, which is charac-

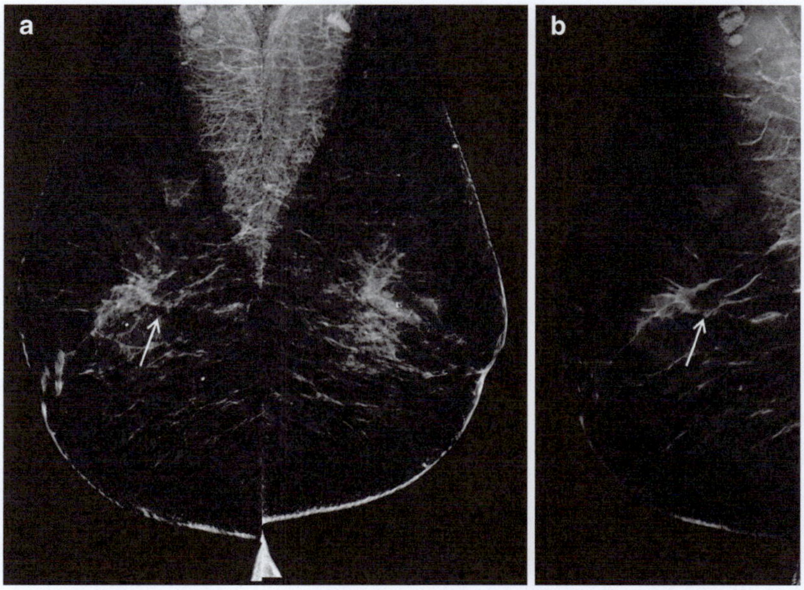

Fig. 5.8 A 56-year-old lady with complaints of right nipple retraction. MLO views of both breasts (**a**) and DBT image (**b**) of the right breast show an area of architectural distortion (arrow) in the upper quadrant with associated retraction of the nipple. Note is also made of circumscribed equal-density masses in the upper quadrant, posterior to the area of architectural distortion

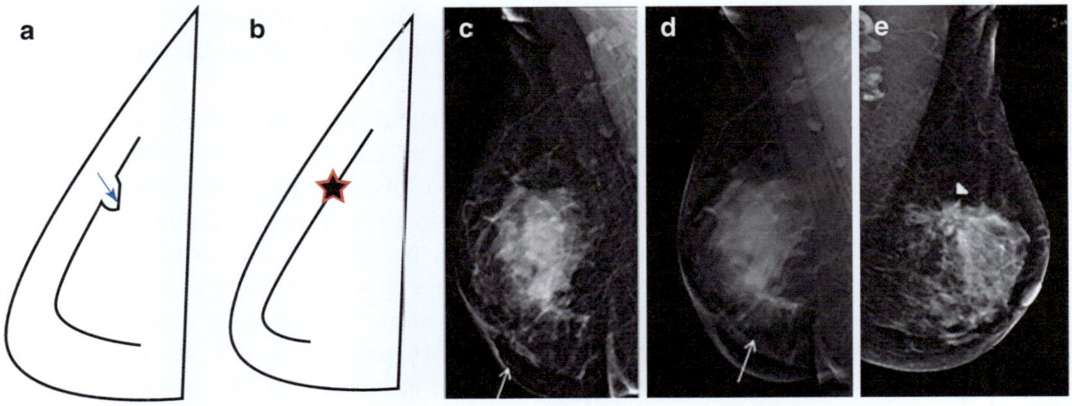

Fig. 5.9 (**a**–**e**). Pictorial representation (**a** and **b**) of abnormal contour at fat-glandular interface manifested as "hook sign" (**a**) and contour bulge (**b**). Right MLO (**c**) and DBT (**d**) images depict the "hook sign (arrow) suggestive of disruption of normal fibroglandular parenchyma. Left MLO (e) image depicts the "contour bulge" (arrowhead) at fat-glandular interface due to the suspicious mass

terized by the replacement of the typically smooth concavity of fibroglandular borders with a convex or "V"-shaped peak, resembling a tent [35]. Additional mammographic spot views and targeted US are needed to identify the hidden lesion, once the "tent sign" is identified. The other spectrum encompasses women with scattered fibroglandular densities or heterogeneously dense breast, who typically have a scalloped or concave margin of the breast tissue. The presence of an outward convex margin along the parenchymal margin may help in identifying the mass (Fig. 5.9c).

Architectural distortion is more often identified on DBT compared to standard MG due to its capability to remove the overlaying parenchymal tissue, as depicted in Fig. 5.10 [15]. By eliminating the obscuring breast tissue, the subtle lines of distortion become more discernible. In some cases where the architectural distortion is visible on only one mammographic view or a few tomosynthesis slices, the localization bar helps in identifying the potential location on the other view. For example, while scrolling through tomosynthesis sections on the CC view, the localization bar moves incrementally, providing a general indication of the direction from the inferior to superior breast and vice versa. This information aids in localizing the abnormality on MLO view and also helps in obtaining the spot compression view, targeted US and localization.

Similarly, the position in the medial-to-lateral plane can be determined from the true lateral 90° view, with approximate information gathered from the MLO view. The localization bar on tomosynthesis images helps in defining the abnormality on both the views. This not only confirms the presence of a minute finding but also assists in pinpointing its precise location, enabling more accurate targeted ultrasound examination.

An underlying mass is often identified on careful scrutiny of architectural distortions on tomosynthesis images that may have been obscured or occult at 2D MG. The architectural distortion may have a mass within the central portion, and the entrapped fat within the malignancies is more frequently identified at tomosynthesis.

The next step in evaluation of architectural distortion involves the correlation of the finding with the patient's clinical status and comparison with the prior imaging studies. In the absence of a prior biopsy or surgical procedure correlate of the architectural distortion, further workup is warranted with targeted US. On US, the imaging findings of architectural distortion include tethering and straightening of Cooper ligaments, with or without a central mass [10]. Despite thorough

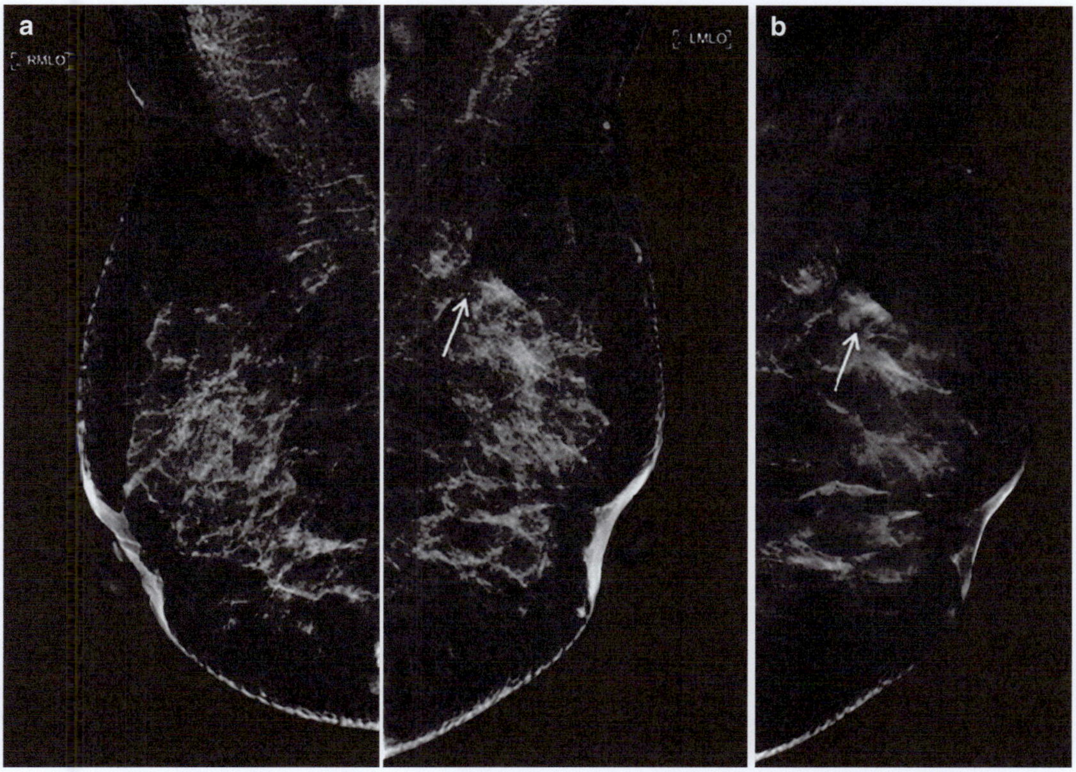

Fig. 5.10 A 56-year-old lady with complaints of mild pain in the left breast. There is architectural distortion in the upper quadrant (arrow) which is more conspicuous on the DBT image as compared to 2D MG

and detailed US evaluation, a US correlate may not be found for all cases of architectural distortion. Architectural distortion with a sonographic correlate is more likely to be malignant, although the absence of a sonographic correlate should not preclude biopsy, as approximately 28% of malignant architectural distortions may not be visualized on US [36].

In certain scenarios, the distortion may be seen on only one view and can be subtle or obscured by the dense breast tissue, questioning its existence. In the absence of a sonographic correlate and tomosynthesis-guided biopsy techniques, breast MRI may be considered for further evaluation. The normal fibroglandular parenchyma is best visualized on T1-weighted images without fat suppression, where findings of tissue distortion with or without skin retraction suggest the presence of architectural distortion. The presence of enhancement within the area of distortion further raises suspicion at MR imaging. MR imaging-guided biopsy could then be performed, with post-biopsy MG of the biopsy marker for confirmation. The lack of enhancement in architectural distortion is reassuring and has a negative predictive value of approximately 98% [37, 38].

CEM is an emerging tool for the evaluation of architectural distortion. By combining functional and morphological assessments, CEM demonstrates high diagnostic accuracy in evaluating malignant architectural distortion with reported sensitivity, specificity, positive predictive value, and NPV of 100%, 42.6%, 48.5%, and 100%, respectively [39]. The absence of enhancement is more frequently seen in the benign causes of architectural distortion. Marked enhancement and enhancing spiculations are considered predictors of malignant architectural distortion. If architectural distortion persists on lesion enhancement images, digital mammogram, and DBT, it should be pursued with a percutaneous biopsy regardless of its enhancement pattern [32].

5.4.2 Percutaneous Biopsy

Architectural distortions seen on MG should be further evaluated with targeted US, and US-guided needle biopsy should be performed in cases of a sonographic correlate. In cases of questionable correlate, a skin marker can be placed over the sonographic finding, and additional MG views can be obtained for confirmation. Though in most cases a US correlation for architectural distortion can be found, in a subset of cases, it cannot be determined requiring tomosynthesis-guided stereotactic percutaneous needle biopsy (10). If adequate nearby landmarks are available at 2D imaging, tissue sampling by means of conventional stereotactic biopsy may be possible. Wire localization followed by surgical excision can also be performed when stereotactic or tomosynthesis-guided biopsy techniques are not available or feasible.

5.5 Causes of Architectural Distortion

There are myriad causes of architectural distortion including various breast interventions, surgeries, and trauma to the breast, or it can be a manifestation of various benign and malignant breast pathologies. It is important to note that architectural distortion can also be falsely perceived due to an overlapping normal breast tissue (Table 5.3) [34, 36, 40].

Table 5.3 Common causes of architectural distortion

Benign	Malignant
Post-breast surgery/breast interventions/reduction mammoplasty	Invasive carcinomas: ductal, lobular, tubular
Breast trauma	DCIS
Complex sclerosing lesions/radial scar	
Sclerosing adenosis	
Fibromatosis	
Diabetic mastopathy	

5.5.1 Secondary Architectural Distortion

The most common non-malignant cause of architectural distortion is post-procedural scar, which typically occurs at the site of intervention or surgery and can persist for years [40]. Histopathologically, changes can range from inflammatory reaction in early cases to stromal fibrosis with prominent collagen in late cases.

On MG, typical features of architectural distortion are observed in the surgical bed, with or without associated fat necrosis, fluid collection, and dystrophic calcifications. Marking of the skin scar prior to MG or identifying surgical staples can facilitate precise correlation between the location of architectural distortion and the surgical bed. Often, post-procedural architectural distortion may appear differently on the two mammographic views, appearing denser and more conspicuous on one view, while less conspicuous on the other view. US may reveal an ill-defined hypoechoic area or line with posterior acoustic shadowing, below the incision site, reaching to the skin surface. However, ultrasound features are often nonspecific and can even mimic malignancy. The secondary architectural distortion typically remains stable or decreases in size and density on serial mammograms. Patients undergoing radiation therapy have radiation-induced changes including architectural distortion, trabecular thickening, and skin edema. Any new finding, including developing asymmetry, suspicious calcifications, or increasing size, warrants further evaluation with US or MRI, and a biopsy is needed to exclude recurrence. MRI is considered the best noninvasive technique to differentiate a post-surgical scar tissue from recurrence, where any enhancement in the post-surgical bed after 12–18 months of surgery is considered suspicious for recurrence and prompts biopsy [41].

Fat necrosis, characterized histologically by saponification of fat resulting from trauma or surgery, may uncommonly manifest solely as architectural distortion and may be associated with skin thickening and retraction. Clinical history can aid in characterizing the architectural distortion, although sampling or short-interval follow-up is warranted in cases of a doubtful clinical scenario. Demonstration of fat within the area of architectural distortion, in an appropriate clinical setting, aids in reaching the diagnosis of fat necrosis [42].

5.5.2 Primary Architectural Distortion

Complex Sclerosing Lesions/Radial Scar

Radial scar/complex sclerosing lesions (CSLs) are idiopathic proliferative breast diseases, histologically characterized by a central fibroelastic core with radiating spokes of elongated ducts and lobules. Due to the elastic component and contraction caused by fibrosis, the ducts and lobules are drawn into a radial configuration, resulting in a "pulled in" stellate appearance. The etiology of CSLs is unclear, but they are believed to arise from localized inflammation with chronic ischemia, leading to sclerosing ductal hyperplasia and subsequent infarction. The myoepithelial cell layer typically remains intact, which can be confirmed through immune-histochemical staining. The term CSL is used for radial scars >1 cm and histologically has more extensive ductal proliferation. CSLs and radial scar can co-exist with other high-risk lesions, including atypical ductal hyperplasia (ADH), ductal carcinoma in situ (DCIS), invasive ductal carcinomas (IDC), and tubular carcinomas, in approximately 30% of cases. Patients are usually asymptomatic with no palpable correlate. On imaging, they typically appear as architectural distortion, with long, gracile spicules radiating from a radiolucent center, giving a "dark star appearance" (Fig. 5.11). This is in contrast to malignant architectural distortion, which usually has a radiodense center with shorter, thicker spicules. However, malignant architectural distortion can resemble a CSL on imaging, especially invasive lobular carcinoma, and may be indistinguishable [40, 42, 43]. On US, architectural distortion is often seen as a non-mass lesion with dense posterior acoustic shadowing, although a sonographic correlate may be absent in many patients. With the introduction of DBT, there is an increased detection rate of these lesions. MRI features remain nonspecific and cannot reliably differentiate between various causes of architectural distortion. The management of CSLs and radial scars remains controversial due to an uncertain upgrade rate and the potential for conversion into malignancy. If isolated without atypia, these lesions may be followed up due to <1% upgradation rate, provided sufficient and accurate sampling has been done. However, excision of these lesions is usually warranted, especially when associated with atypia [44].

Sclerosing Adenosis

Sclerosing adenosis (SA) is a benign proliferative breast disease characterized histologically by an increased number of acini, myoepithelial cells, and connective tissue elements, resulting in compression and distortion of acini while maintaining a normal lobular arrangement. Although it does not pose an increased risk of cancer itself, associated high-risk lesions and cancers can co-exist. It is typically encountered incidentally in perimenopausal women, and some may experience a lump or pain. Architectural distortion with or without calcifications are common imaging manifestations on mammograms. Calcifications can range from tiny amorphous powdery calcifications to fine-pleomorphic calcifications. US and MRI features are nonspecific, and tissue diagnosis is usually needed to exclude malignancy. Isolated SA with no other suspicious features does not require treatment, provided accurate and sufficient sampling has been performed to ensure co-existing lesions have not been missed [40, 42, 45].

DCIS

DCIS is a pre-malignant noninvasive breast condition that commonly presents as suspicious calcifications on MG. However, architectural distortion can also occur in 2–10% of patients with or without calcifications. Unfortunately, no imaging feature can reliably differentiate architectural distortion due to DCIS from other benign causes that can often co-exist. However, the pres-

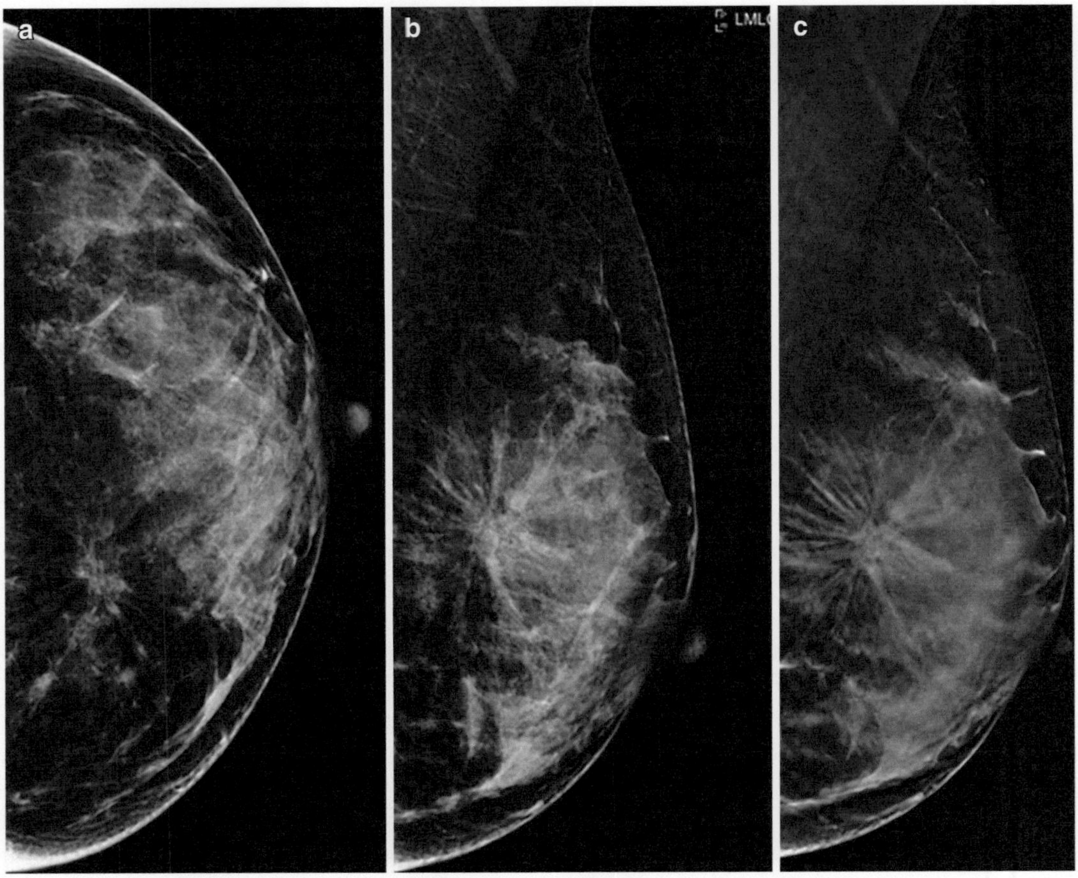

Fig. 5.11 CC (**a**), MLO (**b**), and DBT (**c**) images of left breast mammogram of an 81-year-old lady, showing architectural distortion in the upper inner quadrant of the left breast with long thin radiating spicules from a lucent center with no central mass. Biopsy was suggestive of complex sclerosing lesion

ence of other associated suspicious features increases the likelihood of a malignant cause of architectural distortion [42, 46].

Breast Cancer

IDC, the most common histological type of breast cancer, and ILC, the second most common type, can present as architectural distortion with or without associated findings. ILC typically grows in a single-cell fashion, permeating rather than displacing normal structures. It may manifest as sheet-like architectural distortion, without a definite discernible mass, and may be occult on 2D MG (Fig. 5.12) [47]. Another breast cancer subtype commonly associated with architectural distortion is tubular carcinoma. In cases where patient is asymptomatic and present solely with architectural distortion, there is often a delay in diagnosis of carcinoma.

Other Rare Causes of Benign Architectural Distortion

There are certain rare benign entities that can also present as architectural distortion like granular cell tumors, diabetic mastopathy, focal fibrosis, inflammatory breast pathologies such as tuberculosis or idiopathic granulomastitis, and fibromatosis [34, 42].

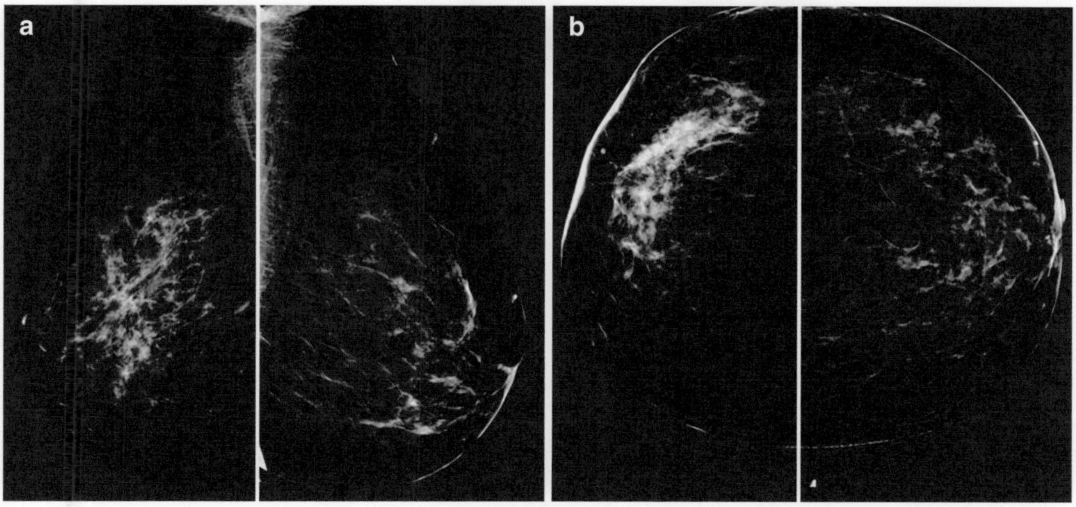

Fig. 5.12 Diagnostic 2D mammogram of a 40-year-old lady with a vague lump in the right breast shows a focal asymmetry with architectural distortion, associated skin thickening, trabecular thickening, and nipple retraction in the upper outer and central quadrant. Biopsy was suggestive of invasive lobular carcinoma

5.6 Potential Challenges and Algorithm for the Workup of Architectural Distortion (Fig. 5.13)

Inevitably, there will be cases where a subtle architectural distortion detected only on 2D MG does not have a corresponding US or MRI finding. Often the subtle distortions are visible on just one mammographic view or very few tomosynthesis slices, making precise needle localization or stereotactic biopsy challenging. It is crucial to consider the patient's clinical status including patient's risk factors when evaluating these distortions, with a lower threshold for biopsy in high-risk scenarios. However, currently, there are no well-established guidelines on how to proceed when faced with questionable subtle architectural distortion without a sonographic or MR imaging correlate.

In low-risk patients without relevant surgical histories, it may be reasonable to consider these lesions as likely benign, with a recommendation for short-interval follow-up. The rationale behind this approach is that these findings may not represent true distortions but rather asymmetries or artifacts. This assessment is supported by negative findings on US and MR imaging, and as such, surveillance under the discretion of the interpreting radiologist may be an appropriate course of action.

However, if architectural distortion is clearly observed on routine MG, it is presumed to be a real finding. In such cases, despite a negative US and/or MR imaging workup, tissue diagnosis should be pursued.

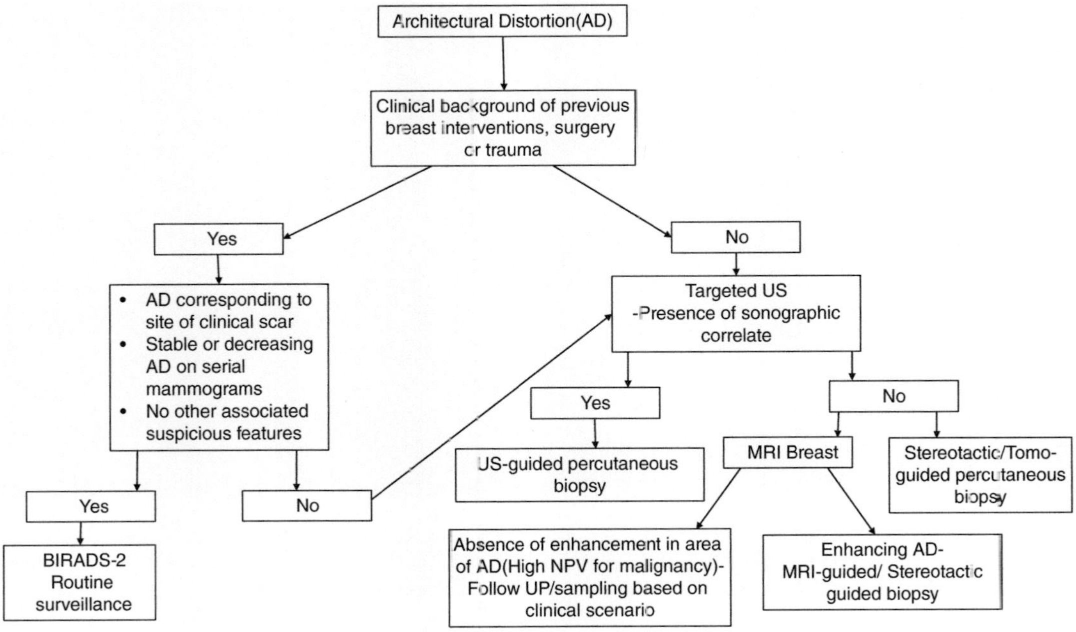

Fig. 5.13 Imaging work up for architectural distortion on mammogram

5.7 Conclusion

Asymmetries and architectural distortion are important early signs of breast cancer that require skillful identification and accurate characterization. A wide range of both benign and malignant causes can give rise to these abnormalities, highlighting the importance of precise clinical-radiological-pathological correlation in establishing a conclusive management plan and recommendation.

References

1. Unger-Saldaña K. Challenges to the early diagnosis and treatment of breast cancer in developing countries. World J Clin Oncol. 2014;5(3):465–77.
2. Venkatesan A, Chu P, Kerlikowske K, Sickles EA, Smith-Bindman R. Positive predictive value of specific mammographic findings according to reader and patient variables. Radiology. 2009;250(3):648–57.
3. Pulappadi VP, Dhamija E, Baby A, Mathur S, Pandey S, Gogia A, Deo SVS. Imaging features of breast cancer subtypes on mammography and ultrasonography: an analysis of 479 patients. Indian J Surg Oncol. 2022;13(4):931–8.
4. Saarenmaa I, Salminen T, Geiger U, Heikkinen P, Hyvärinen S, Isola J, Kataja V, Kokko ML, Kokko R, Kumpulainen E, Kärkkäinen A, Pakkanen J, Peltonen P, Piironen A, Salo A, Talviala ML, Hakama M. The visibility of cancer on previous MGs in retrospective review. Clin Radiol. 2001;56(1):40–3.
5. Goergen SK, Evans J, Cohen GP, MacMillan JH. Characteristics of breast carcinomas missed by screening radiologists. Radiology. 1997;204(1):131–5.
6. Yankaskas BC, Schell MJ, Bird RE, Desrochers DA. Reassessment of breast cancers missed during routine screening mammography: a community-based study. AJR Am J Roentgenol. 2001;177(3):535–41.
7. Lamb LR, Mohallem Fonseca M, Verma R, Seely JM. Missed breast cancer: effects of subconscious bias and lesion characteristics. Radiographics. 2020;40(4):941–60.
8. Majid AS, de Paredes ES, Doherty RD, Sharma NR, Salvador X. Missed breast carcinoma: pitfalls and pearls. RadioGraphics. 2003;23(4):881–95.
9. Giess CS, Frost EP, Birdwell RL. Difficulties and errors in diagnosis of breast neoplasms. Semin Ultrasound CT MR. 2012;33(4):288–99.
10. Sickles EA, D'Orsi CJ, Bassett LW, et al. ACR BI-RADS mammography. In: ACR BI-RADS atlas breast imaging re- porting and data system 2013. 5th ed. Reston: American College of Radiology; 2013. p. 1–175.
11. Youk JH, Kim EK, Ko KH, Kim MJ. Asymmetric mammographic findings based on the fourth edition

of BI-RADS: types, evaluation, and management. Radiographics. 2009;29(1):e33.
12. Chesebro AL, Winkler NS, Birdwell RL, Giess CS. Developing asymmetries at mammography: a multimodality approach to assessment and management. Radiographics. 2016;36(2):322–34.
13. Price ER, Joe BN, Sickles EA. The developing asymmetry: revisiting a perceptual and diagnostic challenge. Radiology. 2015;274(3):642–51.
14. Sickles EA. The spectrum of breast asymmetries: imaging features, work-up, management. Radiol Clin N Am. 2007;45(765-771):v.
15. Dhamija E, Gulati M, Deo SVS, Gogia A, Hari S. Digital breast tomosynthesis: an overview. Indian J Surg Oncol. 2021;12(2):315–29.
16. Hooley RJ, Durand MA, Philpotts LE. Advances in digital breast tomo- synthesis. AJR Am J Roentgenol. 2017;208(2):256–66.
17. Liang A, Baraban E, Myers KS, Mullen LA, Panigrahi B, Oluyemi E, Cimino-Mathews A, Ambinder EB. Developing asymmetries without sonographic correlate at digital breast tomosynthesis. Radiology. 2022;302(3):525–32.
18. Lourenco AP, Barry-Brooks M, Baird GL, Tuttle A, Mainiero MB. Changes in recall type and patient treatment following implementation of screening digital breast tomosynthesis. Radiology. 2015;274(2):337–42.
19. Samardar P, de Paredes ES, Grimes MM, Wilson JD. Focal asymmetric densities seen at mammography: US and pathologic correlation. Radiographics. 2002;22(1):19–33.
20. Moy L, Elias K, Patel V, Lee J, Babb JS, Toth HK, Mercado CL. Is breast MRI helpful in the evaluation of inconclusive mammographic findings? AJR Am J Roentgenol. 2009;193(4):986–93.
21. Chesebro AL, Winkler NS, Birdwell RL, Giess CS. Developing asymmetry at mammography: correlation with US and MR imaging and histopathologic findings. Radiology. 2016;279(2):385–94.
22. Lee CH, Smith RC, Levine JA, Troiano RN, Tocino I. Clinical usefulness of MR imaging of the breast in the evaluation of the problematic mammogram. AJR Am J Roentgenol. 1999;173(5):1323–9.
23. Wessam R, Gomaa MMM, Fouad MA, Mokhtar SM, Tohamey YM. Added value of contrast-enhanced mammography in assessment of breast asymmetries. Br J Radiol. 2019;92(1098):20180245.
24. Jochelson MS, Lobbes MBI. Contrast-enhanced mammography: state of the art. Radiology. 2021;299(1):36–48.
25. Sickles EA. Findings at mammographic screening on only one standard projection: outcomes analysis. Radiology. 1998;208(2):471–5.
26. Evans WP, Warren Burhenne LJ, Laurie L, O'Shaughnessy KF, Castellino RA. Invasive lobular carcinoma of the breast: mammographic characteristics and computer-aided detection. Radiology. 2002;225(1):182–9.
27. Harvey JA, Nicholson BT, Cohen MA. Finding early invasive breast cancers: a practical approach. Radiology. 2008;248(1):61–76.
28. Sickles EA. Periodic mammographic follow-up of probably benign lesions: results in 3,184 consecutive cases. Radiology. 1991;179(2):463–8.
29. Varas X, Leborgne JH, Leborgne F, Mezzera J, Jaumandreu S, Leborgne F. Revisiting the mammographic follow-up of BI-RADS category 3 lesions. AJR Am J Roentgenol. 2002;179(3):691–5.
30. Leung JW, Sickles EA. Developing asymmetry identified on mammography: correlation with imaging outcome and pathologic findings. AJR Am J Roentgenol. 2007;188(3):667–75.
31. Giess CS, Frost EP, Birdwell RL. Interpreting one-view mammographic findings: minimizing callbacks while maximizing cancer detection. Radiographics. 2014;34(4):928–40.
32. Phillips J, Sung J, Lewin J, Newell MS. Contrast-enhanced mammography (A supplement to ACR BI-RADS mammography. System 2013). 5th ed. Reston: American College of Radiology; 2013. p. 1–64.
33. Knutzen AM, Gisvold JJ. Likelihood of malignant disease for various categories of mammographically detected, nonpalpable breast lesions. Mayo Clin Proc. 1993;68(5):454–60.
34. Durand MA, Wang S, Hooley RJ, Raghu M, Philpotts LE. tomosynthesis-detected architectural distortion: management algorithm with radiologic-pathologic correlation. Radiographics. 2016;36(2):311–21.
35. Estrin Y, Drotman M. Re-pitching the tent sign: a case report. Clin Imaging. 2021;72:194–7.
36. Bahl M, Baker JA, Kinsey EN, Ghate SV. Architectural distortion on mammography: correlation with pathologic outcomes and predictors of malignancy. AJR Am J Roentgenol. 2015;205(6):1339–45.
37. Ozcan UA, Ocak F, Altun E. Can breast MRI facilitate decision-making in equivocal mammography and ultrasonography findings? Eur J Radiol. 2012;81(Suppl 1):S112–3.
38. Leung JW. MR imaging in the evaluation of equivocal clinical and imaging findings of the breast. Magn Reson Imaging Clin N Am. 2010;18(2):295–308, ix-x.
39. Goh Y, Chan CW, Pillay P, Lee HS, Pan HB, Hung BH, Quek ST, Chou CP. Architecture distortion score (ADS) in malignancy risk stratification of architecture distortion on contrast-enhanced digital mammography. Eur Radiol. 2021;31(5):2657–66.
40. Gaur S, Dialani V, Slanetz PJ, Eisenberg RL. Architectural distortion of the breast. AJR Am J Roentgenol. 2013;201(5):W662–70.
41. Preda L, Villa G, Rizzo S, Bazzi L, Origgi D, Cassano E, Bellomi M. Magnetic resonance mammography in the evaluation of recurrence at the prior lumpectomy site after conservative surgery and radiotherapy. Breast Cancer Res. 2006;8(5):R53.

42. Shaheen R, Schimmelpenninck CA, Stoddart L, Raymond H, Slanetz PJ. Spectrum of diseases presenting as architectural distortion on mammography: multimodality radiologic imaging with pathologic correlation. Semin Ultrasound CT MR. 2011;32(4):351–62.
43. Ha SM, Cha JH, Shin HJ, Chae EY, Choi WJ, Kim HH, Oh HY. Radial scars/complex sclerosing lesions of the breast: radiologic and clinicopathologic correlation. BMC Med Imaging. 2018;18(1):39.
44. Yan P, DeMello L, Baird GL, Lourenco AP. Malignancy upgrade rates of radial sclerosing lesions at breast cancer screening. Radiol Imaging Cancer. 2021;3(6):e210036.
45. Gill H, Ioffe OB, Berg WA. When is a diagnosis of sclerosing adenosis acceptable at core biopsy? Radiology. 2003;228:50–7.
46. Sekine K, Tsunoda-Shimizu H, Kikuchi M, Saida Y, Kawasaki T, Suzuki K. DCIS showing architectural distortion on the screening mammogram – comparison of mammographic and pathological findings. Breast Cancer. 2007;14(3):281–4.
47. Weaver O, Yang W. Imaging of breast cancers with predilection for nonmass pattern of growth: invasive lobular carcinoma and DCIS-Does imaging capture it all? AJR Am J Roentgenol. 2020;215(6):1504–11.

Indeterminate and High-Risk Lesions

6

Jyoti Arora and Jeevanjot Matharoo

Abstract

Breast lesions with unknown malignant potential (B3) comprise a diverse range of diagnostic abnormalities that may be connected to atypia. Approximately 20–30% of these cases can have associated in situ or invasive cancer; thus these entities are often referred to as high-risk lesions as well. Traditionally, open excision of such lesions was preferred to avoid patients from the needless anxiety or excessive healthcare expenses. However, with advancements in the field of radiological interventions and imaging; there has been emergence of literature regarding minimally invasive procedures/techniques for management of high-risk lesions. Their potential upgradation rates with various types of biopsies and role of multidisciplinary discussions to approach these lesions have also been highlighted by many authors. Thus it becomes imperative for radiologists who interpret breast imaging, to familiarize themselves with B3 lesions, their upgradation rates, and role of imaging in their management. This chapter attempts to discuss these areas of interest along with current recommendations for B3 lesion management.

Keywords

B3 lesions · Mammography · Tomosynthesis
High-risk lesions · Upgradation rates
Papillomas · Phyllodes · Radial scar
Complex sclerosing lesion · Vacuum-assisted biopsy · Vacuum-assisted excision

6.1 Introduction

Breast Imaging Reporting and Data System (BI-RADS) category assignment provides a uniform platform for communication among radiologist, pathologist, and treating physicians. The American College of Radiology provides specific descriptors and definitions to characterize the lesions seen on various imaging modalities that further assists in determining malignant potential of the visible lesions or masses. Imaging plays a vital role in detecting, diagnosing, and delineating the disease extent in addition to the guiding plan for biopsy. Tissue sampling and pathological evaluation are crucial steps for the treatment outline. However, there are certain scenarios which face pathological and clinical dilemma on how to move ahead in patient management, for example, architectural distortions or BI-RADS 4c/5 lesions on imaging which show benign features on histo-

J. Arora (✉)
Apollo Athenaa Women Cancer Centre, New Delhi, Delhi, India

J. Matharoo
Apollo Athenaa Women Cancer Centre, New Delhi, Delhi, India

Scan4Health, Gurgaon, Haryana, India

E. Dhamija, S. V. S. Deo (eds.), *Imaging in Management of Breast Diseases*,
https://doi.org/10.1007/978-981-96-4998-3_6

pathology, etc. Thus, rad-path correlation becomes very important to identify the potential discordant results and take necessary steps. Moreover, there exists a category of breast lesions which carry unknown malignant potential (B3) and is also known as indeterminate or high-risk lesions (HRL). This is a heterogeneous category that includes a variety of lesions that might or might not be related to cytological or architectural atypia. The B3 category includes cellular fibro-epithelial lesions (where phyllodes tumor (PT) is considered), flat epithelial atypia (FEA), lobular in situ neoplasia (including atypical lobular hyperplasia [ALH] and lobular carcinoma in situ [LCIS]), atypical intraductal epithelial proliferation (AIEDP), intraductal papillomas (with and without atypia), and radial scars (with and without atypia). It is recognized that the B3 lesions frequently co-exist with low nuclear grade neoplasia [1]. Other less frequent lesions in this category include bland spindle cell lesions, vascular lesions, apocrine atypia, and myofibroblastomas.

The extensive implementation of screening programs and the introduction of novel imaging modalities have significantly boosted the diagnosis of B3 lesions over the past few decades. B3 lesions are regarded as non-obligatory progenitors of malignancy since they have the potential to progress to higher-grade lesions, primarily ductal carcinoma in situ (DCIS) and less frequently low-grade invasive tumors [2]. Some B3 lesions also serve as risk markers; for instance, women with proliferative breast disease who exhibit atypia have a four- to tenfold increased risk of getting breast cancer in the same or the contralateral breast compared with those who do not. Overall, malignancy risk is low in HRL. However, at surgical specimen, up to 35% of them can get upgraded to DCIS or low-grade carcinoma. These lesions can be categorized based on whether or not there is accompanying atypia. Because of this, several authors proposed further histological classification of B3 lesions into B3a and B3b based on the presence or absence of atypia.

The prime objective of this chapter is to give the reader a thorough summary of the major high-risk breast lesions. In addition to outlining the radiological features of these lesions and their upgrade rates, the most recent research, will also be covered in this chapter, to offer helpful direction for suitable clinical management using vacuum-assisted biopsy (VAB) while minimizing the potential risk associated with surgical removal.

6.2 Atypical Ductal Hyperplasia

Atypical ductal hyperplasia (ADH) is defined as abnormal epithelial proliferation limited to a single terminal ductal lobular unit with a maximum extension of ≤2 mm. Ducts are lined by a single layer of epithelial cells. Proliferation of the epithelial cells takes place, resulting in multiple layers in benign ductal hyperplasia. If nuclear pleomorphism is present, this becomes atypical ductal hyperplasia. If the area of abnormality is greater than 2 mm or more than three ducts are involved or the focus is greater than 1 mm, then it is called low-grade DCIS. ADH can be seen in 12–17% of percutaneous biopsies. This condition is thought to be associated with the highest prevalence of malignant transformation among HRL. Because of this, it is regarded as a voluntary precursor of invasive cancer and a separate risk factor for breast cancer [3].

Pathological Classification and Importance ADH is the term used to describe a specific small lesion (micro-focal, 2 mm, or less than two complete spaces in extent) made up of a uniform, small-cell, atypical epithelial proliferation that is either mixed with a non-uniform process, such as typical epithelial hyperplasia or is too small to be diagnosed as low-grade DCIS. So the only factor differentiating ADH from low-grade DCIS is the size of the lesion. High-grade DCIS usually does not pose a diagnostic dilemma for the pathologist. Some authors prefer the term AIDEP to describe the findings after a percutaneous biopsy that indicate ADH or low-grade DCIS because the sample may represent only part of a larger low-grade DCIS that was not completely sampled.

AIDEP includes lesions that would be classified as ADH on a surgical excision and other types of aberrant epithelial proliferation in duct spaces. Thus it can be inferred that there are different degrees of cytological and architectural atypia in the category of AIDEP which would include the changes that are suspect but don't support a conclusive DCIS diagnosis and also those that merely exhibit a very slight amount of atypia

Imaging Features Although as stated earlier, ADH may be seen with any breast lesion, isolated ADH may present as grouped, linear, or regionally distributed amorphous microcalcifications on mammography (MG). It could be also seen as a mass that contains or lacks microcalcifications (Figs. 6.1 and 6.2). Ultrasound (US) lacks specificity in its detection and may present as an irregular-shaped, small hypoechoic non-mass area. It can also be seen as a mass with microlobulations without posterior acoustic characteristics showing parallel orientation to the parenchymal tissue. These lesions may show a non-mass pattern of enhancement on MRI (Fig. 6.3) [3].

Upgradation Rates A crucial part of managing high-risk lesions effectively is determining the upgrade rate of lesions. In simple terms, it means how worried we should be about overlooking a malignancy when encountering a HRL. Among all HRLs, ADH not only has the highest upgrade rates; it is also the most prevalent high-risk lesion.

According to the available literature, the upgrade rate of AIDEP to malignancy is higher with small samples (e.g., 14 G cores) compared to VAB specimens. The AIDEP upgrade rate

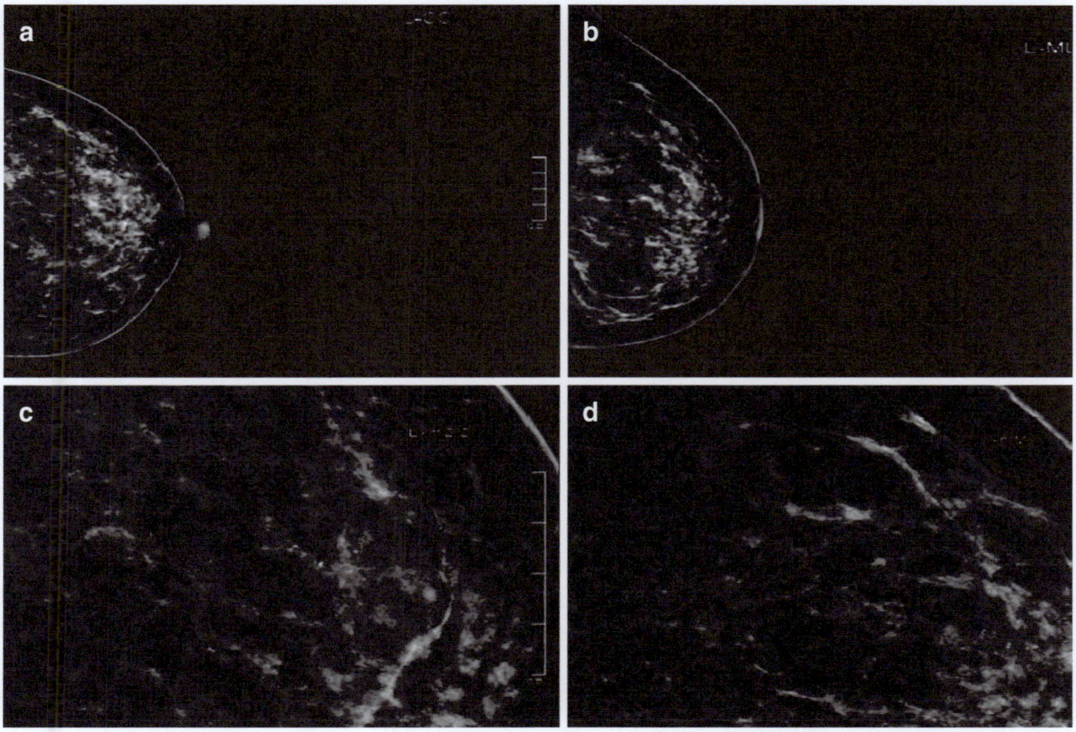

Fig. 6.1 A 45-year-old female came to the hospital with mammograms done outside authors' institute which showed clusters of microcalcifications in the upper outer quadrant of the left breast. Left CC (**a**), lateral (**b**), and CC mag and Lat mag (**c**, **d**) views obtained showed a cluster of variable amorphous and punctate microcalcifications with no tea cupping seen on the lateral view in the upper outer quadrant of the left breast (BI-RADS 4). Stereotactic biopsy revealed ADH

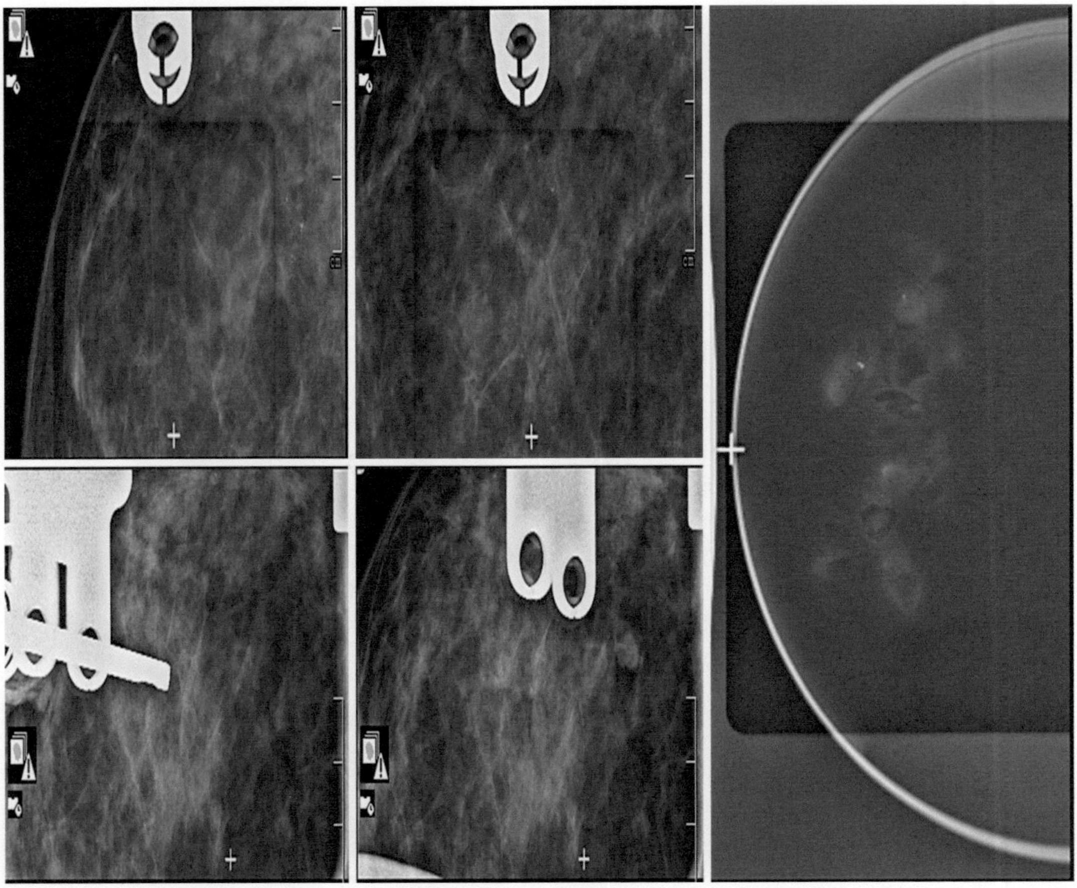

Fig. 6.2 Stereotactic-guided VAB biopsy of the microcalcification in the upper outer quadrant of the left breast was performed using 10 G vacuum probe. Samples had been taken from the suspicious calcifications with residual calcifications still present. Approximately 12–14 cores were obtained through the cluster. Specimen radiograph confirmed microcalcification, and histopathology revealed ADH

ranges from 18% to 87% when using 14 G needles and 10–39% when using 11 or 9 G samples, with a pooled positive predictive value of 21% with the VAB [2]. Consequently, there is a lesser likelihood of "missing" a diagnosis of DCIS or invasive cancer if more tissue has been provided to pathologist. A meta-analysis of 93 studies showed a pooled upgrade rate of ADH to cancer as 29% [4].

Although the upgrade rate to cancer (DCIS and invasive ductal cancer) is high, it's the upgrade to IDC which is more relevant as DCIS is generally low grade and thus does not affect survival significantly. The increased risk of invasive breast carcinoma due to ADH is about four to five times that of the general population and approximately six times in premenopausal women.

Management According to the American Society of Breast Surgeons and National Comprehensive Cancer Network, surgical excision is recommended for most of ADH; however, small volume ADH that is completely removed at biopsy (VAB) may be observed. Authors prefer to do VAB wherever imaging findings are suspicious of ADH/DCIS and, if small, completely remove it at the time of biopsy.

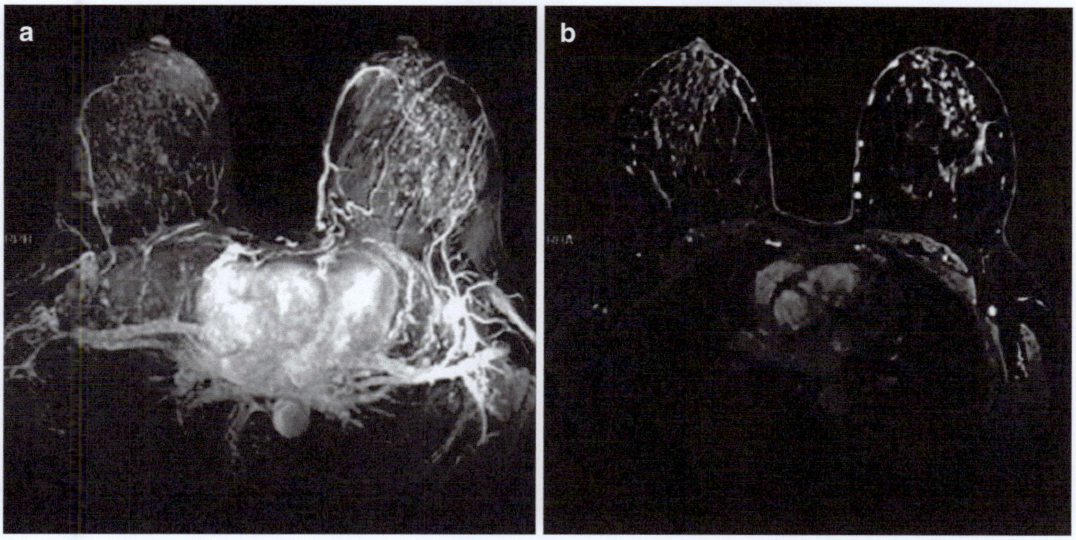

Fig. 6.3 MIP (**a**) and T1 post-contrast fat sat (**b**) images reveal segmental non-clumped non-mass enhancement in the upper half of the left breast which shows heterogeneous internal enhancement (BI-RADS 4). Final mastectomy specimen revealed intermediate DCIS

6.3 Lobular Neoplasia

Classical lobular neoplasia (LN) is a neoplastic proliferation of small dyscohesive epithelial cells within the terminal duct lobular unit (TDLU) of the breast. As per World Health Organization (WHO) classification of breast tumors (2019), classical LN is divided into ALH when TDLU involvement is less than 50% and LCIS when more than 50% TDLU is involved. So ALH and LCIS are physiologically and genetically identical and can be differentiated only on the basis of the amount of TDLU involved which cannot be reliably predicted on core needle biopsy (CNB) specimen. Hence, similar to AIDEP, the name LN is favored in core-biopsy specimens.

LN is considered a risk factor and a potential precursor for breast cancer. LN is found in 0.5–4% of breast biopsies that would otherwise be benign. Although it can occur at any age, premenopausal women are the most susceptible. In 85% of cases, it is regarded as multicentric, and in up to 67% of cases, as bilateral.

Additionally, the WHO classification promotes the usage of the term "intraepithelial lobular neoplasia" (LIN), which can be further classified into three types (LIN1, LIN2, and LIN3).

ALH is referred to as LN1; LCIS as LIN2 and LIN3 comprises non-typical variations of LN that differ from the classic variety by either lacking lobular unit distension (florid form) or cellular atypia (pleomorphic form). Pleomorphic LCIS is characterized by cells that have similar discohesion and growth patterns to those of B5a, malignant in situ, but larger, more diverse nuclei and frequently extensive cytoplasm. This pleomorphic pattern is not seen with LN, but when it has comedo-type necrosis or is mass-forming, it is considered as a variant of pleomorphic LCIS and is classified as B4 (suspicious) [3].

There is currently no evidence to suggest ALH and LCIS having a prognostic significance toward cancer. As a result, they are classified as B3 lesions on both CNB and VAB samples, whereas pleomorphic or florid LN has been classified as a B5a (malignant) lesion.

Imaging Features They are normally occult on mammography but are increasingly found in biopsies of screen-detected lesions. Microcalcifications are detected occasionally in the classical type but are more common in the pleomorphic (B5a) form. Sometimes LN can be seen as a mass, architectural distortion, or asymmetry.

On US, they can appear as an irregular, hypoechoic, avascular mass with shadowing. Because LN rarely presents as a mass on MG or US, a diagnosis of LN does not always adequately explain a mass on imaging. If CNB of a BI-RADS 5 mass reveals LN, it should be considered a discordant finding warranting surgical excision [3].

LCIS may reveal non-mass enhancement on contrast-enhanced MRI imaging (Fig. 6.4). However as differential for NME is wide ranging from benign proliferative lesion to high risk to malignant process, biopsy is a must. Broader sampling is needed to avoid underestimation, and therefore VAB is preferred over CNB.

Upgradation Rates Cases of LN with pathological radiological discordance, pleomorphic cytology, or necrosis, as well as those with accompanying AIDEP, have significantly greater upgrade rates than those with no necrosis and radiological-pathological concordance.

LN is a clonal neoplastic proliferation and a precursor to invasive malignancy, according to molecular studies. Women with LCIS have a

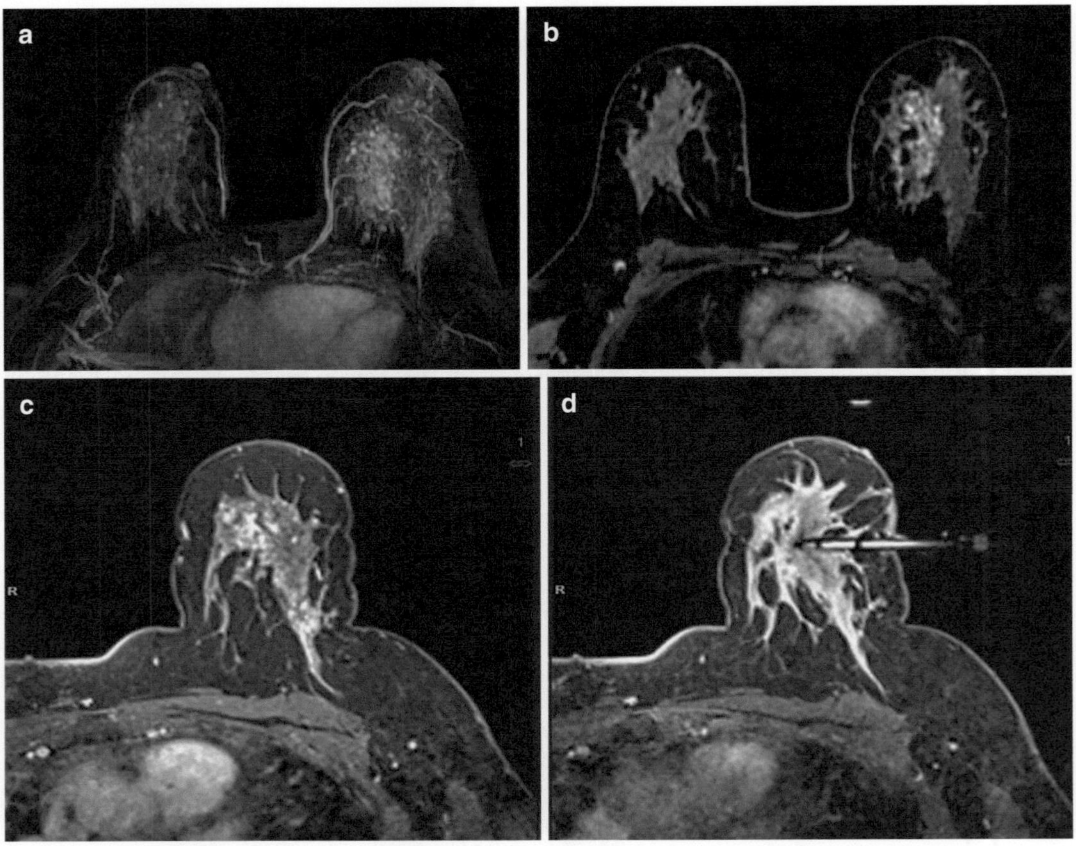

Fig. 6.4 CEMRI breasts of a 47-year-old female had preoperative breast MRI for right breast cancer. MIP and post-contrast T1 WI (**a**, **b**) show an area of non-mass enhancement in the upper inner quadrant of the left breast. As it was mammographically and sonographically occult, MRI-guided VAB with 10 G probe revealed atypical lobular hyperplasia with benign breast changes

4–12 times higher chance of having breast cancer than women without LN, while women with ALH have a 4–5 times higher risk of developing breast cancer than women without LN.

The literature shows that the upgrade rate after surgical excision ranges from 0% to 40%. Murray et al. found a significant difference in the upgrade rate between cases with and without radiologic-pathologic discrepancy (38% vs 3%, respectively) in 85 cases of classic LN [5]. After the LN diagnosis, the relative chance of developing cancer is 1–2% after 1 year, 15–17% after 15 years, and 35% after 35 years, with ipsilateral and contralateral breast cancer rates being nearly equal (8.7 and 6.7%, respectively). When there is the presence of proliferative high-risk lesions combined with a family history of breast cancer, the risk doubles. Although, all types of invasive carcinoma have been recorded following a LN diagnosis, invasive lobular carcinoma or special-type carcinomas are more common than in the general breast cancer population.

Immunophenotypingly and cytogenetically LN, lobular invasive carcinoma and low-grade DCIS are similar revealing estrogen receptor (ER) and progesterone receptor positivity and low Ki-67. However, studies showed that LN is not a precursor of invasive breast cancer. Therefore, it is considered to be a risk marker for breast cancer. Since the pleomorphic variant of LCIS is positive for human epidermal growth factor receptor 2 as well as p53 and the proliferative index Ki-67 but is negative for ER, it is considered a precursor of invasive breast cancer [6].

LCIS can be differentiated from DCIS by the lack of expression of E-cadherin. In very few cases, LCIS can express E-cadherin, and so in histologic samples where differentiation as LCIS or DCIS is difficult, these are classified as "carcinoma in situ with mixed ductal and lobular features."

Management Observation in the setting of small volume lesions completely removed with VAB, rad-path concordance, and absence of other high-risk lesions is suggested. Surgery is recommended for LCIS variants on core biopsy.

6.4 Papillary Lesions

Papillary lesions are characterized by visualization of papillary fronds in an intraductal lesion with central fibrovascular core connecting them to the ductal wall in the lesion, on histopathological assessment (Fig. 6.5). The fibrovascular core is lined by ductal epithelial as well as myoepithelial cells, and the former can undergo variable degree of apocrine metaplasia [3]. Based on the variable appearances on pathological evaluation, the papillary lesions have been classified into four major categories:

(a) Papilloma without atypia.
(b) Papilloma with atypia (ADH or classical LN), both belonging to the B3 category; however the small (<2 mm) papillomas can be categorized as B2 if it is completely surrounded by a duct.
(c) Papilloma with DCIS or papilloma completely involved by DCIS (encapsulated papillary carcinoma).
(d) Solid papillary carcinoma belonging to B4 or B5a category [3].

These papillary lesions can also be classified into central and peripheral groups based on their location. The central papillomas are generally seen in isolation or single lesions arising from the ducts in sub-areolar region, whereas peripheral papillomas are often multiple and develop within the TDLU involving galactophorous ducts.

The pathologist must analyze the extent of the area of atypical epithelial proliferation present while assessing the histopathology of papillary lesions with atypia. If this is present in numerous cores, even if the samples are large, the area cannot be determined, and distinguishing atypical epithelial proliferation inside a papilloma (3 mm in extent) from low-grade DCIS within a papilloma (>3 mm) may be difficult.

Imaging Asymptomatic papillomas can be discovered during routine breast screening. However, in up to 20–50% of cases, they can appear as a palpable lump at the nipple or with

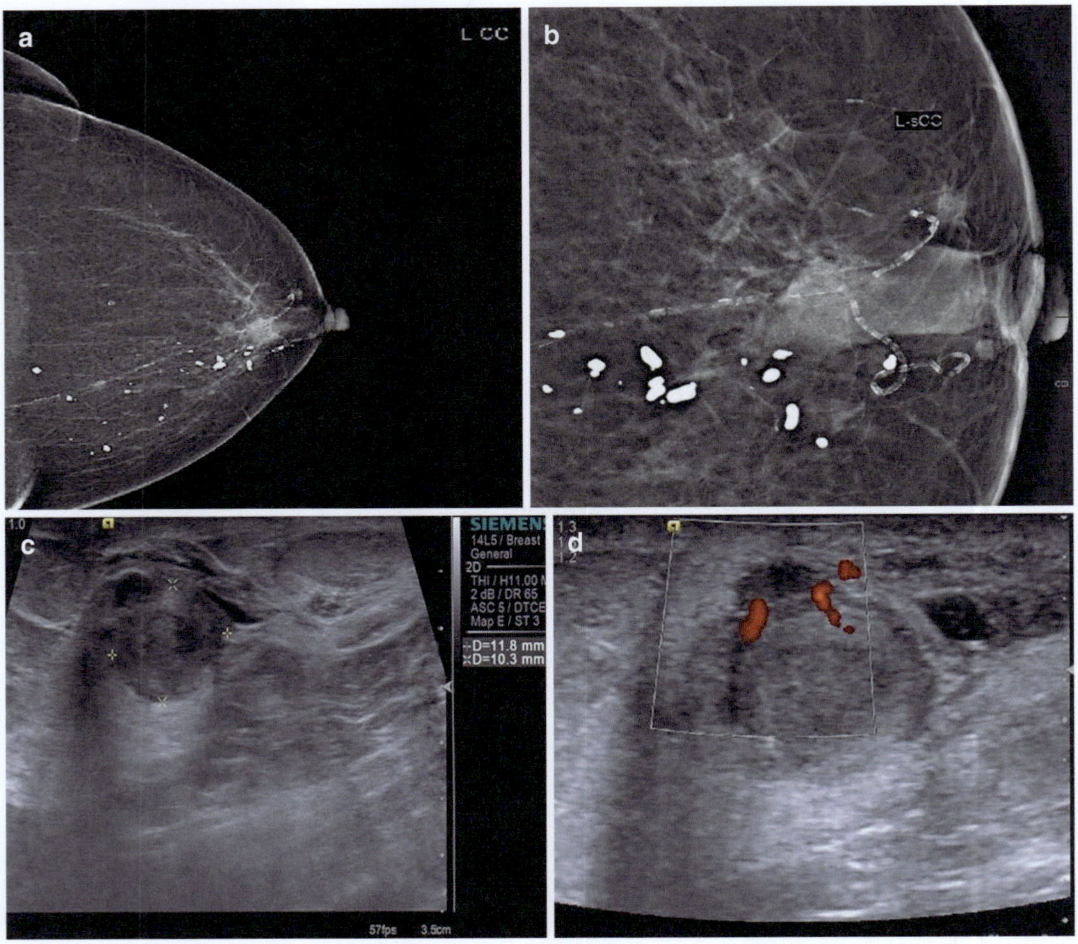

Fig. 6.5 A 51-year-old female presented with a complaint of blood-stained nipple discharge in the left breast with no palpable lump. CC and spot images (**a**, **b**) of mammogram showed a radio dense mass with partially indistinct margins in the left retroareolar region. Benign calcification also noted. Ultrasound images (**c**, **d**) showed dilated ducts in the retroareolar region. There is an isoechoic lesion of size 12 × 10 mm in the retroareolar region with mild peripheral vascularity, which is connected with the dilated duct. Histopathology revealed intraductal papilloma

bloody nipple discharge due to pedicle torsion. Mammography has low sensitivity and specificity; when apparent, mammographic findings may include asymmetric areas of increased density, dilated ducts, or single lesions with accompanying microcalcifications (Fig. 6.5a, b).

Breast USG is quite useful in the identification of papillomas. A solid, round mass with well-circumscribed margins; an intracystic mass; or a hypoechoic, well-defined mass in a dilated duct may be seen on ultrasound (Fig. 6.5c). Color Doppler can be used to assess the fibrovascular stalk of papillomas (Fig. 6.5d). On MRI it can be seen as intraductal enhancing nodule, small linear focus of enhancement solid-enhancing mass, intracystic mass, or as non-mass enhancement. It can be seen as irregular-shaped mass on MRI if its extending into the branch vessel [3].

When the diagnosis of papilloma has already been established, an MRI can be used to determine the extent of the disease in cases of multiple

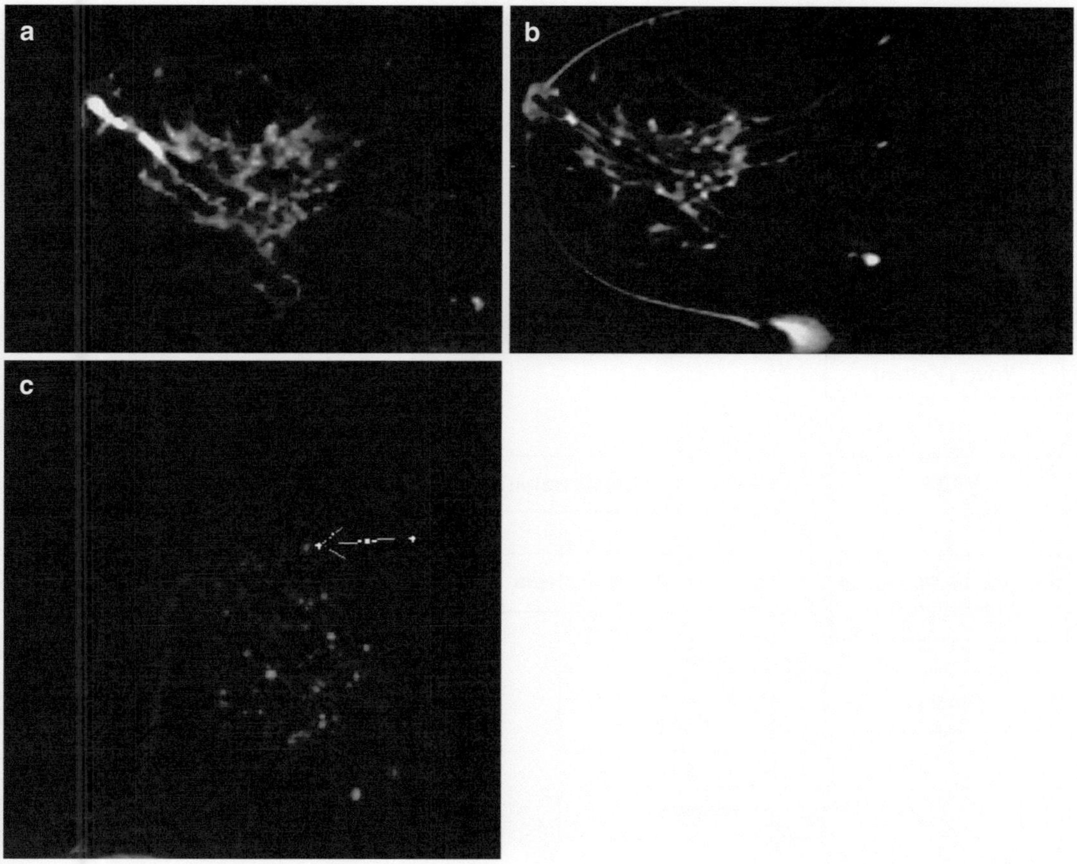

Fig. 6.6 A 60-year-old female patient complained of left breast nipple discharge associated with pain. CEMRI breast (**a**–**c**) revealed a mildly distended duct at 2 o'clock position of the left breast with a couple of tiny 2 to 3 mm intraductal enhancing foci seen within this distended duct (arrow), likely to represent intraductal papilliferous lesions along with marked background enhancement. Major duct excision was performed for this patient which showed intraductal papillomas

papillomatosis or when non-mass findings are noted on US. When histopathological examination reveals malignant papillary lesions, MRI provides for a more precise estimation of disease extent (Fig. 6.6a–c).The ducts are filled with TI hyperintense contents on MRI when there is bloody nipple discharge so subtracted images should be obtained to see for any small enhancing intraductal papilloma which can be easily missed due to TI hyperintense contents.

Upgradation Rates The risk of invasive cancer is two times higher in the central form and three times higher in the peripheral form, with a greater probability of invasive cancer of up to 7.5% in papilloma with atypia. Multiple peripheral papillomas (referred to as "papillomatosis") at CNB further increase the upgrade rates for papillary lesions. The criteria that are most indicative of an upgrade to malignancy are peripheral location, microcalcifications (identified imaging), lesion size (>1 cm), older patient age, and associated HRL like ADH/ALH. In a study by Khan et al., a 7.5% upgrade after surgery was obtained for intraductal papillomas that lacked atypia as compared to 32% for those that contained atypia versus 33% for patients with concurrent ADH/ALH [7].

The upgrade rates are higher when papillomas without atypia are diagnosed on CNB (0–12%) as compared to VAB with no significant upgrade rates [3].

Management **(Figs. 6.7 and 6.8)** It is largely variable as there are low upgrade rates in cases of pure intraductal papillomas and high upgrade rates in papillomas with atypia. According to

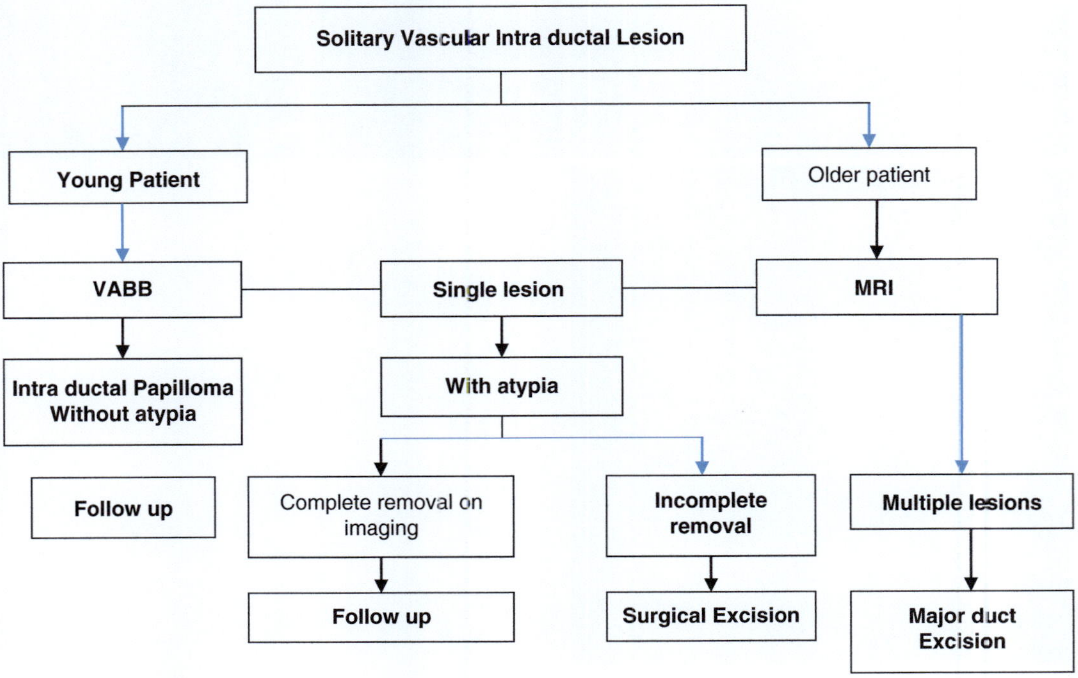

Fig. 6.7 Algorithmic approach to single intraductal papillary lesion

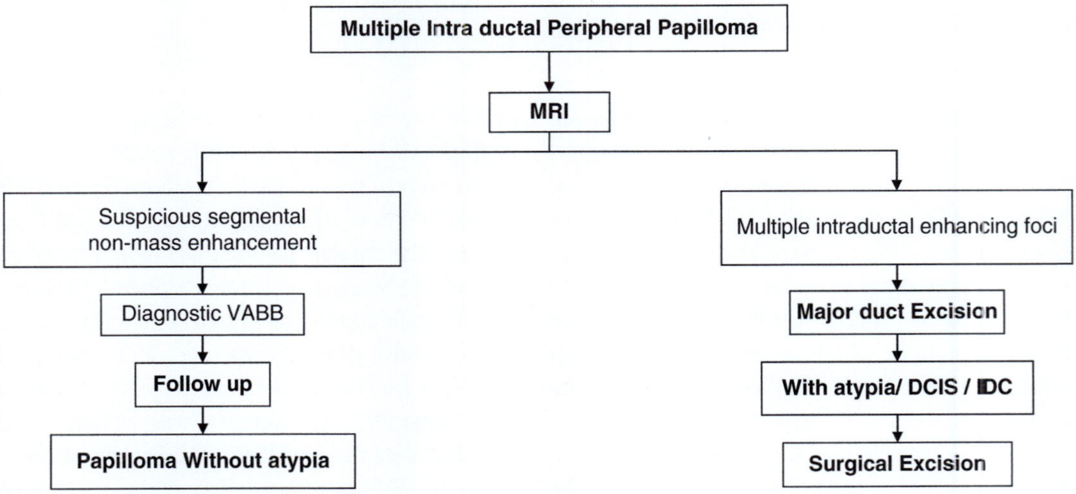

Fig. 6.8 Algorithmic approach to multiple intraductal papillary lesions

National Health Service Breast Screening Programme, papilloma with atypia should undergo surgical excision. According to one school of thought, incidental papilloma without atypia can be observed, if enough sample is obtained and rad-path concordance is established [3]; however the current recommendation from the third International Consensus Conference on lesions of uncertain malignant potential (B3) in CNB-based diagnosis of proliferative lesion without atypia is excision (surgical or vacuum-assisted excision (VAE)) [8]. Surgical excision is preferred for large lesions, while for smaller lesion which can be completely removed, VAE is preferred. For multiple papillomatosis, surgical excision is recommended [3].

6.5 Radial Scar and Complex Sclerosing Lesion (CSL)

The terms radial scar and complex sclerosing lesion are used to describe lesions that are essentially the same in appearance but vary in size, with CSL being larger lesions and radial scarbeing lesions that are not more than 10 mm in size. The central fibroelastic core of RS and CSL is surrounded by elastic fibers and contains one to many inflamed ducts. Other ducts also form a stellate convergence into the scar-like region. The epithelium lining the later ducts may exhibit a wide range of alterations, with benign epithelioid (common ductal hyperplasia) being the most common. On both radiological and histological grounds, the central scar-like area combined with the stellate appearance of the surrounding ducts easily mimics invasive cancer [9].

Because of its stellate configuration, RS is a breast lesion that may resemble invasive cancer. A CSL is a lesion that is greater than 10 mm and has more complicated features than a RS. Traditionally, RS and CSL are not palpable. Women under the age of 30 are less likely to have radial scars than women between the ages of 30 and 60.

Imaging Features A radiolucent star-shaped lesion that generally characterizes a RS/CSL on mammography can be mistaken for an invasive cancer in its presentation. The RS shows the presence of radiolucent linear structures paralleling the radiopaque spicules and is seen as "black stars," while cancers resemble "white stars" with white spicules radiating from radio-opaque center. Asymmetry, lack of a palpable mass and varying appearance of distortion on different mammographic projections are additional characteristic signs (Fig. 6.9a, b). Calcifications are a frequent observation; in certain circumstances, they could be the only doubtful finding that prompts a biopsy.

With the increased use of digital breast tomosynthesis (DBT), the detection rate of RS has increased due to better visualization, characterization, and identification of architectural distortion. RS is the most frequently reported histology among high-risk lesions. Architectural distortion on diagnostic DBT has been reported to demonstrate malignancy in over one-third of cases at pathology.

The sonographic appearance of RS varies from a focal area of shadowing without an accompanying mass to a hypoechoic, irregular mass with indistinct margins [3] (Fig. 6.9c, d). In some instances, RS may exhibit inherent stiffness during elastography.

Similar variations can be seen in RS/CSL's MRI appearance. RS may appear as distortion or spiculate lesion. Since it can closely mimic cancer, further confirmation with biopsy is warranted. If it is not associated with enhancement, malignancy is less likely. At times it can be seen as non-mass enhancement with regional, homogenous enhancement and a type 3 enhancement kinetic curve [10] (Fig. 6.10a–d).

Contrast enhancement is showing an increasing promise in differentiating RS from cancer. For some radiological lesions, the periphery (such as the radial scar) may be the area to target, but for others, there is no proof that any

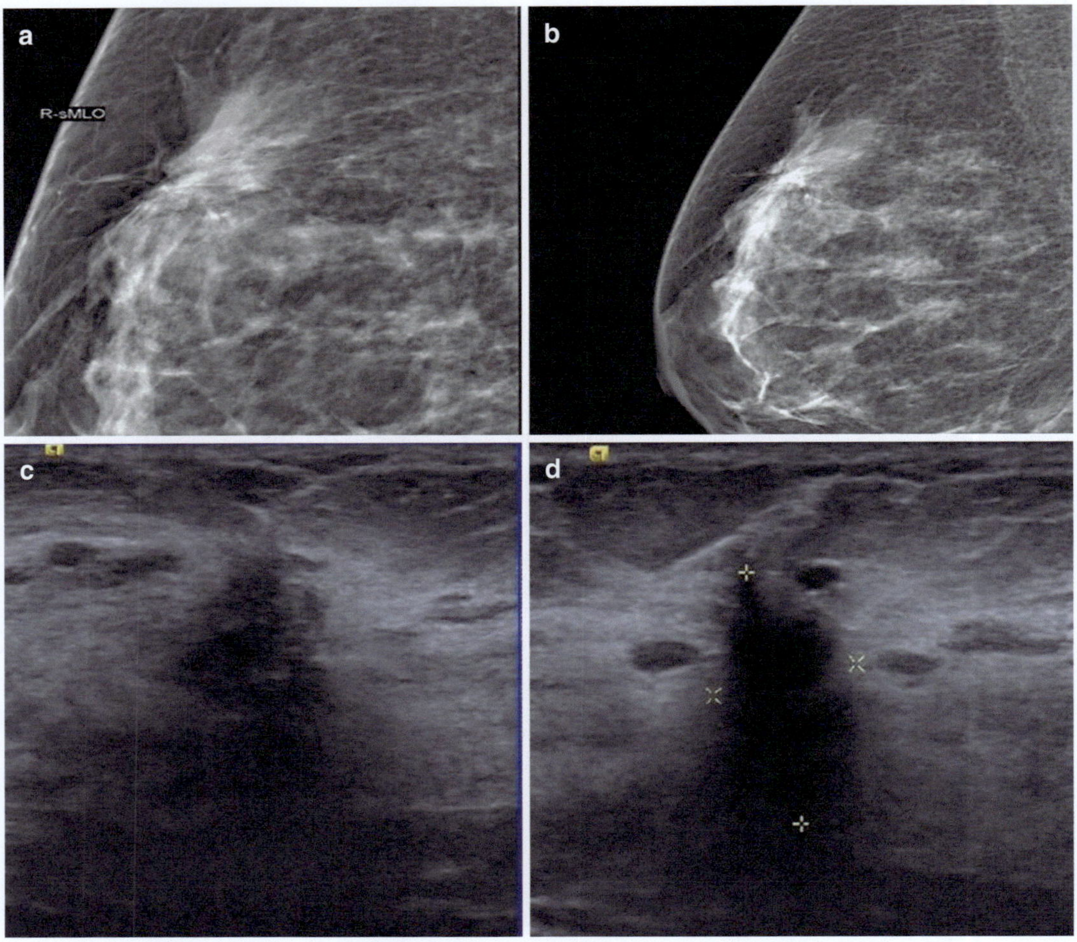

Fig. 6.9 A 37-year-old female presented with a right breast lump. Mammographic images (**a**, **b**) show a focal area of distortion in the upper outer quadrant of the right breast with a lucent center and radiating black line from the center. (**c**, **d**) Ultrasound images revealed an area of marked focal shadowing at 10 o'clock position (BI-RADS 4C). It is associated with a thick echogenic rim and distortion. Multiple small cysts, few of which show internal echoes within, are seen around the lesion

concurrent, undiagnosed cancer is likely to be in a specific zone of the radiological abnormality.

Notably, larger CSLs may be technically challenging to extract with vacuum-assisted technology, and sampling from greater than one site is thought to be the most practical strategy. Overall, the authors believe that sampling is sufficient if a large region of change is reduced by at least one-third. However, even when present, any malignancy associated with such areas is often low-grade (DCIS or invasive) illness. This is most frequently an area of low suspicion microcalcification and may indicate a columnar cell process with flat epithelial atypia as a component.

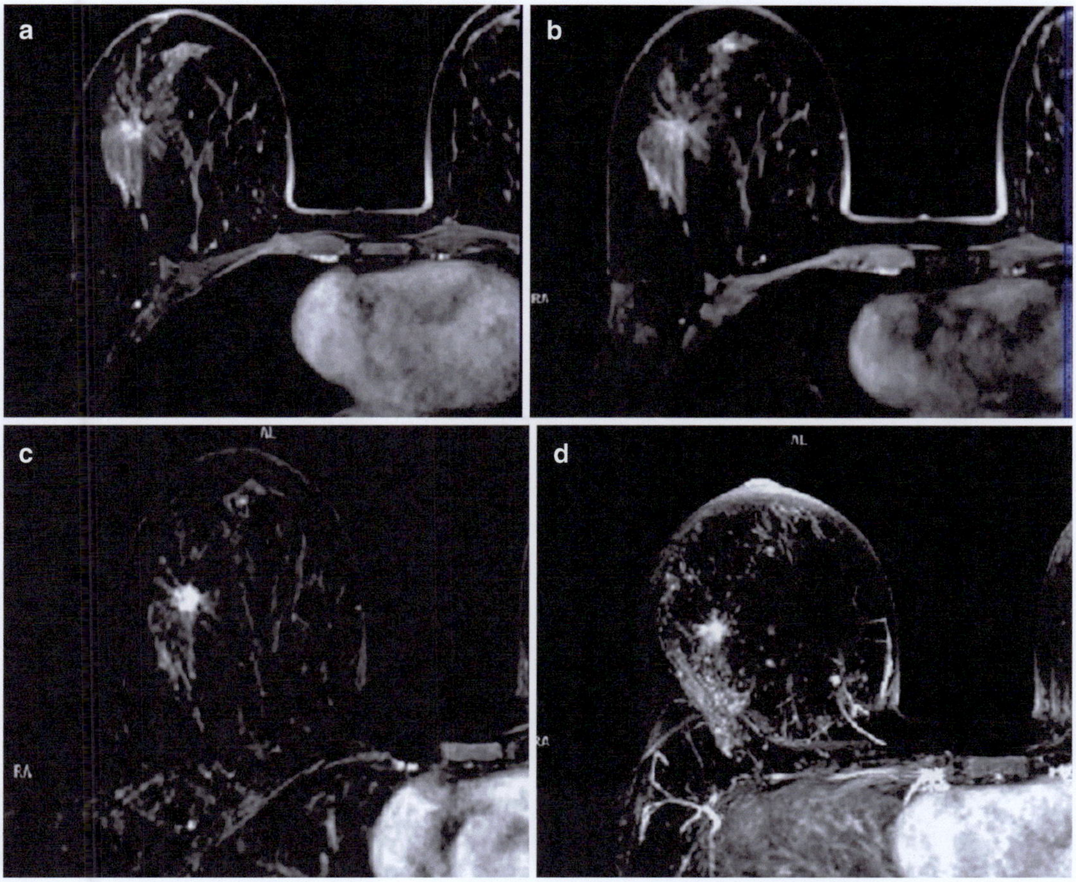

Fig. 6.10 Post-contrast T1 fat sat CEMRI images (**a–c**) and MIP (**d**) images reveal an area of distortion in the outer half of the right breast at 10 o'clock position with central irregular enhancement. Post-biopsy specimen revealed complex sclerosing adenosis

Upgradation Rates In a meta-analysis of 49 studies that included 3163 RS, there were 217 upgrades to malignancies, 71 (32.7%) invasive and 144 (66.4%) DCIS. The pooled estimate was 7%. In RS assessed by 14 G CNB, the upgrade rates were the following: without atypia (5%) and with atypia (29%) (95% CI 20, 38%). For RS assessed by 8–16 G CNB, the respective upgrade rates were 2% and 11% and for RS assessed by 8–11 vacuum-assisted biopsies, 1% and 18% [11].

Management (Fig. 6.11) After the identification of RS (without atypia) on CNB with careful radiological correlation, therapeutic VAE is recommended. If the target lesion was entirely eliminated, after diagnostic VAB imaging, follow-up is recommended. When RS is associated with atypia, surgery is recommended [8].

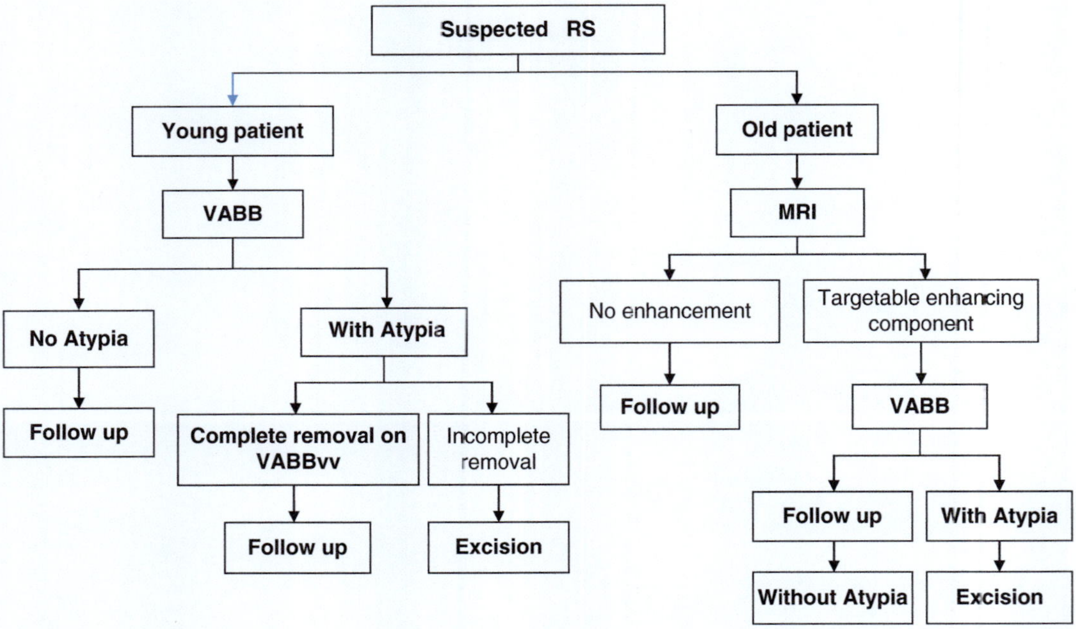

Fig. 6.11 Algorithmic approach in suspicious radial scar on mammography

6.6 Phyllodes

Phyllodes tumors are uncommon breast fibroepithelial lesions that resemble fibroadenomas and hamartomas. From a histological perspective, they can take on benign, borderline, or obviously malignant forms. Sometimes it can be difficult to differentiate a conventional fibroadenoma from a phyllodes tumor. Therefore, for cases that are ambiguous, the WHO suggests to use term "fibroepithelial tumors" to describe the entity. The malignant phyllodes tumors are classified as B5b lesions of the breast; benign and borderline phyllodes tumors are classified as B3 lesions of the breast. Only 20% of all lesions are either borderline or malignant; most often these B3 lesions are benign [3, 8].

Fewer than 1% of all breast cancers and 2–3% of fibroepithelial neoplasms are phyllodes tumors of the breast. It frequently exhibits a huge size and/or quick growth. Despite the average age of incidence being 25 to 30 years in Asian countries, this tumor typically affects women between the ages of 40 and 51 [3].

Histologically, PT exhibit an enhanced stromal intracanalicular growth pattern, with leaf-like projections into variably dilated lumina. These lumina are lined by epithelia and myoepithelial cell layers, stretched into arc-like clefts lining the stromal fronds. This typical histologic analysis differentiates these tumors from fibroadenomas and other stromal sarcomas [8]. Benign phyllodes on histopathology usually exhibit low cellularity, circumscribed borders, less than five mitoses/10 high power field (HPF), monomorphic stromal cell nuclei, and lack stromal overgrowth. On the other hand, malignant phyllodes generally exhibit increased cellularity, infiltrative borders, more than ten mitoses/10 HPF, marked stromal nuclear pleomorphism and stromal overgrowth with or without heterologous stromal malignant elements (such as malignant bone/cartilage/fat). Borderline phyllodes have some but not all features of malignant PT.

Diagnosis and Imaging A phyllodes tumor often appears as a unilateral mass that is often symptomatic in the form of palpable and movable lump which is usually not fixed to deep tissues. By virtue of its large size, it stretches the overlying skin with distension of the superficial veins, and its size ranges from 2 to 5 cm. Rapid growth is a pathognomonic feature for phyllodes tumors, and imaging findings of phyllodes tumors typically overlap with more commonly seen entity of fibroadenoma.

When viewed on a mammogram, phyllodes tumors show as a large, ovoid, highly opaque mass that is lobulated, and because of their rapid growth, coarse calcifications can rarely be visible. It displaces the surrounding fat which can be seen as a lucent halo around its margins that can be better appreciated on digital breast tomosynthesis.

On ultrasonography, it typically appears as a solid mass with moderately heterogeneous internal echotexture, with or without posterior acoustic enhancement, internal microcystic areas, and moderate vascularity.

On MRI, it appears as an oval lobulated mass with internal septations and rapid post-contrast enhancement. These usually show circumscribed margins, low signal on T1-weighted sequences, and variable signal on T2-weighted sequences. The high T2 signal is attributed to fluid-filled slit-like spaces and T2-weighted signal intensity less than or equal to normal breast tissue and low apparent diffusion coefficient indicate a higher risk of associated malignancy. It may present as a solid-cystic lesion with post-contrast images showing enhancement of the solid portion of the tumor [3] (Fig. 6.12).

Prognosis Most phyllodes tumors exhibit a benign nature, and the chance of recurrence ranges

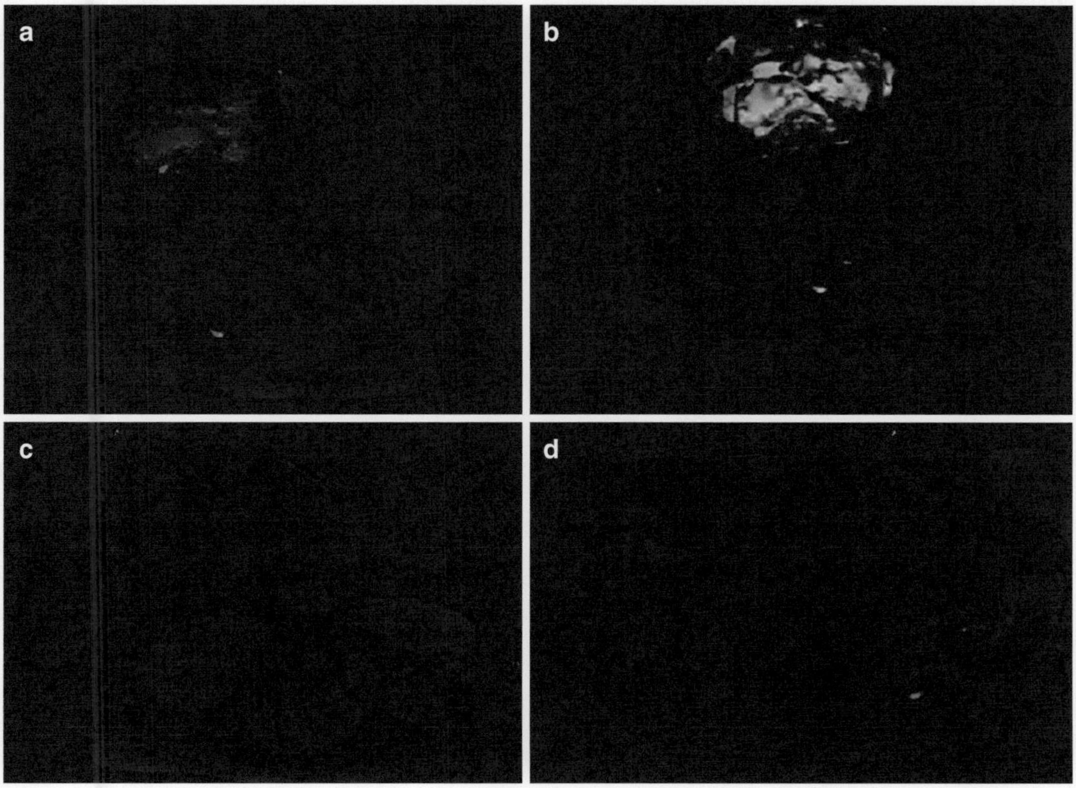

Fig. 6.12 Phyllodes tumor of the right breast: MRI images reveal a large lobulated heterogeneous mass involving an almost entire right breast (**a–d**) in a 37-year-old female. The mass shows a heterogeneous signal on T2 WI (**a**, **b**) with the presence of fluid/cystic areas within and intermediate signal on T1 WI (**c**)

from 10% to 20% for benign lesions and up to 30% for borderline or malignant lesions [8]. Based on histology, malignant phyllodes tumors have a 15–20% chance of metastasizing. Additionally, a number of studies confirmed that involved margins are a significant predictor of recurrence.

Management According to the data that are currently available, surgical excision is the most frequent treatment for phyllodes tumors [12]. When identified at VAB, the likelihood of phyllodes underestimate is only 8%, compared to 20% when diagnosed at CNB [13]. The third International Consensus Conference on lesions of unknown malignant potential (B3) advises open surgical excision with clear margins when a phyllodes tumor is discovered at CNB based on the available information. A benign phyllodes tumor may be monitored if it is unintentionally discovered at the VAB without any associated imaging findings; however borderline and malignant phyllodes tumors must be re-excised in order to achieve clear margins. A surgical excision should be carried out if a lesion that was previously diagnosed as a fibroadenoma experiences fast changes in size [14].

6.7 Flat Epithelial Atypia

The WHO defines FEA as a neoplastic intraductal alteration of the breast characterized by the substitution of native epithelial cells with one layer or three to five layers of moderately atypical cells without architectural atypia. FEA can be seen in 1–2% of benign breast biopsies. Typically, it is discovered secondary to suspicious microcalcifications [15]. These lesions frequently appear on mammography as fine amorphous or branching microcalcifications with accompanying significant duct dilatation because they secrete intraluminal secretions.

Additionally, FEA is frequently found in conjunction with other high-risk breast lesions like ALH, ADH, or LN, though it is now more frequently referred to as a precursor of the latter alteration. It is also thought to be a non-obligatory precursor of invasive carcinoma along with ADH and DCIS as there is a continuum morphological spectrum of ductal proliferations from FEA to ADH and low-grade DCIS [3].

FEA can co-occur in situ or invasive breast cancers, most typically tubular carcinoma. In a meta-analysis by Forester et al., an upgrade rate of 11% was found with FEA lesions to malignancy [16]. ADH and low-grade DCIS are the most common malignant findings found with FEA detected at CNB or VAB, and although invasive carcinoma (often highly differentiated) can occur, it is a less common finding. According to another meta-analysis of 32 studies, the proportion of patients upgraded to cancer ranged from 0% to 42%, with a pooled estimate of 11.1% overall. With the investigation being limited to 16 higher-quality studies, the pooled upgrade rate of 7.5% was seen with cancer, and the invasive cancer rate was 3% [17].

Management According to the guidelines set by the Third International Consensus Conference on B3 lesions, if FEA is diagnosed on core needle biopsy (CNB), surgical excision or vacuum-assisted excision (VAE) is recommended, depending on the clinical presentation and lesion size. However, if more than 90% of the lesion is removed during diagnostic vacuum-assisted biopsy (VAB), radiological surveillance may be considered.

On the other hand, if the lesion is found to represent as a large area of microcalcifications or if pathology and radiology discordance is seen, surgical intervention is required. No additional therapy is advised if FEA is found within surgical resection edges unless microcalcifications have not been entirely removed.

6.8 Importance of Diagnostic Vacuum-Assisted Biopsy and Vacuum-Assisted Excision

In VAB, the standard 14G needle is replaced with a vacuum biopsy needle (typically 11-7G) with application vacuum suction for the specimen/sample from the tissue using single time needle

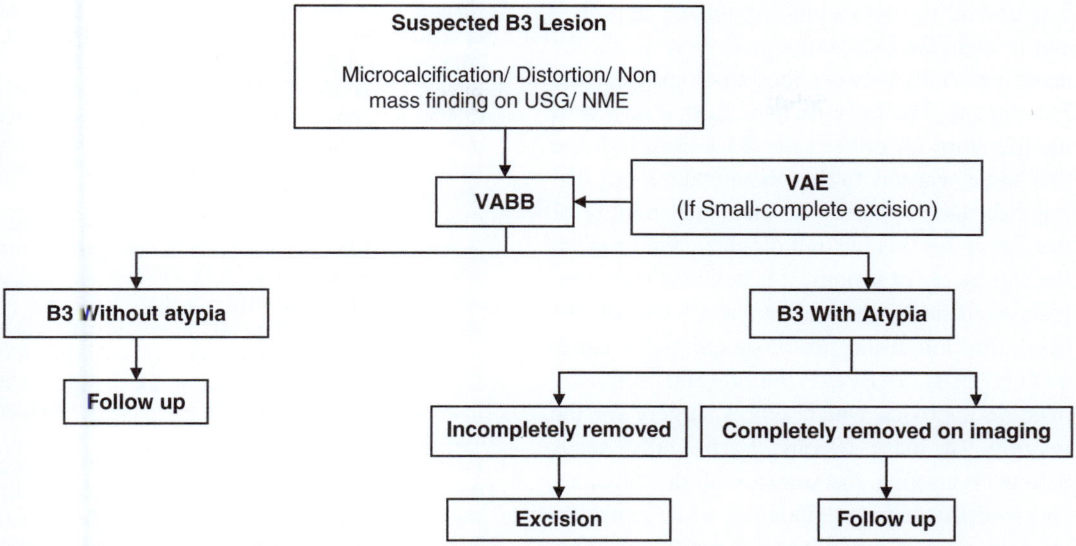

Fig. 6.13 Algorithmic approach to B3 lesions at the author's institute

insertion (Fig. 6.12). In comparison to traditional CNB, VAB enables sampling a larger volume of the tissue to offer enough tissue for pathologists to make a diagnosis. It is by virtue of these advantages that it has comparable accuracy as surgical biopsy. A final B-category is documented, just like a traditional core biopsy.

VAB can remove the entire lesion when the size is less than 15 mm. Thus, for the comprehensive secondary examination of the majority of B3 lesions, whether initially detected on core biopsy or primary diagnostic VAB, VAE can be considered wherever necessary.

When treating large lesions (such as widespread microcalcifications), VAB from multiple sites should be taken and targeted correctly based on the radiological findings. Greater radiological risk areas should be the focus of additional sampling, ideally far from the location of the initial specimen.

Although the technique suggested here for managing B3 lesions by VAE rather than surgical excision has not been widely adopted, there is evidence from some units that this does in fact reduce the number of benign open surgical biopsies and is a safer method. One of the few series included 398 patients with B3 lesions, out of which 321 underwent "second-line" VAB, 24% underwent additional surgery, and 245 in whom surgery was avoided; more importantly, at the 3-year follow-up, it showed no progression or development of cancer at the biopsy site.

Another important step is to place the tumor marker clip at the site of VAB or VAE followed by check mammogram to keep as reference for subsequent follow-up visits.

It is clear that the B3 lesions carry a variety of risks for developing into DCIS or invasive carcinoma, and those that are additionally accompanied by epithelial atypia raise the likelihood that either breast may develop carcinoma in the coming years (Fig. 6.13). All these cases should be discussed in MDT, and further management in terms of surgical excision/VAE or imaging surveillance should be decided for individual cases. The patient's age, presentation, family history, radiology pathology concordance, and patient's choice should be considered prior to taking informed decision regarding management.

6.9 Conclusion

The purpose of this chapter is to provide an overview and recommendations for B3 breast lesions. Regarding these potentially troublesome lesions, it is crucial to use a multidisciplinary approach and to maintain close communication within the team, especially between the pathologists and the radiologists. The upgrade rates from a review of the literature for each of the B3 lesions indicate that these warrant further examination—to distinguish their existence as incidental finding or the cause for visible radiological abnormality. For this group of lesions, it is believed that complete excision by the VAB approach can be utilized after initial diagnostic sampling (by either 14 G or VAB). VAB/VAE is a safe and minimally invasive approach which avoids surgery for the majority of these lesions. Each entity needs patient counseling, discussion with the clinician, and assessment for upgradation while considering follow-up or surveillance as per the available guidelines.

References

1. Clauser P, Kapetas P, Stöttinger A, et al. A risk stratifcation algorithm for lesions of uncertain malignant potential diagnosed by vacuum-assisted breast biopsy (VABB) of mammographic microcalcifcations. Eur J Radiol. 2020;135:109479. https://doi.org/10.1016/j.ejrad.2020.109479.
2. Shaaban AM, Sharma N. Management of B3 lesions—practical issues. Curr Breast Cancer Rep. 2019;11:83–8. https://doi.org/10.1007/s12609-019-0310-6.
3. Catanzariti F, et al. High-risk lesions of the breast: concurrent diagnostic tools and management recommendations. Insights Imaging. 2021;12:63. https://doi.org/10.1186/s13244-021-01005-6.
4. Schiaffino S, Calabrese M, Melani EF. Upgrade rate of percutaneously diagnosed pure atypical ductal hyperplasia: systematic review and meta-analysis of 6458 lesions. Radiology. 2020;294(1):76–86. https://doi.org/10.1148/radiol.2019190748. https://pubmed.ncbi.nlm.nih.gov/31660803/.
5. Murray MP, Luedtke C, Liberman L, et al. Classic lobular carcinoma in situ and atypical lobular hyperplasia at percutaneous breast core biopsy: outcomes of prospective excision. Cancer. 2013;119:1073–9.
6. Fasola CE, Chen JJ, Jensen KC, Allison KH, Horst KC. Characteristics and clinical outcomes of pleomorphic lobular carcinoma in situ of the breast. Breast J. 2018;24:66–9. https://doi.org/10.1111/tbj.12843.
7. Khan S, Diaz A, Archer KJ, et al. Papillary lesions of the breast: to excise or observe? Breast J. 2018;24:350–5. https://doi.org/10.1111/tbj.12907.
8. Elfgen C, et al. Third International Consensus Conference on lesions of uncertain malignant potential in the breast (B3 lesions). Virchows Archiv. 2023;483:5–20. https://doi.org/10.1007/s00428-023-03566-x.
9. Chou WYY, Veis DJ, Aft R. Radial scar on image-guided breast biopsy: is surgical excision necessary? Breast Cancer Res Treat. 2018;170:313–20. https://doi.org/10.1007/s10549-018-47+41-y.
10. Ha SM, Cha JH, Shin HJ, et al. Radial scars/complex sclerosing lesions of the breast: radiologic and clinicopathologic correlation. BMC Med Imaging. 2018;18:39. https://doi.org/10.1186/s12880-018-0279-z.
11. Farshid G, Buckley E. Meta-analysis of upgrade rates in 3163 radial scars excised after needle core biopsy diagnosis. Breast Cancer Res Treat. 2019;174(1):165–77. https://doi.org/10.1007/s10549-018-5040-3. Epub 2018 Nov 20
12. Ouyang Q, Li S, Tan C, et al. Benign phyllodes tumor of the breast diagnosed after ultrasound-guided vacuum-assisted biopsy: surgical excision or wait-and-watch? Ann Surg Oncol. 2016;23:1129–34. https://doi.org/10.1245/s10434-015-4990-5.
13. Youk JH, Kim H, Kim E-K, Son EJ, Kim MJ, Kim JA. Phyllodes tumor diagnosed after ultrasound-guided vacuum-assisted excision: should it be followed by surgical excision? Ultrasound Med Biol. 2015;41:741–7. https://doi.org/10.1016/j.ultrasmedbio.2014.11.004.
14. Pinder SE, Shaaban A, Deb R, et al. NHS breast screening multidisciplinary working group guidelines for the diagnosis and management of breast lesions of uncertain malignant potential on core biopsy (B3 lesions). Clin Radiol. 2018;73:682–92. https://doi.org/10.1016/j.crad.2018.04.004.
15. Schiafno S, Gristina L, Villa A, et al. Flat epithelial atypia: conservative management of patients without residual microcalcifcations post-vacuum-assisted breast biopsy. Br J Radiol. 2018;91(1081):20170484. https://doi.org/10.1259/bjr.20170484.
16. Forester ND, Lowes S, Mitchell E, Twiddy M. High risk (B3) breast lesions: what is the incidence of malignancy for individual lesion subtypes? A systematic review and meta-analysis. Eur J Surg Oncol. 2019;45:519–27. https://doi.org/10.1016/j.ejso.2018.12.008.
17. Rudin AV, Hoskin TL, Fahy A, Farrell AM, Nassar A, Ghosh K, Degnim AC. Flat epithelial atypia on core biopsy and upgrade to cancer: a systematic review and meta-analysis. Ann Surg Oncol. 2017;24(12):3549–58. https://doi.org/10.1245/s10434-017-6059-0. Epub 2017 Aug 22

Benign Mimics of Malignancy

7

Smriti Hari, Shrea Gulati, and Ekta Dhamija

Abstract

Breast cancer is often the first diagnosis that comes to one's mind when a patient presents with complaints related to the breast. However, a variety of benign entities can mimic breast cancer both clinically and radiologically. These entities can be divided into three main categories: inflammatory, proliferative and neoplastic. The radiologist has an armamentarium of investigations such as mammography, ultrasound and magnetic resonance imaging (MRI) available for detailed evaluation. It is of great importance that the radiologist be familiar with the various appearances so that an appropriate differential diagnosis can be considered. Biopsy, which may be ultrasound, mammography, or MRI-guided helps in arriving at a final diagnosis. It is imperative for the radiologist to be familiar with the imaging appearances of these mimics of breast cancer so that they can be more accepting to the seemingly discordant benign histopathological findings on radio-pathological correlation and help guide appropriate management. The purpose of this chapter is to illustrate the spectrum of breast pathologies which may resemble the ominous appearance of breast cancer radiologically.

Keywords

Breast cancer · Breast ultrasound · MRI breast · Mimics · Mastitis · Radial scar Circumscribed masses · Spiculated masses Phyllodes

7.1 Introduction

Breast carcinoma is the gravest diagnosis that comes to one's mind whenever presented with complaints of breast lump, nipple discharge or pain. A gamut of imaging modalities like mammography (MG), ultrasound (US), contrast-enhanced mammography and magnetic resonance imaging (MRI) are present in the armamentarium of the radiologist. The imaging features on each of these modalities lead the radiologist to assess how suspicious the abnormality is for malignancy and accordingly assign the appropriate Breast Imaging Reporting and Data System (BIRADS) category. Lesions which have an irregular shape and indistinct or spiculated margins on mammography indicate aggressiveness and presence of fine pleomorphic or linear branching patterns of microcalcification, and associated findings such as skin thickening and axillary lymphadenopathy imply the presence of

S. Hari · S. Gulati
Radiodiagnosis & Interventional Radiology, AIIMS, New Delhi, India

E. Dhamija (✉)
Department of Diagnostic and Interventional Onco-Radiology, IRCH, AIIMS, New Delhi, India

E. Dhamija, S. V. S. Deo (eds.), *Imaging in Management of Breast Diseases*,
https://doi.org/10.1007/978-981-96-4998-3_7

underlying malignancy. On the other hand, lesions which are round or oval shaped with circumscribed margins are likely to be benign. The caveat here is that some variants of breast carcinoma such as mucinous, medullary and papillary breast carcinoma closely mimic benign entities like fibroadenoma on imaging.

US is an easily available and excellent modality which can differentiate solid from cystic lesions. Amongst the solid lesions, the presence of spiculated margins has the highest positive predictive value for malignancy. Other features which indicate malignancy include lesion appearing taller than wider, microlobulated or angular margins, posterior acoustic shadowing, ductal extension and microcalcifications. Multiparametric breast MRI is a problem-solving modality owing to its high negative predictive value. The presence of high signal intensity (SI) on T2-weighted images (T2WI) indicates that the lesion is likely to be benign, for example, cyst, myxoid fibroadenoma, fat necrosis and lymph nodes [1]. Since most malignant lesions have high cellularity and low water content, they are unlikely to show high signal intensity relative to parenchyma on T2-weighted imaging. However, mucinous carcinoma, necrotic cancer and metaplastic carcinoma also show high signal on T2-weighted images [2]. There are a spectrum of other breast pathologies which can mimic breast carcinoma both clinically and radiologically. These can be classified under inflammatory, proliferative and neoplastic categories (Table 7.1). This chapter aims to discuss the multimodality imaging findings of various benign entities which mimic breast cancer on imaging. It also attempts to highlight the factors that help in differentiating these diseases and assist in appropriate management for the patient.

Table 7.1 Classification of mimics of breast cancer

Category	Pathologies
Inflammatory	Infectious mastitis Granulomatous mastitis Plasma cell mastitis Lymphocytic mastopathy
Proliferative	Fat necrosis Stromal fibrosis Sclerosing adenosis Radial scar/complex sclerosing lesion
Neoplastic	Hamartoma Tubular adenoma PASH Desmoid fibromatosis Granular cell tumour Phyllodes tumour

7.2 Inflammatory Lesions

Benign inflammatory lesions are a heterogeneous group of lesions which can closely resemble the ominous inflammatory breast cancer both clinically and radiologically. Histopathological examination is often essential for establishing a final diagnosis by demonstrating the presence of inflammatory cells and absence of mitotic figures.

7.2.1 Infectious Mastitis

Breast infections or mastitis can present as acute painful breast or recurrent episodes of breast lumps with or without pain. Puerperal, non-puerperal and idiopathic mastitis are the common types, whereas uncommon causes include tuberculosis, filariasis, hydatid and other parasitic infections [3]. Since they often occur in women of the reproductive age group, MG is often not preferred as the first-line investigation due to the high breast density and the painful presentation. However, if done, it can reveal non-specific findings such as asymmetry, architectural distortion and skin and trabecular thickening. The first-line investigation is often ultrasound (US). Sonographic findings include increased parenchymal echogenicity and skin thickening with associated axillary lymphadenopathy. Breast abscess is seen as a hypoechoic collection with moving echoes which may have variable shapes and sizes (Fig. 7.1).

Inflammatory breast cancer is an important differential diagnosis in patients who present with redness, breast tenderness and, thus, closely mimic breast infections. Skin thickening associated with inflammatory breast cancer is usually diffuse in contrast to breast abscess and mastitis which tends to be localized to the involved area.

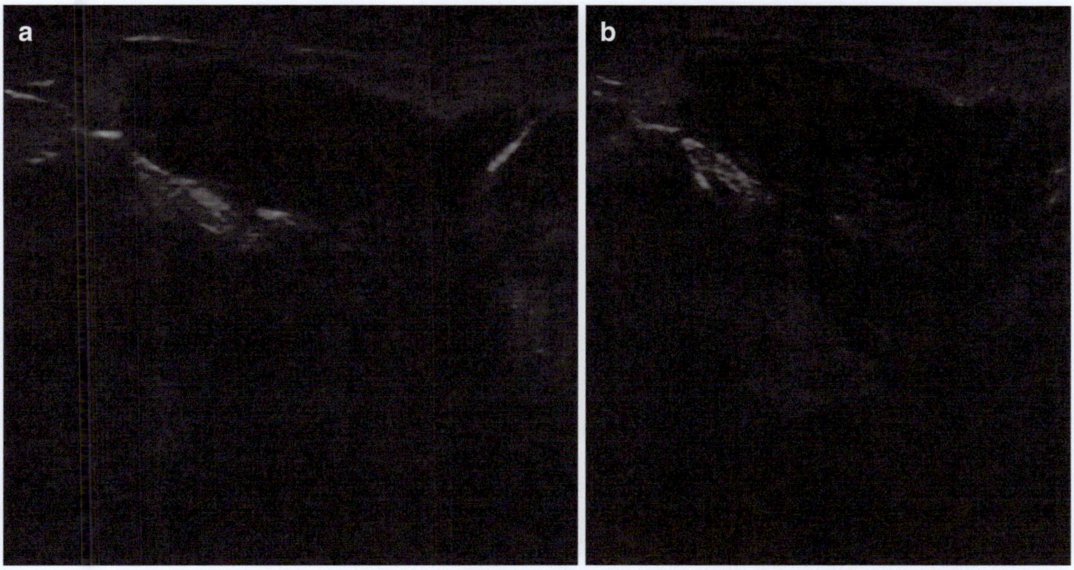

Fig. 7.1 Tubercular abscess: ultrasound images (**a**, **b**) in a female with painful breast lump revealed irregular collections with dense internal echoes within and central anechoic area representing breast abscess

Microcalcifications are the most specific finding for breast cancer in patients with inflammatory breast symptoms of unclear etiology [4]. Lymph node enlargement shows eccentric cortical thickening and loss of fatty hilum in metastatic lymph nodes, while mastitis is usually associated with reactive lymphadenopathy characterized by mild diffuse cortical thickening [5]. MRI in inflammatory breast cancer is more likely to show heterogeneous enhancement with washout kinetics, while breast abscess is more likely to have an increased T2 signal and benign enhancement kinetics [5]. In cases where the diagnosis is unclear, a biopsy is indicated to make a definitive diagnosis.

Zuska's Disease Zuska's disease is a non-puerperal peri-areolar mastitis typically described in middle-aged females who are smokers. Patients can variably present with breast pain, lump or nipple discharge. The pathogenesis is squamous metaplasia of the cuboidal epithelium lining the ducts which leads to keratin plug formation leading to abscess formation and proximal ductal dilatation. Mammography can show skin thickening, asymmetry, architectural distortion or masses, closely mimicking malignancy. US can show areas of skin thickening, ductal dilatation, fistulas, fluid tracking along parenchyma and even circumscribed or irregular masses. The MR kinetic curve has characteristics of a benign disease.

7.2.2 Granulomatous Mastitis

Granulomatous mastitis (GM) is an inflammation of the breast parenchyma with unknown etiology, the pathological hallmark of which is non-caseating granulomas in the absence of any known infectious agent (Fig. 7.2). It is therefore a diagnosis of exclusion and involves ruling out etiologies like plasma cell mastitis, granulomatosis with polyangiitis and sarcoidosis and tuberculosis [6]. An underlying autoimmune etiology is suggested as the underlying cause [7]. The affected population is usually young women of the reproductive age group, often within 6 months of pregnancy [8]. The clinical presentation is usually as a palpable mass which may or may not be associated with erythema or pain, draining sinus tracts and nipple discharge [9]. The absence of clinical signs suggestive of inflammation despite the presence of a palpable mass and enlarged

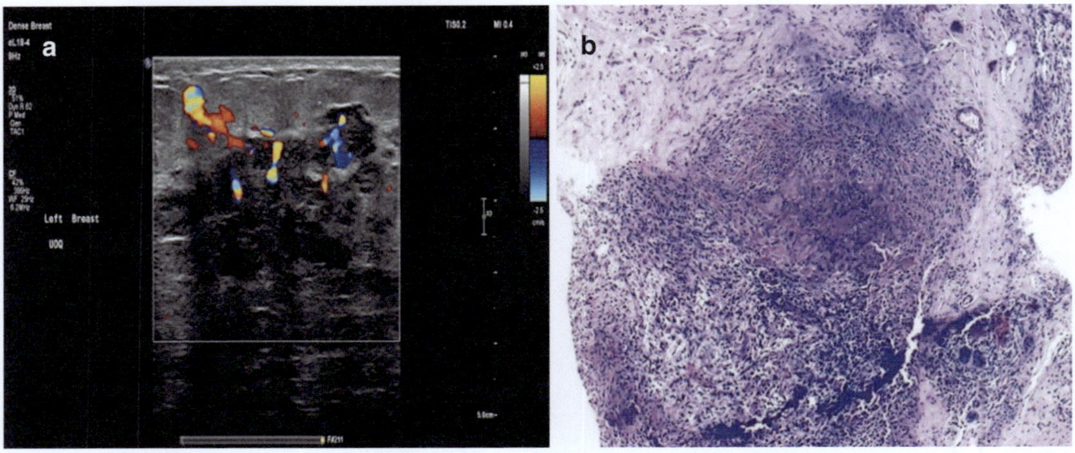

Fig. 7.2 Granulomatous mastitis in a woman with complaints of a hard painless lump since few months: (**a**) Ultrasound shows a hypoechoic tubular mass with lobulated margins and moderately increased vascularity. (**b**) Histopathological examination revealed extensive inflammation with multinucleated giant cells, lymphocytes, plasma cells and eosinophils within and around lobules and absence of caseous necrosis consistent with granulomatous mastitis

axillary lymph nodes in a certain proportion of these subjects may mimic breast cancer [10]. The most common mammographic abnormality is an area of diffuse or focal asymmetry [11]. Other findings include a diffuse increase in breast density, skin and trabecular thickening and nipple retraction [11]. The MG, however, may be normal especially in patients with dense breasts and mild disease [12]. Usually microcalcifications are not seen on MG [13]. The most common finding reported on US in granulomatous mastitis is the presence of multiple tubular hypoechoic masses or interconnected fluid collections which track along the tissue planes with possible formation of sinus opening at the junction of areola and the breast [14]. Colour Doppler shows an increased flow in the periphery of the lesion and in the surrounding breast [15]. There may be reactive axillary lymphadenopathy involving multiple nodes with concentric thickening and maintained fatty hilum in contrast to metastatic lymphadenopathy which shows eccentric cortical thickening and loss of fatty hilum in much fewer nodes [16]. On MRI, most lesions show T2 hyperintense signal and appear heterogeneous on T1-weighted sequences. The most commonly encountered enhancement pattern at dynamic MRI is segmental or regional area of non-mass enhancement with ring-enhancing lesions within, where the central non-enhancing areas represent micro-abscesses [15]. Granulomatous mastitis usually shows benign persistent enhancement kinetics, although washout kinetics may be seen, making MRI unreliable in distinguishing between inflammatory breast cancer and granulomatous mastitis [9]. Since the clinical and radiological features may closely mimic breast cancer, core biopsy is often necessary in establishing a diagnosis. The treatment strategy for GM includes local corticosteroid injections, methotrexate, incision and drainage and/or wide local excision [17]. The disease course is often protracted with bouts of remission and recurrence leading to sinus tracts and scarring. However the overall prognosis is good as the disease is self-limiting in nature [6].

7.2.3 Plasma Cell Mastitis

Plasma cell mastitis often affects non-pregnant and non-lactating females. It is characterized by breast inflammation with breast duct dilatation and plasma cell infiltration. The presentation is in the form of a clinically palpable lump or mass in the breast with ipsilateral breast enlargement, skin thickening and enlarged axillary lymph nodes but the absence of signs of inflammation. In advanced cases there may be nipple discharge and fistula formation. Based on the natural history, the disease can be divided into four stages: duct dilatation, inflammation, abscess and fistula formation. Mammograms show thick rod-like or cigar-shaped calcifications in a bilateral symmetrical in distribution and oriented with long axes pointing toward the nipple [18]. US reveals ductal dilatation with internal debris in the peri-areolar region. There can be marked hypoechogenicity in the region of the nipple with posterior acoustic shadowing indicative of ductal inflammation and thickening [19]. Plasma cell mastitis can closely mimic invasive breast carcinoma as both present with irregular-shaped masses, increased or enlarged adjacent vessels and diffusion restriction on MRI. The differentiation relies on plasma cell mastitis being more localized in the subareolar regions and showing hyperintensity on T2WI, persistent and plateau pattern of time intensity curve, non-mass enhancement and multiple rim enhancements as compared to invasive breast carcinoma which is usually centrally located and is less frequently hyperintense on T2WI [20].

7.2.4 Lymphocytic Mastopathy

Lymphocytic mastopathy is a perivascular and peri-lobular inflammatory disease of the breast characterized by lymphocytic infiltration. It is also referred to as diabetic mastopathy as it is seen in diabetic patients with long-standing type 1 diabetes mellitus [21]. It may however also be seen in other autoimmune diseases like Hashimoto's thyroiditis, Sjogren's syndrome and systemic lupus erythematous. Multicentric and bilateral involvement can occur in the late stages of the disease [22]. The clinical presentation is a painless, mobile, palpable lump closely mimicking malignancy. Various diagnostic criteria have been proposed for making a diagnosis. Logan and Hoffman proposed that the following criteria should be met: (a) long-standing history of diabetes mellitus; (b) unilateral or bilateral painless, hard, irregular poorly demarcated and mobile breast lesions; (c) dense breast tissue on mammography; (d) lesion demonstrating posterior acoustic shadowing on US; and (e) strong resistance to fine needle aspiration or biopsy [23]. Mammography may show a localized increased density, architectural distortion, asymmetry or ill-defined masses which closely mimic malignancy [24]. On US they typically present as an ill-defined hypoechoic mass with posterior acoustic shadowing without any colour flow on Doppler [25]. On MRI, these lesions show a homogenously low enhancement with gradual and progressive enhancement explained by the fibrous tissue [26]. Histopathological examination may be needed in inconclusive cases to make a final diagnosis (Fig. 7.3).

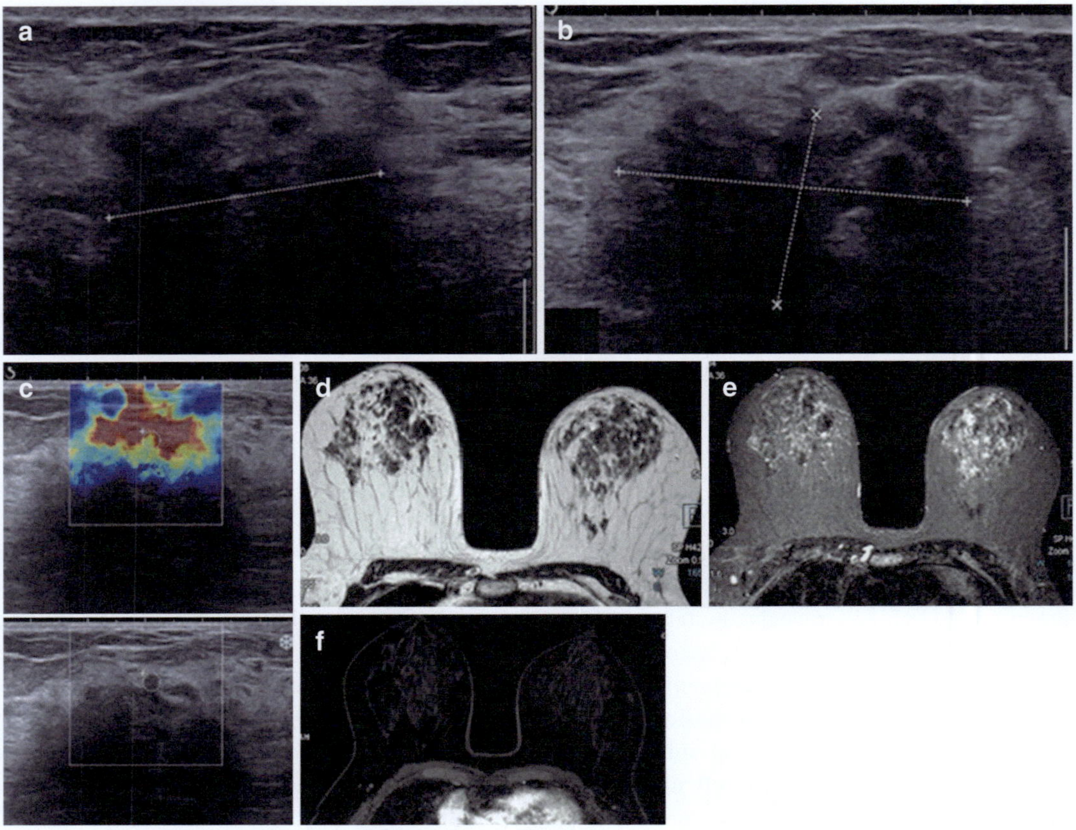

Fig. 7.3 Lymphocytic mastopathy in a diabetic patient: (**a**, **b**) Grey scale US images show irregular-shaped heterogeneously hypoechoic lesions with posterior acoustic shadowing. (**c**) On the shear wave images, the lesions appear hard. (**d**) A T1-weighted image reveals the lesions to be isointense, and (**e**) a T2-weighted image shows the lesions to be hyperintense with (**f**) no contrast enhancement on the post-contrast images. Histopathology confirmed the lesions to be lymphocytic mastopathy

7.3 Proliferative Diseases

A variety of proliferative diseases involving the breast can closely mimic breast carcinoma on mammography. These include fat necrosis, stromal fibrosis, sclerosing adenosis and complex sclerosing scar. Since the imaging appearance of these entities is ominous, often they are misinterpreted for malignancy, and biopsy reveals the final diagnosis. It is of importance to be aware of the radiological findings for these entities so that there is acceptance toward the pathology report during rad-path correlation.

7.3.1 Fat Necrosis

Fat necrosis tends to occur more commonly in fatty and pendulous breasts. Diagnosis is often challenging as it mimics a variety of entities, both clinically and radiologically. Fat necrosis may result from accidental trauma, surgery or post-radiotherapy and can clinically present as a small, painless, ill-defined breast mass [27]. It is commonly seen in the inferior, central breast after reduction mammoplasty and at the periphery of the flap in the reconstructed breasts [28]. The appearance of fat necrosis on mammography depends on the amount of fibrosis. A radiolucent mass or an oil cyst with a peripheral rim of calcification can be seen if there is minimal fibrosis. Infrequently calcifications with suspicious morphology such as branching or rod-like calcifications may be seen. In the presence of fibrosis, the wall of the oil cyst becomes thickened and shows ill-defined or spiculated walls. When there is a significant amount of fibrosis, the entire fat may get replaced giving the appearance of a spiculated mass or focal symmetry on mammography. It is this variety of fat necrosis which can closely mimic breast carcinoma. The appearance of fat necrosis on sonography may be either solid or cystic and also varies based on the extent of fibrosis as discussed earlier. The initial appearance may be non-specific in the form of a focal area of increased echogenicity [29]. Other sonographic appearances may include anechoic mass with posterior acoustic enhancement, anechoic mass with posterior acoustic shadowing, cystic masses with internal echoes and cystic masses with mural nodules [30]. Masses with internal echogenic bands (representing the interface between lipid and serous haemorrhagic components) that show positional changes are considered to be a specific sonographic indicator of fat necrosis [31]. The most common imaging features of fat necrosis on MRI are those of an oil cyst seen as oval, circumscribed T1 hyperintense lesion which correspondingly loses signal on fat-suppressed T1-weighted images. An enhancing rim representing surrounding inflammatory changes and granulation tissue can be seen, the appearance varies based on the proportion of acute and chronic changes [32]. Fat necrosis can show post-contrast enhancement on MRI which may be focal or diffuse and homogenous or heterogeneous varying from slow, gradual to rapid enhancement or even washout [33]. In order to appreciate the enhancement, which may be seen in breast cancer or even fat necrosis, fat-suppressed post-contrast images are essential. The morphology and contrast kinetic curves of fat necrosis can closely mimic malignancy. In these scenarios, where the lesion shows signal intensity similar to that of adjacent fat and doesn't show any contrast enhancement, the diagnosis may be established without sampling; in other cases a biopsy may be required to differentiate it from breast carcinoma [31] (Fig. 7.4).

7.3.2 Stromal Fibrosis

Stromal fibrosis is histopathologically characterized by proliferation of fibrous stroma with atrophy and destruction of normal mammary ductal and acinar architecture, which typically occurs in premenopausal women [34]. It may present as a

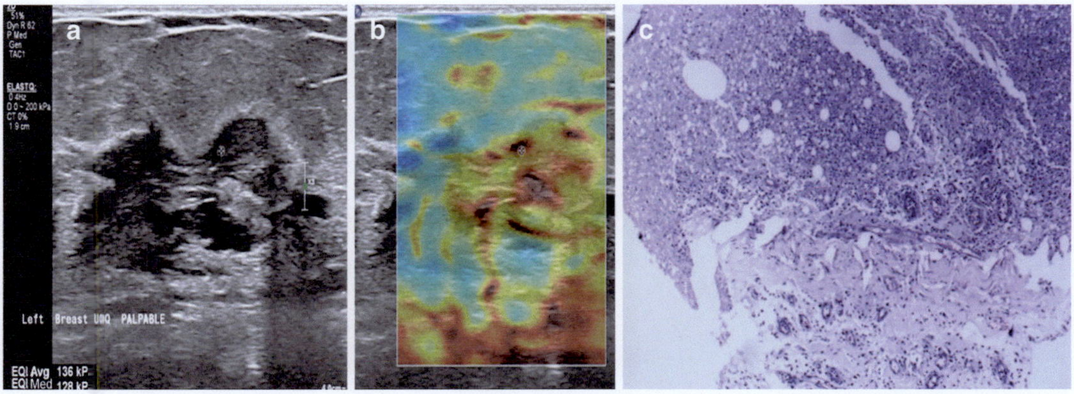

Fig. 7.4 Fat necrosis: (**a**) A grey scale ultrasound image shows an irregular-shaped mass with heterogeneous echotexture and angular margins at places. (**b**) An elastography image shows varying elastography values (highest—136 kPa); this lesion was categorized as BIRADS 4c. (**c**) Ultrasound-guided biopsy revealed lipid-filled spaces surrounded by neutrophils, lymphocytes, plasma cells and histiocytes with foamy cytoplasm consistent with fat necrosis

clinically palpable abnormality; however it may be incidentally detected as an occult, non-palpable abnormality in 65–100% of the patients during screening MG [35]. The most common imaging feature on MG is focal asymmetry and/or irregular-shaped mass [36]. There is no pathognomonic imaging feature for stromal fibrosis on sonography; therefore masses may be hypoechoic, isoechoic or hyperechoic in echogenicity; may be round, oval or irregular-shaped; may have circumscribed, angular, indistinct, microlobulated or spiculated margins; and may show either posterior acoustic enhancement or shadowing [37, 38]. However, patients with dense breasts may have mammographically and sonographically occult disease in which cases MRI may be a useful investigation [34]. MRI findings of this entity can vary from masses with round, oval or irregular-shaped to spiculated margins, and the contrast kinetics patterns may vary from rapid and medium uptake rates with either plateau or washout curves [34]. Non-mass-like enhancement in focal, segmental, regional distributions may also be seen [39]. While apparent diffusion coefficient (ADC) values have been tried in differentiating breast cancer from stromal fibrosis, there exists a considerable overlap with the range of ADC [39]. Owing to a significant clinical and radiological overlap between stromal fibrosis and breast cancer, biopsy is often needed. Establishing radio-pathological concordance is an essential part of the management strategy since a histological diagnosis of stromal fibrosis from a sampled tissue may miss an adjacent underlying breast carcinoma [40]. Cases of radio-pathological discordance require a repeat biopsy or surgical excision [41].

7.3.3 Sclerosing Adenosis

Sclerosing adenosis is a benign disease occurring as an incidental finding in perimenopausal women in which there is hyperplasia involving the epithelial and the mesenchymal component of the breast causing distortion of the normal glandular parenchyma [42]. It is often seen in concurrent existence with benign and malignant breast lesions like ductal epithelial hyperplasia, intraductal papilloma, fibroadenomas, ductal carcinoma in situ (DCIS), and invasive ductal carcinoma (IDC) [43]. Studies have shown 1.7 to 3.7 times the risk of development of invasive breast cancer in patients with sclerosing adenosis [44]. Sclerosing adenosis can closely mimic invasive carcinoma both radiologically and histopathologically, with the discrimination being done on the basis of the presence of an outer myoepithelial layer in adenosis and absence of this layer in invasive breast cancer which is detected by immunostaining for actin protein [45, 46] (Fig. 7.5). The mammographic presentation can

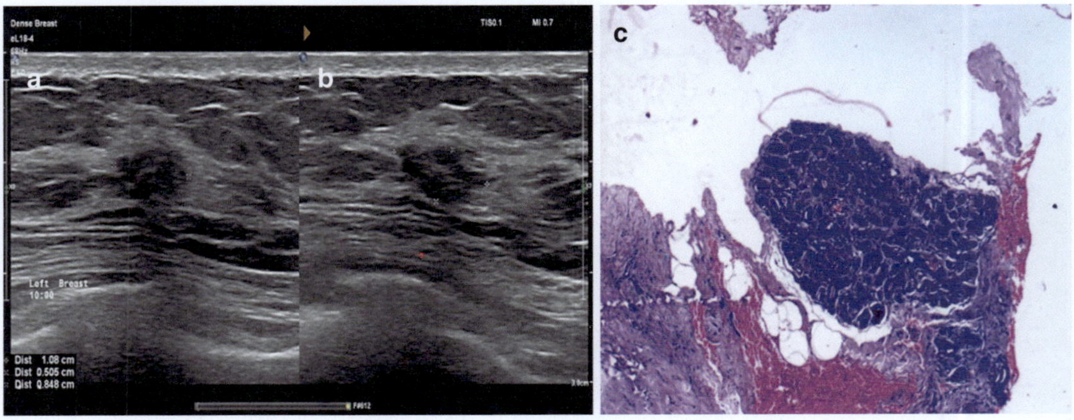

Fig. 7.5 Sclerosing adenosis: (**a**, **b**) Grey scale US images in a woman who complained of a painless lump show an irregularly shaped hypoechoic lesion which is wider than taller and has angular margins. (**c**) Histopathology revealed proliferating tubules which are elongated and have attenuated lumens with preferential preservation of myoepithelial cells in the tubules and epithelial cells are less conspicuous, with lobular fibrosis

be in the form of masses with microcalcification, architectural distortion or focal asymmetry which may be difficult to differentiate from the ominous breast carcinoma [47]. While solid lesions with circumscribed margins are commoner on US, irregular-shaped masses with posterior acoustic shadowing may also be seen in sclerosing adenosis. MRI can show a wide spectrum of morphologic and contrast kinetic features, such as a mass, non-mass enhancement, architectural distortion or non-enhancing lesions with suspicious morphology, with majority of lesions showing enhancement as type I or II curve [48]. The management depends upon establishing radio-pathological concordance as in the case of stromal fibrosis. If the imaging findings are that of circumscribed benign appearing lesion with adequate sample on biopsy, the pathological diagnosis of sclerosing adenosis is considered concordant. Meanwhile, if the radiological findings are that of a suspicious lesion, a repeat biopsy is indicated to rule out an underlying malignancy [9].

7.3.4 Radial Scar/Complex Sclerosing Lesion

Digital breast tomosynthesis is a better modality than standard mammogram than picking up radial scars. The typical mammographic appearance of radial scar/complex sclerosing lesion central radiolucent core with long, thin, radiating spicules arranged parallel to radiolucent linear structures ("black star" appearance) [49]. The appearance varies in different mammographic projections. These can closely mimic invasive malignancies which show the "white star appearance." In contrast to invasive malignancies in which abnormalities are palpable and show overlying skin retraction on mammography, radial scars are not associated with palpable abnormalities and do show overlying skin retraction. Calcifications can be seen in radial scars and are often associated with the proliferative fibrocystic changes and the sclerosing adenosis that exists around the radial scar [50]. The most common appearance on US includes irregular masses with indistinct margins or non-mass features with or without shadowing. This premalignant condition has been discussed in detail in chapter on "high-risk lesions."

7.4 Benign Tumours

A variety of benign tumours like hamartoma, fibroadenoma, phyllodes, pseudoangiomatous stromal hyperplasia (PASH), tubular adenoma, desmoid fibromatosis and granular cell tumour (GCT) can also mimic breast cancer on imaging. It is important to be aware of the atypical imaging features so that there is acceptance toward a benign pathology report.

7.4.1 Complex Fibroadenoma

While classical fibroadenomas are well-circumscribed, oval-shaped and homogenously hypoechoic, these can sometimes have variable appearances and may even closely mimic malignancy. These may present with focal asymmetry on mammography and may display an irregular shape, non-circumscribed margins, heterogeneity and microcalcifications on US (Fig. 7.6). Sampling is needed in order to exclude malignancy.

7.4.2 Hamartoma

Hamartomas, which are also known as fibroadenolipomas, are benign tumours composed of varying proportions of glandular epithelium, adipose tissue and fibrous tissue [51]. They vary in size from small lesions to large masses of 10 to 12 cm. With the increasing use of screening mammography, these lesions are being detected with increasing frequency [52]. They typically appear as circumscribed oval to round masses on MG which have a soft tissue as well as fat foci along with a thin radio-opaque pseudocapsule—the classic description of the breast within a breast appearance [53]. US appearance ranges from well-encapsulated and well-defined isoechoic solid mildly heterogeneous mass to ill-

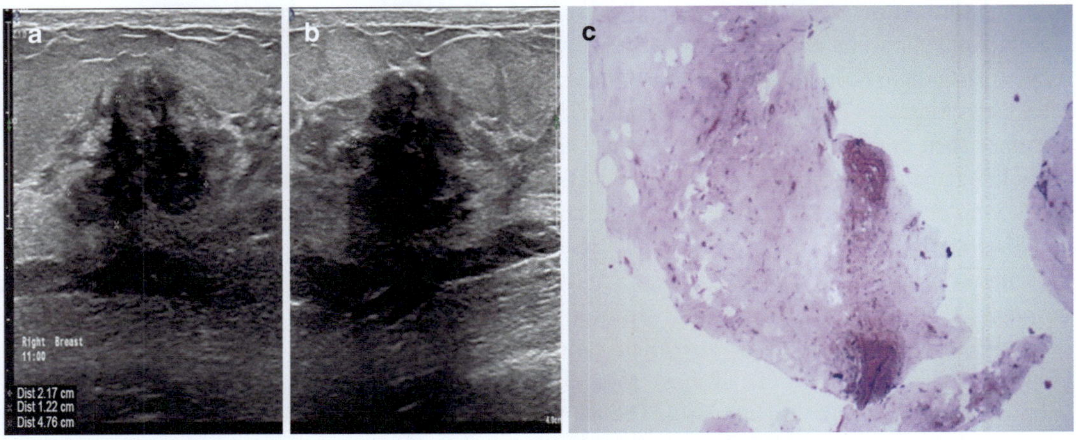

Fig. 7.6 Sclerosed fibroadenoma: (**a**, **b**) A grey scale US image reveals an irregular-shaped hypoechoic lesion with angular margins and anti-parallel orientation and is reaching up to involve the pectoralis muscle posteriorly categorized as BIRADS 4c. (**c**) US-guided biopsy revealed a sclerosed fibroadenoma

defined mass resembling a normal breast tissue with margins difficult to delineate. These are seen as well-demarcated masses with a heterogeneous SI on MRI with a variable degree of intensity on T1WIs and T2WIs based on proportion of the fibrous, glandular and fatty tissue. While hamartomas usually have a typical benign appearance, they may be difficult to differentiate from circumscribed malignant tumours, such as phyllodes tumour or breast sarcoma, especially if large in size or when they show marked heterogeneous enhancement. Though exceedingly rare, case reports of both invasive carcinoma and carcinoma in situ arising in hamartoma have been reported [54, 55]. While hamartomas with typical imaging features do not require sampling, growth of the mass or the presence of atypical features such as axillary lymphadenopathy or suspicious calcifications within the mass warrants a biopsy.

7.4.3 Phyllodes Tumour

Phyllodes tumour of the breast usually occurs in middle-aged females and belongs to the category of fibroepithelial tumours. These vary from a continuum of benign to malignant tumours. They appear as round, lobulated, high-density masses on MG, which can have a radiolucent halo [56]. The malignant spectrum of phyllodes tumours may show spiculated margins and can mimic breast carcinoma; however circumscribed margins are more common [57]. While macrocalcifications may be seen, the presence of microcalcifications is extremely rare [58]. Usually associated lymphadenopathy is not seen, and the presence of lymphadenopathy should prompt consideration of breast carcinoma. On US, most tumours have lobulated margins and a heterogeneous echogenicity. The presence of fluid-filled clefts in a predominantly solid mass is highly suggestive of phyllodes tumour [59]. The differentiation between benign and malignant phyllodes tumours on imaging is difficult with a significant overlap. The features suggesting malignant change include an irregular shape, non-circumscribed margins, marked hypoechogenicity, a surrounding echogenic rim or halo and posterior acoustic shadowing. In contrast, benign tumours usually display a round or oval shape, mildly hypoechoic internal echotexture, smooth borders or a pseudocapsule, homogeneous internal echoes, no central posterior acoustic shadowing, a normal surrounding tissue and a slight change of shape by probe pressure compression [60]. MRI reveals round-shaped tumours with circumscribed margins having a hypointense signal on T1- and hyperintense signal on T2-weighted images. There may be areas of haemorrhage within which can appear bright on T1-weighted

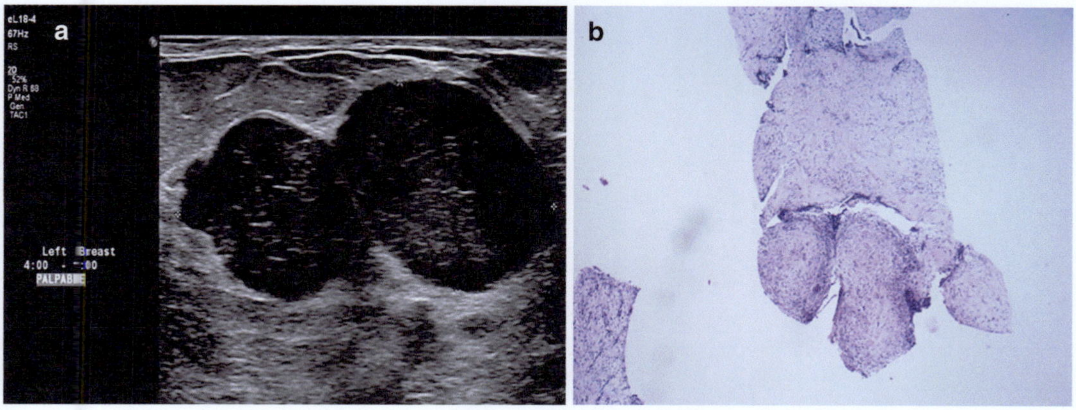

Fig. 7.7 Phyllodes tumour: (**a**) A grey scale US image reveals a hypoechoic solid irregular-shaped lesion with lobulated margins which was wider than taller and showed fluid clefts within (BIRADS 4a). (**b**) Histopathological examination identified it as phyllodes tumour

images and cystic areas appearing T2 bright. Dynamic contrast-enhanced (DCE)-MRI shows slow initial enhancement with persistent enhancement in the delayed phase in benign tumours, whereas malignant tumours can show initial enhancement with plateau or washout phenomenon [61] (Fig. 7.7).

7.4.4 Pseudoangiomatous Stromal Hyperplasia

PASH is a rare benign mesenchymal tumour of the breast that shows dense hyalinized collagen bundles causing intralobular stromal expansion and dissection by slit-like pseudovascular spaces lined by myofibroblasts. Hormonal exposure is considered contributory with the disease being prevalent in those on oral contraceptive pills and hormonal replacement therapy [62]. Although it tends to be focal and unilateral in occurrence, bilateral, diffuse or multifocal patterns are also observed [63, 64]. Patients may present clinically with complaints of a breast lump or be discovered incidentally on screening. It can present as either focal asymmetry or a round/oval -shaped circumscribed mass of variable size with absent microcalcifications. The most common sonographic appearance is a circumscribed, solid, homogenous, oval hypoechoic mass. MRI appearances are non-specific with the lesion appearing isointense on T1- and T2-weighted images with T2 hyperintense cystic areas within. The diagnosis is primarily from histopathological evaluation, with biopsy being preferred over fine needle aspiration because PASH mimics fibroadenoma on cytology in 70% of the cases [65]. After histological diagnosis, it is imperative to establish radio-pathological concordance, and discordant cases may be considered for excisional biopsy. PASH does not have an increased risk for malignancy; however it can coexist with underlying breast malignancies [66]. Post-excision, recurrence may be seen in 5–22% cases of PASH [67] (Fig. 7.8).

7.4.5 Tubular Adenoma

Tubular adenomas are rare benign epithelial tumours of the breast seen in young women. These need to be histologically distinguished from fibroadenomas and show tightly packed tubular or epithelial components with a sparse connective tissue seen in tubular adenomas, in contrast to fibroadenomas which show extensive connective tissue component [9]. On mammography these lesions typically appear as well-circumscribed oval or round lesions without calcifications; however occasionally the margins

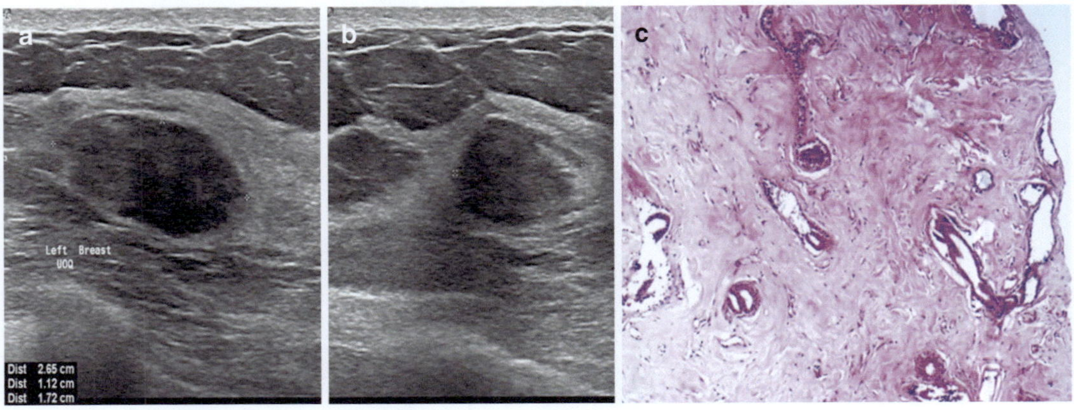

Fig. 7.8 Pseudoangiomatous stromal hyperplasia: Grey scale ultrasound in the (**a**) transverse plane and the (**b**) longitudinal plane shows a solid hypoechoic lesion with circumscribed margins and no microcalcifications seen in the upper outer quadrant of the breast. (**c**) US-guided biopsy revealed diffuse proliferation of compact spindle cells with areas of peri-lobular/periductal accentuation, not showing mitotic activity and atypia

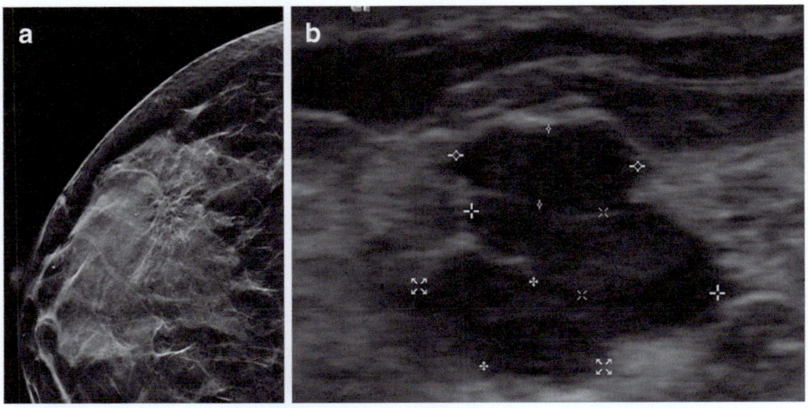

Fig. 7.9 Tubular adenoma in a female with contralateral proven malignancy. (**a**) Diagnostic mammogram revealed a focal area of architectural distortion in the upper central quadrant with spiculations arising from the area. No suspicious microcalcifications noted. (**b**) A corroborative US image shows a hypoechoic irregular mass with lobulated margins. Biopsy confirmed it to be tubular adenoma. The patient underwent modified radical mastectomy for the left breast, and the lesion of the right breast was stable on follow-up during the course of treatment (not shown in this image)

may not be circumscribed, and they may be seen as an area of asymmetry or architectural distortion [68]. US usually shows a circumscribed solid homogenous hypoechoic mass which can have posterior acoustic enhancement (Fig. 7.9). The development of DCIS in tubular adenoma and simultaneous presence of tubular adenoma and IDC have been described [69].

7.4.6 Desmoid Fibromatosis

Desmoid fibromatosis of the breast is a rare slow-growing stromal tumour that comprises <0.2% of all breast tumours [70]. The disease is associated with Gardner's syndrome, familial adenomatous polyposis, surgical trauma and silicone breast implants and occurs in 22–49-year age group [71]. The disease is locally aggressive and recurs locally without distant metastasis. Clinical presentation of mobile nontender masses with associated tethering of the pectoralis muscle and Cooper's ligaments causing skin and nipple retraction has been noted [72]. Mammography may be positive in 33% cases and may show irregular-shaped high-density masses with spiculated margins indistinguishable from breast carcinoma [71]. US findings include solid, spiculated or microlobulated, hypoechoic masses with a thick echogenic rim and posterior shadowing. MRI shows ill-defined, hypo- to isointense masses on T1-weighted images (T1WI) which are correspondingly heterogeneously hyperintense on T2-weighted images. On DCE-MRI, the enhancement patterns vary; however a proportion of these cases can show a type 2 enhancement curve (rapid wash in and plateau) which can mimic malignancy. The morphology of enhancement differs from invasive breast carcinoma which shows peripheral ring enhancement [73]. MRI also plays an important role in determining disease extent and response assessment if the patient receives medical therapy for treatment [74].

7.4.7 Granular Cell Tumour

GCTs are typically benign neoplasms with a myofibroblastic origin. 8.5% of all GCTs arise in the breast, accounting for 0.1% of all cases of breast neoplasms [75]. The occurrence is more frequent in the upper inner quadrant of the breast, along the course of the supraclavicular nerve, which innervates the skin of the breast. This is contrary to breast carcinoma, which is more usually located in the upper outer quadrant [76]. While most breast GCTs are benign, malignant GCTs may also occur, and its possibility should be considered if the size >5 cm, if there is associated lymphadenopathy, heterogeneous signal intensity or rim enhancement on MRI and/or infiltration of the adjacent tissues [77]. Their significance lies in the fact that they closely mimic scirrhous breast malignancies both clinically and radiologically [78]. The presentation on mammography is usually as a focal mass which is an irregular shaped and has spiculated margins mimicking invasive breast carcinoma; however they can also present with benign imaging features such as round lesions with circumscribed margins [79]. US findings are non-specific and may show features like irregular-shaped heteroechoic masses with spiculated margins, which are taller than wider. MRI reveals variable signal intensity on T1- and hyperintensity on T2-weighted image which is less T2 hyperintense as compared to other masses [79]. The mass is round or irregular with non-circumscribed or spiculated margins, exhibits type 1 or type 2 kinetic curve, and has been reported to show ring enhancement [75]. Since imaging features are not specific, the final diagnosis relies on histopathological examination.

7.5 Conclusion

Breast cancer is a grave pathology involving the breast. There are however a spectrum of pathologies which can closely mimic breast cancer on imaging. The morphology of the lesion on mammogram as well as the appearance on T2-weighted imaging can help in arriving at a diagnosis (Flowcharts 7.1 and 7.2). The radiologist must be aware of the diverse imaging features of these pathologies and how to differentiate them from breast cancer. This also helps the radiologist in establishing rad-path correlation so that unnecessary repeat sampling may be avoided when the biopsy results do not reveal breast cancer.

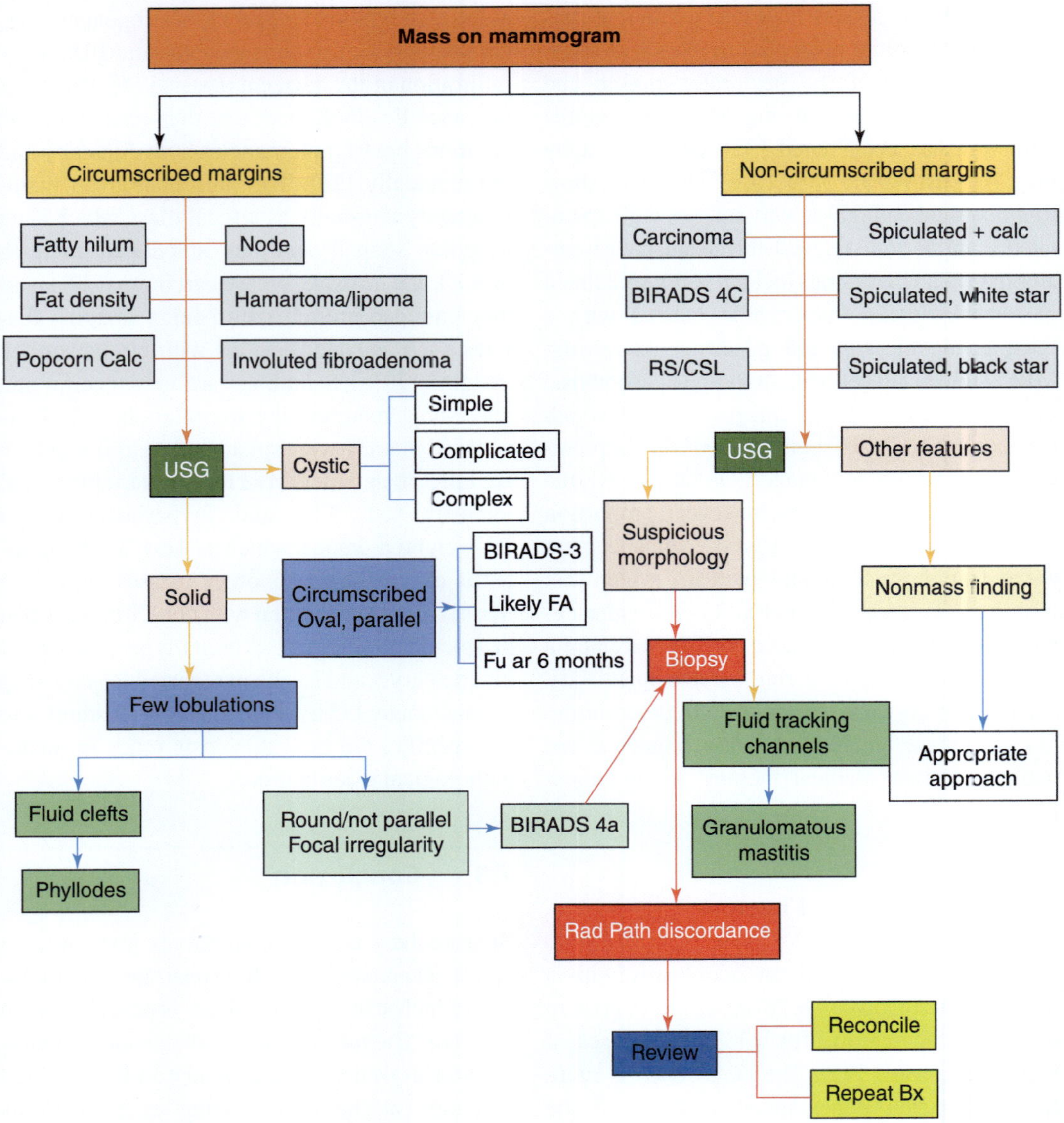

Flowchart 7.1 Approach in masses on mammogram

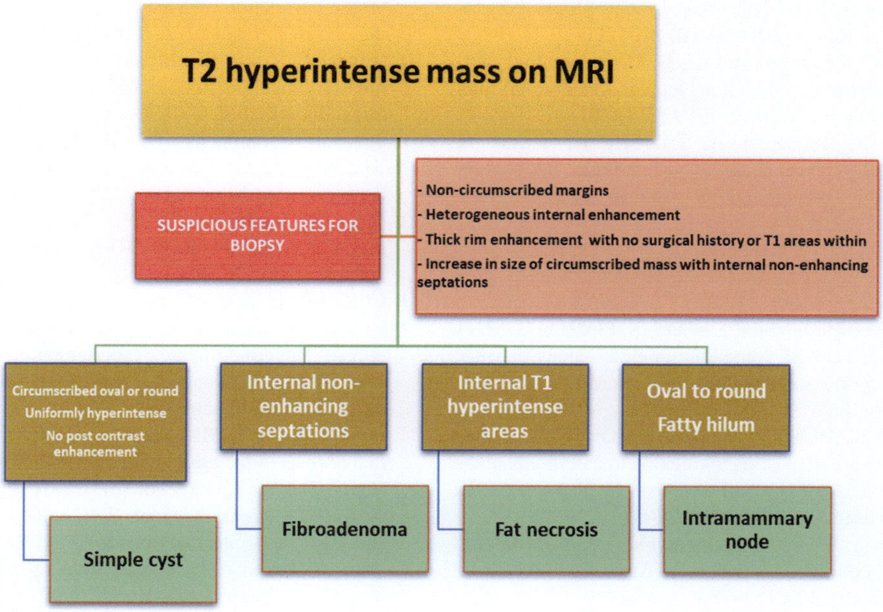

Flowchart 7.2 Approach to T2 hyperintense lesions on MRI

References

1. Westra C, Dialani V, Mehta TS, Eisenberg RL. Using T2-weighted sequences to more accurately characterize breast masses seen on MRI. AJR Am J Roentgenol. 2014;202(3):W183–90.
2. Sardanelli F, Boetes C, Borisch B, Decker T, Federico M, Gilbert FJ, et al. Magnetic resonance imaging of the breast: recommendations from the EUSOMA working group. Eur J Cancer Oxf Engl 1990. 2010;46(8):1296–316.
3. Dhamija E, Gulati S, Hari S. Imaging spectrum in tropical breast infections. Br J Radiol. 2024;97(1154):315–23.
4. Chow CK. Imaging in inflammatory breast carcinoma. Breast Dis. 2005;22:45–54.
5. Trop I, Dugas A, David J, El Khoury M, Boileau JF, Larouche N, et al. Breast abscesses: evidence-based algorithms for diagnosis, management, and follow-up. Radiogr Rev Publ Radiol Soc N Am Inc. 2011;31(6):1683–99.
6. Hovanessian Larsen LJ, Peyvandi B, Klipfel N, Grant E, Iyengar G. Granulomatous lobular mastitis: imaging, diagnosis, and treatment. AJR Am J Roentgenol. 2009;193(2):574–81.
7. Erhan Y, Veral A, Kara E, Ozdemir N, Kapkac M, Ozdedeli E, et al. A clinicopthologic study of a rare clinical entity mimicking breast carcinoma: idiopathic granulomatous mastitis. Breast Edinb Scotl. 2000;9(1):52–6.
8. Ozturk E, Akin M, Can MF, Ozerhan I, Kurt B, Yagci G, et al. Idiopathic granulomatous mastitis. Saudi Med J. 2009;30(1):45–9.
9. Guirguis MS, Adrada B, Santiago L, Candelaria R, Arribas E. Mimickers of breast malignancy: imaging findings, pathologic concordance and clinical management. Insights Imaging. 2021;12:53.
10. Oztekin PS, Durhan G, Nercis Kosar P, Erel S, Hucumenoglu S. Imaging findings in patients with granulomatous mastitis. Iran J Radiol. 2016;13(3):e33900.
11. Gautier N, Lalonde L, Tran-Thanh D, El Khoury M, David J, Labelle M, et al. Chronic granulomatous mastitis: imaging, pathology and management. Eur J Radiol. 2013;82(4):e165–75.
12. Fazzio RT, Shah SS, Sandhu NP, Glazebrook KN. Idiopathic granulomatous mastitis: imaging update and review. Insights Imaging. 2016;7(4):531–9.
13. Handa P, Leibman AJ, Sun D, Abadi M, Goldberg A. Granulomatous mastitis: changing clinical and

imaging features with image-guided biopsy correlation. Eur Radiol. 2014;24(10):2404–11.
14. Engin G, Acunaş G, Acunaş B. Granulomatous mastitis: gray-scale and color Doppler sonographic findings. J Clin Ultrasound. 1999;27(3):101–6.
15. Yildiz S, Aralasmak A, Kadioglu H, Toprak H, Yetis H, Gucin Z, et al. Radiologic findings of idiopathic granulomatous mastitis. Med Ultrason. 2015;17(1):39–44.
16. Al-Khawari HAT, Al-Manfouhi HA, Madda JP, Kovacs A, Sheikh M, Roberts O. Radiologic features of granulomatous mastitis. Breast J. 2011;17(6):645–50.
17. Patel RA, Strickland P, Sankara IR, Pinkston G, Many W, Rodriguez M. Idiopathic granulomatous mastitis: case reports and review of literature. J Gen Intern Med. 2010;25(3):270–3.
18. Naragam AP, Tati SY, Dara H, Kumar VA, Jada M, et al. Plasma cell mastitis mimicking as carcinoma of the breast: a case report and review of the literature. IOSR J Dent Med Sci. 2014;13(2):28–31.
19. Febery A, Bennett I. Sonographic features of inflammatory conditions of the breast. Australas J Ultrasound Med. 2019;22(3):165–73.
20. Chen R, Hu B, Zhang Y, Liu C, Zhao L, Jiang Y, et al. Differential diagnosis of plasma cell mastitis and invasive ductal carcinoma using multiparametric MRI. Gland Surg. 2020;9(2):27890–290.
21. Kudva YC, Reynolds C, O'Brien T, Powell C, Oberg AL, Crotty TB. "Diabetic mastopathy," or sclerosing lymphocytic lobulitis, is strongly associated with type 1 diabetes. Diabetes Care. 2002;25(1):121–6.
22. Bayer U, Horn LC, Schulz HG. Bilateral, tumorlike diabetic mastopathy-progression and regression of the disease during 5-year follow up. Eur J Radiol. 1998;26(3):248–53.
23. Logan WW, Hoffman NY. Diabetic fibrous breast disease. Radiology. 1989;172(3):667–70.
24. Moschetta M, Telegrafo M, Triggiani V, Rella L, Cornacchia I, Serio G, et al. Diabetic mastopathy: a diagnostic challenge in breast sonography. J Clin Ultrasound. 2015;43(2):113–7.
25. Rajasundaram S, Vijayakumar V, Chegu D, Uday Prasad PV, Vimalathithan SN, Saravanan S, et al. Diabetic mastopathy-an uncommon presentation of a common disease. Breast J. 2020;26(7):1409–11.
26. Tuncbilek N, Karakas HM, Okten O. Diabetic fibrous mastopathy: dynamic contrast-enhanced magnetic resonance imaging findings. Breast J. 2004;10(4):359–62.
27. Hogge JP, Robinson RE, Magnant CM, Zuurbier RA. The mammographic spectrum of fat necrosis of the breast. Radiogr Rev Publ Radiol Soc N Am Inc. 1995;15(6):1347–56.
28. Kang BJ, Jung JI, Park C, Park WC, Jeon HM, Hahn ST, et al. Breast MRI findings after modified radical mastectomy and transverse rectus abdominis myocutaneous flap in patients with breast cancer. J Magn Reson Imaging JMRI. 2005;21(6):784–91.
29. Atasoy MM, Ören NC, Ilica AT, Güvenç İ, Günal A, Mossa-Basha M. Sonography of fat necrosis of the breast: correlation with mammography and MR imaging. J Clin Ultrasound. 2013;41(7):415–23.
30. Bilgen IG, Ustun EE, Memis A. Fat necrosis of the breast: clinical, mammographic and sonographic features. Eur J Radiol. 2001;39(2):92–9.
31. Taboada JL, Stephens TW, Krishnamurthy S, Brandt KR, Whitman GJ. The many faces of fat necrosis in the breast. Am J Roentgenol. 2009;192(3):815–25.
32. Daly CP, Jaeger B, Sill DS. Variable appearances of fat necrosis on breast MRI. Am J Roentgenol. 2008;191(5):1374–80.
33. Chala LF, de Barros N, de Camargo Moraes P, Endo E, Kim SJ, Pincerato KM, et al. Fat necrosis of the breast: mammographic, sonographic, computed tomography, and magnetic resonance imaging findings. Curr Probl Diagn Radiol. 2004;33(3):106–26.
34. Lee SJ, Mahoney MC, Khan S. MRI features of stromal fibrosis of the breast with histopathologic correlation. AJR Am J Roentgenol. 2011;197(3):755–62.
35. Nassar L, Baassiri A, Salah F, Barakat A, Najem E, Boulos F, et al. Stromal fibrosis of the breast: a spectrum of benign to malignant imaging appearances. Radiol Res Pract. 2019;2019:5045908.
36. Goel NB, Knight TE, Pandey S, Riddick-Young M, de Paredes ES, Trivedi A. Fibrous lesions of the breast: imaging-pathologic correlation. Radiogr Rev Publ Radiol Soc N Am Inc. 2005;25(6):1547–59.
37. Rosen EL, Soo MS, Bentley RC. Focal fibrosis: a common breast lesion diagnosed at imaging-guided core biopsy. AJR Am J Roentgenol. 1999;173(6):1657–62.
38. You JK, Kim EK, Kwak JY, Kim MJ, Oh KK, Park BW, et al. Focal fibrosis of the breast diagnosed by a sonographically guided core biopsy of nonpalpable lesions: imaging findings and clinical relevance. J Ultrasound Med Off J Am Inst Ultrasound Med. 2005;24(10):1377–84.
39. Yilmaz R, Bayramoglu Z, Kartal MG, Çaliskan E, Salmaslıoglu A, Dursun M, et al. Stromal fibrosis: imaging features with diagnostic contribution of diffusion-weighted MRI. Br J Radiol. 2018;91(1085):20170706.
40. Malik N, Lad S, Seely JM, Schweitzer ME. Underestimation of malignancy in biopsy-proven cases of stromal fibrosis. Br J Radiol. 2014;87(1039):20140182.
41. Venta LA, Wiley EL, Gabriel H, Adler YT. Imaging features of focal breast fibrosis: mammographic-pathologic correlation of noncalcified breast lesions. AJR Am J Roentgenol. 1999;173(2):309–16.
42. Markopoulos C, Kouskos E, Phillipidis T, Floros D. Adenosis tumor of the breast. Breast J. 2003;9(3):255–6.
43. Chen H, Bao L, Yu L, Sun H, Tan Y, Wei P, et al. Value of multimodal imaging in the diagnosis of breast sclerosing adenosis associated with malignant lesions. J Clin Ultrasound. 2023;51(3):485–93.
44. Jensen RA, Page DL, Dupont WD, Rogers LW. Invasive breast cancer risk in women with sclerosing adenosis. Cancer. 1989;64(10):1977–83.

45. Bussolati G, Alfani V, Weber K, Osborn M. Immunocytochemical detection of actin on fixed and embedded tissues: its potential use in routine pathology. J Histochem Cytochem. 1980;28(2):169–73.
46. Gill HK, Ioffe OB, Berg WA. When is a diagnosis of sclerosing adenosis acceptable at core biopsy? Radiology. 2003;228(1):50–7.
47. Tan H, Zhang H, Lei Z, Fu F, Wang M. Radiological and clinical findings in sclerosing adenosis of the breast. Medicine (Baltimore). 2019;98(39):e17061.
48. Pancurgias E, Bourgioti C, Skountzos G, Koutoulidis V, Moulopoulos L. MRI manifestations of sclerosing adenosis of the breast: a single institution experience. Hell J Of Radiol [Internet]. 2020 Dec 23 [cited 2024 Mar 3];5(4). Available from: https://www.hjradiology.org/index.php/HJR/article/view/363
49. Manzar BZ, Phillips J, Dibble EH, Quintana LM, Lourenco AP. Imaging and management of radial scars and complex sclerosing lesions. Radiographics. 2023;43(10):e230022.
50. Orel SG, Evers K, Yeh IT, Troupin RH. Radial scar with microcalcifications: radiologic-pathologic correlation. Radiology. 1992;183(2):479–82.
51. Sonmez FC, Gucin Z, Yildiz P, Tosuner Z. Hamartoma of the breast in two patients: a case report. Oncol Lett. 2013;6(2):442–4.
52. Farrokh D, Hashemi J, Ansaripour E. Breast hamartoma: mammographic findings. Iran J Radiol. 2011;8(4):258–60.
53. Feder JM, de Paredes ES, Hogge JP, Wilken JJ. Unusual breast lesions: radiologic-pathologic correlation. Radiogr Rev Publ Radiol Soc N Am Inc. 1999;19(Spec No):S11–26; quiz S260.
54. Mester J, Simmons RM, Vazquez MF, Rosenblatt R. In situ and infiltrating ductal carcinoma arising in a breast hamartoma. Am J Roentgenol. 2000;175(1):64–6.
55. Tse GMK, Law BKB, Pang LM, Cheung HS. Ductal carcinoma in situ arising in mammary hamartoma. J Clin Pathol. 2002;55(7):541–2.
56. Tan H, Zhang S, Liu H, Peng W, Li R, Gu Y, et al. Imaging findings in phyllodes tumors of the breast. Eur J Radiol. 2012;81(1):e62–9.
57. McCarthy E, Kavanagh J, O'Donoghue Y, McCormack E, D'Arcy C, O'Keeffe SA. Phyllodes tumours of the breast: radiological presentation, management and follow-up. Br J Radiol. 2014;87(1044):20140239.
58. Abdulcadir D, Nori J, Meattini I, Giannotti E, Boeri C, Vanzi E, et al. Phyllodes tumours of the breast diagnosed as B3 category on image-guided 14-gauge core biopsy: analysis of 51 cases from a single institution and review of the literature. Eur J Surg Oncol J Eur Soc Surg Oncol Br Assoc Surg Oncol. 2014;40(7):859–64.
59. Mishra SP, Tiwary SK, Mishra M, Khanna AK. Phyllodes tumor of breast: a review article. ISRN Surg [Internet]. 2013 [cited 2024 Mar 19];2013. Available from: https://www.ncbi.nlm.nih.gov/pmc/articles/PMC3615633/
60. Chao TC, Lo YF, Chen SC, Chen MF. Prospective sonographic study of 3093 breast tumors. J Ultrasound Med Off J Am Inst Ultrasound Med. 1999;18(5):363–70. quiz 371–2
61. Kuhl CK, Mielcareck P, Klaschik S, Leutner C, Wardelmann E, Gieseke J, et al. Dynamic breast MR imaging: are signal intensity time course data useful for differential diagnosis of enhancing lesions? Radiology. 1999;211(1):101–10.
62. Adrada BE, Krishnamurthy S, Carkaci S, Posleman-Monetto FE, Ewere A, Whitman GJ. Unusual benign tumors of the breast. J Clin Imaging Sci. 2015;5:27.
63. Virk RK, Khan A. Pseudoangiomatous stromal hyperplasia: an overview. Arch Pathol Lab Med. 2010;134(7):1070–4.
64. Raj SD, Sahani VG, Adrada BE, Scoggins ME, Albarracin CT, Woodtichartpreecha P, et al. Pseudoangiomatous stromal hyperplasia of the breast: multimodality review with pathologic correlation. Curr Probl Diagn Radiol. 2017;46(2):130–5.
65. Celliers L, Wong DD, Bourke A. Pseudoangiomatous stromal hyperplasia: a study of the mammographic and sonographic features. Clin Radiol. 2010;65(2):145–9.
66. Hargaden GC, Yeh ED, Georgian-Smith D, Moore RH, Rafferty EA, Halpern EF, et al. Analysis of the mammographic and sonographic features of pseudoangiomatous stromal hyperplasia. AJR Am J Roentgenol. 2008;191(2):359–63.
67. Jones KN, Glazebrook KN, Reynolds C. Pseudoangiomatous stromal hyperplasia: imaging findings with pathologic and clinical correlation. AJR Am J Roentgenol. 2010;195(4):1036–42.
68. Rodrigues RA, Azevedo CLAP, Djahjah MCR, Pereira TSS. Tubular adenoma of the breast: radiological and ultrasound findings. Radiol Bras. 2018;51(5):341–2.
69. Saimura M, Anan K, Mitsuyama S, Ono M, Toyoshima S. Ductal carcinoma in situ arising in tubular adenoma of the breast. Breast Cancer Tokyo Jpn. 2015;22(4):428–31.
70. Ng WL, Teoh SY, See MH, Rahmat K, Jayalakshmi P, Ramli MT, et al. Desmoid type fibromatosis of the breast masquerading as breast carcinoma: value of dynamic magnetic resonance imaging and its correlation. Eur J Breast Health. 2021;17(2):197–9.
71. Glazebrook KN, Reynolds CA. Mammary fibromatosis. AJR Am J Roentgenol. 2009;193(3):856–60.
72. Wongmaneerung P, Somwangprasert A, Watcharachan K, Ditsatham C. Bilateral desmoid tumor of the breast: case seriesand literature review. Int Med Case Rep J. 2016;9:247–51.
73. Mesurolle B, Leconte I, Fellah L, Feger C, Nakazono T, Kudo S. Dynamic breast MRI in recurrent fibromatosis. AJR Am J Roentgenol. 2005;184(2):696–7. author reply 697
74. Linda A, Londero V, Bazzocchi M, Zuiani C. Desmoid tumor of the breast: radiologic appearance with a focus on its magnetic resonance features. Breast J. 2008;14(1):106–7.

75. Brown AC, Audisio RA, Regitnig P. Granular cell tumour of the breast. Surg Oncol. 2011;20(2):97–105.
76. Adeniran A, Al-Ahmadie H, Mahoney MC, Robinson-Smith TM. Granular cell tumor of the breast: a series of 17 cases and review of the literature. Breast J. 2004;10(6):528–31.
77. Jardines L, Cheung L, LiVolsi V, Hendrickson S, Brooks JJ. Malignant granular cell tumors: report of a case and review of the literature. Surgery. 1994;116(1):49–54.
78. Fujiwara K, Maeda I, Mimura H. Granular cell tumor of the breast mimicking malignancy: a case report with a literature review. Acta Radiol Open. 2018;7(12):2058460118816537.
79. Jagannathan DM. Benign granular-cell tumor of the breast: case report and literature review. Radiol Case Rep. 2015;10(2):1116.

8 Approach to Non-mass Enhancement on MRI

Malvika Gulati, Sangeeta Taneja, and Ekta Dhamija

Abstract

Enhancement on breast MRI may be classified as focus, mass and non-mass enhancement (NME). Areas of enhancement which do not meet the criteria of a mass, i.e. three-dimensional space-occupying lesions with convex borders, or is not a focus, i.e. a non-space-occupying enhancement <5 mm, and demonstrates intervening fat or normal fibroglandular parenchyma, are referred to as non-mass enhancements. It shows enhancement characteristics distinct from the background parenchymal enhancement and may be spread over a small or wide area in the parenchyma. Description is based on the distribution and internal enhancement characteristics of the NME. Various patterns and enhancement characteristics such as segmental, clumped or clustered ring patterns have a strong positive predictive value for malignancy.

Keywords

Non-mass enhancement · Segmental Clumped · Clustered ring · Ductal carcinoma in situ

8.1 Introduction

Dynamic contrast-enhanced MRI of the breast is becoming increasingly useful in the detection, diagnosis and management of breast cancer. With an increase in the number of breast magnetic resonance imaging (MRI) investigations and its high sensitivity, there has been a rise in the number of detected findings. Since both benign and malignant pathologies can enhance on MRI, there is a need to differentiate various types of enhancement on MR. The extremely high sensitivity of MRI is plagued by low specificity and leads to a large number of false-positive findings.

Enhancing lesions on breast MRI are classified into three main categories: focus, mass and non-mass enhancement (NME).

NME is defined as an enhancing area in the breast distinct from background parenchymal enhancement, is not a focus (i.e. isolated focal enhancement <5 mm in size) and does not exhibit the three-dimensional space-occupying characteristics of a mass (i.e. convex margins and a morphological correlate on non-contrast sequences such as T1 and T2) [1]. NME is usually not discretely

M. Gulati · S. Taneja (✉)
Indraprastha Apollo Hospital, New Delhi, India

E. Dhamija
Department of Diagnostic and Interventional Onco-Radiology, IRCH, AIIMS, New Delhi, India

E. Dhamija, S. V. S. Deo (eds.), *Imaging in Management of Breast Diseases*,
https://doi.org/10.1007/978-981-96-4998-3_8

identified on mammograms and ultrasound (US) due to these being structural modalities.

NME is the most common cause of false positivity on MRI ranging from 40% to 50% because of the substantial overlap among benign, high-risk, and malignant lesions leading to unnecessary biopsies [2]. Thus, there is a need for an evidence-based algorithmic approach for assessing the NME to avoid unnecessary biopsies.

NME is the most common presentation for ductal carcinoma in situ (DCIS) and non-palpable invasive malignancy [3]. When associated with a malignant mass, NME usually indicates an increased extent of the disease which can alter the extent of surgery. Isolated non-mass enhancements can have various benign and malignant differentials.

This chapter aims to discuss the causes, descriptors of NME according to the Breast Imaging Reporting and Data System (BIRADS) lexicon, their association with malignancy and radiologic-pathology correlation of various benign and malignant breast pathologies.

8.2 Background Parenchymal Enhancement Versus NME

Normal fibroglandular tissue enhances on administration of intravenous gadolinium which is referred to as the background parenchymal enhancement (BPE). Both NME and BPE have interspersed areas of a normal fibroglandular tissue or fat [1]. Although symmetric BPE usually does not pose a confusion with NME, asymmetric BPE may often mimic a pathology. It is as important to rule out asymmetric background parenchymal enhancement like in an irradiated breast.

BPE was described under the heading of non-mass enhancement in the initial organization of breast MRI lexicon group; however, it was eventually identified as a separate descriptor. BPE is characteristically affected by the hormonal milieu and hence varies with the phases of the menstrual cycle. It is maximum during the luteal phase of the menstrual cycle, and hence it is recommended to schedule screening MRI early in the cycle, usually in the second week to have minimum confusion from the BPE.

Classically, BPE is bilaterally symmetrical like a mirror image, is diffuse and occasionally may appear as multiple enhancing foci. It shows a gradual type of kinetic curve with a lesser degree of enhancement in the early phases and plateau or rising type of curve. BPE can be predominantly seen in the medial, lateral and posterior inferior parts of the breast forming a 'picture frame' type of appearance [4] (Fig. 8.1).

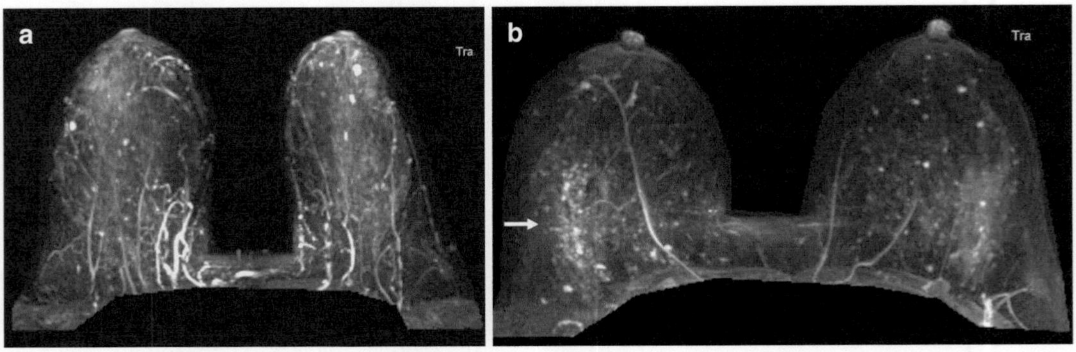

Fig. 8.1 Maximum intensity projection (MIP) images showing (**a**) symmetric moderate BPE with multiple enhancing foci which are considered part of the BPE. The enhancement is symmetrical on both sides. (**b**) On the other hand, an area of enhancement distinct from the moderate BPE (arrow) seen in the outer central quadrant of the right breast would represent a clumped pattern representing NME

8.3 Approach to NME

The first and foremost step is to identify any asymmetrical area of enhancement discrete from the BPE. Any asymmetrical area of NME then needs to be classified based on its morphological descriptors according to the MR BIRADS lexicon. Further evaluation of the contrast kinetics and its appearance on diffusion images and their corresponding apparent diffusion coefficient (ADC) maps help improve the specificity of MRI. This multiparametric approach helps assign an appropriate BIRADS category to the lesion.

The next step would be to perform a second-look US. US performed on lesions newly detected on MRI that were not selected for close scrutiny on first-look US is referred to as 'MRI second-look US'. In contrast to the reported rate of US correlation for masses (49–92%), most previous studies have reported that the yield for NME-US correlation is low and variable (0–54%) in second-look settings [5]. Hsu et al. reported that second-look US identified 43% of NME lesions, with a correlation rate of 76% in malignant lesions compared with 18% in benign lesions [6].

For all suspicious BIRADS 4 and 5 NME lesions, if an US correlate is found, it is biopsied under ultrasound guidance, or else an MRI-guided biopsy is imperative.

Steps for Assessment of NME:

1. *Identification of NME.*
2. *Assign appropriate morphological descriptors.*
3. *Kinetic curve assessment.*
4. *Assessment of DWI images.*
5. *Assign a BIRADS category.*
6. *Second-look ultrasound for BIRADS 4 and 5 lesions*

8.4 MR BIRADS Descriptors for Non-mass Enhancement

8.4.1 Morphological Assessment

According to the fifth edition of BIRADS, any NME is described on the basis of its distribution and internal enhancement characteristics (Table 8.1; Fig. 8.2).

8.4.2 Kinetic Curve Assessment

The kinetic analysis of contrast enhancement is performed in the same way as done for masses. The most suspicious curve pattern derived from the fastest enhancing part of the lesion is chosen to describe the enhancement curve. The initial enhancement phase that is enhanced within the post 2 minutes of contrast injection indicates the contrast inflow and is described as slow, medium or rapid. The delayed phase may show persistent, plateau or washout contrast kinetics. Based on this, we can get three curves: persistent (type I), plateau (type II) and washout (type III) curve.

The kinetics assessment in NME is much more heterogeneous than in masses because of volume of interest averaging resulting from the intervening normal fibroglandular parenchyma or fat and hence the size and placement of region of interest are crucial. Colour-coded maps obtained from computer-aided detection software are of particular importance in NME.

There are, however, conflicting reports over the reliability of kinetic analysis in the assessment of non-mass enhancements. For example, DCIS, which most often presents as NME, is shown to exhibit any type of curve, and hence kinetic curve assessment cannot be solely relied upon [7, 8]. A study performed by Jansen et al. and Newell et al. did not find a statistically significant difference in kinetic curve assessment while differentiating benign vs malignant NME [9, 10].

Table 8.1 Descriptors for non-mass enhancement on MRI [1]

Distribution of NME [1]	
Focal	A small area of enhancement corresponding to <25% of a quadrant and within a single ductal system. This appears as a small area of enhancement with an interspersed normal fibroglandular tissue and not having any T2 correlate Needs to be differentiated from focus which is a single enhancing dot <5 mm A small mass will have convex borders and will have space-occupying characteristics
Linear	Enhancement is seen along a line and mostly denotes an abnormality along a single duct. It may be seen with or without branching
Segmental	The enhancement is typically in a triangular or wedge shape with apex pointing towards the nipple. The segmental enhancement would mean that the underlying pathology or process is following an entire ductal system
Regional	This distribution spans to involve >25% of a quadrant of a breast without any specific ductal morphology. It may be a geographic distribution lacking convex margins
Multiple regions	These represent at least two geographic areas of enhancement with a normal intervening fat or parenchyma
Diffuse	It refers to evenly scattered enhancement in the entire breast showing similar characteristics throughout the breast
Internal enhancement pattern [1]	
Homogeneous	It represents a uniform area of enhancement
Heterogeneous	Seen as a non-uniform pattern of enhancement with random areas of normal non-enhancing breast parenchyma interspersed with enhancing areas
Clumped	Appears as small and large aggregates of enhancement in a cobblestone fashion
Clustered ring	Appears as small enhancing rings which are closely placed and denote ductal enhancement. This implies enhancement in the duct wall and periductal stroma

Nevertheless, lesions with rapid or medium initial enhancement followed by a delayed phase plateau or washout have a positive predictive value (PPV) of 77% for malignancy [11].

Washout kinetics are significantly associated with invasive malignancy and persistent curves with benign etiology in certain studies [12].

8.4.3 Evaluation of Diffusion-Weighted Images

Diffusion-weighted image (DWI) is becoming a routine part of breast MRI protocol, and several studies have demonstrated the effectiveness of DWI in the detection of NME lesions wherein it significantly increases the specificity of MRI in distinguishing between benign and malignant breast tumours avoiding unnecessary breast biopsies [13].

Lower ADC values have been seen in malignant NME with a cut-off of $<1.3 \times 10^{-3}$ mm^2/s showing a sensitivity and specificity of 83.9% and 43% for malignancy [14]. However, the evaluation of NME on DWI may often be limited due to inherent susceptibility artefacts on DWI leading to poor image quality. DWI/ADC could distinguish between invasive disease and DCIS; however, there may be an overlap between in situ and benign disease. DWI may be of particular use in suspected cases of mastitis as microabscesses exhibit central diffusion restriction.

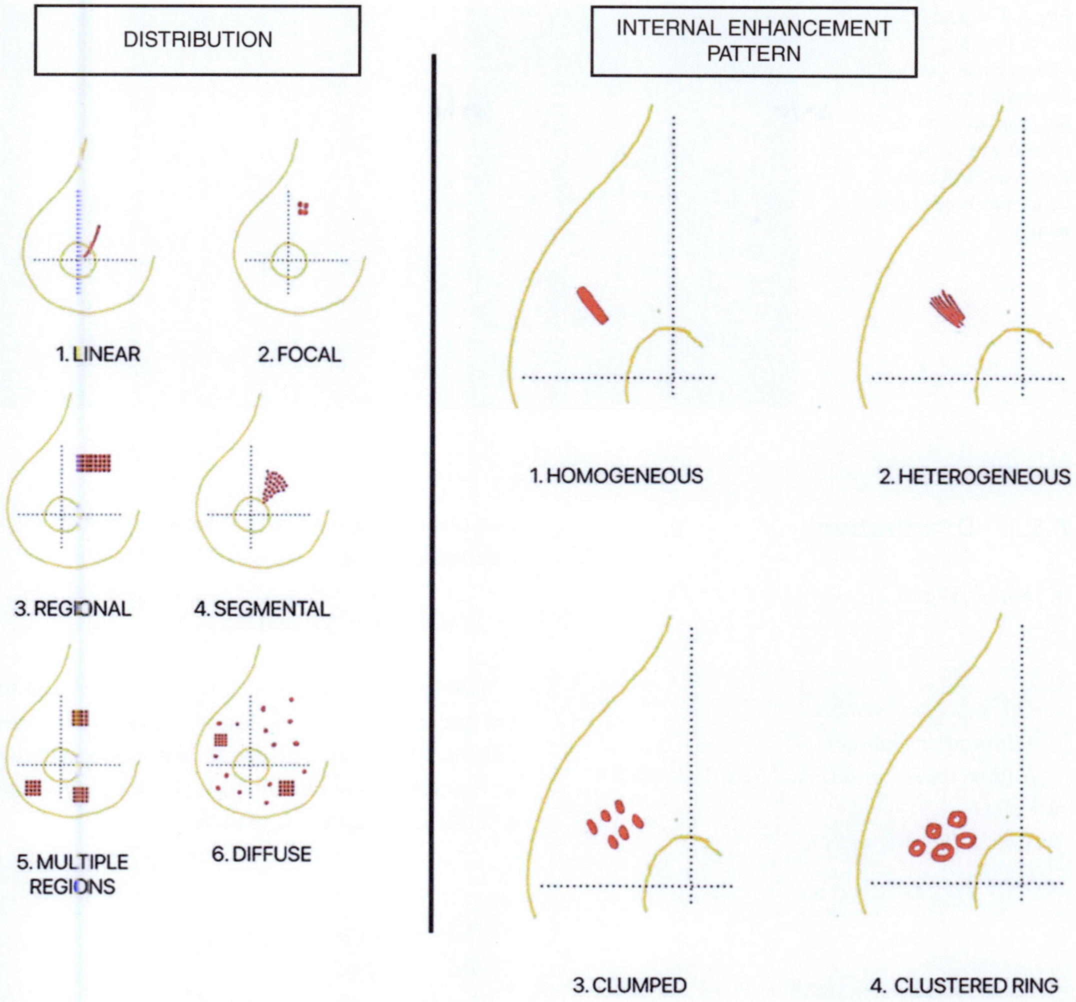

Fig. 8.2 Schematic diagram depicting the NME descriptors [1]

8.5 Morphological Descriptors of NME and Their Histopathological Differentials

NME is evaluated and described based on its distribution, enhancement characteristics and symmetry in both breasts [1]. Although certain features like segmental distribution and clumped pattern of enhancement strongly favour malignancy, there is a substantial overlap between the imaging picture of benign, high-risk and malignant pathologies, and tissue diagnosis is often necessary for the final diagnosis [14].

It is of utmost importance to establish clinico-pathological-radiological concordance which forms the cornerstone of breast imaging. Excision is warranted in cases of radiological-pathological discordance as followed in the other breast imaging modalities.

The American College of Radiology-BIRADS document does not clearly classify the exact MRI characteristic of NME into BIRADS categories due to limited experience compared to mammography and ultrasonography (USG) [1]. The following section shall discuss the various differential diagnoses of distribution and internal enhancement patterns of NME.

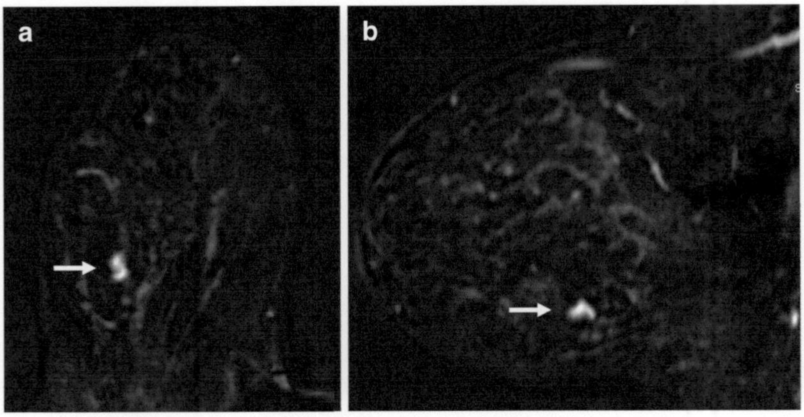

Fig. 8.3 Focal NME: (**a**, **b**) Focal enhancement (arrow) in the right-lower outer quadrant in a low-risk female was stable on follow-up MRIs and hence presumed to be benign

8.5.1 Distribution

1. *Focal* (Fig. 8.3)

*D/Ds of Focal NME***:**
Fibrocystic changes
Radial scars/complex sclerosing lesions
PASH
Sclerosing Adenosis
DCIS

Focal NME is a small area of enhancement which occupies <25% of the volume of a breast quadrant and has a fat or normal glandular tissue between the abnormally enhanced components. These usually do not have any morphological T1/T2 correlate. Also, they neither have an ultrasound nor mammographic correlate except if they are associated with microcalcifications on mammography. This type of enhancement usually manifests as clumped, irregular contrast enhancement. It may also represent a cluster of foci which are small enhancing dots <5 mm. It is more likely to be associated with benign lesions. Differentials of focal NME may vary from benign pathologies such as fibrocystic changes (wherein there are associated small interspersed cysts) to high-risk lesions such as radial scars and sclerosing adenosis. Focal NME usually harbours a low risk of malignancy but if associated with microcalcifications may represent DCIS [14–16].

2. *Linear* (Figs. 8.4 and 8.5)

Linear NME known as ductal enhancement in the previous BIRADS lexicon usually denotes enhancement that is arranged in a non-branching or branching line and denotes abnormality along a single duct and/or its branches.

D/Ds of Linear NME:
Intraductal papilloma
Atypical ductal hyperplasia
Radial scars/complex sclerosing lesions
DCIS

NME lesions with a linear pattern that are smaller than 1 cm and linear enhancement in non-ductal distribution with type I/II curve and no diffusion restriction are more likely to be benign. They can reliably be assigned a BIRADS 3 and followed up [17]. According to some studies, ~6.7% of linear enhancement are associated with malignancy [15]. Linear NME with branching is a significantly stronger predictor of malignancy.

When linear NME is associated with a malignant mass, it usually denotes an in situ component of the malignancy.

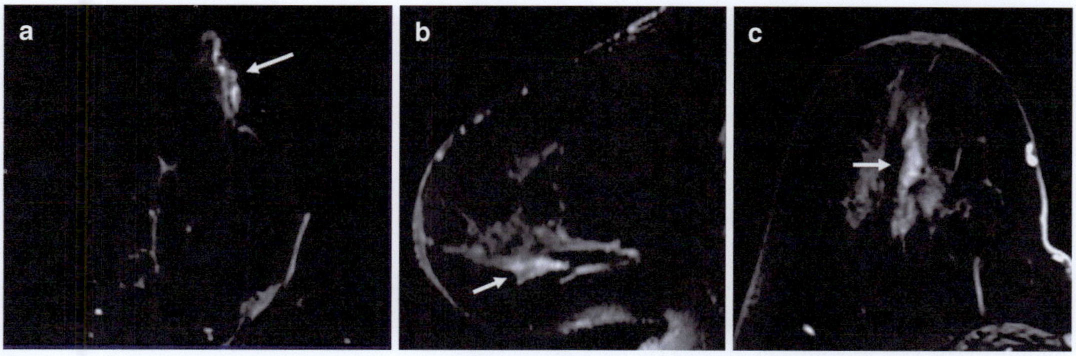

Fig. 8.4 Linear enhancement. (**a**) Linear clumped enhancement in a case of intraductal papilloma. MRI in a screen-detected linear microcalcifications on mammography (not shown) revealed (**b**, **c**) Linear clumped non-branching enhancement (arrow) at a 6 o'clock position at the site of microcalcifications. Stereotactic-guided biopsy revealed atypical ductal hyperplasia. Linear clumped enhancement in (**a**) intraductal papilloma and (**b**, **c**) ADH

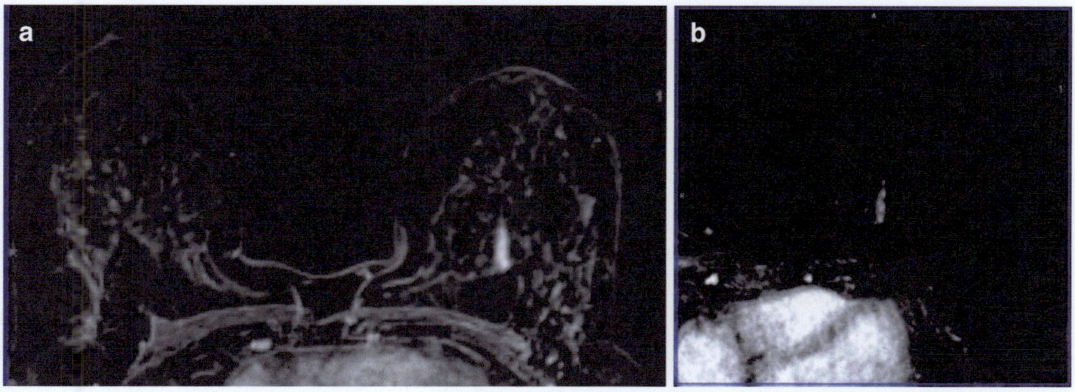

Fig. 8.5 Linear non-branching enhancement stable on scans done at an interval of 1 year: benign

Occasionally linear NME may be associated with microcalcifications in the same distribution on mammography making a stereotactic biopsy feasible.

Ultrasound may reveal one or more dilated ducts with an intraductal vascular soft tissue or periductal/ductal thickening and hence can guide a biopsy. In case there is no correlate on mammogram or ultrasound, MR-guided biopsy is needed in suspicious linear NME.

Histopathological differentials associated with linear or branching NME include intraductal papilloma (IDP), radial scars/complex sclerosing lesions, atypical ductal hyperplasia (ADH) and DCIS.

3. *Segmental* (Fig. 8.6)

D/Ds of Segmental NME:
PASH
Sclerosing adenosis
ADH
DCIS (low/intermediate/high grade)
IDC
Papillary neoplasms

Segmental enhancement is typically seen in a triangular or wedge shape with apex pointing towards the nipple and indicates pathology or process involving an entire single branching ductal system. This distribution has the highest association with malignancy especially if seen exhibiting a clumped or clustered ring type of internal enhancement. The PPV of malignancy with this distribution pattern ranges from 67% to 100% in certain studies [3, 15, 18].

According to Lui et al., 42.9% of the malignant cases presented with segmental NME [14]. Asada et al. and Lunkiewicz et al. showed similar findings [16, 19]. Machida et al. and Hahn et al. concluded that segmental distribution and clustered ring pattern were significantly more common in invasive disease than DCIS [20, 21].

Segmental NME, be it with any kind of internal enhancement, definitely warrants sampling. This can be done under USG or stereotactic guidance if correlates are present. In the absence of any correlate on USG and mammogram, an MRI-guided biopsy is mandatory.

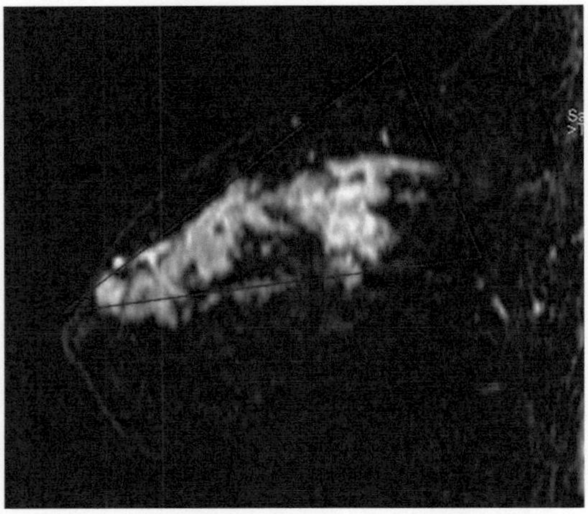

Fig. 8.6 Segmental NME in a case of invasive carcinoma with high-grade DCIS

The segmental distribution of enhancement may be associated with ductal carcinoma in situ, invasive ductal cancer, atypical ductal hyperplasia, papillary neoplasm or sclerosing adenosis [22].

4. *Regional* (Fig. 8.7)

Regional enhancement is geographical, neither ductal nor segmental, and larger than focal and involves more than 25% of one quadrant of a breast. This may be associated with benign or malignant causes and likely to be associated with cancer in 21%.

Homogenous regional enhancements with type I kinetics and no diffusion restriction are assigned BIRADS 2, whereas heterogeneous enhancements in regional distribution with type II and III kinetics with diffusion restriction need to be addressed with biopsy.

These may or may not be associated with mammographic or ultrasound correlates in which case they need to be addressed with MR-guided biopsy.

Benign causes include mastitis particularly idiopathic granulomatous mastitis (IGM) which can show a clumped or clustered ring pattern of enhancement. DWI and their corresponding

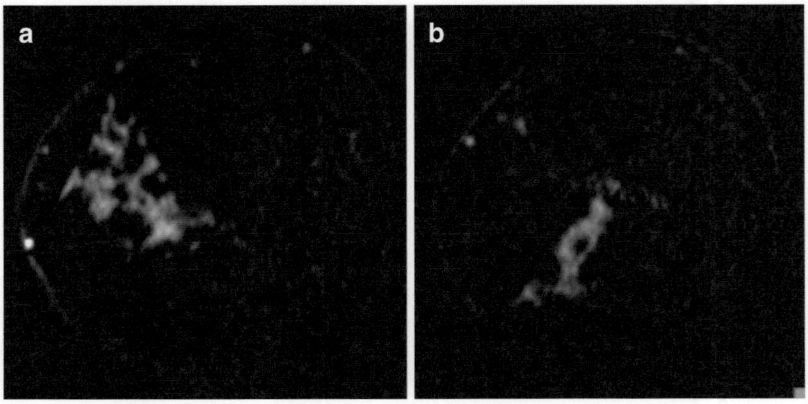

Fig. 8.7 (**a**, **b**) Regional clumped NME in a case presenting with bloody nipple discharge. Pathology revealed low- to intermediate-grade DCIS

ADC maps may reveal central diffusion restriction corresponding with the non-enhancing component within the ducts suggesting microabscesses. Malignant causes of regional NME may include DCIS and invasive lobular carcinoma (ILC).

5. *Multiple Regions*

> *D/Ds of Regional and Multiple Regional NME:*
> *Mastopathic changes*
> *Hormone induced changes*
> *Invasive lobular carcinoma*

These represent involvement of more than one geographical segment of the breast with normal intervening fat or parenchyma and no discernible ductal or segmental distribution. They can be found in both benign and malignant processes in the breast like multicentric IDC, ILC or granulomatous mastitis.

Multiple regional enhancement if symmetrical and seen in similar areas bilaterally usually represents benign proliferative or hormonally mediated breast changes. Asymmetric distribution might be a pointer to sinister pathology such as ILC and should be sampled [23–25].

6. Diffuse

> *D/Ds of Diffuse NME:*
> *Invasive ductal carcinoma*
> *Benign fibrocystic changes*

This refers to uniform enhancement of the entire breast parenchyma showing similar characteristics throughout the breast and is usually associated with benign processes or normal fibroglandular tissue.

It is important to differentiate diffuse NME from BPE. BPE in most cases will be bilateral and symmetrical; however diffuse NME, although widely spread, is usually unilateral. Diffuse NME mostly denotes benign disease, however when associated with a known malignancy, it more likely represents invasive than in situ disease [14].

8.5.2 Internal Enhancement

1. *Homogeneous*

Homogeneous NME represents a confluent uniform area of enhancement and is usually seen in benign pathologies, viz. fibroadenosis [26, 27].

2. *Heterogeneous* (Figs. 8.8 and 8.9)

Heterogeneous NME is seen as non-confluent mixed enhancement with random areas of normal

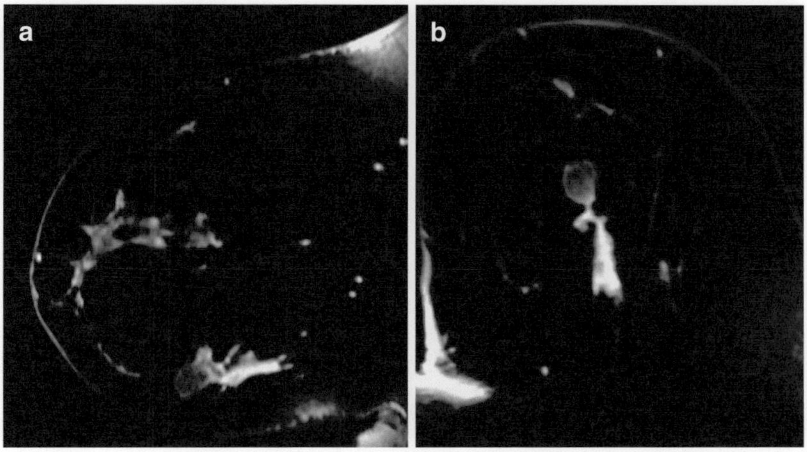

Fig. 8.8 (**a**, **b**) Linear heterogeneous enhancement in biopsy-proven case of DCIS

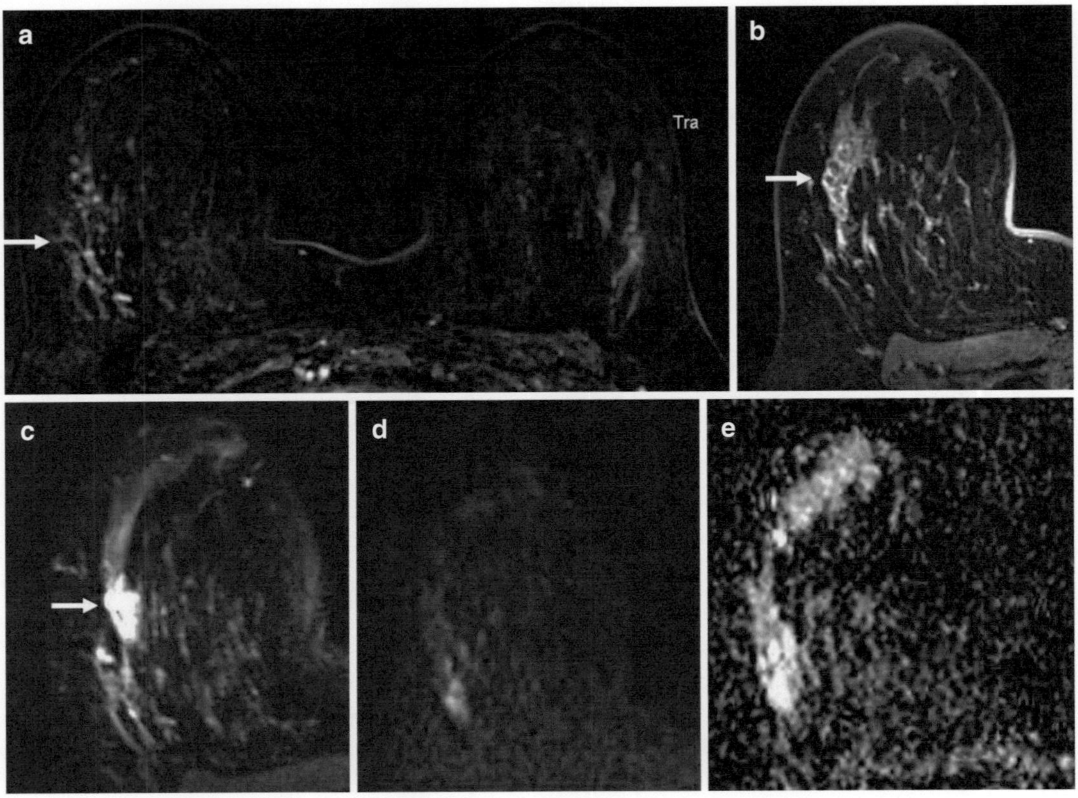

Fig. 8.9 In a patient with right breast pain, MRI revealed (**a**, **b**) regional heterogeneous non-mass enhancement (arrow) in the right outer breast. (**c**) On T2 images, multiple cysts (arrow) were seen associated with the area of NME. (**d**, **e**) No diffusion restriction was demonstrated in the area. Hence a diagnosis of focal fibrocystic changes was established

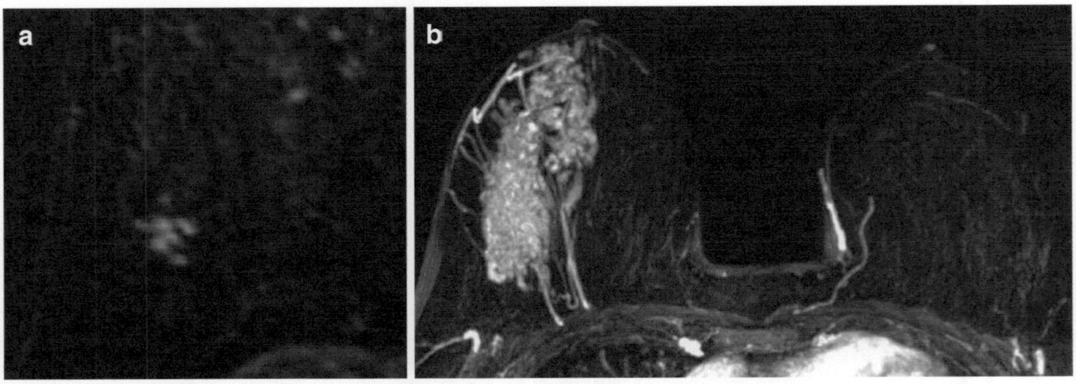

Fig. 8.10 (**a**) Focal clumped NME in a case of DCIS. (**b**) Segmental clumped enhancement in high-grade DCIS

non-enhancing breast parenchyma interspersed between the enhancing areas and is more commonly seen with malignancies [28].

3. *Clumped* (Fig. 8.10)

Clumped NME refers to small and large aggregates of enhancement in a cobblestone fashion. It is frequently seen with malignancies; however, no statistically significant difference has been seen in its prevalence in benign and malig-

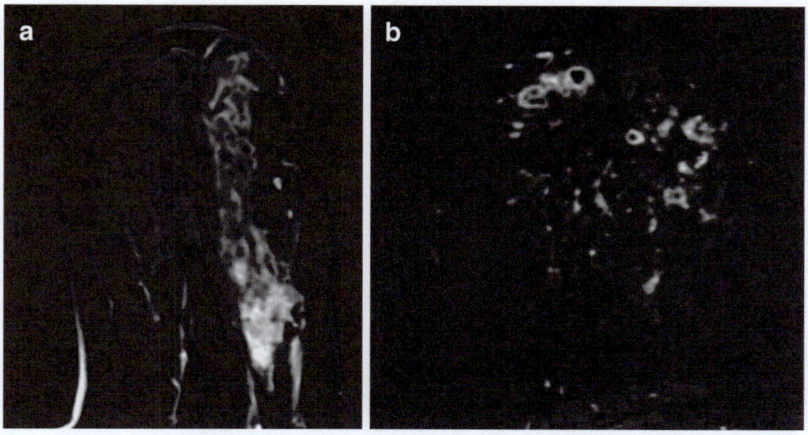

Fig. 8.11 Clustered ring enhancement in a case of (**a**) high-grade DCIS and (**b**) granulomatous mastitis

nant pathologies [15]. Linear clumped and segmental clumped patterns of enhancement have more often been associated with malignancies.

4. *Clustered Ring* (Fig. 8.11)

Clustered ring pattern typically appears as small enhancing rings which are closely placed and implies enhancement in the duct wall and/or periductal stroma. Clustered ring enhancement has been reported to have a PPV of 41% reaching up to 61% if seen in a segmental distribution [15, 28, 29]. Both invasive and in situ carcinomas and granulomatous mastitis are two important differential diagnoses demonstrating this type of enhancement.

8.6 Pathological Correlates of Various Benign and Malignant Breast Diseases Presenting as NME on MRI

Pseudoangiomatous stromal hyperplasia (PASH) PASH is usually detected as an incidental finding on biopsies in premenopausal females and is a benign entity [30]. Presenting as a circumscribed oval noncalcified mass on mammogram, it may also appear as a focal or developing asymmetry. MRI often shows focal or segmental clumped non-mass enhancement with type I or II curves. It is possible to detect T2 hypointense linear fibrous stroma and T2 hyperintense cystic spaces within the area which mimics the histological picture consisting of slit-like vascular spaces [31]. These do not require surgical excision unless there is a significant increase in size [32].

Idiopathic granulomatous mastitis (IGM) is a common benign differential in cases of regional NME which mimics malignancy clinically and radiologically. It is commonly seen in premenopausal females with a recent history of childbirth and lactation [33]. A chronic noninfectious mastitis, it is characterized by remitting relapsing course and may be complicated by discharging sinuses on the breast skin [34]. Ultrasound reveals multiple dilated ducts with internal nonvascular contents and surrounding inflammatory changes. Multiple collections with finger-like extensions into the surrounding breast parenchyma are also seen [35, 36]. MRI works as a problem-solving modality in cases where ultrasound is equivocal. MRI reveals a segmental or regional area of NME showing a clustered ring pattern. Delineation of small T2 bright peripherally enhancing collection representing microabscesses in the correct clinical background clinches the diagnosis [37]. Biopsy is usually required to confirm the diagnosis. Aspiration is usually not helpful due to the nondrainable nature of these collections. Management options include conservative, medical management with surgical options resorted to in nonresponsive cases [38, 39] (Fig. 8.12).

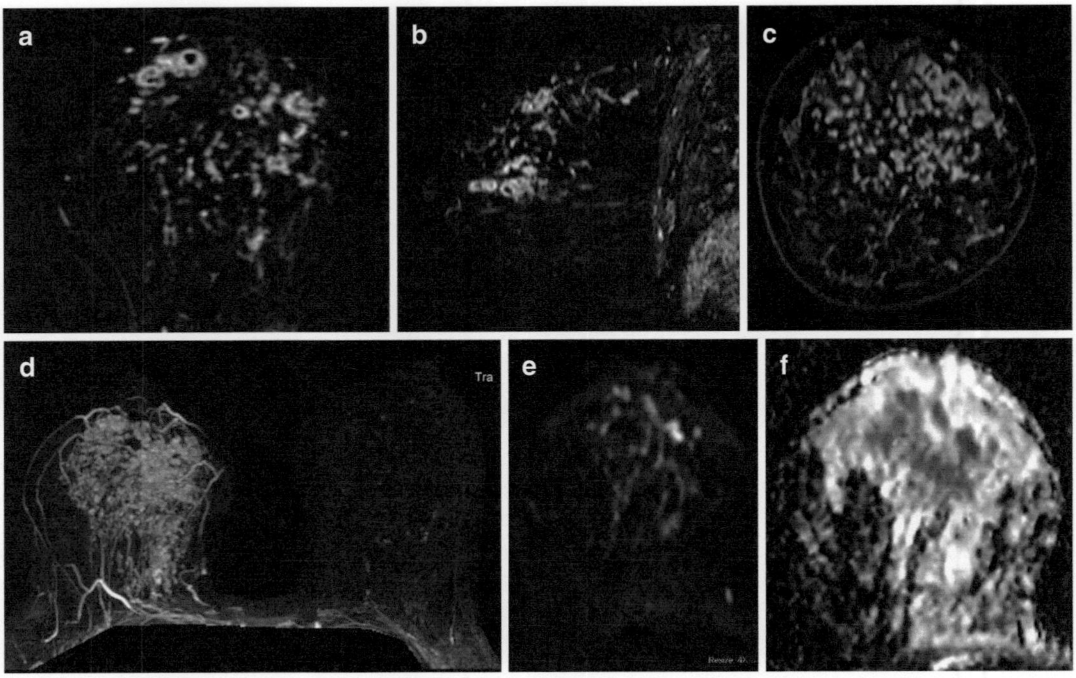

Fig. 8.12 A high-risk patient presented with a palpable lump in the right breast. Mammogram (not shown) showed extremely dense breasts and was inconclusive. MRI showed (**a**–**c**) regional clustered ring enhancement in the right upper inner and upper outer quadrants. (**d**) MIP image demonstrates the large area of NME with prominent vessels. (**e**, **f**) Diffusion-weighted images revealed areas of central diffusion restriction in the clustered enhancing rings. BIRADS 4b was assigned to the imaging. An USG-guided biopsy was performed, and the final diagnosis was idiopathic granulomatous mastitis

Radial scars/complex sclerosing lesions are usually detected incidentally on mammograms as isolated areas of architectural distortion often with low-density centre and thin long spicules [40]. Such an imaging appearance warrants a biopsy to rule out the alternate ominous diagnosis of ductal carcinoma in situ. MRI may be done to further investigate a mammogram-detected lesion. Lesions may appear as focal or linear clumped non-mass enhancement with early rapid enhancement with type 2 or 3 kinetic curve [32]. These lesions per say are not pre-malignant but may have associated foci of in situ and invasive carcinoma, and hence excision is the classical teaching [41]. However recent studies have shown that excision can be avoided in select cases not exhibiting any atypia and where sampling is done by vacuum-assisted biopsy [42].

Complex sclerosing lesions may appear as linear or clumped nonmass enhancement with early rapid enhancement and type 2 or 3 kinetic curve [32]. These lesions per say are not pre-malignant but may have associated foci of in situ and invasive carcinoma, and hence excision is the classical teaching [41]. However recent studies have shown that excision can be avoided in select cases not exhibiting any atypia and where sampling is done by vacuum-assisted biopsy [42].

Intraductal papillomas One of the most common pathologies presenting with linear NME is *intraductal papilloma*. Papillary lesions of the breast encompass a spectrum including benign intraductal papillomas without and with atypia and papillary carcinomas. Papillomas are the most common cause of unilateral spontaneous bloody nipple discharge. These are usually occult on mammograms or may appear as a solitary dilated duct with or without microcalcifications. Ultrasound shows a dilated duct with an internal echogenic soft tissue typically with a vascular core. MRI may show an enhancing focus or lin-

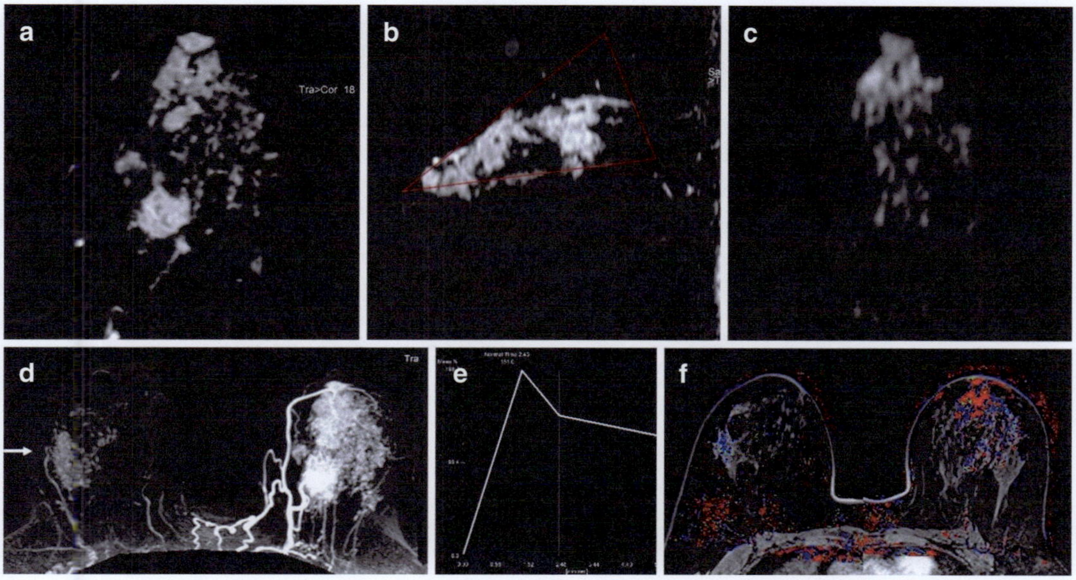

Fig. 8.13 NME in a patient presenting with a left breast palpable lump. MRI showed (**a**, **b**) segmental mass and non-mass enhancement with a heterogeneous pattern in the left upper breast. (**c**) Diffusion restriction was seen on DWI images. (**d**) MIP images showed additional regional clumped NME in the right outer breast (arrow). The left breast NME showed a (**e**, **f**) washout pattern, and the right NME showed a plateau type of kinetics as seen in the curve and colour maps. The final diagnosis was invasive ductal carcinoma with high-grade DCIS in the left breast and isolated intermediate-grade DCIS in the right breast

ear non-mass enhancement mostly in the retroareolar region [43]. Management varies from institute to institute with some advocating excision for all papillary lesions due to nearly 40% upgrade to malignancy, while others advocating close follow-up in cases of small, asymptomatic adequately sampled lesions [44, 45].

Atypical ductal hyperplasia ADH is a high-risk lesion having one of the highest upgrade rates to malignancy on surgical excision varying from 7% to 54% and may present as linear or segmental NME [46]. These are lesions showing ductal proliferation with atypia falling below the criteria for diagnosis of ductal carcinoma in situ. The possible reason of upgrade could be due to underrepresentation of the disease because of limited sampling on core biopsy. Hence, detection of these lesions warrants excisional biopsy. These appear to be grouped suspicious microcalcifications on mammograms and show a variety of non-mass enhancement or a mass on MRI. Studies have shown that it is not possible to reliably predict upgrade rate by studying MRI characteristics [47].

Ductal carcinoma in situ (Fig. 8.13) DCIS is one of the most important differential diagnoses of non-mass enhancement which needs to be ruled out. It is often a screen-detected lesion appearing as suspicious linear branching or segmental microcalcifications or area of architectural distortion on mammogram [48]. MRI is done to delineate the exact extent of the lesion due to the presence of noncalcified components of DCIS. Segmental or linear clustered ring or clumped enhancement is the most common finding [49]. These lesions are managed with breast conservation surgery and radiation therapy.

Invasive ductal carcinoma (IDC) (Fig. 8.13) This is the most common variety of breast cancer and may develop de novo or in a preexisting focus of DCIS. It classically presents as an irregular high-density spiculated mass on mammogram with or without calcifications. Suspicious microcalcifications may extend beyond the mass and represent the intraductal extension of the malignancy. MRI mirrors the mammographic findings showing an enhancing mass with spiculated margins. Associated non-mass enhancement of variable patterns may be associated with the primary mass and represent the associated DCIS component, thus impacting the management. Rarely, IDC may primarily present as an area of non-mass enhancement with variable distribution and enhancement pattern [50].

Invasive lobular cancer ILC is the rarer variety of breast cancers comprising 10–15% of the cases. They are notorious for being mammographically occult and appearing as asymmetries and masses with indistinct margins without associated architectural distortion. They usually present as palpable abnormality, and ultrasound reveals non-mass areas with posterior shadowing. MRI is invariably recommended in all diagnosed cases of ILC due to its strong association with multifocality, multicentricity and bilaterality. Lesions commonly show a focal or regional type of non-mass enhancement with washout kinetics rarely seen [23–25].

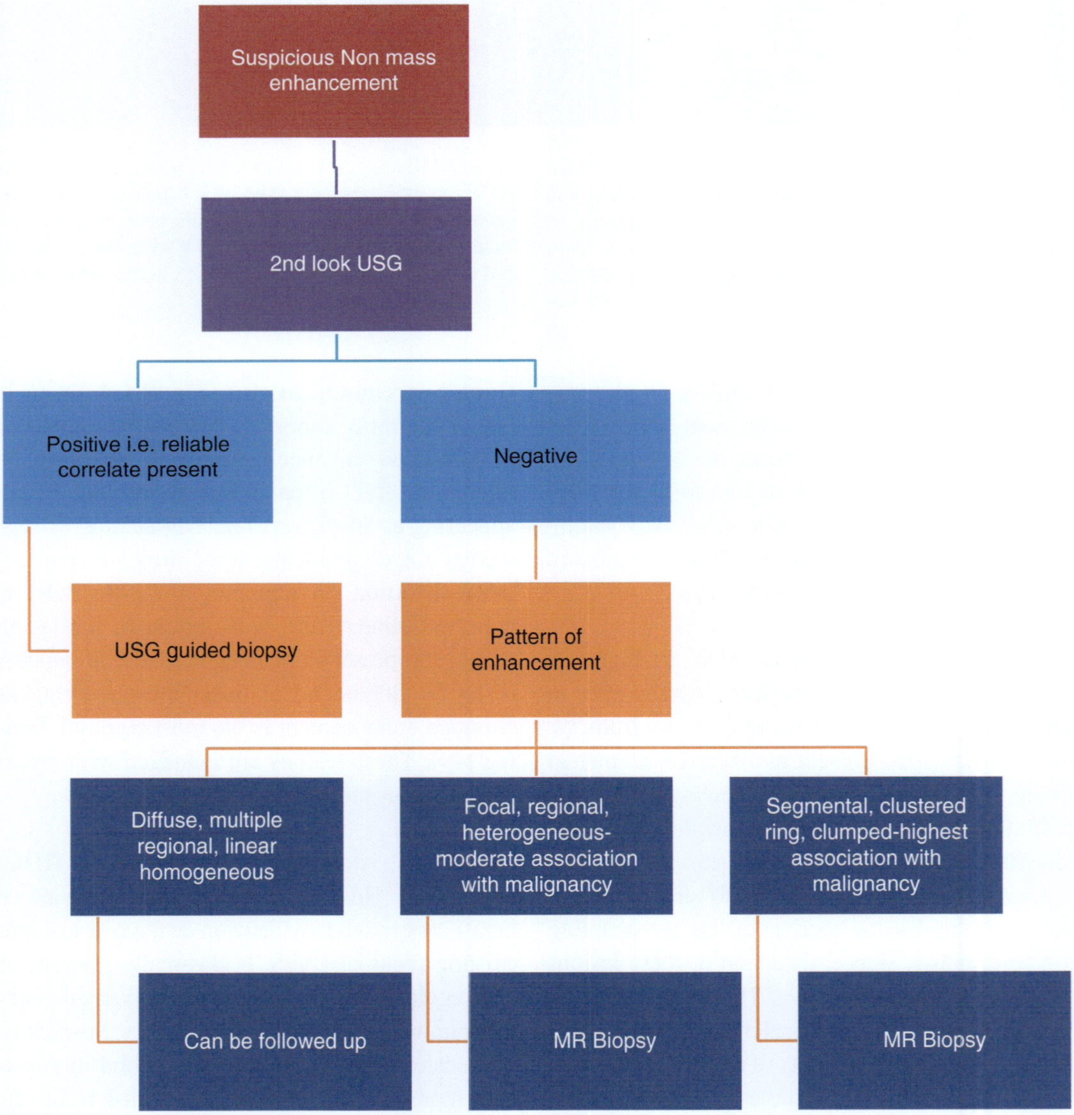

Fig. 8.14 Algorithmic approach to NME on MRI

8.7 Algorithmic Approach to NME

Figure 8.14 illustrates a general approach to NME seen on MRI.

The entity of fibrocystic changes might be often confused with DCIS as both present with non-mass enhancement on MRI. Some imaging pointers such as the presence of small T2 bright cystic areas within, plateau or late wash in of contrast may suggest fibrocystic changes and avoid a biopsy. In contrast signs like adjacent vessel washout pattern of enhancement point towards DCIS [51].

8.8 Role of Newer Breast MRI Techniques in Assessment of NME

There is paucity of data on the impact of newer breast MRI techniques such as abbreviated and ultrafast MRI on diagnosis of NME. Abbreviated breast MRI only comprises a single early post-contrast image and hence does not provide any kinetic information regarding enhancing lesions [52]. A study by Moriki et al. showed that kinetic information derived from ultrafast and dynamic contrast MRI was comparable to the morphological features in differentiating benign and malignant NME [12]. However more studies are needed to validate these relatively newer techniques.

8.9 Conclusion

Non-mass enhancement has various patterns of distribution and internal enhancement. Certain features like segmental clumped and clustered ring patterns have a significant association with malignancy. It is preferable to do the MRI scans in the correct phase of the menstrual cycle to avoid confusion with background parenchymal enhancement. Kinetic and diffusion characteristics are complementary to the morphology of the NME; however, there is a wide overlap between the imaging appearance of benign and malignant pathologies, and hence a biopsy is needed in most cases.

References

1. Morris EA, Comstock CE, Lee CH, et al. ACR BI-RADS® magnetic resonance imaging. In: ACR BI-RADS® atlas, breast imaging reporting and data system. Reston: American College of Radiology; 2013.
2. Baltzer PA, Benndorf M, Dietzel M, Gajda M, Runnebaum IB, Kaiser WA. False-positive findings at contrast-enhanced breast MRI: a BI-RADS descriptor study. AJR Am J Roentgenol. 2010;194:1658–63.
3. Yang QX, Ji X, Feng LL, Zheng L, Zhou XQ, Wu Q, et al. Significant MRI indicators of malignancy for breast non-mass enhancement. J Xray Sci Technol. 2017;25:1033–44. https://doi.org/10.3233/XST-17311.
4. Liao GJ, Henze Bancroft LC, Strigel RM, Chitalia RD, Kontos D, Moy L, Partridge SC, Rahbar H. Background parenchymal enhancement on breast MRI: a comprehensive review. J Magn Reson Imaging. 2020;51(1):43–61. https://doi.org/10.1002/jmri.26762. Epub 2019 Apr 19. PMID: 31004391; PMCID: PMC7207072
5. Newburg AR, Chhor CM, Young Lin LL, Heller SL, Gillman J, Toth HK, et al. Magnetic resonance imaging-directed ultrasound imaging of non-mass enhancement in the breast: outcomes and frequency of malignancy. J Ultrasound Med. 2017;36:493–504.
6. Hsu HH, Chang TH, Chou YC, Peng YJ, Ko KH, Chang WC, et al. Breast non-mass enhancement detected with MRI: utility and lesion characterization with second-look ultrasonography. Breast J. 2015;21:579–87.
7. Kim JA, Son EJ, Youk JH, et al. MRI findings of pure ductal carcinoma in situ: kinetic characteristics compared according to lesion type and histopathologic factors. AJR. 2011;196:1450–6.
8. Rosen EL, Smith-Foley SA, DeMartini WB, Eby PR, Peacock S, Lehman CD. BI-RADS MRI enhancement characteristics of ductal carcinoma in situ. Breast J. 2007;13:545–55.
9. Newell D, Nie K, Chen JH, et al. Selection of diagnostic features on breast MRI to differentiate between malignant and benign lesions using computer-aided diagnosis: differences in lesions presenting as mass and non-mass-like enhancement. Eur Radiol. 2010;20:771–81.

10. Jansen SA, Fan X, Karczmar GS, et al. DCEMRI of breast lesions: is kinetic analysis equally effective for both mass and nonmass-like enhancement? Med Phys. 2008;35:3102–9.
11. Kuhl CK, Mielcareck P, Klaschik S, et al. Dynamic breast MR imaging: are signal intensity time course data useful for differential diagnosis of enhancing lesions? Radiology. 1999;211:101–10.
12. Mori N, Sheth D, Abe H. Nonmass enhancement breast lesions: diagnostic performance of kinetic assessment on ultrafast and standard dynamic contrast-enhanced MRI in comparison with morphologic evaluation. Am J Roentgenol. 2020;215(2):511–8.
13. Yabuuchi H, Matsuo Y, Kamitani T, Setoguchi T, Okafuji T, Soeda H, et al. Non-mass-like enhancement on contrast enhanced breast MR imaging: lesion characterization using combination of dynamic contrast-enhanced and diffusion weighted MR images. Eur J Radiol. 2010;75:e126–32. https://doi.org/10.1016/j.ejrad.2009.09.013.
14. Liu G, Li Y, Chen SL, Chen Q. Non-mass enhancement breast lesions: MRI findings and associations with malignancy. Ann Transl Med. 2022;10(6):357. https://doi.org/10.21037/atm-22-503. PMID: 35433999; PMCID: PMC9011203
15. Aydin H. The MRI characteristics of non-mass enhancement lesions of the breast: associations with malignancy. Br J Radiol. 2019;92(1096):20180464. https://doi.org/10.1259/bjr.20180464. Epub 2019 Jan 29. PMID: 30673299; PMCID: PMC6540851
16. Asada T, Yamada T, Kanemaki Y, et al. Grading system to categorize breast MRI using BI-RADS 5th edition: a statistical study of non-mass enhancement descriptors in terms of probability of malignancy. Jpn J Radiol. 2018;36:200–8.
17. Amarnath C, Patel H, Rama Murthy BS, Raghavan B, Jhankaria B, Chotai N, editors. Comprehensive textbook of clinical radiology. Volume V: Obstetrics and breast-eBook. Elsevier Health Sciences; 2023.
18. Thomassin-Naggara I, Trop I, Chopier J, David J, Lalonde L, Darai E, et al. Nonmasslike enhancement at breast MR imaging: the added value of mammography and US for lesion categorization. Radiology. 2011;261:69–79. https://doi.org/10.1148/radiol.11110190.
19. Lunkiewicz M, Forte S, Freiwald B, et al. Interobserver variability and likelihood of malignancy for fifth edition BI-RADS MRI descriptors in non-mass breast lesions. Eur Radiol. 2020;30:77–86.
20. Machida Y, Shimauchi A, Tozaki M, et al. Descriptors of malignant non-mass enhancement of breast MRI: their correlation to the presence of invasion. Acad Radiol. 2016;23:687–95.
21. Hahn SY, Han BK, Ko EY, et al. MR features to suggest microinvasive ductal carcinoma of the breast: can it be differentiated from pure DCIS? Acta Radiol. 2013;54:742–8.
22. Liberman L, Morris EA, Dershaw DD, et al. Ductal enhancement on MR imaging of the breast. AJR. 2003;181:519–25.
23. Mann RM. The effectiveness of MR imaging in the assessment of invasive lobular carcinoma of the breast. Magn Reson Imaging Clin N Am. 2010;18:259–76.
24. Mann RM, Hoogeveen YL, Blickman JG, Boetes C. MRI compared to conventional diagnostic workup in the detection and evaluation of invasive lobular carcinoma of the breast: a review of existing literature. Breast Cancer Res Treat. 2008;107:1–14.
25. Lopez JK, Bassett LW. Invasive lobular carcinoma of the breast: spectrum of mammographic, US, and MR imaging findings. Radiographics. 2009;29:165–76.
26. Mahoney MC, Gatsonis C, Hanna L, DeMartini WB, Lehman C. Positive predictive value of BI-RADS MR imaging. Radiology. 2012;264:51–8. https://doi.org/10.1148/radiol.12110619.
27. Uematsu T, Kasami M. High-spatial-resolution 3-T breast MRI of nonmasslike enhancement lesions: an analysis of their features as significant predictors of malignancy. AJR Am J Roentgenol. 2012;198:1223–30. https://doi.org/10.2214/AJR.11.7350.
28. Tozaki M, Igarashi T, Fukuda K. Breast MRI using the VIBE sequence: clustered ring enhancement in the differential diagnosis of lesions showing non-masslike enhancement. AJR Am J Roentgenol. 2006;187(2):313–21. https://doi.org/10.2214/AJR.05.0881. PMID: 16861532
29. Yuen S, Uematsu T, Masako K, Uchida Y, Nishimura T. Segmental enhancement on breast MR images: differential diagnosis and diagnostic strategy. Eur Radiol. 2008;18:2067–75. https://doi.org/10.1007/s00330-008-0980-3.
30. Ibrahim RE, Sciotto CG, Weidner N. Pseudoangiomatous hyperplasia of mammary stroma: some observations regarding its clinicopathologic spectrum. Cancer. 1989;63:1154–60.
31. Jones KN, Glazebrook KN, Reynolds C. Pseudoangiomatous stromal hyperplasia: imaging findings with pathologic and clinical correlation. AJR. 2010;195:1036–42.
32. Chadashvili T, Ghosh E, Fein-Zachary V, Mehta TS, Venkataraman S, Dialani V, Slanetz PJ. Nonmass enhancement on breast MRI: review of patterns with radiologic-pathologic correlation and discussion of management. Am J Roentgenol. 2015;204(1):219–27.
33. Bani-Hani KE, Yaghan RJ, Matalka II, et al. Idiopathic granulomatous mastitis: time to avoid unnecessary mastectomies. Breast J. 2004;10:318–22.
34. Tse GMK, Poon CSP, Ramachandram K, et al. Granulomatous mastitis: a clinicopathological review of 26 cases. Pathology. 2004;36:254–7.
35. Pluguez-Turull CW, Nanyes JE, Quintero CJ, et al. Idiopathic granulomatous mastitis: manifestations at multimodality imaging and pitfalls. Radiographics. 2018;38:330–56.
36. Yildiz S, Aralasmak A, Kadioglu H, et al. Radiologic findings of idiopathic granulomatous mastitis. Med Ultrason. 2015;17:39–44.
37. Dursun M, Yilmaz S, Yahyayev A, et al. Multimodality imaging features of idiopathic granulomatous masti-

tis: outcome of 12 years of experience. Radiol Med. 2012;117:529–38.
38. Erozgen F, Ersoy YE, Akaydin M, et al. Corticosteroid treatment and timing of surgery in idiopathic granulomatous mastitis confusing with breast carcinoma. Breast Cancer Res Treat. 2010;123:447–52.
39. Ahmed YS, Abd El Maksoud W. Evaluation of therapeutic mammoplasty techniques in the surgical management of female patients with idiopathic granulomatous mastitis with mild to moderate inflammatory symptoms in terms of recurrence and patients' satisfaction. Breast Dis. 2016;36(1):37–45.
40. Tabar L, Dean PB. Teaching atlas of mammography. Fortschr Geb Rontgenstrahlen Nuklearmed Erganzungsbd. 1983;116:1–222.
41. Andacoglu O, Kanbour-Shakir A, Teh YC, et al. Rationale of excisional biopsy after the diagnosis of benign radial scar on core biopsy: a single institutional outcome analysis. Am J Clin Oncol. 2013;36:7–11.
42. Resetkova E, Edelweiss M, Albarracin CT, Yang WT. Management of radial sclerosing lesions of the breast diagnosed using percutaneous vacuumassisted core needle biopsy: recommendations for excision based on seven years' of experience at a single institution. Breast Cancer Res Treat. 2011;127:335–43.
43. Kurz KD, Roy S, Saleh A, Diallo-Danebrock R, Skaane P. MRI features of intraductal papilloma of the breast: sheep in wolf's clothing? Acta Radiol. 2011;52:264–72.
44. Rozentsvayg E, Carver K, Borker S, Mathew M, Enis S, Friedman P. Surgical excision of benign papillomas diagnosed with core biopsy: a community hospital approach. Radiol Res Pract. 2011;2011:679864.
45. Ashkenazi I, Ferrer K, Sekosan M, et al. Papillary lesions of the breast discovered on percutaneous large core and vacuum-assisted biopsies: reliability of clinical and pathological parameters in identifying benign lesions. Am J Surg. 2007;194:183–8.
46. Eby PR, Ochsner JE, DeMartini WB, Allison KH, Peacock S, Lehman CD. Frequency and upgrade rates of atypical ductal hyperplasia diagnosed at stereotactic vacuum-assisted breast biopsy: 9- versus 11-gauge. AJR. 2009;192:229–34.
47. Crystal P, Sadaf A, Bukhanov K, McCready D, O'Malley F, Helbich TH. High-risk lesions diagnosed at MRI-guided vacuum-assisted breast biopsy: can underestimation be predicted? Eur Radiol. 2011;21:582–9.
48. Slanetz PJ, Giardino AA, Oyama T, et al. Mammographic appearance of ductal carcinoma in situ does not reliably predict histologic subtype. Breast J. 2001;7:417–21.
49. Rosen EL, Smith-Foley SA, DeMartini WB, Eby PR, Peacock S, Lehman CD. BI-RADS MRI enhancement characteristics of ductal carcinoma in situ. Breast J. 2007;13:545–50.
50. Liberman L, Morris EA, Lee MJ, et al. Breast lesions detected on MR imaging: features and positive predictive value. AJR. 2002;179:171–8.
51. Dietzel M, Kaiser CG, Wenkel E, Clauser P, Uder M, Schulz-Wendtland R, Baltzer PA. Differentiation of ductal carcinoma in situ versus fibrocystic changes by magnetic resonance imaging: are there pathognomonic imaging features? Acta Radiol. 2017;58(10):1206–14.
52. Gao Y, Heller SL. Abbreviated and ultrafast breast MRI in clinical practice. Radiographics. 2020;40(6):1507–27.

Ductal Carcinoma In Situ: Imaging and Management

9

Seema Sud, Rakesh Kaul, and Seema Rao

Abstract

Ductal carcinoma in situ (DCIS) is a preinvasive malignancy and a nonobligate precursor to invasive carcinoma. DCIS shares common risk factors with invasive carcinoma in terms of age, hormonal influence, and genetic factors; hence it is thought to be a precursor to invasive carcinoma. There is proliferation of malignant cells within the terminal ductal lobular unit and can spread into the lactiferous ducts or involve the nipple without invasion of the basement membrane or myoepithelial layer. It is crucial to detect malignancy in this early stage for providing optimal patient management. DCIS rarely presents as a palpable mass and thus mostly detected in asymptomatic women on screening mammography. The commonest presentation is with fine pleomorphic calcification, which is best detected by mammography. The noncalcified DCIS can be better delineated on contrast-enhanced magnetic resonance imaging. Mammography along with ultrasonography are the imaging modalities used for detection followed by tissue sampling. Contrast-enhanced spectral mammography has added a new dimension to the delineation of extent of the disease by demonstrating the enhancing component along with the visualization of microcalcification. Magnetic resonance imaging stays as the gold standard by virtue of its better resolution and illustration as nonmass enhancement for DCIS. This chapter provides a comprehensive review of the various imaging modalities available for diagnosis, pathological evaluation, and management of DCIS.

Keywords

Ductal carcinoma in situ · Invasive carcinoma Nonmass enhancement · Dynamic contrast-enhanced MRI · Microcalcification · Digital mammography

9.1 Introduction

DCIS is a preinvasive carcinoma limited to the terminal ductal lobular unit without stromal invasion [1]. It is a stage between benign breast diseases like atypical ductal hyperplasia and malignancy, that is, invasive ductal carcinoma (IDC). DCIS shares common risk factors with IDC in terms of age, hormonal influence, and

S. Sud (✉)
Department of CT & MRI, Sir Ganga Ram Hospital, New Delhi, India

R. Kaul
Department of Surgical Oncology, Sir Ganga Ram Hospital, New Delhi, India

S. Rao
Department of Pathology, Sir Ganga Ram Hospital, New Delhi, India

E. Dhamija, S. V. S. Deo (eds.), *Imaging in Management of Breast Diseases*,
https://doi.org/10.1007/978-981-96-4998-3_9

genetic factors; hence it is thought to be a precursor to IDC. It involves proliferation of malignant cells within the terminal ductal lobular unit that can spread into the lactiferous ducts or involve the nipple without invasion of the basement membrane or myoepithelial layer.

With the advent of screening mammography in the 1980s, detection and diagnosis of DCIS significantly has increased as DCIS rarely presents with a palpable mass. The commonest imaging presentation as fine pleomorphic calcification is best detected by mammography (MG). The noncalcified DCIS can be better delineated on contrast-enhanced magnetic resonance imaging (CE-MRI).

9.2 Clinical Features and Risk Factors

Most (50–70%) of DCIS are clinically occult and thus often incidentally detected on either screening MG or diagnostic MG for unrelated indications. Rarely, in 2–3% patients, they can present as small palpable masses which are less than a cm in size or are associated with Paget's disease of the nipple or pathological nipple discharge.

The risk factors for DCIS are similar to IDC, which include germ line mutations (e.g., BRCA1/BRCA2), family history, nulliparity, late age at first childbirth, late menopause, elevated body mass index, and hormone replacement therapy [2]. The lifetime risk of DCIS for a BRCA mutation carrier is about sixfold higher vs a noncarrier [3]. High levels of genomic alterations are seen in high-grade DCIS in comparison to low-grade DCIS [4].

Women diagnosed with DCIS have tenfold higher risk of developing ipsilateral IDC, if remain untreated [5, 6]. Although the proportion of developing IDC in untreated high-grade and low-grade DCIS is similar, the time interval to the development of recurrence varies. Low-grade DCIS has longer interval (>15 years), whereas rapid progression has been observed in high-grade DCIS (<5 years) [6, 7]. Meta-analysis study of long-term outcome in DCIS showed a 15-year total local recurrence rate of 40%, with 28% recurring as invasive disease [8]. Positive surgical margins, high nuclear grade, large lesion size, comedo necrosis, and young age (<45 years) are the most important clinicopathologic predictors associated with local recurrence and prognosis [9].

9.3 Histopathological Features of DCIS

DCIS is a noninvasive proliferation of neoplastic epithelial cells confined within mammary duct-lobular system, without any evidence of tumor spread into surrounding breast tissue. It encompasses a heterogeneous group of lesions that differ with regard to their genetic abnormalities, histopathological features and risk for progression.

Gross appearance Most DCIS detected by MG cannot be appreciated visually and may require specimen radiograph for localization. On sectioning, DCIS are poorly defined; however, prominent comedo-type necrosis may be seen as small cystic ducts exuding pale material within poorly defined fibrous areas. A small proportion of high-grade DCIS may present as multiple ill circumscribed, firm, gritty areas. The sampling method used depends on the size and location of the DCIS lesion. In general, the entire lesion should be sampled sequentially, if possible. If the lesion is very large or involves multiple quadrants of the breast, multiple sections should be taken. All margins should be documented similar to IDC.

Microscopic features DCIS is a segmental disease characteristically limited to a single duct system but can show lobular involvement. DCIS shows various architectural patterns, namely, solid, cribriform, comedo, micropapillary, papillary, and flat types, where the terminology is sufficiently self-explanatory (Fig. 9.1 a-g). However, the use of cytonuclear morphology has been recommended for histological grading of DCIS over architectural patterns as the former has more homogeneity [10]. According to the nuclear grading [11, 12], DCIS can be categorized as low, intermediate, or high nuclear grade using defined criteria (Figs. 9.2a, 9.3a, b, and 9.4a, b).

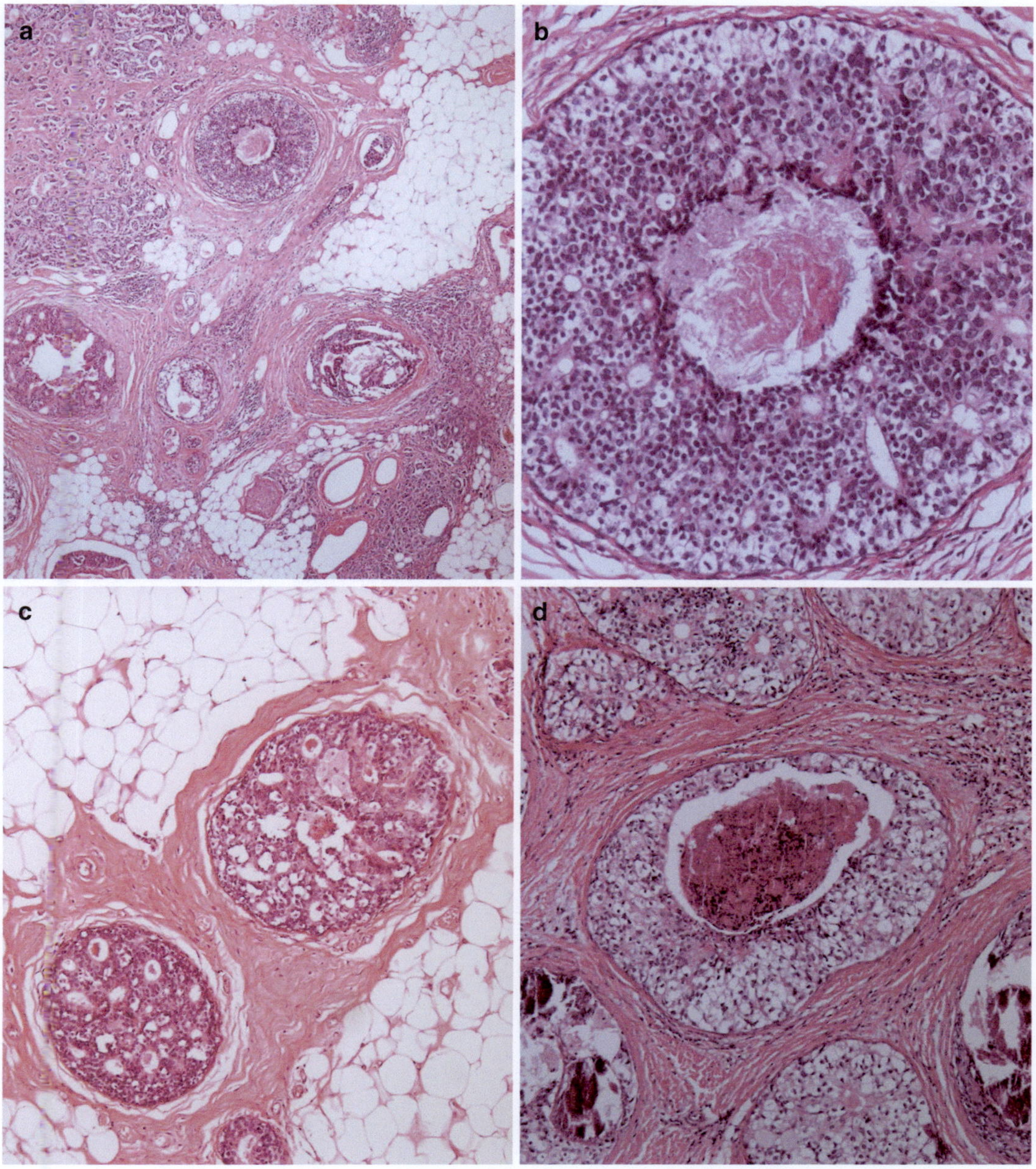

Fig. 9.1 (**a**) DCIS arranged in solid and cribriform pattern at the edge of invasive breast carcinoma, H&E, 100X. (**b**) Solid pattern: Lumen of duct filled with sheets of cohesive cells; pseudoacinar arrangement evident in this example of low-grade solid DCIS, H&E, 200X. (**c**) Cribriform DCIS showing fenestrated proliferation with multiple, round, rigid extracellular lumens with punched out appearance, H&E, 100X. (**d**) DCIS with central comedonecrosis and focal dystrophic calcification, H&E, 100X. (**e**) Micropapillary DCIS, showing small papillary fronds lacking fibrovascular cores projecting into duct lumen, H&E, 100X. (**f**) Papillary DCIS, composed of true papillary fronds containing fibrovascular septa projecting into duct lumen, papillary cores generally lack myoepithelial cell layer, H&E, 100X. (**g**) Flat DCIS, composed of 1–2 layers of high-grade malignant cells lining a gland, H&E, 100X

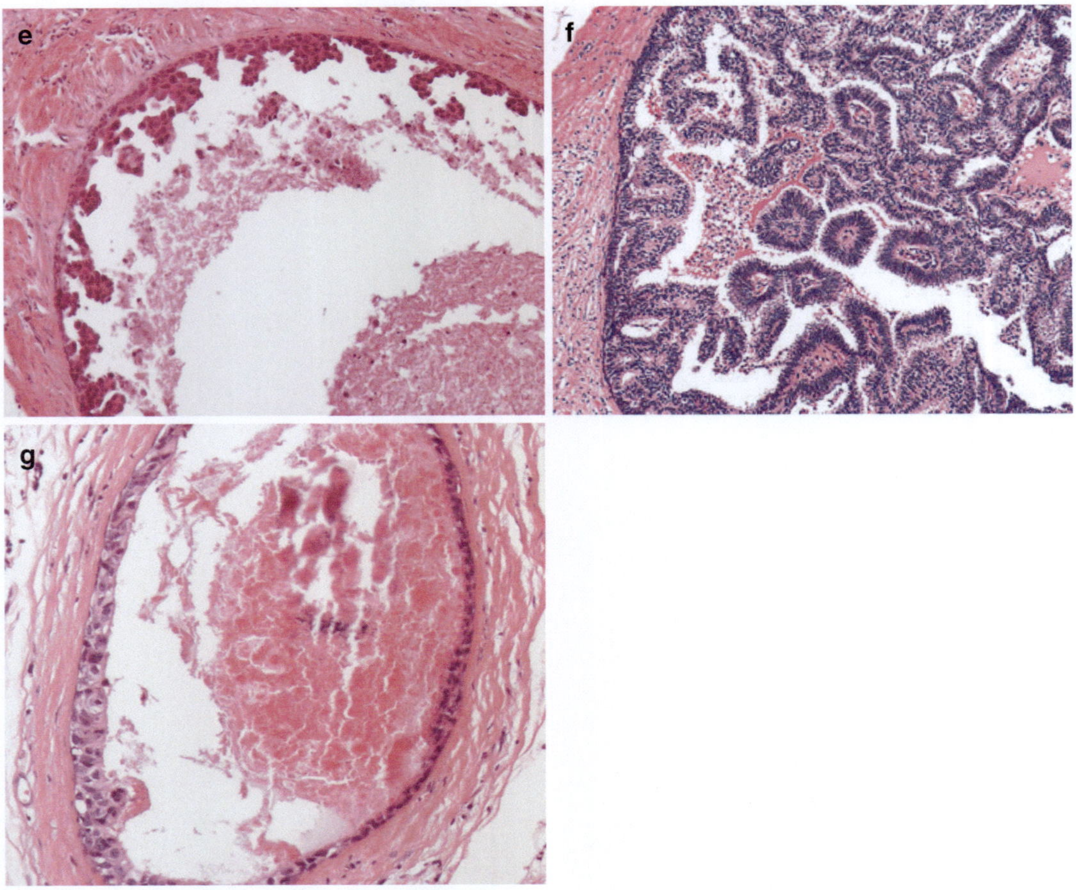

Fig. 9.1 (continued)

Fig. 9.2 (**a**) DCIS showing low-grade nuclear features with uniform bland nuclei, H&E, 100X. (**b**) P63 demonstrates absence of myoepithelial layer inside the lesion, whereas preserved myoepithelial layer is present at the periphery of tumor lobules (arrow), IHC, 200X. (**c**) Diffuse ER positivity is seen in this case, IHC, 200X. (**d**) Diffuse membranous positivity for Her2, IHC, 200X. (**e**): CK5/CK6 is negative in the tumor cells, with only peripheral myoepithelial layer showing positive expression, IHC, 200X

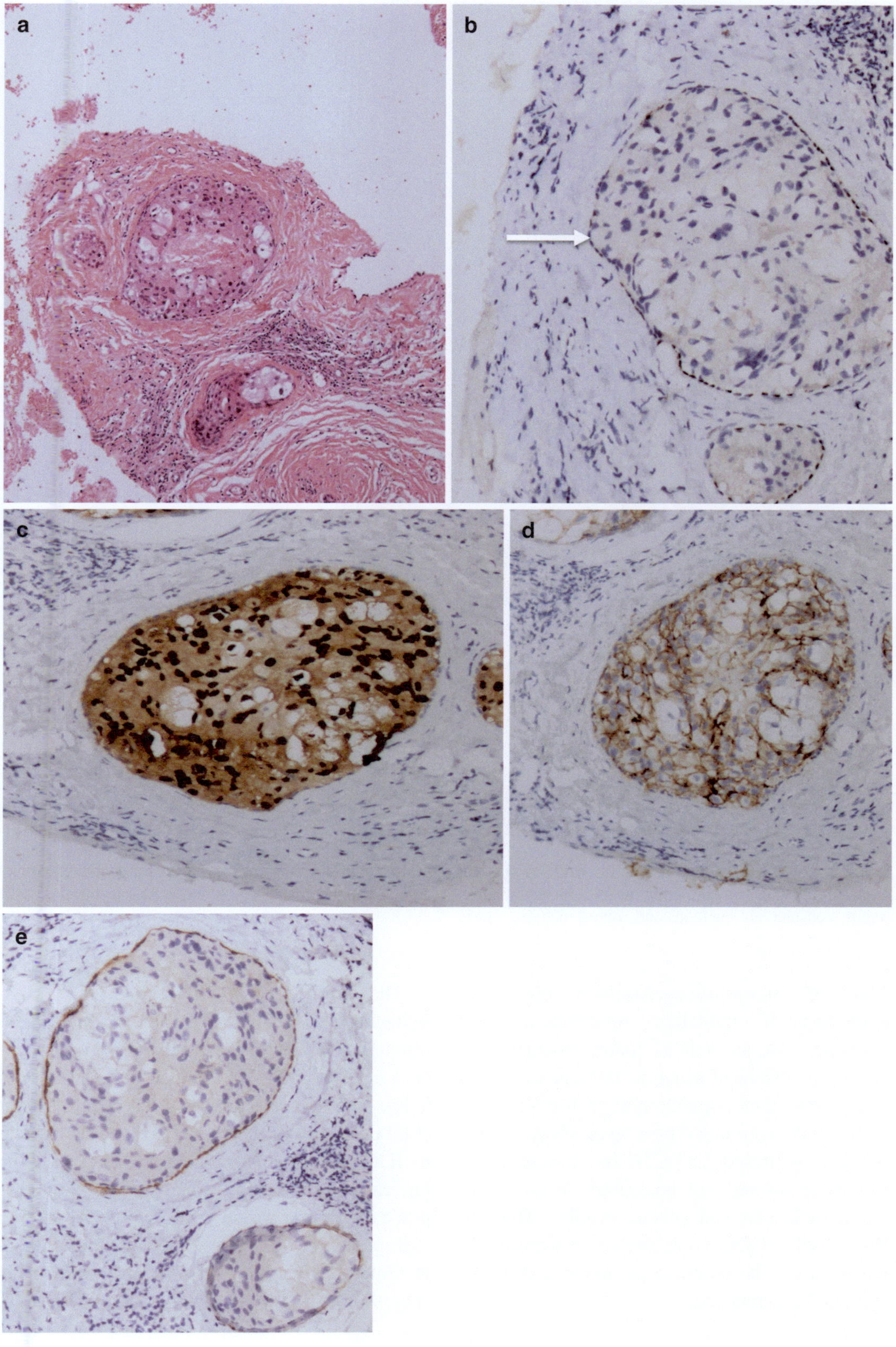
a
b
c
d
e

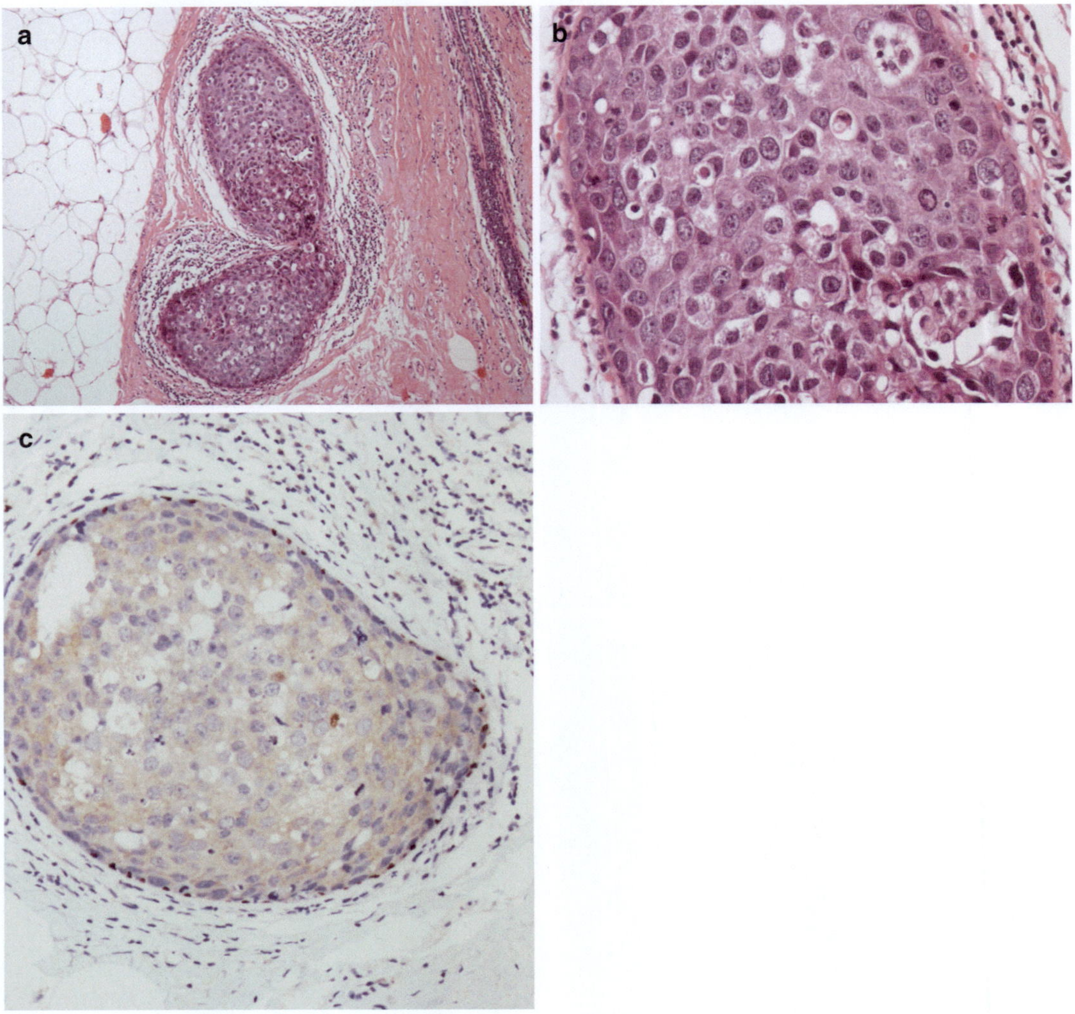

Fig. 9.3 (**a**) High-grade solid DCIS, H&E, 100X. (**b**) High-grade DCIS showing large nuclei with coarse chromatin, conspicuous nucleoli, and mitotic activity, H&E, 400X. (**c**) P63 demonstrates preserved myoepithelial layer at the periphery of tumor lobule (nuclear positivity), IHC, 200X

Role of immunohistochemistry (IHC) An admixture of epithelial, myoepithelial, and apocrine cells as well as foamy histiocytes is present in lesions of usual ductal hyperplasia. As against this, pure population of proliferating epithelial cells surrounded by a layer of myoepithelial cells is present in DCIS. In addition, DCIS lesions of low and high nuclear grade harbor different molecular and genetic profiles. Thus the IHC profile of DCIS lesions varies accordingly, which has to be assessed in myoepithelial and epithelial components.

The intact myoepithelial cell layer is highlighted by p40, p63, SMMS, calponin, and CK5/6 immunostains/markers, which might be attenuated in high-grade DCIS (Figs. 9.2b, 9.3c, and 9.4c). The acinar cells show estrogen receptor (ER) positivity in more than 70% cases, similar to IDC, and expression is correlated with the nuclear grade—being strongly positive in low-grade DCIS and variably positive to negative in high-grade DCIS (Fig. 9.2c). Expression of Her2neu is frequently found in acinar cells (Fig. 9.2d), while basal cytokeratins (CK5/CK6,

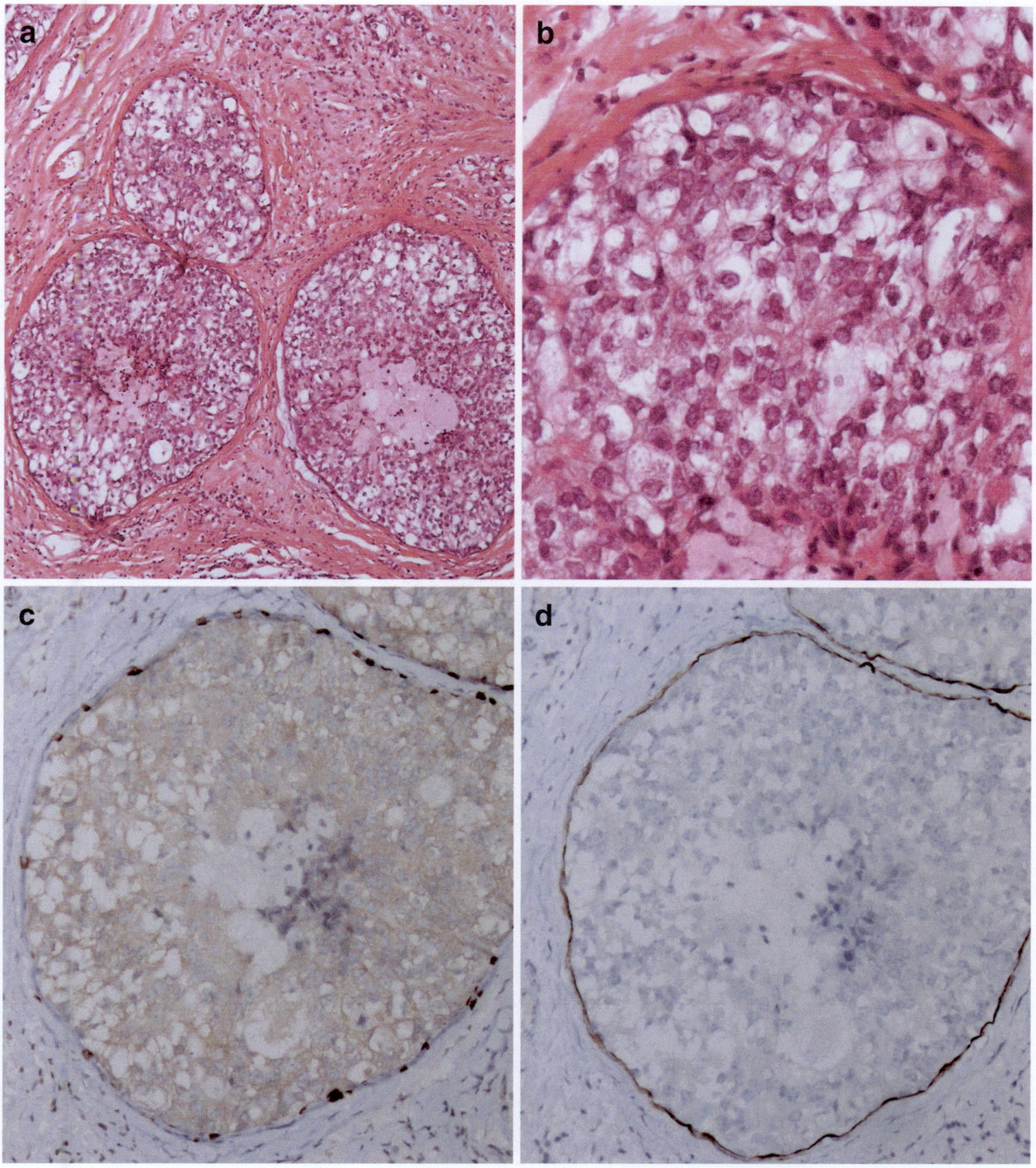

Fig. 9.4 (**a**) Solid DCIS of intermediate nuclear grade, H&E, 100X. (**b**) Nuclei show mild pleomorphism, variably coarse chromatin, and small nucleoli, H&E, 400X. (**c**) P63 demonstrates attenuated myoepithelial layer at periphery of lobule, IHC, 200X. (**d**) CK5/CK6 is negative in the tumor cells, IHC, 200X

CK14, 34betaE12) are usually negative (Figs. 9.2e and 9.4d) in DCIS.

Histological reports of DCIS should note the cytonuclear grade, the presence/absence of necrosis, the architectural pattern, the size of the lesion, and the distance to margins. Information about the presence and site of microcalcifications is valuable for radiopathological correlation. DCIS cannot be distinguished from IDC on cytology because comment on basement membrane breach and stromal invasion is not possible on fine needle aspiration smear examination.

Currently ER is the only immunohistochemical biomarker recommended for routine clinical use, and progesterone receptor is considered optional [12]. In coherence with IDC, around 75% of DCIS show ER positive status, which determines the potential benefit of the hormonal therapy in these patients [13]. On the other hand, nonexpression of estrogen receptor indicates risk of ipsilateral recurrence [14]. Her2neu (epidermal growth factor receptor family member 2) is more frequently expressed in DCIS than invasive carcinoma and is reported to correlate with increased recurrence risk [14]. High Ki67 proliferation index has also reported to correlate with increased recurrence risk [14].

The differential diagnosis for DCIS includes usual ductal hyperplasia and atypical ductal hyperplasia at one end of the spectrum and invasive and microinvasive carcinoma at the other. There are morphological clues, which help in differentiating various lesions; however, IHC plays a crucial role in making this distinction.

Usual ductal hyperplasia (UDH) UDH shows heterogeneous proliferation of cells that are irregularly distributed with haphazard orientation of nuclei, nonrigid peripheral slit-like fenestrations with nuclei parallel to the lumina (Fig. 9.5a, b). It can mimic low- to intermediate-grade DCIS. However, it shows variable or mosaic pattern of expression of CK5/CK6 and ER, in comparison to negative CK5/CK6 and strong ER seen in DCIS.

Atypical ductal hyperplasia (ADH) ADH and low-grade DCIS share similar cytoarchitectural details; however, the distinction is based on the size of the lesion with a cutoff of two completely involved membrane-bound spaces or equivalent, that is, < 2 mm [15].

Lobular cancerization and involvement of sclerosing adenosis DCIS may involve the lobular units, or it may extend into sclerosing lesions; both presentations may mimic invasive carcinoma. Careful examination for small, irregular (*rather than rounded*) clusters of cells should be undertaken to exclude microinvasion. Myoepithelial cell markers can be helpful to demonstrate an intact myoepithelial layer around involved lobules or sclerosing adenosis.

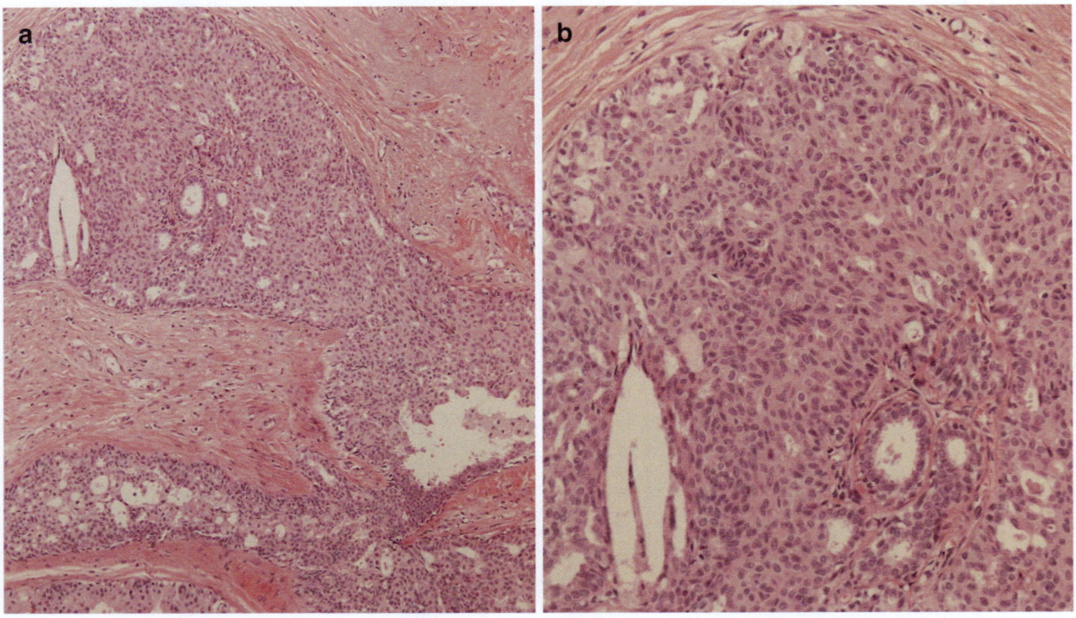

Fig. 9.5 (**a**) Usual ductal hyperplasia, H&E, 100X. (**b**) UDH shows haphazard orientation of benign epithelial cells admixed with myoepithelial cells and presence of secondary lumina, H&E, 200X

Invasive cribriform carcinoma It shows infiltrative growth pattern, stromal reaction, and lack of circumscription by myoepithelial markers.

Solid papillary carcinoma It shows a solid growth pattern punctuated by delicate fibrovascular cores, extracellular mucin and, neuroendocrine features (*Synaptophysin positive)* and lacks circumscription by myoepithelial markers.

Paget's disease of breast Mammary Paget's disease is characterized by an intraepidermal proliferation of malignant glandular epithelial cells in the nipple areolar region (adenocarcinoma in situ of skin) which can be associated with underlying DCIS or IDC.

Macroscopically, the nipple can show redness, scaling, crusting, pigmentation, and erosion or may appear normal. The histological hallmark is the presence of intraepidermal large tumor cells having abundant pale cytoplasm and pleomorphic nuclei with prominent nucleoli and variable mitotic activity (Fig. 9.6a, b). Paget cells occur singly or in small clusters usually at the dermoepidermal junction, rarely forming acinar structures as well [16]. Paget cells may also show phagocytosed melanin, mimicking melanocytes. Not infrequently, prominent lymphocytic infiltrate and numerous melanophages can be seen in the superficial dermis. Dermal invasion by Paget cells has been reported in 4–8% of cases Paget's disease [17–19]. It should be diagnosed only when clusters or isolated Paget cells are seen invading through the basement membrane, having similar cytological features as the Paget cells, and there is a clear separation of the invading Paget cells from the underlying breast carcinoma [17]. It can be diagnosed in scrape preparations from the nipple, although diagnosis is challenging.

On immunohistochemistry, Paget cells are positive for low-molecular-weight cytokeratins (CK7 and CAM5.2), HER2 (Fig. 9.6c), and GATA3 [20, 21]. ER and PR are positive in approximately 40% and 30% of them, respectively [20, 22]. High-molecular-weight cytokeratin (CK5/CK6) is negative.

The differential diagnoses for mammary Paget's disease include squamous cell carcinoma in situ (Bowen disease) and melanoma in situ, although these diseases only rarely involve the nipple. IHC plays the decisive role in clinching the accurate diagnosis. Squamous cell carcinoma in situ is positive for CK5/CK6 and negative for CK7 as well as Her2neu [23]. GATA3 can show variable positivity. Melanoma in situ is positive for S100, melan-A, SOX10, and MITF and negative for keratins and Her2neu [23]. Toker cells resemble Paget cells and when prominent become an important diagnostic consideration. Toker cells are also positive for CK7 and CAM5.2 to compound the confusion; however, they lack atypical nuclear features and are HER2-negative [24].

If there is no underlying carcinoma or only presence of DCIS, mammary Paget's disease is to be categorized as Tis according to the Union for International Cancer Control (UICC) TNM classification [25]. However, if invasive carcinoma is present in underlying breast, the staging will be based on the extent of invasive carcinoma.

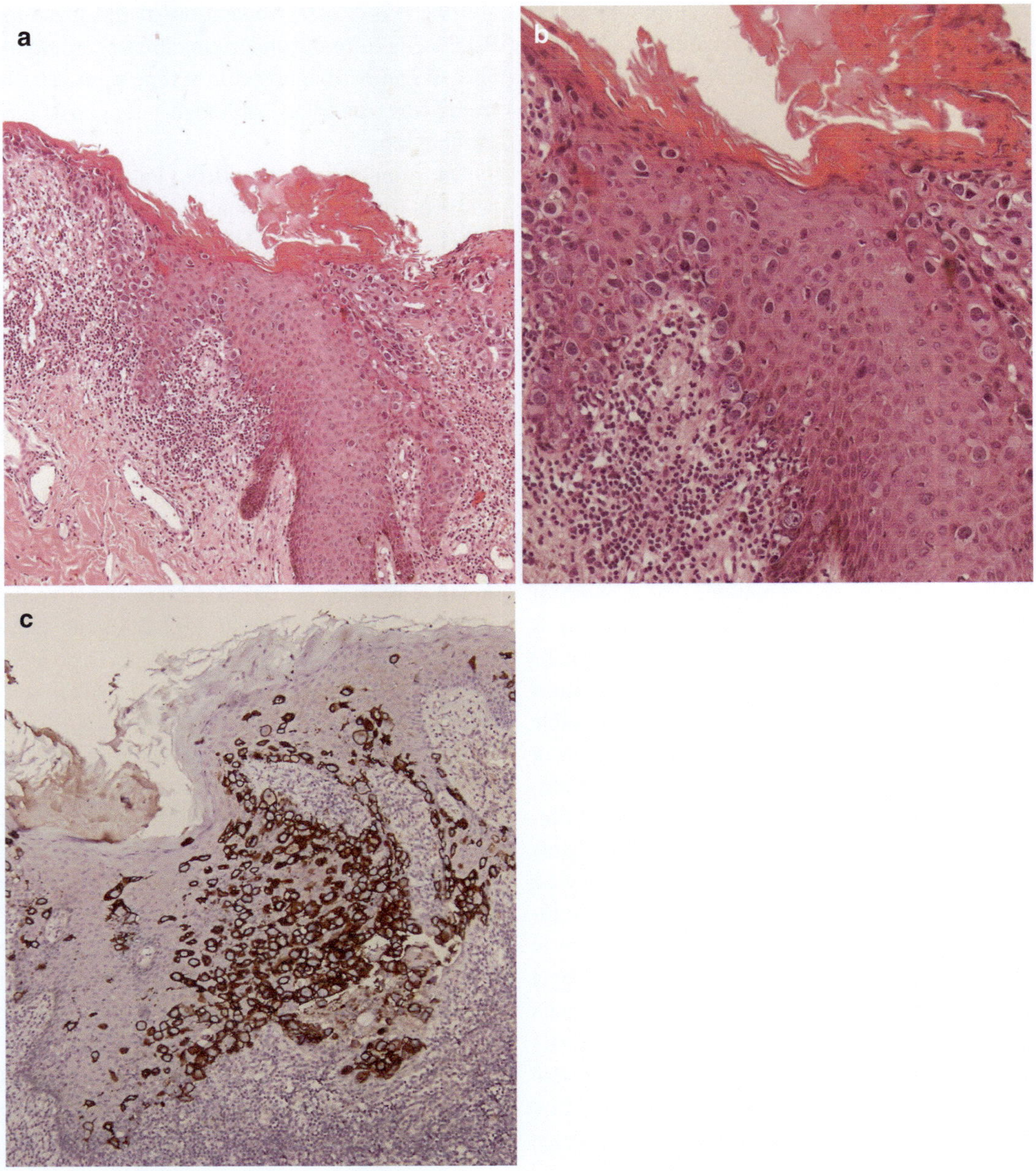

Fig. 9.6 (**a**) Involved epidermis is hyperkeratotic, with dermis showing dense lymphocytic infiltrate, H&E, 100X. (**b**) Tumor cells are large with clear cytoplasm and hyperchromatic nuclei, H&E, 200X. (**c**) Strong Her2 positivity in tumor cells, IHC, 200X

9.4 Imaging Modalities

DCIS is usually detected incidentally on screening and does not present as a palpable mass; hence imaging plays a vital role. It usually presents as groups of pleomorphic microcalcifications and is commonly seen on MG. The DCIS which shows absence of calcification is better evaluated by ultrasonography (US) & CE-MRI. CE-MRI is the modality of choice to determine the true extent of DCIS. Contrast-enhanced spectral mammography is a relatively new imaging technique which not only shows the calcifications but also the enhancing component of the disease. The role and limitations of each imaging modality have been described in the following sections.

9.4.1 Digital Mammography and Digital Breast Tomosynthesis

MG plays a pivotal role in the detection and diagnosis of DCIS. It is the primary imaging modality utilized in breast screening and is highly effective in diagnosing DCIS. Microcalcification is the most reliable mammographic feature of DCIS followed by architectural distortion (Fig. 9.7a, b). They can also present as an area of asymmetry (Fig. 9.8) or a mass (Fig. 9.9). Only a few patients present with nipple discharge and associated changes, the latter being more common with Paget's disease (Fig. 9.7a–f) [26].

Microcalcifications can be fine, linear branching, amorphous, or coarse heterogenous. The distribution of the calcification plays a crucial role in categorizing into the right BI-RADS category.

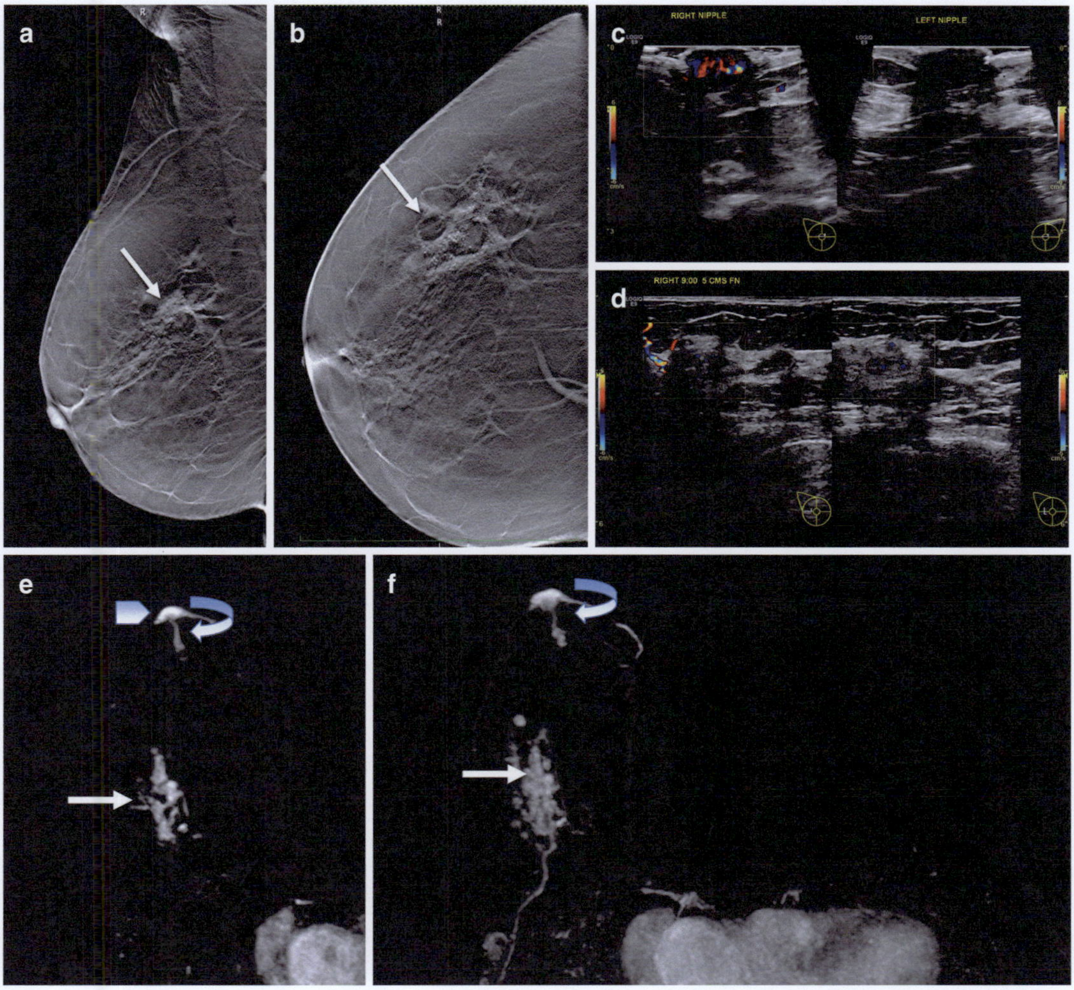

Fig. 9.7 (**a**, **b**) Right MLO (**a**) and CC (**b**) DBT showing segmental fine pleomorphic and linear branching microcalcifications from the 8–11 o'clock segments (arrows). (**c**, **d**) USG showing hypervascularity in the right nipple as compared to the left (**c**). Nonmass findings in the right 9 o'clock segment with increased vascularity and hyperechoic foci suggestive of microcalcifications. (**e**) CE-MRI axial and (**f**) maximum intensity projection (MIP) axial images, showing segmental, clumped NME (arrows) with thickened enhancing right nipple with intense enhancement (arrowhead). Linear NME is seen in the subareolar region (curved arrow) which on HPE revealed Paget's disease of the nipple with DCIS in subareolar region and DCIS with invasive component in the area of segmental NME

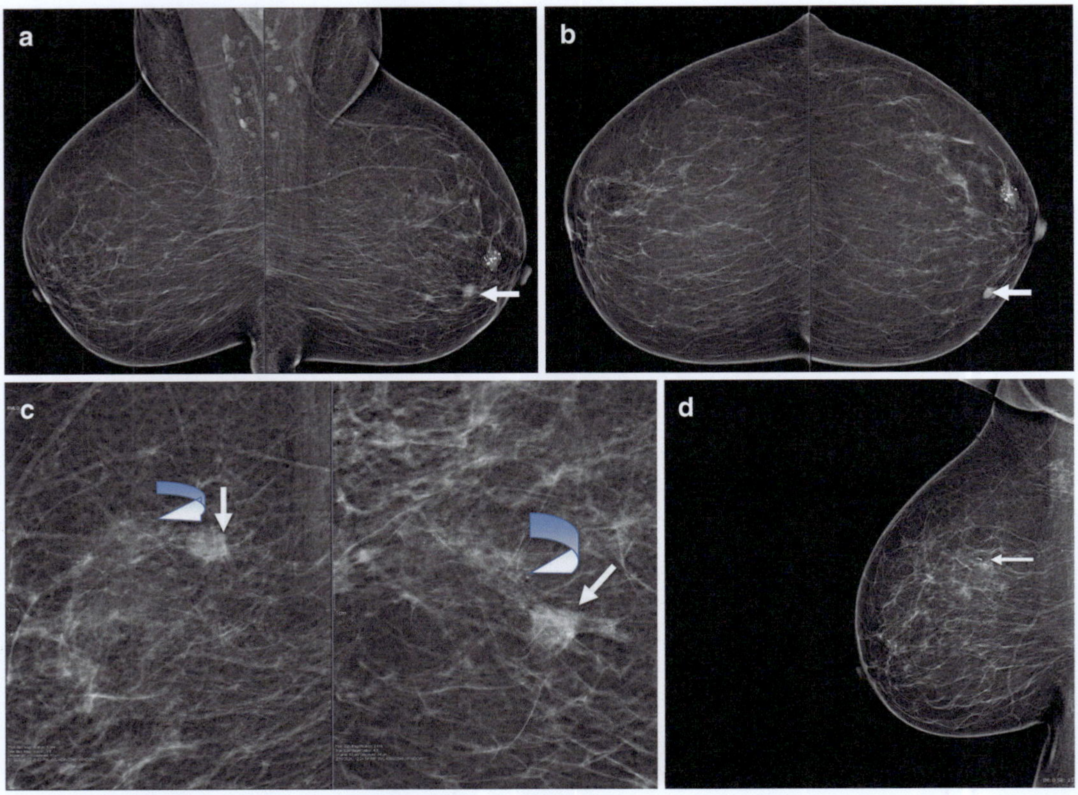

Fig. 9.8 Bilateral MLO (**a**) and CC mammogram (**b**) and magnified MLO and CC showing an irregular, high-density mass (arrow) with adjoining asymmetry (curved arrow in (**c**). Biopsy of the asymmetry revealed DCIS and the solid mass was invasive carcinoma. (**d**) Postbiopsy clips were placed in the area of asymmetry, prior to surgery (arrow)

The most suspicious microcalcification is the fine, linear branching which has a high PPV (positive predictive value) for DCIS and hence is placed in the BIRADS 4C category (Fig. 9.10). If the distribution is grouped, linear or segmental, then it can be upgraded to BIRADS 5 category (Fig. 9.7). Amorphous calcification in a grouped, linear, or segmental distribution has a PPV of 20% for malignancy and hence should be placed in BIRADS 4B category. A single group of coarse heterogenous calcification is suspicious for malignancy and has a PPV of approximately 15%, so these should also be placed in BI-RADS 4B category [27]. The distribution pattern and architectural features of the calcifications can provide valuable information regarding the extent and severity of the disease. It has however been found that correlation of MG with extent on pathology is not accurate.

The histological subtype (*solid*, *papillary*, *cribriform) of DCIS* does not correlate well with type of microcalcifications; however, the MG features can vary depending on the histological grade. High-grade DCIS tends to demonstrate linear or segmental, fine, branching pleomorphic microcalcifications with irregular shape and sizes, whereas low-grade DCIS often exhibits round/punctate grouped calcifications [27].

Local recurrence of DCIS is more commonly seen with ER negative, HER2 positive, and a high Ki-67 index [28].

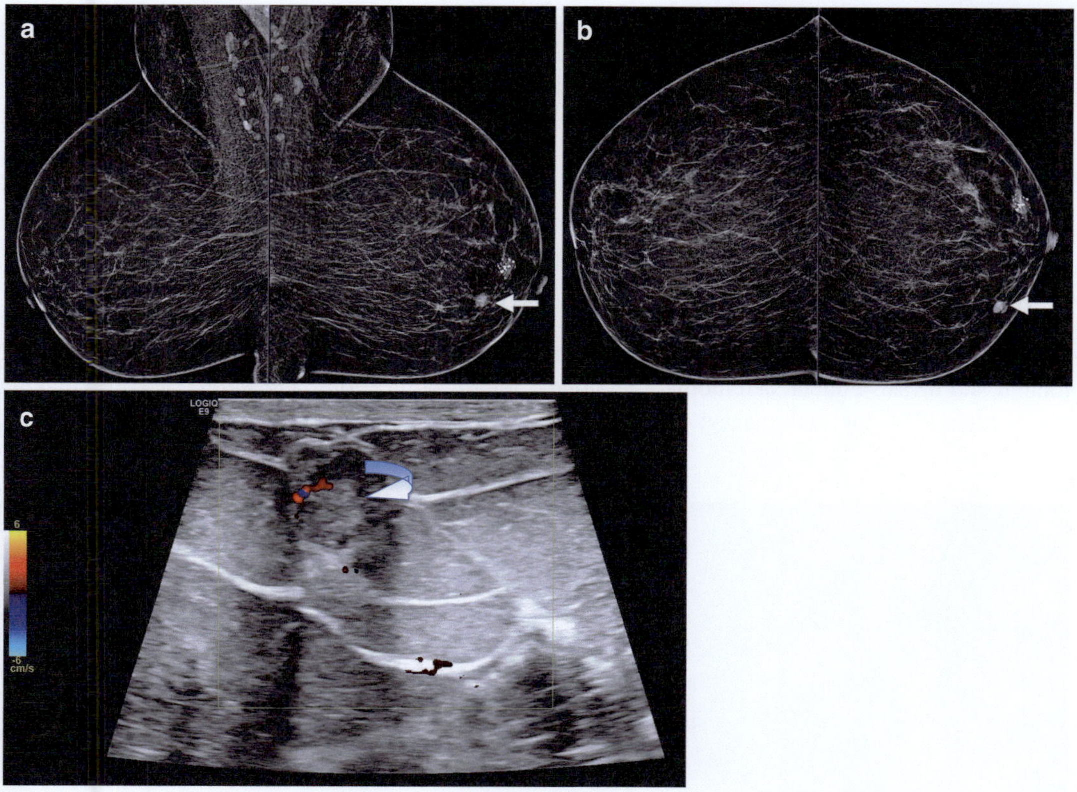

Fig. 9.9 Bilateral MLO (**a**) and CC mammogram (**b**) and usg (**c**)showing an irregular, high density mass with microlobulated margins (arrow). Correlative ultrasound (**c**) shows a heterogenous, almost isoehoic, irregular mass with microlobulated margins and significant hypervascularity. Biopsy of the mass revealed DCIS

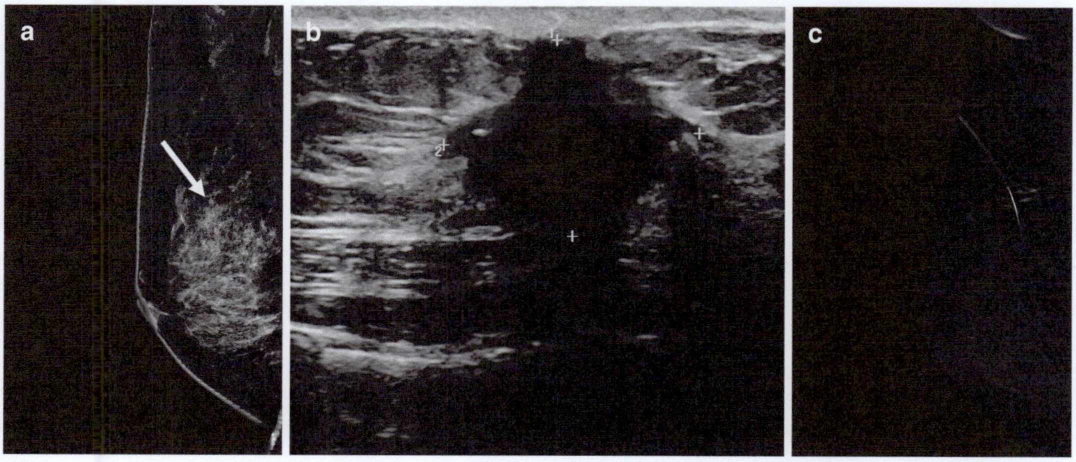

Fig. 9.10 (**a**) Right mammogram MLO view showing fine pleomorphic calcification in a linear distribution (arrow); (**b**) ultrasound showing an irregular hypoechoic mass, taller than wider with posterior shadowing; and (**c**) Hookwire localization on DBT. No correlative enhancement was seen on MRI.HPE suggestive of low-grade DCIS

Occasionally, low-grade DCIS can be missed on mammography. as they can be noncalcified. They present commonly as masses on US and rarely as an area of architectural distortion (AD) or focal asymmetry on MG [27].

AD on MG is defined as an area of focal retraction, straightening of the anterior or posterior edge of the breast parenchyma or radiating spicules from a point. It can be due to benign or malignant causes, and the malignant lesions that commonly present as AD are DCIS and invasive lobular and invasive ductal carcinoma. AD alone has a high PPV for malignancy; hence tissue sampling is recommended (Fig. 9.11) [27, 28]. The management of AD on mammography should be managed as shown in Flow Chart 9.1.

Noncalcified DCIS with a mass seen on US and occult on MG are usually low nuclear grade, whereas calcified DCIS with a mass seen on US is more likely to be an invasive cancer [27].

Women with dense breasts have a higher risk of developing breast cancer and have a higher proportion of missed cancers on MG. Dense breast tissue can obscure the visualization of microcalcifications and subtle lesions. making the interpretation challenging.

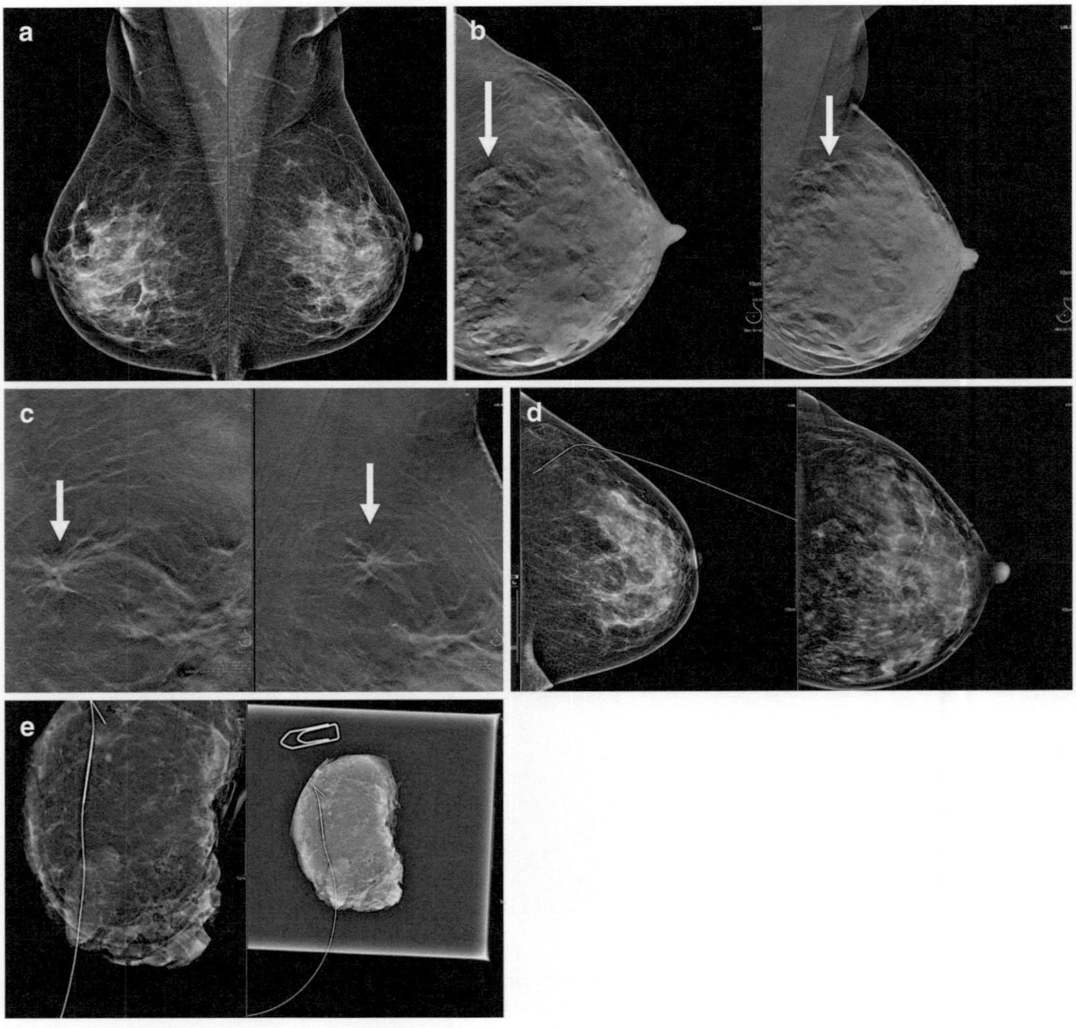

Fig. 9.11 Bilateral MLO (**a**) and CC and MLO DBT (**b**) zoom CC and MLO DBT (**c**) showing an area of AD. Radiating spicules seen on DBT (arrow). No correlate was seen on ultrasound or MRI. (**d**) In view of interval change on MG, hookwire localization of the area of AD was performed followed by excision which revealed low-grade DCIS. Mammogram of postexcision specimen (**e**)

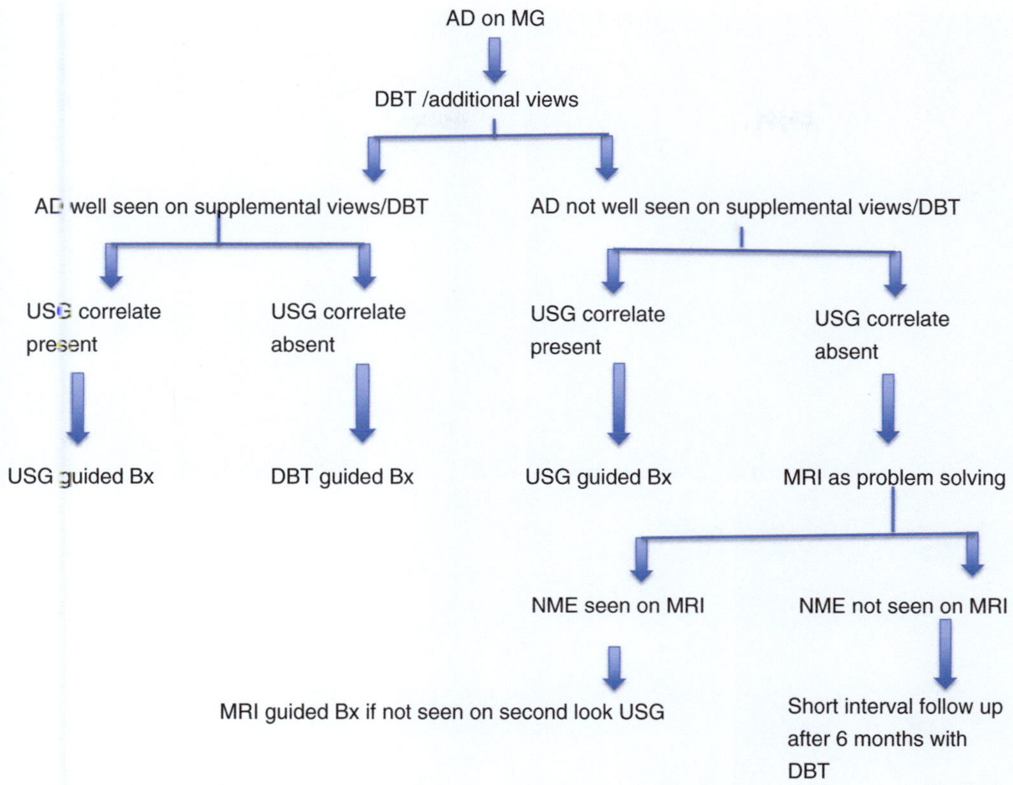

Flow Chart 9.1 Imaging approach in a suspected case of DCIS. AD—Architectural distortion; DBT—Digital breast tomosynthesis; NME—Non-mass enhancement

As MG is very sensitive in picking up microcalcifications, it will also diagnose lesions which are low grade, which will never progress to invasive cancer and results in overtreatment (Fig. 9.8) [5, 29].

9.4.2 Contrast-Enhanced Spectral Mammography (CESM)

It is a relatively new imaging technique in the field of digital mammography based on dual-energy principle—the low energy spectral images show the microcalcification and the subtracted or recombined images show the enhancement representing neoangiogenesis of the lesion.

Since it highlights the areas of increased blood supply due to neoangiogenesis, this technique has potential to illustrate the extent of DCIS as there can be tumor beyond the areas of microcalcification seen on MG (Fig. 9.12). Low-grade DCIS may not show enhancement and can be missed on CESM. Significant background parenchymal enhancement can obscure masses as well as nonmass enhancement (NME) [30, 31].

9.4.3 Ultrasonography (US)

US is a valuable adjunct to MG in the evaluation of DCIS. DCIS on US can be seen as either a mass, a nonmass finding, abnormalities of the ducts or it can be occult on US. In a retrospective study carried out by Hwajin Cha et al. *in 2018*, DCIS was seen as a mass in 53.2% patients, nonmass findings in 39.7% and no US correlate in 7% of the patients [32].

Whenever seen as mass, it can be solid or mixed solid cystic. Solid masses are usually hypoechoic, noncircumscribed, antiparallel with or without increase in vascularity on color dop-

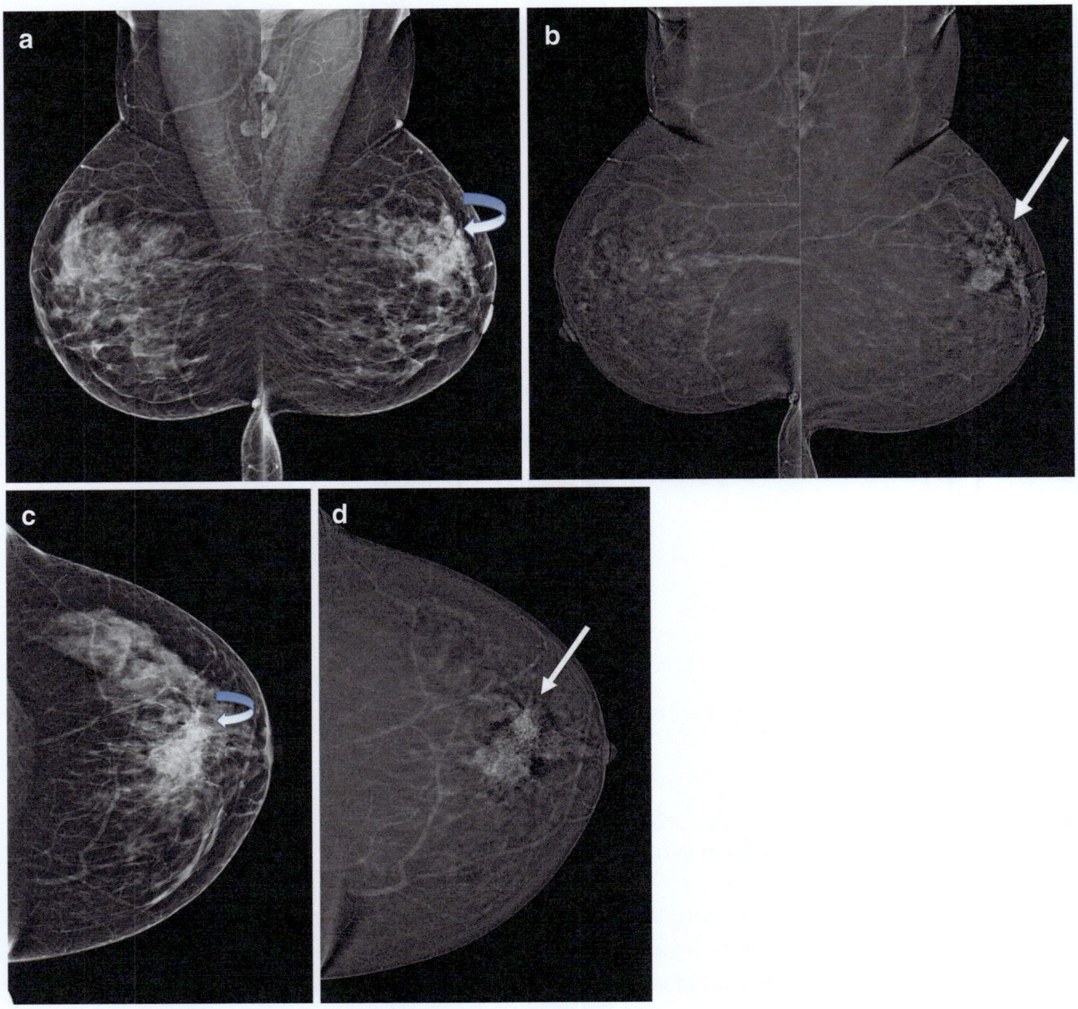

Fig. 9.12 Bilateral MLO mammogram (**a**) and CESM (**b**) showing heterogenous segmental enhancement in the left breast (arrow) correlating to the area of clustered microcalcification with architectural distortion seen on conventional mammogram (curved arrow). (**c**, **d**) CC mammogram and CEDM of the left breast showing the same findings

pler (Fig. 9.10b). They may or may not be associated with microcalcifications. DCIS primarily develops in the terminal duct lobular unit (TDLU) and then spreads into the subsegmental and segmental ducts. When the disease is limited to the TDLU or in the peripheral ducts, it results in unfolding of the TDLU and that is what is seen as a solid or mixed solid hypoechoic mass, with or without ductal extension on US. US findings of a mass have no correlation to the grade of tumor except for internal vascularity that suggests a higher-grade tumor. As the disease progresses into the central ducts, abnormality of the ducts starts appearing on US. These are seen as dilated ducts with inhomogeneous hypoechoic masses upstream of the lactiferous duct, giving it a "pipe-like" appearance on US. A dilated duct in DCIS may also be because of necrosis in tumor cells or lumen of the duct. A lymph-forming reaction around the duct can also result in dilatation of the duct [33].

On the other hand, as the disease progresses to the peripheral ducts, hypoechoic nonmass findings are seen US (Fig. 9.13). The nonmass

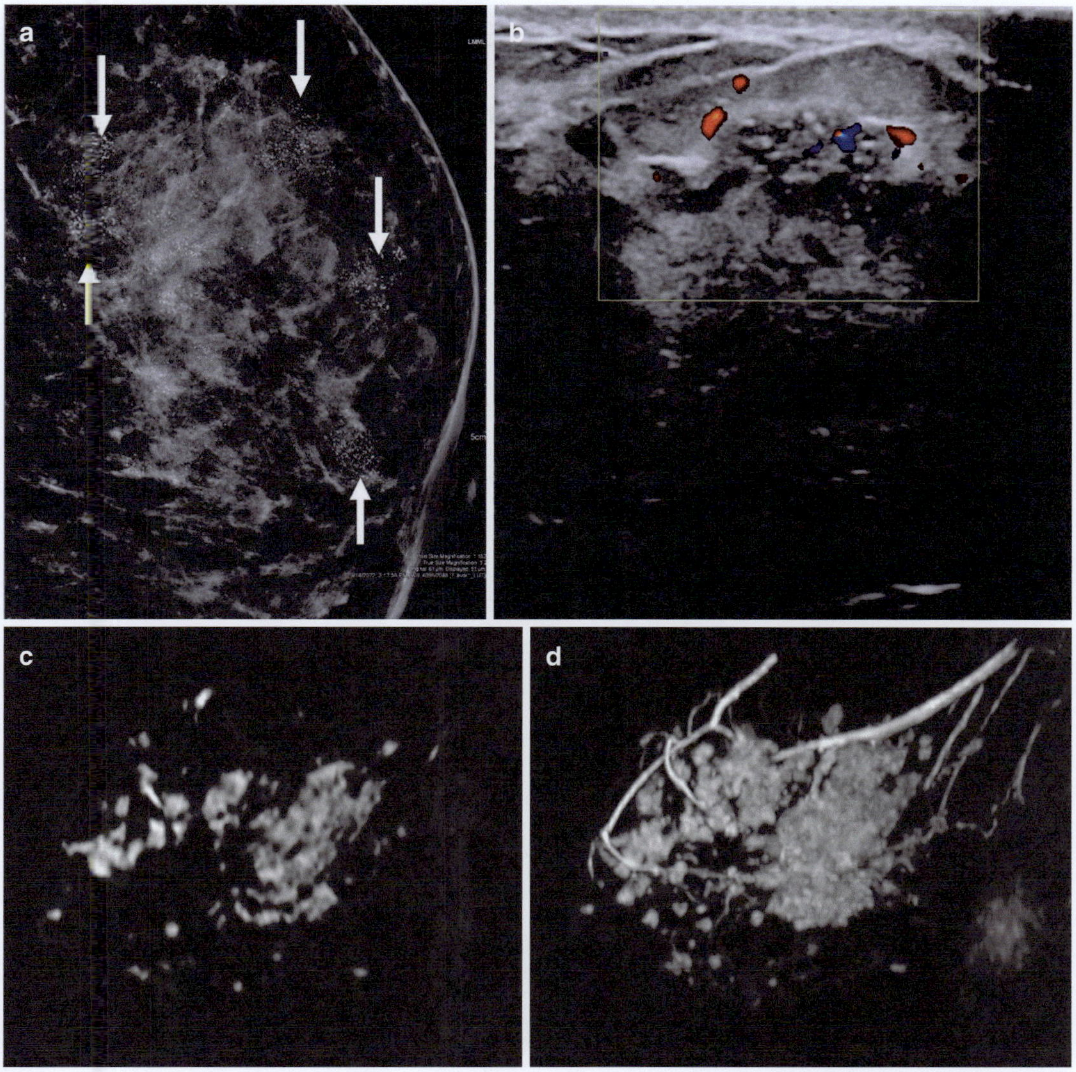

Fig. 9.13 Magnified CC MG (**a**) showing multiple clusters of grouped, fine, pleomorphic microcalcifications (arrows). US (**b**) showing dilated ducts with echogenic foci with increase in vascularity. CE-MRI (**c**) and MIP (**d**) images in the sag plane reveal multiregional areas of clumped NME, HPE suggestive of multicentric high-grade DCIS

findings are often associated with architectural distortions (AD) and duct changes [34]. Hypoechoic areas in the mammary gland are seen which are in a ductal or segmental distribution unlike masses which do not follow any distribution pattern.

Echogenic foci within a duct or in hypoechoic areas in the mammary gland are commonly seen in DCIS. Not all echogenic foci (especially those seen in isolation without hypoechoic areas) are seen as microcalcifications on MG or by histology; hence the term echogenic foci should be used instead of microcalcifications on US (Fig. 9.14) [34].

9.4.4 Magnetic Resonance Imaging

Dynamic contrast-enhanced MRI (DCE-MRI) is the modality of choice for detection and demonstration of the extent of DCIS (Fig. 9.15). In addi-

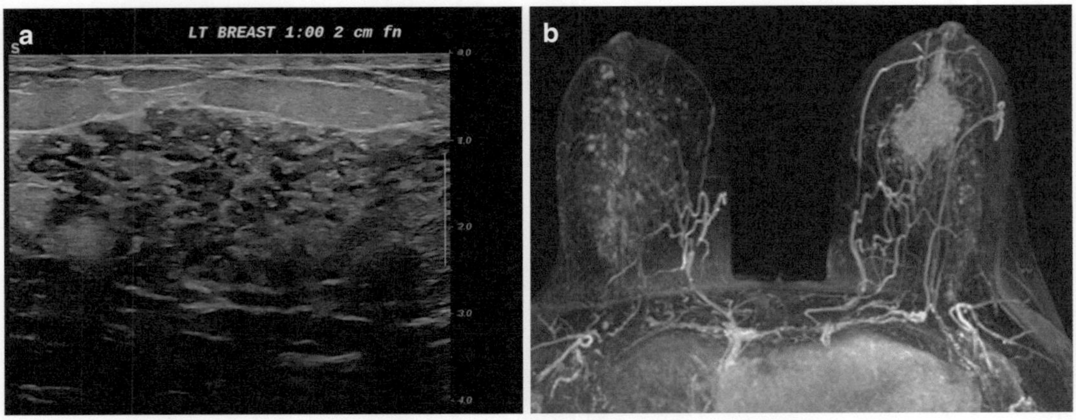

Fig. 9.14 USG showing NMLs with echogenic foci suggestive of microcalcifications (**a**) and CE-MRI MIP images (**b**) showing linear NME in the left subareolar region and segmental NME in the central breast

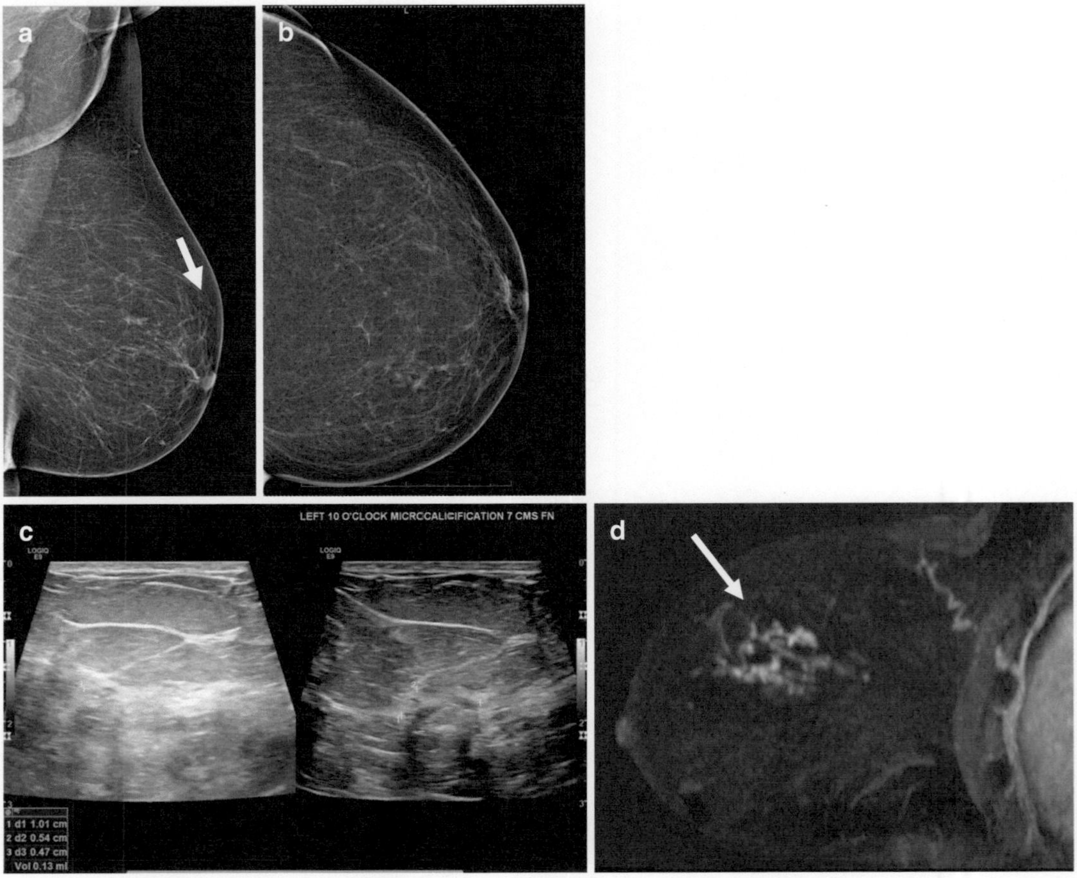

Fig. 9.15 MLO and CC view of the left breast showing fine linear branching microcalcification (arrows) (**a**, **b**). USG showing ill-defined shadowing in the same region (**c**) CE-MRI in the sag plane (**b**) reveals more extensive tumor seen as clumped segmental NME (arrow in **d**) with MRI showing the true extent of disease

tion, the performance of CE-MRI is not limited by breast density in tumor detection. It should be performed on a 1.5/3 T magnet with a dedicated breast coil using intravenous contrast. Ultrafast DCE-MRI can be done along with the conventional DCE-MRI. Ultrafast DCE-MRI has the added advantage of no background parenchymal enhancement; however, it is limited in the detection of low-grade DCIS as those enhance later.

DCIS may be seen as a mass or NME on DCE-MRI (Fig. 9.13). Studies have shown that DCIS may present as NME in a linear or segmental distribution (60–81%), followed by a mass (1421%) and rarely as a focus (1–12%) [35, 36]. Low-grade DCIS can be seen as segmental or regional NME. The morphological appearance of NME can be described as clumped internal enhancement or clustered ring-like enhancement (Fig. 9.13) [36–38].

DCIS can also present as a mass with irregular margins and heterogeneous enhancement. Intratumoral high signal intensity and peritumoral oedema are predictors for invasive carcinoma and frequently encountered in the histological upgrade groups rather than pure DCIS (Fig. 9.16). Studies have shown that the reason for central hyperintensity is because of necrosis as they outgrow their blood supply, suggesting aggressive tumors [39–41].

A wide variation in the kinetic curve analysis can be found in DCIS, with a rapid initial washin of contrast being the most common. On the delayed contrast images, all three types of kinetic curves, washout, plateau, and persistent enhancement, can be seen. Due to overlap in the enhancement kinetics, it is imperative to understand and follow the morphology to approach a pathology on MRI.

The predictors for worrisome features for histopathology upgrade in masses are irregular shape, noncircumscribed margins, intratumoral edema, intratumoral hyperintensity on T2W images, and clumped or clustered ring NME pattern [42–44].

Over the recent years, DCE-MRI has been found to be more sensitive in the detection of DCIS as compared to US and MG. MRI has higher sensitivity in detection of high-grade DCIS vs low- to intermediate-grade DCIS. The sensitivity of DCE MRI for detection of DCIS is 89–92% which is comparable to that of US; however, the sensitivity of MG is only 55–56% [45–48].

Kuhl et al. reported a sensitivity of 92% for MRI as compared to 56% for MG in detection of DCIS. They also reported a higher sensitivity of 98% in detection of high-grade DCIS as compared to 85% for intermediate- and low-grade

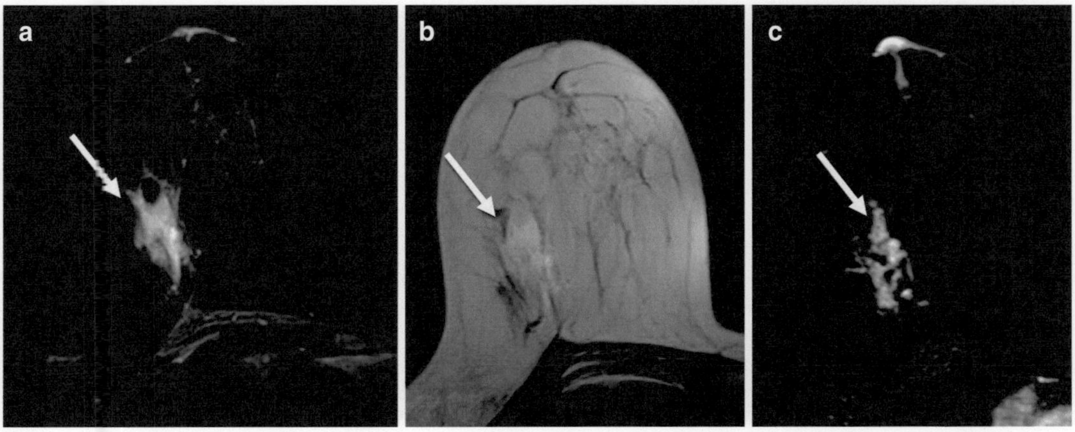

Fig. 9.16 (**a**) Turbo inversion recovery magnetization (TIRM) axial, (**b**) T2W axial images show intramammary oedema (arrow), a predictor of Invasive Carcinoma on HPE, sub CE axial image (**c**) shows segmental NME which was IDC on pathology

DCIS. On the other hand, they found that MG has less sensitivity for detection of high-grade (52%) as compared to low-grade DCIS (60%) [46].

A study conducted by Baur et al. found contradictory results to Kuhl et al. They reported decreasing sensitivity of detection of DCIS with nuclear grade, being highest- with low-grade (100%) as compared to 84.6% with intermediate-grade and 66.7% with high-grade DCIS [48]. They also found no statistical difference in the sensitivity of MRI vs mammography in detecting pure DCIS. Despite these contradictory reports, it is universally accepted that MRI detects all clinically significant cancers which can impact patient outcome. Since angiogenesis seen on MRI is a biomarker of protease and angiogenic activity, protease is required for the tumor to penetrate the basement membrane; hence lesions that enhance on MRI are the ones that have potential to progress to invasive cancers and not the ones that do not enhance [49]. It has been suggested that MRI may detect the more clinically relevant cases of DCIS. With increasing grades of DCIS, vascularity increases. DCIS lesions that enhance on MRI are therefore more likely to progress to invasive carcinoma as compared to those detected on MG [43].

The role of MRI in evaluating DCIS in the clinical setting is focused both on early detection in screening high-risk patients as well as preoperative evaluation of the extent of disease. In addition, new research studies are using MRI for assessing treatment response as well as for the purpose of active surveillance in patients not undergoing surgical management of DCIS [45, 47].

Heterogenous ductal and segmental NME seen on CE-MRI should be biopsied as it has high PPV for malignancy. NME seen on MRI should be reevaluated by second-look ultrasound, and biopsied on the modality, it is best visualized. Homogenous focal or regional enhancement with no correlate on MG and US may be followed up especially if associated with a cluster of microcysts [44, 45].

9.5 Treatment

DCIS can be treated with local or systemic therapy. Local therapy includes surgery (mastectomy or breast conservation surgery/BCS) and radiotherapy (RT). Systemic therapy includes the endocrine/hormonal therapy.

Both mastectomy and BCS are equally appropriate options for most women with DCIS. However, for BCS, certain set of criteria need to be met with. In an observational study of 100,000 patients of DCIS in Surveillance, Epidemiology, and End Results (SEER) database, both BCS (with or without RT) and mastectomy resulted in a similar 10-year breast cancer-specific mortality [50–52].

Mastectomy is curative in 98% of patients with DCIS [53] and has a recurrence rate of 1–2% [54]. RT is not routinely indicated for DCIS after mastectomy because RT reduces only the chances of local recurrences without changing the odds of distant metastasis and mortality; and after mastectomy, risk of local recurrences is already negligible.

Patients undergoing mastectomy for DCIS should undergo sentinel lymph node biopsy (SLNB) procedure in the same sitting as conducting the same at a later date is impossible in case the final histopathology report turns out to be invasive [55].

Women with unilateral DCIS have approximately 1%/year risk of developing either invasive breast cancer or DCIS in the contralateral breast [56, 57]. So some women choose contralateral prophylactic mastectomy [58], though without claimed survival benefit. Those women who do not want prophylactic mastectomy can benefit from chemoprevention by using endocrine therapy [59, 60]. Women who have undergone bilateral mastectomy do not benefit from chemoprevention.

BCS is the wide local excision of the DCIS presenting either as a palpable lump or as only image detected lesion, to ensure negative margins and maintaining the breast cosmesis at the same time. It, in conjunction with adjuvant radiotherapy, is associated with almost 50% reduction of local recurrence compared to the lumpectomy alone [61]. Wide local excision ensures a negative margin, that is, absence of tumor on inked margin or minimum 2 mm of free margin. Image-guided localization is crucial for image-detected malignancy with no palpable correlate. This is usually done with hookwire placement using appropriate imaging modality (Fig. 9.16). Most of the times, localization with one wire is enough for lesion localization and facilitation of surgery; however, for scenarios where there is segmental or linear distribution of the disease, placement of more than one wire may be required to obtain tumor-free margins. The latter is also called as "hookwire bracketing" (Fig. 9.17), and to ascertain the adequacy of margins, post excision specimen MG should be considered and reexcision performed where it is warranted [62].

Absolute contraindications to BCT include multicentric disease, during pregnancy as RT should be avoided, persistently positive margins in spite of repeated resections and profusely dispersed microcalcifications. Multifocal disease is however a relative contraindication for BCS [63].

Since DCIS is rarely associated with positive axillary lymph nodes, SLNB is not performed along with BCS. However, it can be performed as a second procedure if the final histopathology of the resected specimen turns out to be invasive carcinoma which occurs in 10–20% of cases [64, 65].

Patients undergoing BCS for DCIS should be followed by adjuvant RT to the ipsilateral whole breast as it decreases the long-lasting risk of local breast recurrence without affecting the chances of distant metastasis or survival advantage [66]. Radiotherapy reduces the risk of invasive and noninvasive recurrences by about 50% [61]. It should preferably be used "within eight weeks after surgery," as a part of standard care protocol. In an observational study of 1323 women with a median follow-up of 6.6 years, initiation of adjuvant RT before/within 8 weeks after surgery was associated with lower incidence of ipsilateral breast tumor recurrences than those who initiated it 12 weeks after surgery [67].

The conventional dose of radiotherapy is 1.8–2 Gy daily fractions over a period of 4.5–5.0 weeks to a total of 45–50 Gy. In an analysis of two single institution trials, 145

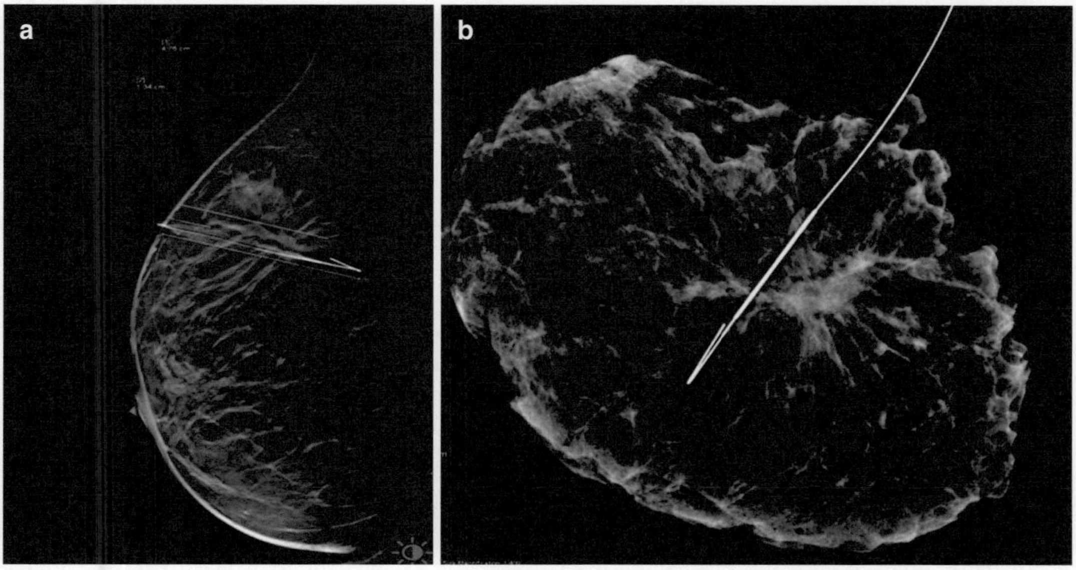

Fig. 9.17 Hookwire localization of lesion (**a**) and postexcision specimen mammogram (**b**)

patients with DCIS were enrolled. They underwent BCS followed by accelerated partial breast radiotherapy, delivering 41–42 Gy in 15 fractions. The recurrence rate after 5 years was 4%, and it was almost equivalent to those employing conventional dose radiotherapy to whole breast in NSABP B-17 trial. The understanding is that with APBI, higher dose of RT can be administered in shorter span of time and with lesser side effects and almost equivalent outcomes [68].

Low-risk DCIS have been described as those with low- or intermediate-grade DCIS on pathology, less than 2.5 cm in size and widely resected margins, >1 cm. Two trials, ECOG 5194 [69] and RTOG 9804 [70], addressed to the possibility of the omission of adjuvant RT in low-risk DCIS, but both the trials have not convincingly assured of the same as the locoregional recurrences were not low enough to justify the omission of RT. In ECOG trial, the locoregional recurrence for low and intermediate DCIS at 5 years was 6.1% which at 12 years increased to 14.4% and 24.6% for low and intermediate groups, respectively. Gene expression analysis and utilizing data from oncotype Dx, DCIS is being evaluated to find out the recurrence score of patients and in whom radiotherapy can be convincingly omitted after lumpectomy [71].

Key pathological components that influence treatment and its outcome include the margin width (distance between the edge of the DCIS and the inked margins). It reflects the completeness of excision (2 mm) and is an important determinant of local recurrence in DCIS. Size of the lesion, the nuclear grade and necrosis, the expression of the estrogen receptor, and HER 2 Neu receptors also influence the treatment. Status of the estrogen receptor expression guides the role of systemic therapy; however, the role of HER 2neu receptor is still evolving, and at present guidelines do not recommend routine testing of this receptor in pure DCIS cases. At present Her2neu status does not have any influence or alter treatment in cases of DCIS. However, it needs to be done in case the histopathology is upgraded to invasive one where it has an important bearing on the treatment.

Approximately, 75% of DCIS lesions express estrogen receptors (ER) and/or progesterone receptors (PR) [72]. Choice of endocrine therapy between tamoxifen and the aromatase inhibitors will depend upon the menopausal status of the patient. For premenopausal women, tamoxifen is used but for postmenopausal ones; both tamoxifen and aromatase inhibitors are acceptable options. Meta-analysis of two randomized controlled trials including *NSABP B-24* and UK, Australia, and New Zealand DCIS, enrolling 3375 cases of DCIS, revealed that the addition of tamoxifen to BCS reduces the recurrence of ipsilateral and contralateral DCIS [60].

9.6 Approach to Recurrent DCIS

Approximately 50% of all locoregional recurrences are invasive irrespective of the modality employed to treat DCIS [73, 74]. Both noninvasive and invasive recurrences after the completion of treatment for DCIS will present either on imaging during follow-up or as palpable lumps. Some of the presentations of invasive recurrences may be as distant metastasis ones.

All recurrences should be subjected to core needle biopsy as true recurrences need to be differentiated from second primary tumors. Typically, but not mandatorily, the estrogen, progesterone, and Her 2 neu receptor assays of a true recurrence match to that of its original tumor. Changed receptor status assays of the local tumor may in fact represent a true second primary tumor. Other useful differentiating features will be based upon histologic subtype, mammographic appearance, discordant DNA flow cytometry, length of disease-free interval, and tumor arising from other quadrants of the breast [73, 75, 76].

All invasive recurrences need to be managed just like recurrence after the treatment of invasive breast carcinoma and should include the metastatic workup, including PET scan as well. Recurrence in patients of DCIS having undergone BCS plus radiotherapy earlier will in all probability end up in mastectomy rather than repeat BCS as administering local radiotherapy again may not be feasible in them. However, a few selected patients who have received whole breast irradiation earlier may be the candidates for accelerated partial breast irradiation, preferably in patients with prolonged disease-free interval [77].

For patients having undergone previous wide local excision without adjuvant radiation for DCIS, options of repeat BCS with radiation and mastectomy exist for the pure DCIS recurrence, depending upon the extent of disease recurrence and the preference of the patient and the treatment provider [78]. Recurrence of pure DCIS in the mastectomy flap should be considered for its wide local excision and possible role of radiation after excision should be discussed with the radiation oncologist.

Role of continuing tamoxifen in patients of pure DCIS recurrence while already on this drug is not clear. Some prefer to continue with the tamoxifen but others switch to the aromatase inhibitors. In the presence of the paucity of data regarding the preferred option, the role of endocrine therapy for chemoprevention should be discussed.

9.7 Conclusion

DCIS is a disease limited to the ducts with no disruption of the basement membrane. It can be confined to a single or multiple ducts. It can be segmental in distribution and involve the terminal ductal lobular unit. Commonly pure DCIS on biopsy is upgraded to invasive carcinoma post-surgery in approximately 20% cases. Presence of tumor necrosis, peritumoral edema, and masses with irregular margins on MRI have higher pathological grade. NME showing clustered ring or clumped enhancement are also predictors of higher grade of tumor on pathology.

The key pathological components that influence treatment include the margin width, size of the lesion, nuclear grade, and necrosis and receptor expression. Systemic treatments in DCIS lesions that express ER and PR are tamoxifen and the aromatase inhibitors depending upon the menopausal status of the patient.

Treatment modalities are local which include surgery and RT. Surgical modalities can be mastectomy or BCS. BCS is routinely followed by RT. Hormonal treatment by tamoxifen or aromatase inhibitors (depending upon the menopausal status of the patient) is the systemic treatment of choice.

Acknowledgments We would like to thank Dr. Madhavi Chandra, (Department of Breast Imaging, Sir Ganga Ram Hospital, New Delhi), Dr Shelly Sharma (Department of Breast Imaging, Apollo Hospital, New Delhi) and Dr. Rupa Renganathan (Department of Breast Centre, Kovai Medical Centre & Hospital, Coimbatore) for their contribution in providing the US, MG, DBT, and CEM images.

References

1. Page DL, Dupont WD. Anatomic indicators (histologic and cytologic) of increased breast cancer risk. Breast Cancer Res Treat. 1993;28(2):157–66. https://doi.org/10.1007/BF00666428. PMID: 8173068
2. Kerlikowske K. Epidemiology of ductal carcinoma in situ. J Natl Cancer Inst Monogr. 2010;2010(41):139–41. https://doi.org/10.1093/jncimonographs/lgq027. PMID: 20956818; PMCID: PMC5161058
3. Mazzola E, Cheng SC, Parmigiani G. The penetrance of ductal carcinoma in situ among BRCA1 and BRCA2 mutation carriers. Breast Cancer Res Treat. 2013;137(1):315–8. https://doi.org/10.1007/s10549-012-2345-5. Epub 2012 Nov 27. PMID: 23184082; PMCID: PMC3836600
4. Ellsworth RE, Ellsworth DL, Love B, Patney HL, Hoffman LR, Kane J, Hooke JA, Shriver CD. Correlation of levels and patterns of genomic instability with histological grading of DCIS. Ann Surg Oncol. 2007;14(11):3070–7. https://doi.org/10.1245/s10434-007-9459-8. Epub 2007 Jun 5. PMID: 17549568
5. Burstein HJ, Polyak K, Wong JS, Lester SC, Kaelin CM. Ductal carcinoma in situ of the breast. N Engl J Med. 2004;350(14):1430–41. https://doi.org/10.1056/NEJMra031301. PMID: 15070793
6. Page DL, Dupont WD, Rogers LW, Landenberger M. Intraductal carcinoma of the breast: follow-up after biopsy only. Cancer. 1982;49(4):751–8. https://doi.org/10.1002/1097-0142(19820215)49:4<751::aid-cncr2820490426>3.0.co;2-y. PMID: 6275978
7. Collins LC, Tamimi RM, Baer HJ, Connolly JL, Colditz GA, Schnitt SJ. Outcome of patients with ductal carcinoma in situ untreated after diagnostic biopsy: results from the Nurses' Health Study. Cancer. 2005;103(9):1778–84. https://doi.org/10.1002/cncr.20979. PMID: 15770688
8. Stuart KE, Houssami N, Taylor R, Hayen A, Boyages J. Long-term outcomes of ductal carcinoma in situ

of the breast: a systematic review, meta-analysis and meta-regression analysis. BMC Cancer. 2015;15:890. https://doi.org/10.1186/s12885-015-1904-7. PMID: 26555555; PMCID: PMC4641372
9. EORTC Breast Cancer Cooperative Group; EORTC Radiotherapy Group, Bijker N, Meijnen P, Peterse JL, Bogaerts J, Van Hoorebeeck I, Julien JP, Gennaro M, Rouanet P, Avril A, Fentiman IS, Bartelink H, Rutgers EJ. Breast-conserving treatment with or without radiotherapy in ductal carcinoma-in-situ: ten-year results of European Organisation for Research and Treatment of Cancer randomized phase III trial 10853—a study by the EORTC Breast Cancer Cooperative Group and EORTC Radiotherapy Group. J Clin Oncol. 2006;24(21):3381–7. https://doi.org/10.1200/JCO.2006.06.1366. Epub 2006 Jun 26. PMID: 16801628
10. Lester SC, Bose S, Chen YY, Connolly JL, de Baca ME, Fitzgibbons PL, Hayes DF, Kleer C, O'Malley FP, Page DL, Smith BL, Weaver DL, Winer E, Members of the Cancer Committee, College of American Pathologists. Protocol for the examination of specimens from patients with ductal carcinoma in situ of the breast. Arch Pathol Lab Med. 2009;133(1):15–25. https://doi.org/10.5858/133.1.15. PMID: 19123730
11. The Consensus Conference Committee. Consensus conference on the classification of ductal carcinoma in situ. Cancer. 1997;80(9):1798–802. https://doi.org/10.1002/(sici)1097-0142(19971101)80:9<1798::aid-cncr15>3.0.co;2-0. PMID: 9351550.
12. Allison KH, Hammond MEH, Dowsett M, McKernin SE, Carey LA, Fitzgibbons PL, Hayes DF, Lakhani SR, Chavez-MacGregor M, Perlmutter J, Perou CM, Regan MM, Rimm DL, Symmans WF, Torlakovic EE, Varella L, Viale G, Weisberg TF, McShane LM, Wolff AC. Estrogen and progesterone receptor testing in breast cancer: ASCO/CAP guideline update. J Clin Oncol. 2020;38(12):1346–66. https://doi.org/10.1200/JCO.19.02309. Epub 2020 Jan 13. PMID: 31928404
13. Tamimi RM, Baer HJ, Marotti J, Galan M, Galaburda L, Fu Y, Deitz AC, Connolly JL, Schnitt SJ, Colditz GA, Collins LC. Comparison of molecular phenotypes of ductal carcinoma in situ and invasive breast cancer. Breast Cancer Res. 2008;10(4):R67. https://doi.org/10.1186/bcr2128. Epub 2008 Aug 5. PMID: 18681955; PMCID: PMC2575540
14. Lari SA, Kuerer HM. Biological markers in DCIS and risk of breast recurrence: a systematic review. J Cancer. 2011;2:232–61. https://doi.org/10.7150/jca.2.232. PMID: 21552384; PMCID: PMC3088863
15. Tozbikian G, Brogi E, Vallejo CE, Giri D, Murray M, Catalano J, Olcese C, Zee V, Kimberly J, Wen HY. Atypical ductal hyperplasia bordering on ductal carcinoma in situ. Int J Surg Pathol. 2016;25(2):100–7.
16. Shousha S. Glandular Paget's disease of the nipple. Histopathology. 2007;50(6):812–4. https://doi.org/10.1111/j.1365-2559.2007.02643.x. Epub 2007 Mar 21. PMID: 17376174.
17. Duan X, Sneige N, Gullett AE, et al. Invasive Paget disease of the breast: clinicopathologic study of an underrecognized entity in the breast. Am J Surg Pathol. 2012;36(9):1353–8. PMID: 22895267.
18. Lee HW, Kim TE, Cho SY, Kim SW, Kim WH, Lee JE, Nam SJ, Cho EY. Invasive Paget disease of the breast: 20 years of experience at a single institution. Hum Pathol. 2014;45(12):2480–7. https://doi.org/10.1016/j.humpath.2014.08.015. Epub 2014 Sep 7. PMID: 25288235.
19. Sanders MA, Dominici L, Denison C, Golshan M, Wiecorek T, Lester SC. Paget disease of the breast with invasion from nipple skin into the dermis: an unusual type of skin invasion not associated with an adverse outcome. Arch Pathol Lab Med. 2013;137(1):72–6. https://doi.org/10.5858/arpa.2011-0611-OA. PMID: 23276177
20. Caliskan M, Gatti G, Sosnovskikh I, Rotmensz N, Botteri E, Musmeci S, Rosali dos Santos G, Viale G, Luini A. Paget's disease of the breast: the experience of the European Institute of Oncology and review of the literature. Breast Cancer Res Treat. 2008;112(3):513–21. https://doi.org/10.1007/s10549-007-9880-5. Epub 2008 Feb 1. PMID: 18240020.
21. Ozerdem U, McNiff JM, Tavassoli FA. Cytokeratin 7-negative mammary Paget's disease: a diagnostic pitfall. Pathol Res Pract. 2016;212(4):279–81. https://doi.org/10.1016/j.prp.2016.01.004. Epub 2016 Jan 22. PMID: 26944832
22. Bhargava R, Dabbs DJ. Use of immunohistochemistry in diagnosis of breast epithelial lesions. Adv Anat Pathol. 2007;14(2):93–107. https://doi.org/10.1097/PAP.0b013e31803244d5. PMID: 17471115.
23. Elbendary A, Xue R, Valdebran M, Torres KMT, Parikh K, Elattar I, Kwon EJ, Elston DM. Diagnostic criteria in intraepithelial pagetoid neoplasms: a histopathologic study and evaluation of select features in Paget disease, Bowen disease, and Melanoma in situ. Am J Dermatopathol. 2017;39(6):419–27. https://doi.org/10.1097/DAD.0000000000000704. PMID: 28525420.
24. Garijo MF, Val D, Val-Bernal JF. An overview of the pale and clear cells of the nipple epidermis. Histol Histopathol. 2009;24(3):367–76. https://doi.org/10.14670/HH-24.367. PMID: 19130406
25. Brierly JD, Gospodarowicz MK, Wittekind C, editors. TNM classification of malignant tumours. 8th ed. Wiley Blackwell: Oxford (UK); 2017.
26. Sripathi S, Ayachit A, Kadavigere R, Kumar S, Eleti A, Sraj A. Spectrum of imaging findings in Paget's disease of the breast-a pictorial review. Insights Imaging. 2015;6(4):419–29. https://doi.org/10.1007/s13244-015-0415-z. Epub 2015 Jul 5. PMID: 26142549; PMCID: PMC4519816
27. Shehata M, Grimm L, Ballantyne N, Lourenco A, Demello LR, Kilgore MR, Rahbar H. Ductal carcinoma in situ: current concepts in biology, imaging, and treatment. J Breast Imaging. 2019;1(3):166–76. https://doi.org/10.1093/jbi/wbz039. Epub 2019 Aug 18. PMID: 31538141; PMCID: PMC6735611

28. Salvatorelli L, Puzzo L, Vecchio GM, Caltabiano R, Virzì V, Magro G. Ductal carcinoma in situ of the breast: an update with emphasis on radiological and morphological features as predictive prognostic factors. Cancers (Basel). 2020;12(3):609. https://doi.org/10.3390/cancers12030609. PMID: 32155777; PMCID: PMC7139619
29. Allred DC. Ductal carcinoma in situ: terminology, classification, and natural history. J Natl Cancer Inst Monogr. 2010;2010(41):134–8. https://doi.org/10.1093/jncimonographs/lgq035. PMID: 20956817; PMCID: PMC5161057
30. Cozzi A, Schiaffino S, Sardanelli F. The emerging role of contrast-enhanced mammography. Quant Imaging Med Surg. 2019;9(12):2012–8. https://doi.org/10.21037/qims.2019.11.09. PMID: 31929976; PMCID: PMC6942965
31. Sudhir R, Sannapareddy K, Potlapalli A, Krishnamurthy PB, Buddha S, Koppula V. Diagnostic accuracy of contrast-enhanced digital mammography in breast cancer detection in comparison to tomosynthesis, synthetic 2D mammography and tomosynthesis combined with ultrasound in women with dense breast. Br J Radiol. 2021;94(1118):20201046. https://doi.org/10.1259/bjr.20201046. Epub 2020 Dec 2. PMID: 33242249; PMCID: PMC7934319
32. Cha H, Chang YW, Lee EJ, Hwang JY, Kim HJ, Lee EH, Ryu JK. Ultrasonographic features of pure ductal carcinoma in situ of the breast: correlations with pathologic features and biological markers. Ultrasonography. 2018;37(4):307–14. https://doi.org/10.14366/usg.17039. Epub 2017 Oct 13. PMID: 29169230; PMCID: PMC6177689
33. Wang LC, Sullivan M, Du H, Feldman MI, Mendelson EB. US appearance of ductal carcinoma in situ. Radiographics. 2013;33(1):213–28. https://doi.org/10.1148/rg.331125092. PMID: 23322838
34. Choe J, Chikarmane SA, Giess CS. Nonmass findings at breast US: definition, classifications, and differential diagnosis. Radiographics. 2020;40(2):326–35. https://doi.org/10.1148/rg.2020190125. PMID: 32125954
35. Jansen SA, Newstead GM, Abe H, Shimauchi A, Schmidt RA, Karczmar GS. Pure ductal carcinoma in situ: kinetic and morphologic MR characteristics compared with mammographic appearance and nuclear grade. Radiology. 2007;245(3):684–91. https://doi.org/10.1148/radiol.2453062061. PMID: 18024450
36. Chan S, Chen JH, Agrawal G, Lin M, Mehta RS, Carpenter PM, Nalcioglu O, Su MY. Characterization of pure ductal carcinoma in situ on dynamic contrast-enhanced MR imaging: do nonhigh grade and high grade show different imaging features? J Oncol. 2010;2010:431341. https://doi.org/10.1155/2010/431341. Epub 2010 Sep 21. PMID: 20885929; PMCID: PMC2946595
37. Rosen EL, Smith-Foley SA, DeMartini WB, Eby PR, Peacock S, Lehman CD. BI-RADS MRI enhancement characteristics of ductal carcinoma in situ. Breast J. 2007;13(6):545–50. https://doi.org/10.1111/j.1524--4741.2007.00513.x. PMID: 17983393
38. Greenwood HI, Heller SL, Kim S, Sigmund EE, Shaylor SD, Moy L. Ductal carcinoma in situ of the breasts: review of MR imaging features. Radiographics. 2013;33(6):1569–88. https://doi.org/10.1148/rg.336125055. PMID: 24108552
39. Baltzer PA, Yang F, Dietzel M, Herzog A, Simon A, Vag T, Gajda M, Camara O, Kaiser WA. Sensitivity and specificity of unilateral edema on T2w-TSE sequences in MR-Mammography considering 974 histologically verified lesions. Breast J. 2010;16(3):233–9. https://doi.org/10.1111/j.1524-4741.2010.00915.x. PMID: 20565468
40. Uematsu T, Kasami M, Yuen S. Triple-negative breast cancer: correlation between MR imaging and pathologic findings. Radiology. 2009;250(3):638–47. https://doi.org/10.1148/radiol.2503081054. PMID: 19244039.
41. Goto M, Yuen S, Akazawa K, Nishida K, Konishi E, Kajihara M, Shinkura N, Yamada K. The role of breast MR imaging in pre-operative determination of invasive disease for ductal carcinoma in situ diagnosed by needle biopsy. Eur Radiol. 2012;22(6):1255–64. https://doi.org/10.1007/s00330-011-2357-2. Epub 2011 Dec 30. PMID: 22205445.
42. Hahn SY, Han BK, Ko EY, Shin JH, Hwang JY, Nam M. MR features to suggest microinvasive ductal carcinoma of the breast: can it be differentiated from pure DCIS? Acta Radiol. 2013;54(7):742–8. https://doi.org/10.1177/0284185113484640. Epub 2013 Apr 30. PMID: 23588154.
43. Mori N, Ota H, Mugikura S, Takasawa C, Tominaga J, Ishida T, Watanabe M, Takase K, Takahashi S. Detection of invasive components in cases of breast ductal carcinoma in situ on biopsy by using apparent diffusion coefficient MR parameters. Eur Radiol. 2013;23(10):2705–12. https://doi.org/10.1007/s00330-013-2902-2. Epub 2013 Jun 4. PMID: 23732688.
44. Machida Y, Shimauchi A, Tozaki M, Kuroki Y, Yoshida T, Fukuma E. Descriptors of malignant non-mass enhancement of breast MRI: their correlation to the presence of invasion. Acad Radiol. 2016;23(6):687–95. https://doi.org/10.1016/j.acra.2016.01.014. Epub 2016 Mar 11. PMID: 26976623
45. Lehman CD. Magnetic resonance imaging in the evaluation of ductal carcinoma in situ. J Natl Cancer Inst Monogr. 2010;2010(41):150–1. https://doi.org/10.1093/jncimonographs/lgq030. PMID: 20956821; PMCID: PMC5161071
46. Kuhl CK, Schrading S, Bieling HB, Wardelmann E, Leutner CC, Koenig R, Kuhn W, Schild HH. MRI for diagnosis of pure ductal carcinoma in situ: a prospective observational study. Lancet. 2007;370(9586):485–92. https://doi.org/10.1016/S0140-6736(07)61232-X. PMID: 17693177

47. Berg WA, Gutierrez L, NessAiver MS, Carter WB, Bhargavan M, Lewis RS, Ioffe OB. Diagnostic accuracy of mammography, clinical examination, US, and MR imaging in preoperative assessment of breast cancer. Radiology. 2004;233(3):830–49. https://doi.org/10.1148/radiol.2333031484. Epub 2004 Oct 14. PMID: 15486214
48. Baur A, Bahrs SD, Speck S, Wietek BM, Krämer B, Vogel U, Claussen CD, Siegmann-Luz KC. Breast MRI of pure ductal carcinoma in situ: sensitivity of diagnosis and influence of lesion characteristics. Eur J Radiol. 2013;82(10):1731–7. https://doi.org/10.1016/j.ejrad.2013.05.002. Epub 2013 Jun 3. PMID: 23743052
49. Jansen SA, Paunesku T, Fan X, Woloschak GE, Vogt S, Conzen SD, Krausz T, Newstead GM, Karczmar GS. Ductal carcinoma in situ: X-ray fluorescence microscopy and dynamic contrast-enhanced MR imaging reveals gadolinium uptake within neoplastic mammary ducts in a murine model. Radiology. 2009;253(2):399–406. https://doi.org/10.1148/radiol.2533082026. PMID: 19864527; PMCID: PMC2770112
50. Narod SA, Iqbal J, Giannakeas V, et al. Breast cancer mortality after a diagnosis of ductal carcinoma in situ. JAMA Oncol. 2015;1:888.
51. Meijnen P, Olden HS, Peterse JL, et al. Clinical outcome after selective treatment of patients diagnosed with ductal carcinoma in situ of breast. Ann Surg Oncol. 2008;15:235.
52. Chatterjee A, Pyfer B, Czerniecki B, Rosenkranz K, Tchou J, Fisher C. Early postoperative outcomes in lumpectomy versus simple mastectomy. J Surg Res. 2015;198(1):143–8. https://doi.org/10.1016/j.jss.2015.01.054. Epub 2015 Feb 4. PMID: 26070497
53. Kinne DW, Petrek JA, Osborne MP, Fracchia AA, DePalo AA, Rosen PP. Breast carcinoma in situ. Arch Surg. 1989;124(1):33–6. https://doi.org/10.1001/archsurg.1989.01410010039008. PMID: 2535929
54. Hwang ES. The impact of surgery on ductal carcinoma in situ outcomes: the use of mastectomy. J Natl Cancer Inst Monogr. 2010;2010:197.
55. Virnig BA, Tuttle TM, Shamliyan T, Kane RL. Ductal carcinoma in situ of the breast: a systematic review of incidence, treatment, and outcomes. J Natl Cancer Inst. 2010;102:170.
56. Fisher B, Land S, Mamounas E, et al. Prevention of invasive breast cancer in women with ductal carcinoma in situ: an update of the National Surgical Adjuvant Breast and Bowel Project Experience. Semin Oncol. 2001;28(4):400–18. https://doi.org/10.1016/s0093-7754(01)90133-2. PMID: 11498833
57. Gao X, Fisher SG, Emami B. Risk of second primary cancer in the contralateral breast in women treated for early-stage breast cancer: a population-based study. Intl J Radiat Oncol Biol Phys. 2003;56(4):1038–45. https://doi.org/10.1016/s0360-3016(03)00203-7. PMID: 12829139
58. Tuttle TM, Jarosek S, Habermann EB, Arrington A, Abraham A, Morris TJ, Virnig BA, et al. Increasing rates of contralateral prophylactic mastectomy among patients with ductal carcinoma in situ. J Clin Oncol. 2009;27(9):1362–7. https://doi.org/10.1200/JCO.2008.20.1681. Epub 2009 Feb 17. PMID: 19224844
59. Fisher B, Dignam J, Wolmark N, Wickerham DL, Fisher ER, Mamounas E, Smith R, Begovic M, Dimitrov NV, Margolese RG, Kardinal CG, Kavanah MT, Fehrenbacher L, Oishi RH. Tamoxifen in treatment of intraductal breast cancer: National Surgical Adjuvant Breast and Bowel Project B-24 randomised controlled trial. Lancet. 1999;353(9169):1993–2000. https://doi.org/10.1016/S0140-6736(99)05036-9. PMID: 10376613
60. Staley H, McCallum I, Bruce J. Postoperative tamoxifen for ductal carcinoma in situ. Cochrane Database Syst Rev. 2012;10:CD007847. https://doi.org/10.1002/14651858.CD007847.pub2. PMID: 23076938
61. Wapnir IL, Dignam JJ, Fisher B, Mamounas EP, Anderson SJ, Julian TB, Land SR, Margolese RG, Swain SM, Costantino JP, Wolmark N. Long-term outcomes of invasive ipsilateral breast tumor recurrences after lumpectomy in NSABP B-17 and B-24 randomised clinical trials for DCIS. J Natl Cancer Inst. 2011;103(6):478–88. https://doi.org/10.1093/jnci/djr027. Epub 2011 Mar 11. PMID: 21398619; PMCID: PMC3107729
62. Aref A, Youssef E, Washington T, et al. The value of post lumpectomy mammogram in the management of breast cancer patients presenting with suspicious microcalcifications. Cancer J Am. 2000;6:25.
63. Rakovitch E, Pignol JP, Hanna W, et al. Significance of multifocality in ductal carcinoma in situ: outcomes of women treated with breast-conserving therapy. J Clin Oncol. 2007;25:5591.
64. Brennan ME, Turner RM, Ciatto S, Marinovich ML, French JR, Macaskill P, Houssami N. Ductal carcinoma in situ at core needle biopsy: meta-analysis of underestimation and predictors of invasive breast cancer. Radiology. 2011;260(1):119–28. https://doi.org/10.1148/radiol.11102368. Epub 2011 Apr 14. PMID: 21493791
65. Allen A, Cauthen A, Dale P, et al. Evaluating the frequency of upgrade to malignancy following surgical excision of high-grade breast lesions and ductal carcinoma in situ identified by core needle biopsy. Breast J. 2019;25:103.
66. Goodwin A, Parker S, Ghersi D, Wilcken N. Postoperative radiotherapy for ductal carcinoma in situ of breast-a systematic review of randomised trials. Breast. 2009;18:143.
67. Shurell E, Olcese C, Patil S, McCormick B, Van Zee KJ, Pilewskie ML. Delay in radiotherapy is associated with an increased risk of disease recurrence in women with ductal carcinoma in situ. Cancer. 2018;124(1):46–54. https://doi.org/10.1002/cncr.30972. Epub 2017 Sep 28. PMID: 28960259; PMCID: PMC5734990

68. Ciervide R, Dhage S, Guth A, Shapiro RL, Axelrod DM, Roses DF, Formenti SC. Five-year outcome of 145 patients with ductal carcinoma in situ (DCIS) after accelerated breast radiotherapy. Int J Radiat Oncol Biol Phys. 2012;83(2):e159–64. https://doi.org/10.1016/j.ijrobp.2011.11.025. PMID: 22579378. Effects of chemotherapy and hormonal therapy for early breast cancer on recurrence and 15- year survival: an overview of the randomized trials. Lancet. 2005;365:1687–717
69. Hughes LL, Wang M, Page DL, Gray R, Solin LJ, Davidson NE, Lowen MA, Ingle JN, Recht A, Wood WC. Local excision alone without irradiation for ductal carcinoma in situ of the breast: a trial of Eastern Cooperative Oncology Group. J Clin Oncol. 2009;27(32):5319–24. https://doi.org/10.1200/JCO.2009.21.8560. Epub 2009 Oct 13. PMID: 19826126; PMCID: PMC2773217
70. McCormick B, Winter K, Hudis C, Kuerer HM, Rakovitch E, Smith BL, Sneige N, Moughan J, Shah A, Germain I, Hartford AC, Rashtian A, Walker EM, Yuen A, Strom EA, Wilcox JL, Vallow LA, Small W Jr, Pu AT, Kerlin K, White J. RTOG 9804: a prospective randomised trial for good-risk ductal carcinoma in situ comparing radiotherapy with observation. J Clin Oncol. 2015;33(7):709–15. https://doi.org/10.1200/JCO.2014.57.9029. Epub 2015 Jan 20. Erratum in: J Clin Oncol. 2015;33(26):2934. PMID: 25605856; PMCID: PMC4334775.
71. Rakovitch E, Sutradhar R, Nofech-Mozes S, et al. 21-Gene Assay and Breast Cancer Mortality in Ductal Carcinoma in Situ. J Natl Inst. 2021;113:572.
72. Selim AG, El-Ayat G, Wells CA. Androgen receptor expression in ductal carcinoma in situ of the breast: relation to oestrogen and progesterone receptors. J Clin Pathol. 2002;55:14.
73. Kerlikowske K, Molinaro A, Cha I, Ljung BM, Ernster VL, Stewart K, Chew K, Moore DH 2nd, Waldman F. Characteristics associated with recurrence among women with ductal carcinoma in situ treated by lumpectomy. J Natl Cancer Inst. 2003;95(22):1692–702. https://doi.org/10.1093/jnci/djg097. PMID: 14625260
74. Solin LJ, Fourquet A, Vicini FA, et al. Long term outcome after breast conservation treatment with radiation for mammographically detected ductal carcinoma in situ of the breast. Cancer. 2005;103:1137.
75. Haffty BG, Carter D, Flynn SD, et al. Local recurrence versus new primary: clinical analysis of 82 breast relapses and potential applications of genetic finger printing. Int J Radiat Oncol Biol Phys. 1993;27:575.
76. Huang E, Buchholz TA, Meric F, et al. Classifying local disease recurrences after breast conservation therapy based on location and histology: new primary tumors have more favorable outcomes than true local disease recurrences. Cancer. 2002;95:2059.
77. Arthur DW, Winter KA, Kuerer HM. Effectiveness of breast-conserving surgery and 3-dimensional conformal partial breast reirradiation for recurrence of breast cancer in the ipsilateral breast: the NRG oncology/RTOG 1014 phase 2 clinical trial. JAMA Oncol. 2020;6(1):75.
78. McCready DR, Fish EB, Hiraki GY, et al. Total mastectomy is not always mandatory for the treatment of recurrent breast cancer after lumpectomy alone. Can J Surg. 1992;35(5):485.

Paget's Disease

10

Dhritiman Maitra, Srineil Vuthaluru, and Seenu Vuthaluru

Abstract

This chapter deals with Paget's disease of the breast, a rare presentation of underlying breast malignancy. The lesions are usually unilateral, and very rarely bilateral, and may also develop on accessory nipples or ectopic breasts. A vast majority of patients diagnosed with Paget's disease have an underlying neoplasm associated with it, making diagnosis and treatment of the disease a controversy.

Keywords

Paget's disease · Paget cells · Toker cells

10.1 Introduction

Paget's disease of the breast is a rare and often misdiagnosed manifestation of breast cancer seen in approximately 1–4% cases. It is a noninvasive cutaneous malignancy of the breast involving the nipple areola complex, commonly mistaken for benign breast conditions leading to delay in diagnosis. Mammary Paget's disease (PD) occurs almost exclusively in women; involvement of the male breast is rarely reported and may be more aggressive [1].

Patients present with unilateral, erythematous, pruritic eruption with scaly crusting over the nipple and adjacent areolar skin, which may often be mistaken for eczema and thus overlooked. In patients with clinically PD, the mammographic findings vary from nipple areola skin thickening and nipple retraction to diffuse, malignant microcalcifications [2].

A similar disease involving external genitalia (vulva, glans penis) is known as extramammary Paget's disease, the histologic features being similar to mammary PD. This chapter deals with description of PD of breast with its association with breast cancer, workup, management, and prognosis.

10.2 History

The first clinical description of Paget's disease (PD) was by Velpeau in 1840, when he described eczematous lesions in two of his patients [3], but it was Sir James Paget, an English surgeon who first described the association of PD with an underlying breast malignancy in 1874. He identified 15 women with chronic nipple lesions, all of whom developed breast cancer later on. They had

D. Maitra
Department of General Surgery, Medical College & Hospital, Kolkata, India

S. Vuthaluru
Department of Surgery, University of Nebraska, Omaha, NE, USA

S. Vuthaluru (✉)
Department of Surgery, AIIMS, New Delhi, India

E. Dhamija, S. V. S. Deo (eds.), *Imaging in Management of Breast Diseases*,
https://doi.org/10.1007/978-981-96-4998-3_10

been described as ulcerative or vesicular lesions present over the nipple and areola with clear yellowish exudates. It was subsequently discovered that these skin lesions consist of malignant cells and this entity was described as mammary Paget's disease [4]. George Thin illustrated the first histologic description of PD in 1881 and he postulated the theory of Pagetoid spread.

10.3 Etiopathogenesis

Epidermotropic theory: The tumor cells, namely, Paget cells, are intraepidermal extension of an underlying ductal carcinoma of the breast. They migrate up via the lactiferous ducts and invade the epidermis (epidermotropism) [5]. These malignant Paget cells infiltrate the epidermis, causing thickening of the nipple areolar skin. They disrupt the normal epithelial barrier, allowing extracellular fluid to seep out onto the nipple surface as exudate. This view was supported by the fact that more than 90% of the patients with PD have an underlying breast carcinoma which is of ductal origin. IHC staining properties were found to be common between Paget cells and ductal epithelial cells in many case series [6]. Many molecular markers discovered in Paget cells were also found in parenchymal breast tumors like amplification or overexpression of the gene for HER2. Heregulin alpha, a mobility factor released by normal epidermal keratinocytes, binds to Her2 neu receptors expressed on the Paget cells resulting in chemotaxis of breast ductal carcinoma cells [7].

Transformation theory: It proposes that PD arises from epidermal keratinocytes and actually represents an epidermal carcinoma in situ. This was proposed by George Thin in 1881; he claimed that secretions from breast ducts continuously damage the epithelium leading to malignant transformation. This alternate theory, though less reliable than the former, was supported by an observation that some patients of mammary PD did not have an underlying parenchymal cancer. Moreover, if an underlying malignancy was present, it was situated peripheral to the nipple, suggesting two independent neoplastic processes [8].

10.4 Histopathology

The histologic hallmark of mammary PD is the presence of Paget cells. These are spherical cells occurring singly or in clusters in the rete pegs of epithelium of the nipple, larger than epidermal cells, with pale to clear vacuolated cytoplasm and nuclei with prominent nucleoli. They stain positively with mucicarmine and PAS. They do not invade the dermal basement membrane (which is continuous with the basement membrane of lactiferous sinuses) and are therefore categorized as carcinoma in situ. It has been speculated that the cells may be derived from glandular stem cells or epidermal Toker cells. Toker cells are benign cells found in the epidermis of nipples in 10% of both males and females. Like Paget cells, they have clear vacuolated cytoplasm and are considered a benign counterpart of Paget cells [9]. They may sometimes proliferate resulting in a condition known as clear cell papulosis. Though distinct from Paget cells, IHC studies have implicated them as possible source of PD. Both Toker cells and Paget cells are positive for CK7, epithelial membrane antigen and negative for P63. Toker cells are positive for ER and PR, while Paget cells are negative for ER and PR. Paget cells also express tumor markers CEA and CA15–3.

Paget's disease may be confused with superficially spreading melanoma since Paget cells can phagocytose melanin from adjacent melanocytes. It can be differentiated by positive S100 and HMB4 5 immunostaining in melanoma, which is usually negative in PD.

10.5 Epidemiology and Clinical Presentation

In the USA, about 1–4% of female breast carcinoma patients have associated PD. Less than 2% PD are seen in males [10].In female patients with mammary PD, age ranges from 24 to 84 years with a mean age of diagnosis at 55 years.

Majority of patients with PD present with usually unilateral eczematous eruption of the nipple which may be subtle or may evolve to an ulcerated weeping lesion. The disease may lead to complete destruction of the nipple and may spread centrifugally to involve the areola (Fig. 10.1). A palpable lump may be present in up to 50% of the cases [6]. Although bilateral PD has been reported, it is usually unilateral.

In addition to PD, clinical differential diagnoses of scaling skin and pruritic, erythematous nipple areola complex include eczema, contact dermatitis, psoriasis, and postradiation dermatitis (Table 10.1). Bilaterality and good response to topical steroids are more consistent with eczema or contact dermatitis.

Table 10.1 Clinical differentials of Paget's disease of the breast

Eczema	Mammary PD	Contact dermatitis
May be bilateral, similar itchy lesions may be present elsewhere too	Usually unilateral	Bilateral
Nipple remains intact	Nipple usually distorted	Nipple remains intact
No underlying lump	Underlying limp may be present	No underlying lump
Itchy	Nonitchy	Itchy
Responsive to steroids	Nonresponsive to steroids	Responsive to steroids

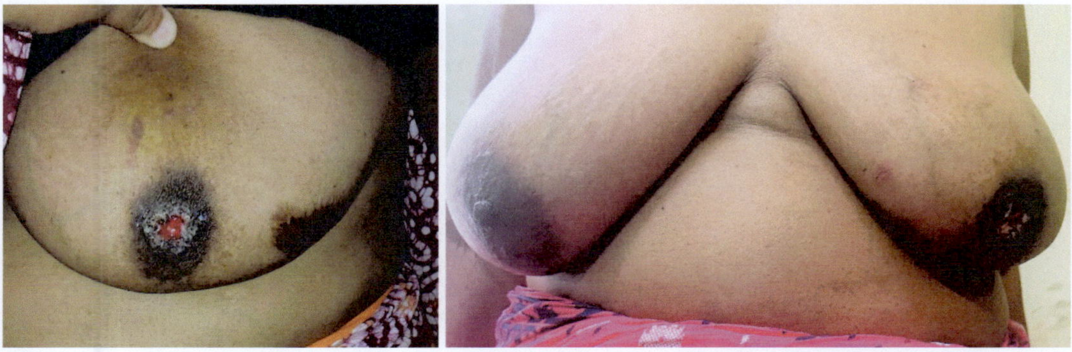

Fig. 10.1 Clinical presentation of Paget's disease: Nipple ulceration with exudates in two different patients, with no underlying lump or mammographic abnormality

10.6 Imaging Evaluation

The aim of radiological evaluation is to ascertain presence of underlying malignancy (Fig. 10.2). Bilateral mammography (MG) should be done to look for underlying mass. In 20% cases, a mammographic abnormality may be present without a palpable lump. Findings include thickening of areolar skin, nipple retraction, subareolar or more diffuse microcalcification, and discrete mass or architectural distortion. It sometimes cannot map the true distribution of an underlying pathology, if present [2]. Therefore, a normal mammography does not rule out an underlying malignancy. USG can describe in details, the characteristics of any underlying lump in females with palpable lump or mass detected on MG.

CEMRI breast being a more sensitive imaging tool can demonstrate an occult cancer in some patients with PD; however, negative preoperative MRI cannot reliably exclude underlying occult malignancy. The findings on MRI include mass or nonmass enhancement along with enhancing nipple-areolar complex region.

10.7 Tissue Analysis

Scrape cytology—noninvasive rapid diagnostic screening method for mammary PD, where the affected area is scraped with a glass slide and stained.

Biopsy—incisional biopsy (punch or wedge biopsy) of the lesional skin of the NAC to include adequate epidermis to provide Paget cells and lactiferous duct is recommended.

USG-guided core needle biopsy from any underlying lump, if present, is mandatory. IHC staining of nipple biopsy—helpful to differentiate from other similar lesions.

The usual diagnostic panel consists of CK 7 and CK 20, CEA, ER, PR, HER2, and S-100. PD is usually positive for CEA and CK 7 and negative for S-100. Most cases of PD show the absence of expression of hormone receptor (estrogen/progesterone), and over 80% are positive for Her2 receptors [11].

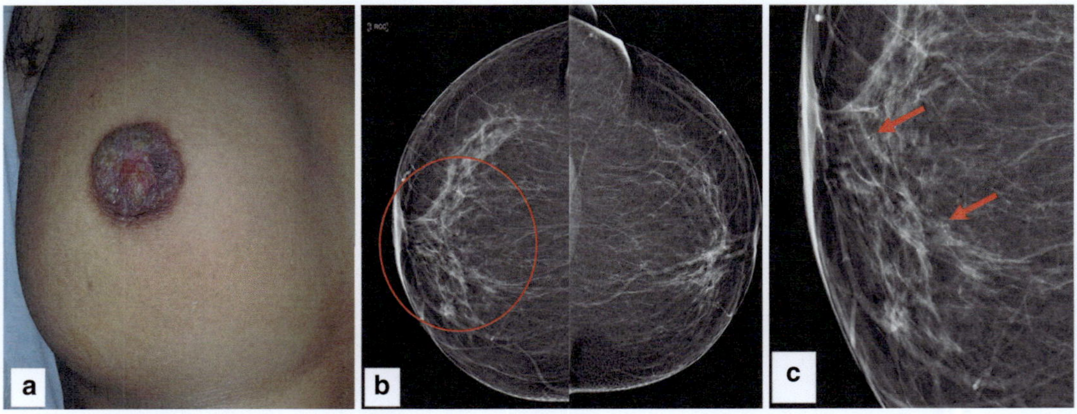

Fig. 10.2 Mammography of patient with Paget's disease: A 55-year-old female presented with itching and nipple discharge since 1.5 years (**a**). (**b**) Craniocaudal views of bilateral breasts reveal thickening of nipple-areola complex on the right side with the presence of pleomorphic calcification in linear distribution (circled area and arrows in zoomed image, **c**). The patient underwent mastectomy which confirmed Paget's disease of the nipple and DCIS along the calcification showing comedonecrosis

10.8 Management

PD of the breast is classified as Tis (Paget). If there is an underlying lump which is diagnosed as invasive duct carcinoma (IDC) on core biopsy, then TNM staging is done according to that of invasive carcinoma.

Various treatment options have been described in literature over the years for management of mammary PD, including nipple excision, radiotherapy alone, central core excision with or without addition of radiotherapy, and mastectomy. Concerns for underlying malignancy and potential for multifocal or multicentric disease had led to mastectomy with or without axillary lymph node dissection (ALND) to be the standard of care for PD in the past. However, role of BCS without any form of axillary assessment (sentinel lymph node biopsy/axillary sampling/ALND) is now established as an acceptable form of treatment for PD with no underlying lump.

Complete removal of the NAC is a mandate in patients undergoing breast conservation regardless of the extent of NAC involvement. However, breast conservation alone (without radiotherapy) is associated with a high local failure rate and is therefore not recommended.

Polgar et al. reported 33% local recurrence in 33 women with mammary PD who underwent breast conservation without adjuvant radiation. Of these 33, 30 had an underlying Ductal carcinoma in situ (DCIS), and three had no underlying malignancy. With a median of 6 years of follow-up, 11 developed local recurrence of which 10 were invasive [12].

Dixon et al. evaluated ten women with PD with no underlying malignancy documented by imaging. NAC was excised with an underlying cone biopsy. All were found to have underlying DCIS with negative margins on HPE. At a median follow-up of 56 months, 40% had a local recurrence [13].

If breast conservation is to be considered, central lumpectomy (central core excision) should be followed by postoperative radiation. Bijker et al. evaluated 61 patients with PD of which 97% did not have any underlying lump and 84% had a normal mammography. They underwent central core excision, and it was observed that 93% of them had DCIS, all with free resection margins. They were followed with whole breast irradiation. After 6.4 years, a 5-year local recurrence was 5.2% [14].

Several studies confirmed that for a mammary PD with no palpable lump or mammographic abnormality, breast conservation with central lumpectomy followed by radiation therapy provides excellent local control, disease-free survival, and overall survival [15–19]. If conservative therapy is adopted, patient must be followed up with mammography on a regular basis and mastectomy done should a relapse occur.

If there is an underlying lump, then surgical and adjuvant therapy should be planned as per standard protocol for DCIS/IDC as the case may be. When mammary PD is associated with a palpable breast lump or a definite mammographic abnormality, the associated breast cancer tends to be of a more advanced stage with higher risk of axillary lymph node positivity or multifocal disease or invasive disease. The underlying lesion has to be removed along with NAC. Also, the axilla needs to be evaluated. Clinically suspicious axilla should be investigated preoperatively with a US-guided FNA or core needle biopsy; if disease is confirmed histologically, full ALND is recommended. On the other hand, if negative, sentinel lymph node biopsy (SLNB) should be done if breast lump is present [20].

If wide local excision (WLE) can be performed with negative resection margins and good cosmesis, then BCS followed by whole breast irradiation is appropriate [18].Role of SLNB is controversial in DCIS, and therefore patients undergoing breast conservation therapy for PD without a known invasive carcinoma need not undergo SLNB. Some surgeons await final histopathology report and only proceed with SLNB if invasive disease is found.

Patients with diffuse calcifications or multicentric disease should be treated with mastectomy and axillary evaluation by SLNB. In all cases being planned for mastectomy, it is reasonable to perform SLNB in order to prevent an unnecessary ALND in case an invasive component is identified in operative specimen as once mastectomy is performed, SLNB becomes difficult to execute in future.

PD is associated with an underlying malignancy in most cases of which a substantial amount of patients may have invasive carcinoma. Lymph node metastasis is considered the most important prognostic factor in invasive carcinoma, and therefore, all patients with invasive component should be offered axillary evaluation. SLNB being less invasive has replaced ALND in clinically negative axilla.

Patients with PD are more likely to have cancer which is ER/PR negative and of high histologic grade. There is no supporting evidence of tamoxifen or aromatase inhibitors reducing risk of local recurrence in patients with PD without an underlying DCIS/invasive carcinoma, who underwent breast conservation therapy.

With better reconstructive options available to patients, the loss of NAC can be managed by several techniques with excellent cosmesis (Figs. 10.3 and 10.4). Chung et al. reconstructed

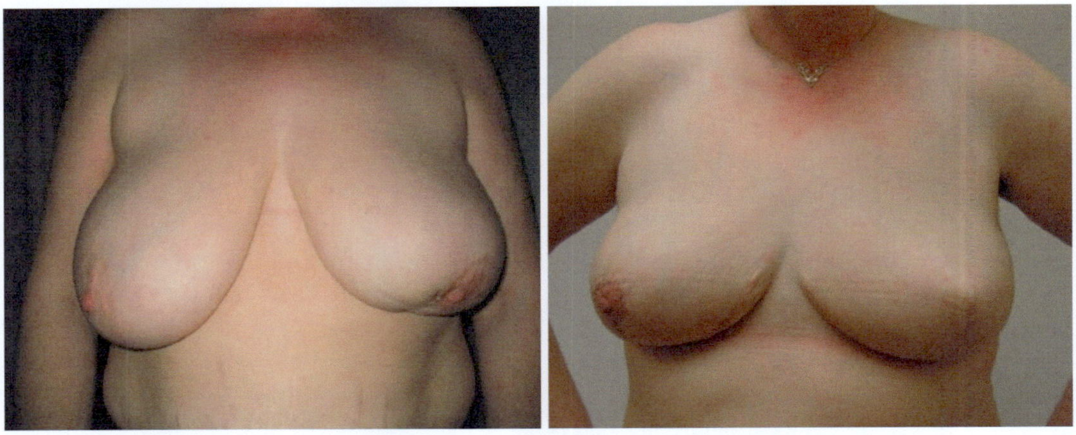

Fig. 10.3 Surgical planning in Paget's disease—preoperative picture of left-sided Paget's disease (left); inverted T mammoplasty done bilaterally (right). The NAC is encompassed between the incision which has to be removed. On the contralateral side, standard Wise incision made and reduction mammoplasty done to preserve the symmetry of breasts

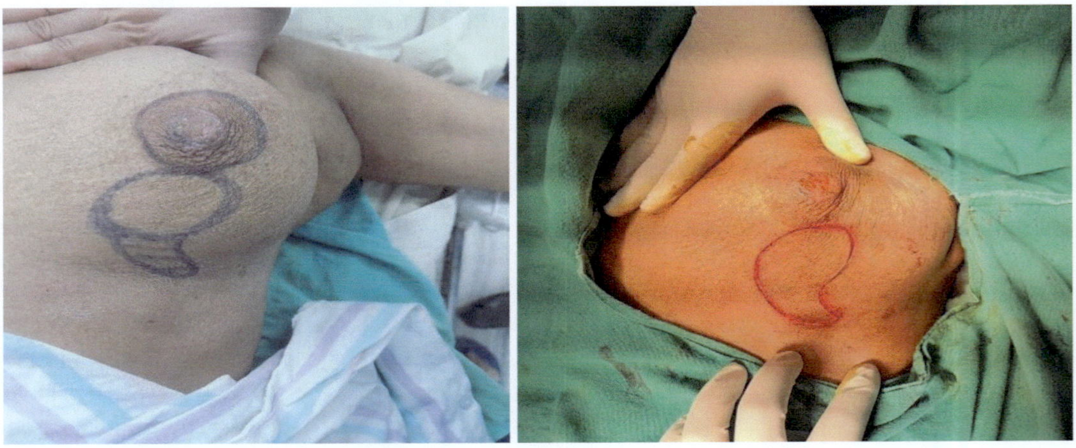

Fig. 10.4 Surgical technique—marking of the NAC with another small circle with equal radius as NAC just inferior to the NAC within an inverted comma-shaped area

NAC immediately in 29 women with PD by using a standard Wise pattern incision for reduction mammoplasty, central lumpectomy, and removal of NAC. The central defect was filled by the inferior pedicle which was deepithelialized and advanced or rotated. Breast and skin flaps were mobilized and approximated to midline and then inframammary fold closed. After completion of radiotherapy, reconstruction of the nipple was done [21].

Another technique to restore the central breast area is placement of a Grisotti flap. It is a local rotational dermoglandular flap to fill the central defect. The Grisotti flap uses tissues from the inferior pole to create a deepithelialized pedicled flap with a circular skin island and pushes it up to fill the central defect.

Prognosis and Outcome Outcome of PD depends on the presence or absence of underlying in situ or invasive cancer. In the presence of invasive cancer, TNM stage of the cancer determines prognosis.

PD of the nipple that has not spread beyond the lactiferous ducts (stage 0) has excellent outcome following completion of treatment. The overall reported 5-year survival rates range from 81% to 98% [22, 23].

Conclusion Paget's disease of the breast is a rare entity. In the absence of underlying in situ or invasive cancer, local treatment in the form of central core excision with radiation or mastectomy with sentinel node biopsy is associated with excellent prognosis.

Acknowledgments We express our sincere thanks to Dr. Adrija Basak, Junior Resident, Department of Surgery, Kolkata, who helped in the compilation of this chapter.

References

1. Valdes EK, Feldman SM. Paget's disease of the breast. Breast J. 2006;12(1):83.
2. Gunhan BI, Oktay A. Paget's disease of the breast: clinical, mammographic, sonographic, and pathologic findings in 52 cases, ear. J Radiol. 2006;60(2):256–63.
3. Velpeau A. On disease of the mammary areola preceding cancer of the mammary region. London: Sydenham Society; 1856.
4. Paget J. On disease of the mammary areola preceding cancer of the mammary gland. St Barts Hosp Rep. 1874;10:87–9.
5. Muir R. Further observation on Paget's disease of the nipple. J Pathol Bacteriol. 1939;49:299.
6. Chaudhary MA, Millis RR, Lane EB, Miller NA. Paget's disease of the nipple: a ten-year review including clinical, clinical, pathological, and immunohistochemical findings. Breast Cancer Res Treat. 1986;8(2):139–46.
7. Schelfhout VR, Coene ED, Delaey B, Thys S, Page DL, De Potter CR. Pathogenesis of Paget's disease: epidermal heregulin alpha, motility factor and the HER receptor family. J Natl Cancer Inst. 2000;92(8):622–8.
8. Yim JH, Wick MR, Philpott GW, Norton JA, Doherty GM. Underlying pathology in mammary Paget's disease. Ann Surg Oncol. 1997;4:287–92.
9. Van der Putte SC, Toonstra J, Hennioman A. Mammary Paget's disease confined to areola and associated with multifocal Tokercell hyperplasia. Am J Dermatopathol. 1995;17(5):487–93.
10. Mooer SA, Notgrass HM, Vadergriff TW, Sahoo S. Mammary Paget's disease of the Male Breast: a rare case with an unusual immunohistochemical profile. Int J Surg Pathol. 2020;28(2):210–5.
11. Kothari AS, Beechay-Newman N, Hamed H, Fentiman IS, D'Arrigo C, Hanby AM, Ryder K. Paget disease of the nipple: a multifocal manifestation of higher risk disease. Cancer. 2002;95(1):1–7.
12. Polgar C, Orosz Z, Kovacs T, et al. Breast conservation therapy for Paget disease of the nipple: a prospective European Organisation for Research and Treatment for Cancer study of 61 patients. Cancer. 2001;94:1904–5.
13. Dixon AR, Galea MH, Ellis IO, et al. Paget's disease of the nipple. Br J Surg. 1991;78:722–3.
14. Bijker N, Rutgers NJ, Duchateau L, er al. Breast conserving therapy for Paget disease of the nipple: a prospective European Organisation for research and treatment of cancer study of 61patients. Cancer. 2001;91:472–7.
15. Marshall JK, Griffith KA, Haffty BG, et al. The conservative management of Paget disease of the breast with radiotherapy: 10-and 15-year results. Cancer. 2003;97(9):2142–9.
16. Dalberg K, Hellborg H, Warnberg F. Paget disease of the nipple in a population based cohort. Breast Cancer Res Treat. 2008;111(2):313–9.
17. Kawase K, Dimaio DJ, Tucker SL, et al. Paget's disease of the breast: there is a role for breast conservation surgery. Ann Surg Oncol. 2005;12(5):391–7.
18. Zakaria S, Pantvaidya G, Ghosh K, et al. Pagets' disease of the breast: accuracy of preoperative assessment. Breast Cancer Res Treat. 2007;102(2):137–42.

19. Caliskan M, Gatti G, Sosnovskikh I, et al. Paget's disease of the breast: the experience of the European institute of oncology and review of the literature. Breast Cancer Res Treat. 2008;112(3):513–21. PMID18240020
20. Sukumvanich P, Benrem DJ, Cody HS, Brogi E, Fey JV, Borgen PI, Gemignani ML. The role of sentinel lymph node biopsy in Paget's disease of the breast. Ann Surg Oncol. 2007;14(3):1020–3.
21. Chung TL, Schnaper L, Silverman RP, et al. A novel reconstructive technique following central lumpectomy. Plast Reconstr Surg. 2006;118:23–7.
22. Oritz-Pagan S, Cunto-Amesty G, Narayan S. Effect of Paget's disease of breast on survival in breast cancer: an exploratory study. Arch Surg. 2011;46:1267–70.
23. American Cancer Society (ACS). Cancer facts and figures. 2006. Web site http://www.cancer.org.

11 Approach to Nipple Discharge

Jwala Srikala, Supraja Laguduva Mohan, and Nisha Hariharan

Abstract

Nipple discharge is the third most common clinical complaint among females with breast-related symptoms which often is due to benign causes like duct ectasia or papilloma. However, the risk of associated malignancy increases if the discharge is spontaneous, bloody or serous, persistent, or unilateral, from a single duct and with associated lump. The most common associated malignancy is ductal carcinoma in situ (DCIS).

The clinical examination aims to determine when imaging assessment should be included in the patient workup. Although mammography (MG) is routinely performed first, it has low sensitivity in detecting the cause of nipple discharge especially if the lesion is small, in retroareolar location, and has no internal microcalcifications. On the other hand, ultrasound (USG) has variable sensitivity and specificity as it is an operator-dependent technique and needs various maneuvers to assess retroareolar location. Magnetic resonance imaging (MRI) has been used for patients with suspicious nipple discharge but no abnormality on MG or USG, to rule out DCIS which is seen as nonmass enhancement on MRI.

The treatment approach for nipple discharge includes microdochectomy, vacuum-assisted excision, or surgical excision, based on specific scenarios. This chapter aims to highlight all these concerns related to diagnosis and management of patients with nipple discharge.

Keywords

Nipple discharge · Solitary dilated duct Breast ultrasound · Mammography Ductography · MRI breast · Intraductal papilloma · DCIS · VAE · Microdochectomy

11.1 Introduction

More than 80% of females experience some form of nipple discharge in life, including lactational, physiological, or pathological conditions [1]. Approximately, 4.8–7.4% patients present with symptomatic nipple discharge in the breast clinic and underlying malignancy is the cause in 5–12% of patients [2]. Physiological nipple discharge is seen in lactation, pregnancy, medical or endocrinological conditions, hypothalamic or pituitary masses, long-term consumption of few medica-

J. Srikala (✉)
KIMS, Hyderabad, India

S. L. Mohan
Department of Radiodiagnosis and Interventional Radiology, AIIMS, New Delhi, India

N. Hariharan
Basavatarakam Indo American Cancer Hospital and Research Institute, Hyderabad, India

E. Dhamija, S. V. S. Deo (eds.), *Imaging in Management of Breast Diseases*,
https://doi.org/10.1007/978-981-96-4998-3_11

tions, postsurgery, or trauma. Pathological nipple discharge can be associated with intraductal masses, duct ectasia, and carcinomas. Although most breast carcinomas present as a palpable lump, mastalgia, nipple retraction, discharge, or overlying skin changes, nipple discharge may be the only sign of breast malignancy in smaller carcinomas and in situ carcinoma. Mammography (MG) with or without digital breast tomosynthesis (DBT) is the first step in evaluation of most patients with nipple discharge, while ultrasound is complimentary and preferred in younger patients with dense breasts. MRI can serve as a problem-solving tool and identify additional lesions that are not seen by mammography or sonography [3]. Techniques like galactography and galactoscopy are unpopular due to their invasive nature and may be useful only for localizing the trigger duct preoperatively [4]. Given the wide range of causes and differences in their management, an algorithmic approach is needed for tailoring the appropriate radiological investigation and treatment strategy for such patients.

11.2 Anatomy of the Duct Lobular Unit and Nipple-Areola Complex of the Breast

The breast is comprised of 15–20 lobes or segments, the smallest functional units of which are called "acini." About 10–100 acini form a lobule, which drains into a common terminal duct. Around 20–40 terminal ducts drain into subsegmental and segmental ducts, which join to form the main duct [5]. A fusiform dilatation of the main duct called the lactiferous sinus is seen just before narrowing and terminating into the external opening on the surface of the nipple. All the duct walls are formed by surface epithelium, covered by a discontinuous layer of myoepithelium and connective tissue [5]. The areola is made of projections of sebaceous glands, which later enlarge in pregnancy when they are called tubercles of Montgomery. The nipple is a cylindrical projection from the center of the areola, comprised of circular muscle fibers of Sappey and radial fibers of Meyerholz. It has no subcutaneous tissue or sebaceous glands. These muscle fibers extend contiguously to surround the ductal system of the breast, and their contraction causes mild secretion into the lactiferous sinuses [6]. The nipple-areolar complex (NAC) is supplied predominantly by the perforating branches of the internal mammary artery. Additional blood supply is from the intercostal arteries, which mainly supply the deeper part of the breast. The NAC drains through a superficial venous plexus of Haller that radiates just below the areola and a deep venous system, which eventually drains into axillary, internal mammary, and intercostal veins. Similarly, an areolar lymphatic plexus drains into the subareolar plexus of Sappey, which further drains lymph into the deep system and axillary lymph nodes [6].

11.3 Types and Causes of Nipple Discharge

Nipple discharge is the third most common breast complaint following pain and lump in the breast [2]. It can be categorized into physiological and pathological discharge. Lactational nipple discharge refers to normal milk production, which happens in pregnancy and up to 1 or 2 years postpartum. During pregnancy, mammogenesis starts at 6–8 weeks of gestation, when the breasts increase in size and volume; there is an increase in vascularity, and the nipples become pigmented and erectile [7]. Estrogen induces duct development and arborization, while progesterone causes growth of the lobules and secretory differentiation of alveolar cells, starting from midtrimester. By the end of pregnancy, the alveoli get filled with colostrum. Full-fledged milk production starts after childbirth through positive feedback by prolactin secretion, when the inhibitory effects of estrogen and progesterone on milk secretion are no longer present [7, 8]. Unilateral or bilateral discharge can also occur well before parturition, from the second trimester onward.

Physiological nipple discharge, including lactation, can be white, clear, straw-colored, yellow, green, or brown. It is usually bilateral, involving multiple pores, and associated with breast compression or stimulation of the nipple [9]. Milky white discharge in nonpregnant/nonlactating women, also called galactorrhoea, can be due to hyperprolactinemia induced by hypothalamic-pituitary axis dysfunction (pituitary adenoma, hypothyroidism) or certain medications (conventional antipsychotics, antidepressants, opiates, metoclopramide, H2-blockers, and antihypertensives including reserpine, methyldopa, verapamil, and oral contraceptives) [10]. Chest wall injury in the form of burns, intercostal nerve damage, Herpes zoster infection, or surgery (thoracotomy) can also induce nonpuerperal galactorrhoea [2].

Pathological nipple discharge is usually spontaneous and unilateral, from single pore; can be clear, bloody, or serous in nature; or is associated with a mass. The most common causes are intraductal papilloma (35–62%), duct ectasia (15–20%), and carcinoma (7–15%) [10]. Intraductal papilloma is a localized hyperplasia of the duct epithelium, with a central fibrovascular stalk. Up to 60–80% intraductal papillomas can be associated with spontaneous or induced nipple discharge. It usually occurs in middle-aged women, can be single or multiple (papillomatosis), and is usually nonpalpable [11]. They are a part of the spectrum of papillary lesions of breast, which includes lesions of the large ducts (solitary intraductal papilloma, papillary carcinoma) which present as nipple discharge and small ducts of the terminal ductal lobular unit (multiple papillomatosis, papillary ductal carcinoma in situ), which are often incidental [12]. Differentiation of such benign from malignant papillary lesions is an important diagnostic challenge.

Duct ectasia, defined as dilatation of one or more ducts over 2 mm or the ampullary portions over 3 mm [13], is the second most common cause of pathological nipple discharge. It is usually seen in perimenopausal females and is associated with inflammation and periductal fibrosis of retro areolar ducts, with accumulation of cheese like secretions within the ducts. There can be serous, white, or green nipple discharge, and in later stages, there may be nipple inversion and calcification. It can present as a firm mass just below the nipple, mimicking malignancy [11]. Central duct ectasia is usually benign, while peripheral duct ectasia, particularly with irregular walls and focal wall thickening, favors malignancy [13]. Duct ectasia can also be associated with apocrine metaplasia, a benign condition where the epithelium of the lobular cells around the ducts are transformed into apocrine glandular cells, resulting in the formation of periductal cysts [13]. Fibrocystic changes, which are areas of cysts, adenosis, or fibrosis with or without ductal or lobular hyperplasia, are another cause of multiple duct-nipple discharge. They can be focal, regional, or diffuse and are seen as simple, clustered, complicated, complex cysts, or calcifications [14]. Other benign conditions causing nipple discharge are mastitis and discharge after biopsy or breast conservative surgery [15].

The most common types of malignancy to be associated with nipple discharge are ductal carcinoma in situ (DCIS) and papillary carcinoma. Discharge from malignancies can be serous or serosanguinous and usually from a single duct. When nipple discharge is accompanied by the presence of a palpable mass or a visible lesion on imaging, especially in older age groups, the risk of malignancy increases [15]. Nipple discharge from male breast is rare, but when present, it is strongly associated with carcinoma [16].

11.4 Clinical Evaluation of Nipple Discharge

The aim of clinical evaluation is to differentiate physiological from pathological discharge. A thorough history of the presenting complaints should include the onset, duration of nipple discharge, color, quantity, and frequency of discharge, whether it is spontaneous or induced, unilateral or bilateral, and presence or absence of lump or other associated symptoms (redness, cyclical or noncyclical mastalgia, fever). A history of visual disturbance, headache, polyuria, or polydipsia can point to an underlying pituitary or hypothalamic pathology. Documentation of recent pregnancy or lactation, history of drug intake, hypothyroidism, endocrine or menstrual abnormalities, recent trauma, or surgery and family history of breast cancer can aid in distinguishing physiological from pathological causes [17].

Physical examination should include inspection for asymmetry, contour changes, visible lump or nipple discharge, nipple inversion, ulcers, or skin thickening. Inspection should ideally be done under a magnifying lamp. Causes of pseudodischarge such as eczema, dermatosis, and erosive adenomatosis of the nipple need to be excluded [18]. The site and color of nipple discharge are to be ascertained. This is followed by palpation in full day light, in sitting, followed by supine position. The entire breast and axilla are palpated for masses or lymph nodes and their consistency. Centripetal or radial approach is used in each quadrant in search of any palpable mass or trigger point that induces the discharge. Single or multiple duct origin and the clock position of nipple discharge can be tested by pressing gently on the areola, between the thumb and index finger [18]. Systematic examination should also be done for evaluation of ocular, thyroid, or other endocrine abnormalities, to exclude physiological causes [2, 19]. A thorough hormonal profile workup should follow in case of suspected endocrinological cause of discharge.

Nipple discharge cytology from smears is no longer recommended due to their low sensitivity and specificity for both benign and malignant causes [20]. It is performed by direct imprint from the nipple in spontaneous discharge or by expression through gentle pressure on the areola. The smeared slides are fixed by dipping them in 95% ethyl alcohol and stained with Papanicolaou stain, which is examined by a cytopathologist for the presence of any atypical cells. This may be useful only in a small subset of patients, in whom there are no detectable lesions by palpation or imaging, particularly in those with single pore and bloody discharge. The result is valid only if it is malignant, as the false-negative rate is as high as 50% [18, 21].

11.5 Radiological Evaluation

The imaging modalities that are initially used in the workup of nipple discharge include ultrasound (US) and digital mammography (MG) with or without digital breast tomosynthesis (DBT). Ductography was previously used in US and MG negative cases but has been replaced now by breast magnetic resonance imaging (MRI). Nuclear medicine modalities including Tc-99m Sestamibi molecular breast imaging and 18F—FluoroDeoxyGlucose Positron Emission Mammography (18F—FDG PEM) can detect smaller noninvasive malignancies [3].

The ACR appropriateness criteria recommendations in imaging evaluation of nipple discharge [3, 22] have been summarized as follows:

1. *Physiological nipple discharge*—There is no need for additional imaging apart from the routine screening MG.
2. *Pathological nipple discharge, in men or in women over 40 years of age*—MG ± DBT with spot compression or magnification views for better evaluation of the retroareolar region. US is a complementary tool. MRI or ductography is not appropriate and is done only when initial screening is negative.
3. *Pathological discharge in women between 30 and 39 years of age*—US is the initial step instead of MG. MRI or ductography is not appropriate and is done only when initial screening is negative.
4. *Pathological discharge in women less than or equal to 30 years of age*—US is the initial step and MG is complementary, in patients with high-risk genetic mutations or suspicious findings on ultrasound.
5. *Pathological discharge in men between 25 and 30 years of age*—MG should be done as the initial step; US is complimentary.
6. *Pathological discharge in men less than or equal to 25 years of age*—US is the initial step; MG is complimentary and can be done if needed.

11.6 Imaging Modalities with Their Indication and Utility

Mammography Digital mammography (MG) is the initial diagnostic modality of choice in women over 40 years of age. Standard craniocaudal and mediolateral oblique views are obtained, and if needed, additional spot compression or magnification views are done. It has a low sensitivity (20–25%) in detecting malignant lesions associated with nipple discharge as most of these lesions are small, may not contain calcifications, or may be completely intraductal [3, 23]. The utility of MG in evaluation of pathological nipple discharge lies in picking up suspicious calcifications, especially in DCIS, which is one of the most common malignant causes of nipple discharge. DCIS can be associated with amorphous, coarse, or fine pleomorphic or fine linear calcifications, in suspicious linear or segmental distribution [24].

Amorphous calcifications are small (2–300 microns), seen in 20% of DCIS cases [25]. Fine pleomorphic calcifications are more conspicuous, irregular in shape, and of similar size as amorphous calcifications. Coarse pleomorphic calcifications are larger than fine pleomorphic and amorphous calcifications but less than 1 mm. Fine linear calcifications constitute thin, discontinuous calcifications, individually less than 0.5 mm [24]. Linear distribution is due to calcifications within a duct, while segmental distribution is due to calcifications within a duct and its branches; and both patterns (Figs. 11.1 and 11.2) are highly associated with malignancy [24, 25]. The calcifications associated with DCIS are also larger at presentation and show a higher growth rate than benign breast diseases [26]. On the other hand, round or rim calcifications can be seen in papilloma, while rod-like calcifications can be associated with duct ectasia [18].

MG can also depict masses (which could represent papilloma, papillary carcinoma, or infil-

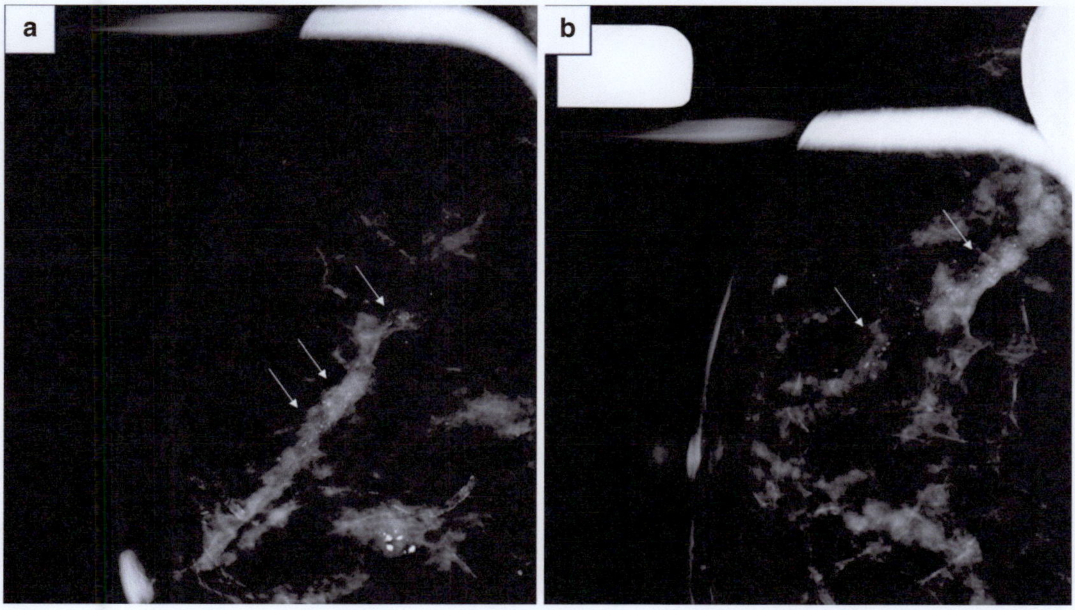

Fig. 11.1 Calcifications in ductal carcinoma in situ (DCIS). Magnified views of the right upper and outer quadrant of the right breast show microcalcifications in a linear distribution (arrows) with an associated ductal density in a 40-year-old lady presenting with unilateral (right) spontaneous bloody nipple discharge. Histopathological examination revealed intermediate-grade DCIS

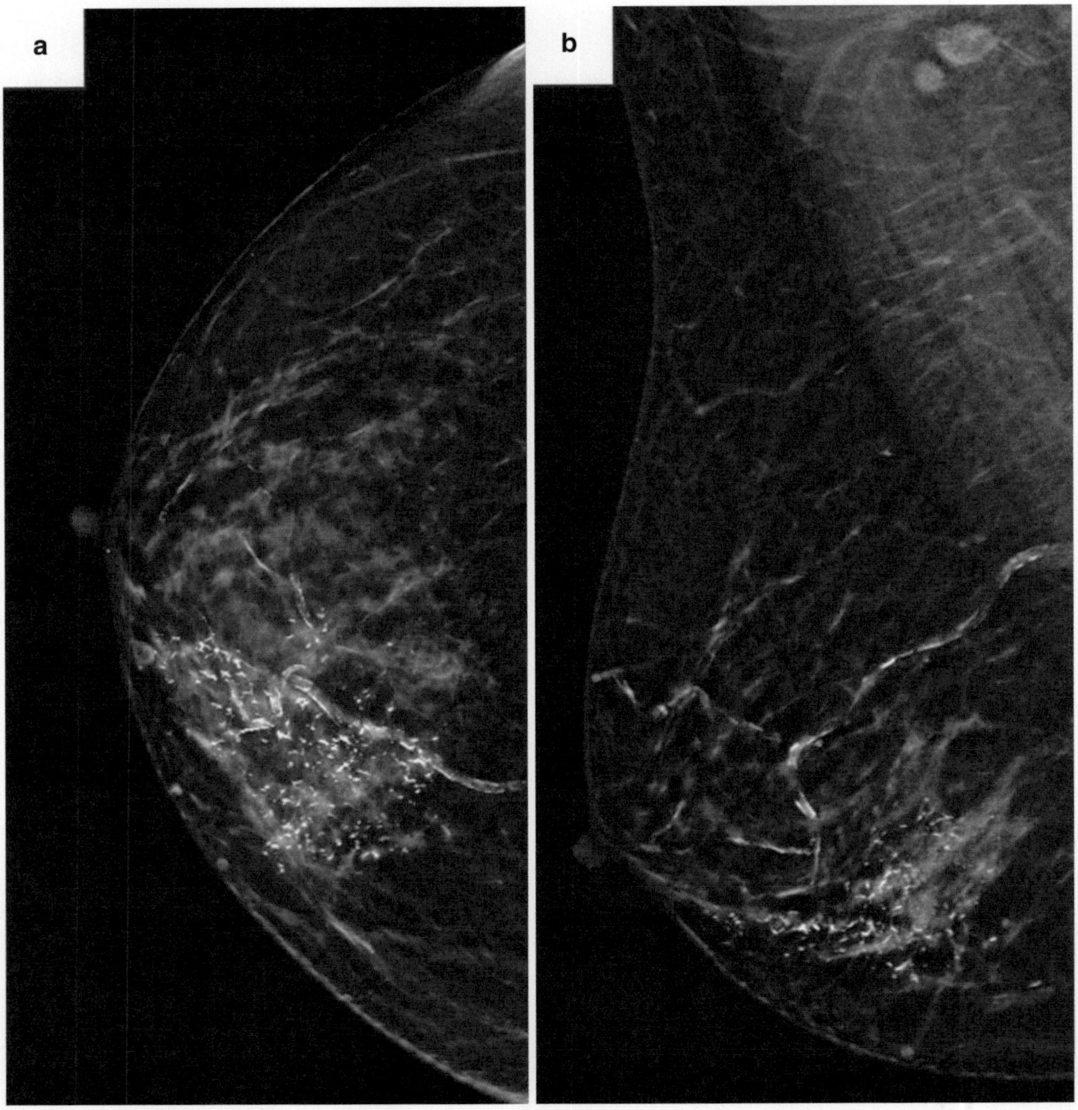

Fig. 11.2 Calcifications in ductal carcinoma in situ (DCIS). Craniocaudal (**a**) and mediolateral oblique (**b**) views of the right breast showing pleomorphic microcalcification in a segmental distribution in the medial and lower quadrant of the right breast

trating ductal carcinoma), focal asymmetry, architectural distortions, or duct ectasia in patients with nipple discharge (Fig. 11.3). Dilated ducts appear as retroareolar tubular or branching structures (Fig. 11.4). The subareolar region normally shows increased density; hence, duct ectasia may also appear as focal asymmetries and may need further spot compression, tomosynthesis, or US for a conclusive diagnosis. Asymmetric duct ectasia is most often diagnosed by MG initially [27]. It may be associated with suspicious microcalcification, nonsubareolar location, or the presence of beaded contour of ducts raising concern for malignancy [27, 28]. Nevertheless, further evaluation with US or MRI is needed to find out the underlying cause.

The application of DBT can improve the diagnosis of smaller lesions by overcoming the effect of superimposition of glandular parenchyma, with better depiction of mass margins and spicu-

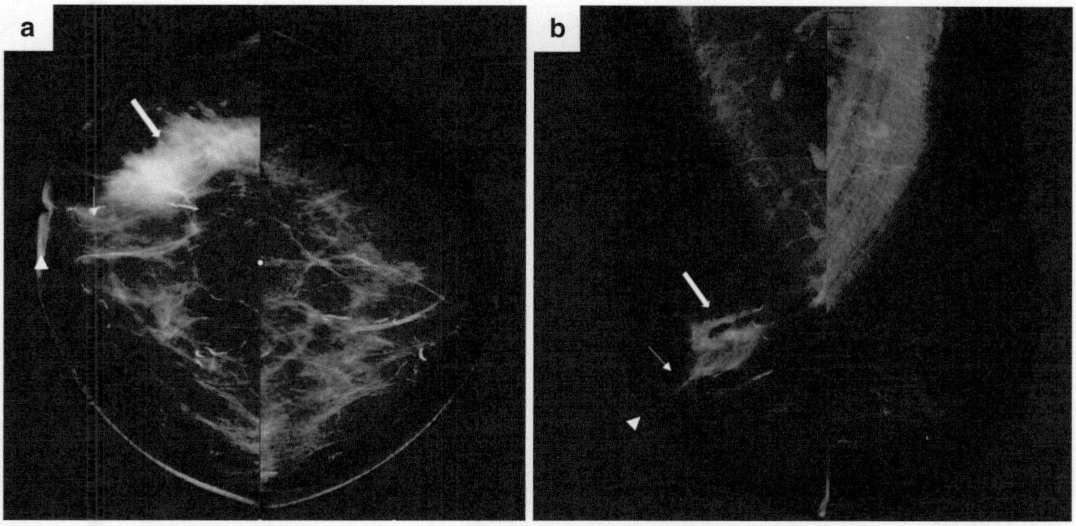

Fig. 11.3 Mass and duct ectasia in mammography in a case of DCIS. Craniocaudal (**a**) and mediolateral oblique (**b**) views of the right breast in a 70-year-old lady with bloody nipple discharge show a dilated duct (thin arrow) with a large asymmetry (thick arrow) in the upper and outer quadrant of the right breast. There is associated retraction and thickening of the right nipple (arrow head). The final diagnosis was grade 2 ductal carcinoma in situ (DCIS)

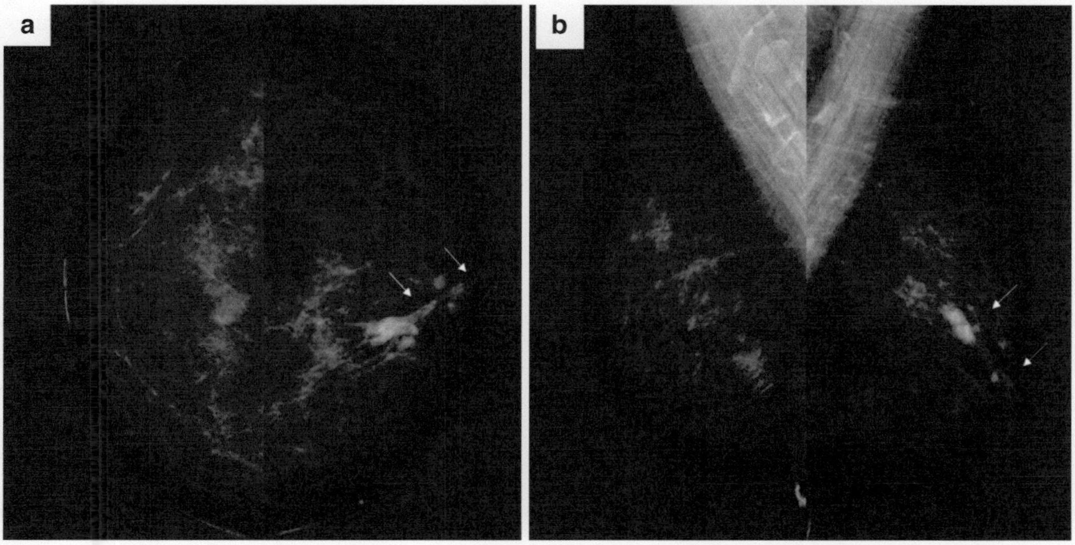

Fig. 11.4 Duct ectasia on mammography. Craniocaudal (**a**) and mediolateral oblique (**b**) views of the left breast in a 58-year-old lady with spontaneous bloody nipple discharge show dilated ducts seen as retroareolar tubular and branching structures (arrows)

lations [29]. However, magnification imaging may still be needed to characterize calcifications, in view of better spatial resolution (Fig. 11.5). Another useful technique to improve conspicuity of smaller masses and detection of multifocal or multicentric lesions is contrast-enhanced spectral mammography (CESM). It involves two acquisitions—high and low energy, after injection of

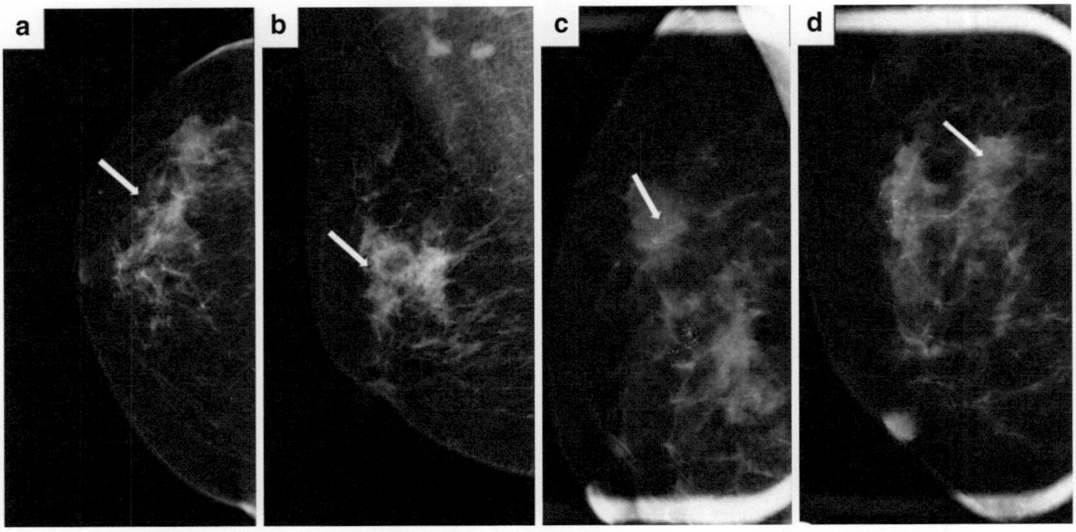

Fig. 11.5 Magnification imaging for calcifications. Cluster of suspicious pleomorphic microcalcifications (arrows) are seen in the upper and outer quadrant of right breast on craniocaudal (**a**) and mediolateral oblique (**b**) views. Magnified views (**c**, **d**) show the morphology and extent of the calcifications much better and reveal presence of additional amorphous microcalcifications in the adjacent breast (arrows)

iodinated contrast. The low-energy image appears like routine MG, while the high-energy image, by virtue of the K edge effect of iodine, can depict the tumor neovascularity [30]. CESM is comparable to MRI in detection of malignancies, besides the added advantages such as low cost, speed of acquisition, accessibility of equipment, and detection of suspicious calcifications [30–32].

Ultrasound (US) Breast US is predominantly a complimentary tool to mammography in the initial workup of patients with nipple discharge. It is however the initial modality of choice in women less than 40 years of age due to increased breast density. With the advantages of real-time imaging and assessment of vascularity by doppler, it can help in further characterization of abnormalities picked up on MG and aid in guiding biopsies. The use of US along with MG can lead to detection of additional malignancies and high-risk lesions in patients with nipple discharge [33, 34]. Small intraductal pathologies are better picked up on US particularly with high-resolution probes. The common causes of nipple discharge including duct ectasia (Fig. 11.6) and intraductal papilloma are easily visualized by US. As per the American College of Radiology Breast Imaging Reporting and Data System (ACR BI-RADS), duct changes are considered associated features. They include cystic dilatation or irregular caliber/branching of ducts, extension of dilated ducts from suspicious masses, and intraductal mass, debris, or thrombus [35]. Intraductal masses have 8% risk of malignancy and hence characterized as BIRADS 4a and need biopsy [35, 36].

Duct masses are better visualized during radial orientation of the ultrasound probe, bringing the duct in line with the mass. Subareolar ultrasound can be difficult due to the posterior shadowing from the air gap created between the probe and nipple. This can be overcome by using a stand-off pad or a thick layer of ultrasound gel or through few maneuvers [36]:

1. Peripheral compression—Radial orientation over nipple areolar complex parallel to long axis of duct followed by compression of the lateral end of the transducer.
2. Rolled nipple—Nipple is fixed between the index finger of the free hand and the transducer held in radial orientation to the duct, and the transducer is gradually slide toward

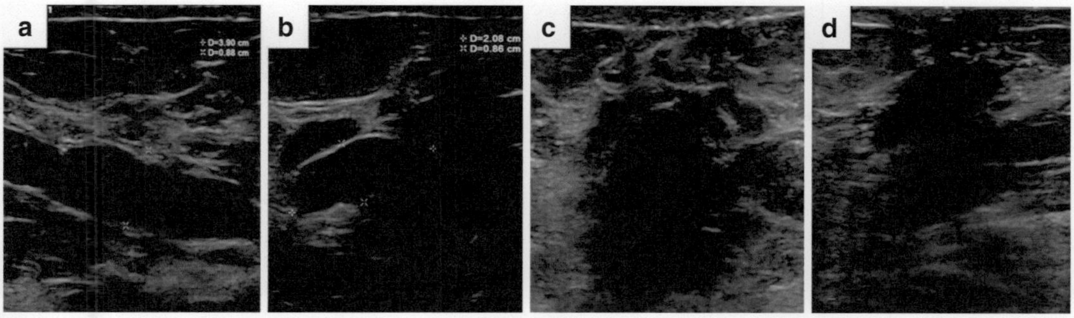

Fig. 11.6 Duct ectasia on ultrasonography. Ultrasound of a 35-year-old lady with bilateral spontaneous nipple discharge showing multiple dilated ducts with inspissated secretions in the retroareolar region of left breast (**a**, **b**) and mildly dilated ducts with anechoic fluid in the retroareolar region of the right breast (**c**, **d**), suggestive of bilateral duct ectasia

the nipple, which gets rolled over the index finger.

3. Two-hand compression—The transducer is in radial orientation and both the transducer and free hand are used to compress the NAC, to differentiate mobile debris from fixed masses. Dynamic compression can also be combined with doppler for diagnosis of ductal debris, as the movement of intraductal debris on compression produces artefactual color flow during compression. If an intraductal mass is identified, its size, clock position, distance from the nipple, distance between the mass and base of nipple, and extent of duct involvement are to be noted.

Intraductal papillary neoplasms can be seen on ultrasound as intraductal mass, intracystic mass or a solid mass (Fig. 11.7). A solitary dilated duct, even without an identifiable mass, is highly suggestive of an intraductal papilloma, as opposed to multiple sectorally dilated ducts in duct ectasia. They are very vascular and may bleed spontaneously, creating fluid debris levels in the dilated duct. A central vascular pedicle with branching vessels can be identified on doppler [37]. Ultrasound is however less sensitive in picking up small malignancies or in situ carcinomas which originate from the terminal ductal lobular unit and peripheral ducts rather than the central ducts and are negative in 80% malignant causes of nipple discharge [38]. Suspicious microcalcifications are not commonly seen on ultrasound compared to mammography, but when seen, there are more frequently malignant [39]. Elastography, with a combination of qualitative and quantitative measurements, can be an alternative tool in differentiation of benign and malignant masses causing nipple discharge; it can be used as a screening tool before invasive techniques like ductoscopy or duct excision are done [40]. Contrast enhanced ultrasound (CEUS) of the breast can also guide in predicting malignant ductal lesions and small carcinomas. An area of peripheral enhancement beyond the confines of the hypoechoic lesion visualized on B mode US is seen with malignancies. Rapid washout, which is considered as sign of malignancy, can be seen in benign papilloma as well as papillary or ductal carcinomas and does not help in patients with nipple discharge, wherein most of the cases are due to intraductal papilloma [41].

MRI MG and US can be negative in up to half the patients with pathological nipple discharge [4]. MRI has a high negative predictive value and is useful in peripheral duct lesions, which are not easily picked up on ultrasound. It can also help in locating the lesions on second-look ultrasound for the lesions that were missed initially. It provides good visualization of the subareolar region, imaging of which is often difficult with MG and US. The imaging protocol includes noncontrast T2 fat saturated sequence/short Tau inversion

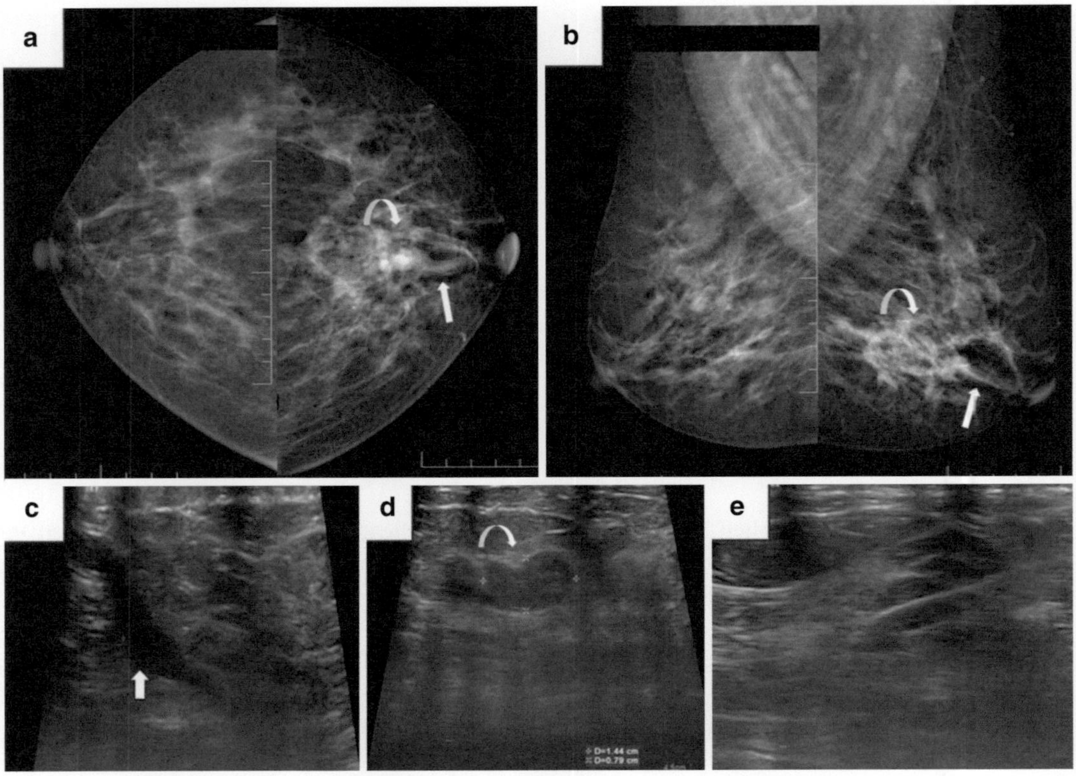

Fig. 11.7 Papillary neoplasm on mammography and ultrasound. Craniocaudal (**a**) and mediolateral oblique (**b**) mammogram views show dilated tortuous duct (straight white arrow) in the retroareolar region extending into the central left breast leading to an irregular mass (curved white arrow) in the central left breast with multiple adjacent smaller dilated tortuous ducts. Ultrasound of the left breast (**c**, **d**) showing single large dilated duct (straight white arrow) in the retroareolar region with a large intraductal mass lesion (curved white arrow) measuring 1.4 × 0.8 cm in size at about 5 o' clock position in the periareolar region. USG-guided core biopsy (**e**) from the mass revealed papillary lesion with sclerotic stroma and atypia on histopathological examination

recovery sequence, noncontrast T1-weighted sequence with and without fat saturation, up-to-five dynamic postcontrast T1-weighted sequences after injection of gadolinium contrast, and subtraction images. Proper positioning of the breast and nipples is necessary. The breasts should hang down freely, with nipples pointing downward. If the nipple appears to be pointing medially, the medial breast tissue should be pulled down and outward, away from the sternum. Common positioning-related artefacts to be aware of include [42] (1) poor superior or medial positioning that can lead to inhomogeneous signal intensities or poor fat suppression, (2) skin folds which can also cause inhomogeneity, and (3) compression of anterior breast tissue and nipple in large breasts, which can reduce the blood flow anteriorly and change the contrast dynamics of retro areolar lesions.

Normal nipple enhancement is bilaterally symmetrical, equal, or less than that of the background parenchymal enhancement. There are three layers of enhancement (Fig. 11.8): a superficial linear enhancement (SLE) from a vascular epidermis, which enhances more than the nearby skin, a nonenhancing zone (NEZ) made of connective tissue beneath the epidermis, and a deeper layer of patchy or linear internal nipple enhancement (INE) from ductal structures [43, 44]. Normal ducts are not seen on MRI unless dilated. Duct ectasia can be seen as T1 hyperintense signals filling the ducts due to proteinaceous contents or blood within. Subtraction sequences can be helpful in differentiating duct wall or intraductal enhancement from inspissated secretions [44].

One of the common imaging features picked up on MRI in patients with nipple discharge is nonmass enhancement, which is commonly focal or linear, followed by regional and segmental (Fig. 11.9) [45]. Mass lesions could be papilloma, invasive ductal, or lobular carcinoma, nipple adenoma, Paget's disease, or DCIS. Papilloma can be central or peripheral—central lesions occur in the major subareolar ducts, are solitary, and are more likely to cause nipple discharge, whereas peripheral lesions are seen in the TDLU, about 5 cm from the nipple, are multiple and bilateral, and show high risk for malignancy. Papilloma can be seen as well-circumscribed round or oval masses, with type 2 or 3 dynamic enhancement curves. Papillomatosis and papillary malignancies present as nonmass enhancement [44]. Periductal mastitis associated with duct ectasia can also present as nonmass enhancement or an enhancing mass, with additional findings of skin thickening, abnormal nipple orientation, enlarged blood vessels, and increase in breast size. They may also be associated with breast abscesses, which show peripheral rim of enhancement and surrounding T2 hyperintense edema [44].

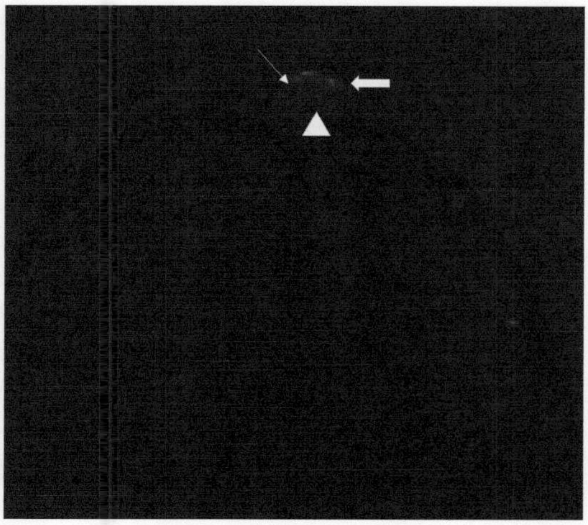

Fig. 11.8 Layers of normal nipple enhancement. Axial first postcontrast T1-weighted breast MR image shows a thin rim of smooth superficial linear enhancement, SLE (thick arrow) at the level of the skin, nonenhancing zone, NEZ (thin arrow) without enhancement seen immediately beneath the SLE; and internal nipple enhancement, INE (arrowhead) seen as an area of patchy enhancement below the NEZ and above the base of the nipple

DCIS is commonly seen as nonmass enhancement, less commonly as a mass or focus of enhancement with variable dynamic enhancement pattern. Clustered ring enhancement (Fig. 11.10) has high specificity for DCIS, seen in up to 63% cases. There may be false negatives on MRI in patients with DCIS, due to reduced angiogenesis within the lesion or due to low spatial resolution of MRI [44, 46]. On the other hand, invasive ductal carcinomas (IDC) or inva-

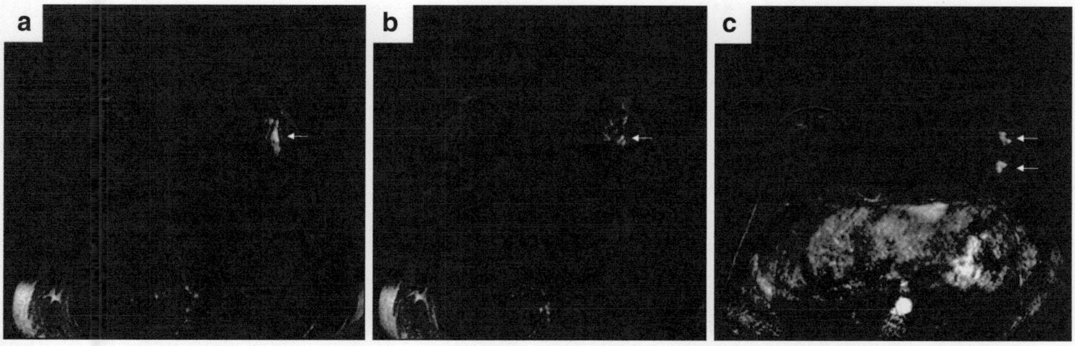

Fig. 11.9 MRI in nipple discharge. In a 30-year-old lady with spontaneous bloody nipple discharge from the left breast, with ultrasound showing dilated duct with no intraductal mass, MRI reveals hyperintense intraductal contents on precontrast T1 fat saturated images (**a**, **b**) likely hemorrhage. Postcontrast subtracted image (**c**) shows focal areas of clumped pattern of nonmass enhancement in the outer and lower quadrant of the left breast. Final diagnosis was multifocal invasive ductal carcinoma (IDC)

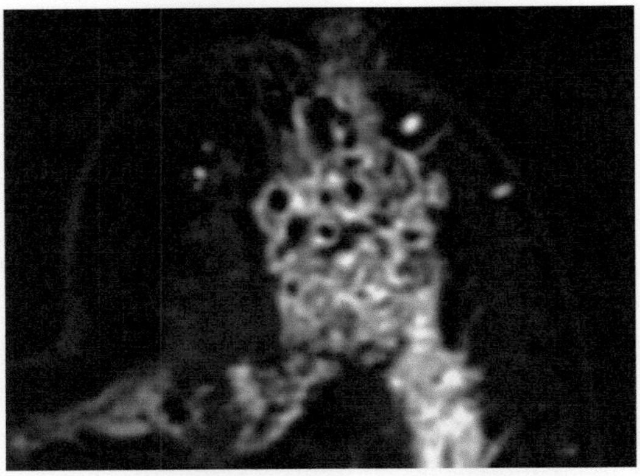

Fig. 11.10 Clustered ring enhancement in DCIS. Postcontrast subtracted MRI of a 53-year-old lady diagnosed with high-grade DCIS in the central left breast shows extensive clustered ring pattern of nonmass enhancement

sive lobular carcinomas (ILC) can be identified with high sensitivity on MRI. Both are commonly seen as irregular masses with spiculated margins, with type 2 or 3 dynamic enhancement curves. Less commonly, they can present as nonmass enhancement, particularly with multiple enhancing foci around a dominant lesion, and architectural distortion in ILC [44]. Local causes of pathological nipple discharge such as nipple adenoma or Paget's disease can also be seen well with MRI—the former showing nipple enlargement, with homogeneous or rim enhancement, rapid uptake, and washout, and the latter seen as asymmetric irregular thickening and enhancement of the nipple [44].

Alternative techniques like MR ductography employ the use of a heavily weighted T2 sequence, which can help to localize lesions within ducts. However, the presence of debris can reduce the T2 weighing of the fluid in the ducts, and the imaging plane should also be tangential to the long axis of the duct to get an adequate image [47]. Direct MRI galactography has also been explored, by injection of gadolinium into the ducts followed by a T1 sequence. But this is an invasive technique, causing patient discomfort just like in conventional galactography and is not usually recommended [48].

Ductography Conventional ductography or galactography was previously the gold standard investigation. It is an invasive test, done by cannulation of the discharging duct followed by injection of 0.5–1 ml of iodinated contrast. Standard craniocaudal and mediolateral oblique mammography views are obtained. At the end of the procedure, as much of the injected contrast as possible is aspirated and the rest is attempted to be expressed out manually. Having history of contrast allergy and nipple surgery, inverted nipples are contraindications [34]. Findings that can be picked up on ductography include duct ectasia, ducts communicating with cysts (fibrocystic changes), or intraductal filling defect (papilloma, carcinoma) or irregular contour/stricture. In papilloma, the duct downstream to the lesion (toward nipple) is dilated due to increased secretions from the lesion, while peripheral ducts are normal in caliber [49]. It can also be used for guiding preoperative wire localization. Very proximal obstructions can cause immediate reflux of contrast into the cannula, and if combines with rapid injection of contrast, this can lead to extravasation into the breast parenchyma or lymphatics. The presence of air bubbles can cause false-positive appearance of intraductal masses. On the other hand, a normal ductography does not exclude malignancy [50]. The use of DBT with galactography can increase the sensitivity of detection of intraductal lesions and shows higher diagnostic accuracy than conventional FFDM galactography [51]. However, due to the invasive nature of galactography causing patient discomfort and with increased availability of MRI, MRI has replaced galactography as the next step in MG and US-negative cases.

Nuclear medicine Techniques like Tc 99m Sestamibi imaging and FDG PEM use high-resolution cameras to detect small and in situ carcinomas [52]. The cancer detection rate of PEM is almost ten times greater than that of PET/CT in screening population; however, the sensitivity of detection of smaller malignancies is still higher with MRI, and there are no conclusive studies exploring the utility of PEM or breast-specific gamma imaging in evaluation of nipple discharge. [22, 53, 54]

11.7 Ductoscopy and Biopsy Techniques

Ductoscopy involves direct visualization of lesions through a microendoscope (0.9 mm diameter). Saline solution is injected into the working channel for ductal lavage. The microendoscope can reach up to 5–6 cm depth from the nipple. Smaller, peripheral ducts cannot be evaluated [55]. Though not always possible, ductoscopic extraction of intraductal lesions is one of its advantages, obviating the need for surgery [56]. MRI and ductoscopy have comparable sensitivity in evaluation of patients with nipple discharge, while both techniques are superior to ultrasound [57]. Invasive nature of the test, limited availability of equipment, and experienced personnel are hindrances for the routine use of this technique.

Once lesions are identified on imaging, histopathological diagnosis is needed for the confirmation of their benign or malignant nature. Image-guided biopsy can be done with the help of stereotactic mammography, ultrasound, or MRI. Core needle biopsy (CNB) is preferred over fine needle aspiration cytology (FNAC), to get better quantity of the samples. In particular, vacuum-assisted biopsy (VAB) can be useful in intraductal lesions, with therapeutic advantages of incidental removal of the whole lesion [22, 58]. This however cannot be completely relied on if lesions are high risk or DCIS and surgery is needed. Placement of a marker can be done in the same sitting after biopsy, to help in locating the lesion for subsequent surgery. An alternative to CNB in papillomas would be excisional biopsy, which can be done if there is a strong suspicion of malignancy on imaging [22].

11.8 Management and Surgical Perspectives

Surgery is now primarily reserved for women with suspicious or pathologic nipple discharge. This includes women with a single duct spontaneous or copious discharge, bloody or blood-stained nipple discharge, or any nipple discharge with an underlying clinical or imaging abnormality. The risk of malignancy in such cases is estimated to be between 5% and 23% [59, 60], both in situ and invasive carcinoma have been documented, and it is crucial that the affected duct is excised for confirmation.

Various techniques for surgical removal of pathologic mammary ducts have been described. Of these, the commonly employed techniques include microdochectomy and a total duct excision also known as Hadfield's surgery. The choice of procedure depends upon the extent of excision required, the location of the intraductal lesion, the patient's age, and her plan for lactation in future. Typically, microdochectomy is preferred in situations where there is a single isolated discharging duct. This procedure has the advantage of allowing a targeted excision of the desired duct while preserving the remaining normal ducts to retain the ability to breastfeed from that nipple and limit the loss of sensation. In contrast, a major duct excision is useful in scenarios of multiple duct involvement or intraductal papilloma affecting multiple ducts simultaneously.

Microdochectomy is a procedure which removes a single abnormal duct while preserving the surrounding normal ductal tissue. After surgical draping, the surgeon exerts circumferential pressure around the areola to trigger the discharge from the affected duct. A prior review of the imaging reports can be immensely useful localizing the affected duct during surgery. The duct is then cannulated with a lacrimal probe for a targeted excision. As an alternative, methylene blue dye can be injected into the ductal system, and the affected duct is identified by the blue-stained tissue [61]. A radial transareolar incision is taken traversing the nipple, and a careful dissection is done and the affected ductal system is removed along with any other underlying pathology. Surgeons who have access to a ductoscope can use the endoscope for direct visualization of the duct as a guide during microdochectomy.

A total duct excision or Hadfield's surgery can be performed through a circumareolar incision or a radial one. After the incision is made, all the ducts are encircled and tied off as they enter the nipple. Following that, the subareolar tissue is coned out for several centimeters to ensure removal of all ductal tissue. If any abnormality was documented in the imaging, the excision is extended to include this abnormality in the specimen. It is important to take care to avoid any cautery burn to the undersurface of the nipple to reduce the possibility of nipple necrosis. This extensive subareolar tissue resection may leave the patient with numbness, nipple retraction, and an inability to nurse on the affected side [62].

Papillary neoplasms deserve a special mention with respect to their management, as many of these lesions arise within or close to a duct and present with variable nipple discharge. These neoplasms comprise a broad spectrum of breast diseases ranging from a benign solitary intraductal papilloma to invasive papillary carcinoma. An accurate diagnosis depends on the morphology and architecture of the lesion along with myoepithelial markers [63], and in these cases, a routine core needle biopsy may prove to be insufficient for a diagnosis. Traditionally, these lesions were subjected to a diagnostic surgical biopsy along with an excision of the affected ductal system. A promising alternative in recent times is vacuum-assisted excision (VAE) [64, 65]. The Third International Consensus Conference on lesions of uncertain

malignant potential in the breast almost equally suggested open excision or therapeutic VAE.

following a CNB-based diagnosis of PL without atypia [66]. The European guidelines recommend that intraductal papilloma without concomitant ADH can be managed safely with VAE, and if fully excised, imaging surveillance is sufficient. In intraductal papilloma with concomitant ADH, surgical excision is recommended [67]. VAE is a minimally invasive technique which involves specialized probe under guidance of ultrasound or mammogram. The probe is positioned in the suspicious area and a vacuum draws the tissue into the probe which is then collected for further analysis. This process can be repeated several times until the entire lesion is removed, followed by insertion of a marker clip. VAE has the distinct advantage of avoiding a surgical procedure and gives an excellent cosmetic outcome.

11.9 Postop/Treatment Follow-Up and Surveillance

Treated patients may be followed up with an annual mammogram with/without ultrasound. The postoperative changes may be seen as focal areas of distortion in the central retroareolar regions with mild thickening of the areola. In patients undergoing VAE, the site of excision can be identified by the postprocedural marker clip. The signs of recurrence may be seen as a focal mass or new microcalcifications particularly in patients with final histology of ADH or DCIS.

11.10 Conclusion

Evaluation of nipple discharge starts with exclusion of physiological causes (Fig. 11.11). Mammography and ultrasonography are the initial investigations of choice, followed by MRI, which has replaced galactography. Image-guided biopsy is done for identifiable lesions, while surgical management such as central or single duct excision are done if no cause is identified. Although benign causes amount to nipple discharge most of the times, malignancies associated with nipple discharge are usually smaller or in situ carcinomas, which are associated with a good prognosis. Hence, vigilant imaging workup is essential and those with no identifiable cause can undergo a short-term follow-up.

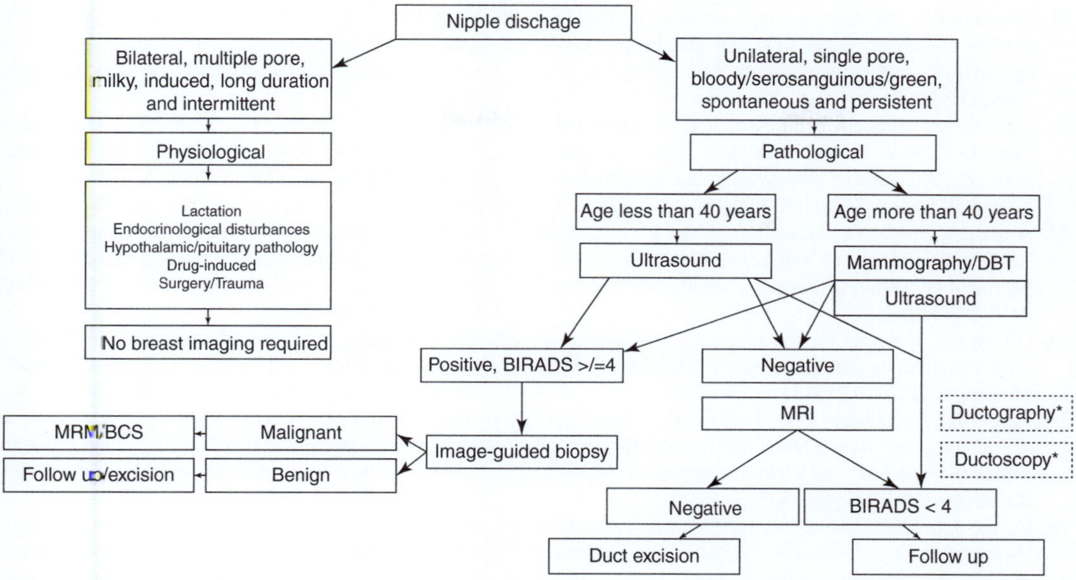

Fig. 11.11 Flow chart depicting an algorithmic approach to imaging in nipple discharge. *Not routinely used

References

1. Morrogh M, Park A, Elkin EB, King TA. Lessons learned from 416 cases of nipple discharge of the breast. Am J Surg. 2010;200:73–80.
2. Hussain AN, Policarpio C, Vincent MT. Evaluating nipple discharge. Obstet Gynecol Surv. 2006;61:278–83.
3. Expert Panel on Breast Imaging, Lee SJ, Trikha S, Moy L, Baron P, diFlorio RM, et al. ACR appropriateness criteria® evaluation of nipple discharge. J Am Coll Radiol JACR. 2017;14:S138–53.
4. Berger N, Luparia A, Di Leo G, Carbonaro LA, Trimboli RM, Ambrogi F, et al. Diagnostic performance of MRI versus galactography in women with pathologic nipple discharge: a systematic review and meta-analysis. AJR Am J Roentgenol. 2017;209:465–71.
5. Henrot P, Leroux A, Barlier C, Génin P. Breast microcalcifications: the lesions in anatomical pathology. Diagn Interv Imaging. 2014;95:141–52.
6. Zucca-Matthes G, Urban C, Vallejo A. Anatomy of the nipple and breast ducts. Gland Surg. 2016;5:32–6.
7. Buhimschi CS. Endocrinology of lactation. Obstet Gynecol Clin N Am. 2004;31:963–79, xii
8. Vashi R, Hooley R, Butler R, Geisel J, Philpotts L. Breast imaging of the pregnant and lactating patient: physiologic changes and common benign entities. AJR Am J Roentgenol. 2013;200:329–36.
9. Patel BK, Falcon S, Drukteinis J. Management of nipple discharge and the associated imaging findings. Am J Med. 2015;128:353–60.
10. Mazzarello S, Arnaout A. Nipple discharge. CMAJ Can Med Assoc J. 2015;187:599.
11. Zervoudis S, Iatrakis G, Economides P, Polyzos D, Navrozoglou I. Nipple discharge screening. Womens Health Lond Engl. 2010;6:135–51.
12. Rakha EA, Ellis IO. Diagnostic challenges in papillary lesions of the breast. Pathology (Phila). 2018;50:100–10.
13. Ferris-James DM, Iuanow E, Mehta TS, Shaheen RM, Slanetz PJ. Imaging approaches to diagnosis and management of common ductal abnormalities. Radiographics. 2012;32:1009–30.
14. Cho SH, Park SH. Mimickers of breast malignancy on breast sonography. J Ultrasound Med. 2013;32:2029–36.
15. Gupta D, Mendelson EB, Karst I. Nipple discharge: current clinical and imaging evaluation. Am J Roentgenol. 2021;216:330–9.
16. Morrogh M, King TA. The significance of nipple discharge of the male breast. Breast J. 2009;15:632–8.
17. Salzman B, Collins E, Hersh L. Common breast problems. Am Fam Physician. 2019;99:505–14.
18. Lippa N, Hurtevent-Labrot G, Ferron S, Boisserie-Lacroix M. Nipple discharge: the role of imaging. Diagn Interv Imaging. 2015;96:1017–32.
19. McDonald S, Saslow D, Alciati MH. Performance and reporting of clinical breast examination: a review of the literature. CA Cancer J Clin. 2004;54:345–61.
20. Das DK, Al-Ayadhy B, Ajrawi MT, Shaheen AA, Sheikh ZA, Malik M, et al. Cytodiagnosis of nipple discharge: a study of 602 samples from 484 cases. Diagn Cytopathol. 2001;25:25–37. Available from: https://pubmed.ncbi.nlm.nih.gov/11466810/.

21. Kooistra BW, Wauters C, van de Ven S, Strobbe L. The diagnostic value of nipple discharge cytology in 618 consecutive patients. Eur J Surg Oncol. 2009;35:573–7.
22. Sanford MF, Slanetz PJ, Lewin AA, Baskies AM, Bozzuto L, Branton SA, et al. ACR appropriateness criteria® evaluation of nipple discharge: 2022 update. J Am Coll Radiol. 2022;19:S304–18.
23. Ashfaq A, Senior D, Pockaj BA, Wasif N, Pizzitola VJ, Giurescu ME, et al. Validation study of a modern treatment algorithm for nipple discharge. Am J Surg. 2014;208:222–7.
24. D'Orsi CJ. Imaging for the diagnosis and management of ductal carcinoma in situ. J Natl Cancer Inst Monogr. 2010;2010:214–7.
25. Berg WA, Arnoldus CL, Teferra E, Bhargavan M. Biopsy of amorphous breast calcifications: pathologic outcome and yield at stereotactic biopsy. Radiology. 2001;221:495–503.
26. Grimm LJ, Miller MM, Thomas SM, Liu Y, Lo JY, Hwang ES, et al. Growth dynamics of mammographic calcifications: differentiating ductal carcinoma in situ from Benign breast disease. Radiology. 2019;292:77–83.
27. Lee SJ, Sobel LD, Shamis M, Mahoney MC. Asymmetric ductal ectasia: an often overlooked sign of malignancy. Am J Roentgenol. 2019;213:473–81.
28. Huynh PT, Parellada JA, de Paredes ES, Harvey J, Smith D, Holley L, et al. Dilated duct pattern at mammography. Radiology. 1997;204:137–41.
29. Dhamija E, Gulati M, Deo SV, Gogia A, Hari S. Digital breast tomosynthesis: an overview. Indian J Surg Oncol. 2021;12(2):315–29.
30. Xing D, Lv Y, Sun B, Xie H, Dong J, Hao C, et al. Diagnostic value of contrast-enhanced spectral mammography in comparison to magnetic resonance imaging in breast lesions. J Comput Assist Tomogr. 2019;43:245–51.
31. Łuczyńska E, Heinze-Paluchowska S, Hendrick E, Dyczek S, Ryś J, Herman K, et al. Comparison between breast MRI and contrast-enhanced spectral mammography. Med Sci Monit. 2015;21:1358–67.
32. Hegazy R, Adel L, Yasin R. The value of CESM in the evaluation of intraductal breast papilloma: a comparative study with DCE-MRI. Egypt J Radiol Nucl Med. 2020;51:27.
33. Yoon H, Yoon JH, Kim EK, Moon HJ, Park BW, Kim MJ. Adding ultrasound to the evaluation of patients with pathologic nipple discharge to diagnose additional breast cancers: preliminary data. Ultrasound Med Biol. 2015;41:2099–107.
34. Panzironi G, Pediconi F, Sardanelli F. Nipple discharge: the state of the art. BJR Open. 2018;1:20180016.
35. Mendelson EB, Böhm-Vélez M, Berg WA, Whitman G, Feldman M, Madjar H. ACR BI-RADS® ultrasound. In: ACR BI-RADS® atlas breast imaging report data system. Reston: American College of Radiology; 2013. p. 149.
36. Yoon JH, Yoon H, Kim EK, Moon HJ, Park YV, Kim MJ. Ultrasonographic evaluation of women with pathologic nipple discharge. Ultrasonography. 2017;36:310–20.
37. Ganesan S, Karthik G, Joshi M, Damodaran V. Ultrasound spectrum in intraductal papillary neoplasms of breast. Br J Radiol. 2006;79:843–9.
38. Rissanen T, Reinikainen H, Apaja-Sarkkinen M. Breast sonography in localizing the cause of nipple discharge: comparison with galactography in 52 patients. J Ultrasound Med Off J Am Inst Ultrasound Med. 2007;26:1031–9.
39. Soo MS, Baker JA, Rosen EL. Sonographic detection and sonographically guided biopsy of breast microcalcifications. AJR Am J Roentgenol. 2003;180:941–8.
40. Guo X, Liu Y, Li W. Diagnostic accuracy of shear wave elastography for prediction of breast malignancy in patients with pathological nipple discharge. BMJ Open. 2016;6:e008848.
41. Wang B, Yang D, Zhang X, Gong X, Xu T, Han J, et al. The diagnostic value of contrast-enhanced ultrasonography in breast ductal abnormalities. Cancer Imaging. 2023;23:25.
42. Yeh ED, Georgian-Smith D, Raza S, Bussolari L, Pawlisz-Hoff J, Birdwell RL. Positioning in breast MR imaging to optimize image quality. Radiographics. 2014;34:E1–17.
43. Gao Y, Brachtel EF, Hernandez O, Heller SL. An analysis of nipple enhancement at breast MRI with radiologic-pathologic correlation. Radiographics. 2019;39:10–27.
44. Samreen N, Madsen LB, Chacko C, Heller SL. Magnetic resonance imaging in the evaluation of pathologic nipple discharge: indications and imaging findings. Br J Radiol. 2021;94:20201013.
45. Tokuda Y, Kuriyama K, Nakamoto A, Choi S, Yutani K, Kunitomi Y, et al. Evaluation of suspicious nipple discharge by magnetic resonance mammography based on breast imaging reporting and data system magnetic resonance imaging descriptors. J Comput Assist Tomogr. 2009;33:58–62.
46. Greenwood HI, Heller SL, Kim S, Sigmund EE, Shaylor SD, Moy L. Ductal carcinoma in situ of the breasts: review of MR imaging features. Radiogr Rev Publ Radiol Soc N Am Inc. 2013;33:1569–88.
47. Hirose M, Otsuki N, Hayano D, Shinjo H, Gokan T, Kashiwase T, et al. Multi-volume fusion imaging of MR ductography and MR mammography for patients with nipple discharge. Magn Reson Med Sci MRMS Off J Jpn Soc Magn Reson Med. 2006;5:105–12.
48. Wenkel E, Janka R, Uder M, Doellinger M, Melzer K, Schulz-Wendtland R, et al. Does direct MR galactography have the potential to become an alternative diagnostic tool in patients with pathological nipple discharge? Clin Imaging. 2011;35:85–93.
49. Slawson SH, Johnson BA. Ductography: how to and what if? Radiographics. 2001;21:133–50.
50. Sheiman LS, Levesque PH. The In's and Out's of ductography: a comprehensive review. Curr Probl Diagn Radiol. 2016;45:61–70.

51. Moschetta M, De Ruvo V, Drago A, Troiano N, Paolicelli S, Rubini G, et al. DBT-galactography: a promising tool for improving the diagnostic workup of nipple discharge. Eur Radiol Exp. 2020;4:40.
52. Brem RF, Fishman M, Rapelyea JA. Detection of ductal carcinoma in situ with mammography, breast specific gamma imaging, and magnetic resonance imaging: a comparative study. Acad Radiol. 2007;14:945–50.
53. Yanai A, Itoh M, Hirakawa H, Yanai K, Tashiro M, Harada R, et al. Newly-developed positron emission mammography (PEM) device for the detection of small breast cancer. Tohoku J Exp Med. 2018;245:13–9.
54. Berg WA, Madsen KS, Schilling K, Tartar M, Pisano ED, Larsen LH, et al. Breast cancer: comparative effectiveness of positron emission mammography and MR imaging in presurgical planning for the ipsilateral breast. Radiology. 2011;258:59–72.
55. Fisher CS, Margenthaler JA. A look into the ductoscope: its role in pathologic nipple discharge. Ann Surg Oncol. 2011;18:3187–91.
56. Waaijer L, van Diest PJ, Verkooijen HM, Dijkstra NE, van der Pol CC, Borel Rinkes IHM, et al. Interventional ductoscopy in patients with pathological nipple discharge. Br J Surg. 2015;102:1639–48.
57. Yılmaz R, Bender Ö, Çelik Yabul F, Dursun M, Tunacı M, Acunas G. Diagnosis of nipple discharge: value of magnetic resonance imaging and ultrasonography in comparison with ductoscopy. Balk Med J. 2017;34:119–26.
58. Dennis MA, Parker S, Kaske TI, Stavros AT, Camp J. Incidental treatment of nipple discharge caused by Benign intraductal papilloma through diagnostic mammotome biopsy. Am J Roentgenol. 2000;174:1263–8.
59. Sabel MS, Helvie MA, Breslin T, Curry A, Diehl KM, Cimmino VM, et al. Is duct excision still necessary for all cases of suspicious nipple discharge? Breast J. 2012;18:157–62.
60. Chen L, Zhou WB, Zhao Y, Liu XA, Ding Q, Zha XM, et al. Bloody nipple discharge is a predictor of breast cancer risk: a meta-analysis. Breast Cancer Res Treat. 2012;132:9–14.
61. Tan WT, Lim TC. Transareolar dye-injection microdochectomy. Am Surg. 1992;58:404–8.
62. Srivastava A, Griwan MS, Samaiyar SS, Sharma LK. A safe technique of major mammary duct excision. J R Coll Surg Edinb. 1995;40:35–7.
63. Wang Y, Song EC. Papillary neoplasm of the breast–a review and update. Hum Pathol Rep. 2021;26:300581.
64. Bicchierai G, Pugliese F, Amato F, De Benedetto D, Boeri C, Vanzi E, et al. Percutaneous vacuum-assisted excision (VAE) of breast lesions of uncertain malignant potential (B3 lesions): a preliminary single-centre Italian experience. Radiol Med (Torino). 2023;128:528–36.
65. Watson JF, Radic R, Frost R, Paton S, Kessell MA, Dessauvagie BF, et al. Vacuum-assisted excision biopsy for definitive diagnosis of breast lesions of uncertain malignant potential (B3 lesions) on core biopsy – a single centre Western Australian experience. J Med Imaging Radiat Oncol. 2023;67:365–76.
66. Elfgen C, Leo C, Kubik-Huch RA, Muenst S, Schmidt N, Quinn C, et al. Third International Consensus Conference on lesions of uncertain malignant potential in the breast (B3 lesions). Virchows Arch. 2023;483:5–20.
67. Rubio IT, Wyld L, Marotti L, Athanasiou A, Regitnig P, Catanuto G, et al. European guidelines for the diagnosis, treatment and follow-up of breast lesions with uncertain malignant potential (B3 lesions) developed jointly by EUSOMA, EUSOBI, ESP (BWG) and ESSO. Eur J Surg Oncol J Eur Soc Surg Oncol Br Assoc Surg Oncol. 2024;50:107292.

12 Mastitis

Janaki P. Dharmarajan, D. K. Vijayakumar, and Jyotsna Yesodharan

Abstract

Mastitis means inflammation of the breast that affects both lactating and nonlactating women across a wide age group ranging from 15 to 67 years. The inflammation may or may not be associated with infection. Lactational mastitis is the most common form accounting for about 10–30% of breastfeeding women and is invariably bacterial in origin. Most common forms of nonlactational mastitis are periductal mastitis and granulomatous mastitis. Periductal mastitis can be attributed to duct obstruction due to squamous metaplasia leading to recurrent infection and is more common in smokers. Granulomatous mastitis has a strong association with previous pregnancy and other conditions causing prolactin elevation. The treatment varies from watchful expectancy to oral medications like antibiotics, steroids, and immune modulators in resistant cases. Response has been observed by a combination of conservative approach and oral medication in 90% of the women within two years of symptom onset. The resistant ones consisting of less than 10% of cases might need intervention in the form of incision and drainage of the abscess or guided aspiration with injection of steroids in the abscess cavity.

Keywords

Mastitis · Infectious mastitis · Granulomatous mastitis · Tubercular mastitis

12.1 Introduction

Mastitis is an inflammation of the breast tissue that may or may not be accompanied by infection. Mastitis occurring most commonly during lactation is always accompanied by microbial infection and may resolve with antibiotics. Clinical presentation is usually with pain, redness, and swelling. Fever may be present. However, not all lactational mastitis cases respond to antibiotics. The other spectrum of chronic inflammatory diseases of the nonlactating breasts cause considerable difficulty in diagnosis and treatment. In cases of nonlactational mastitis, inflammation usually starts in the ducts. Etiological factors range from infection to autoimmune disorders. The disease causes consider-

J. P. Dharmarajan (✉)
Lisie Advanced Breast Imaging Centre, LIRRIS, Lisie Hospital, Ernakulam, Kerala, India

D. K. Vijayakumar
Department of Breast and Gynac Oncology, Amrita Institute of Medical Sciences, Kochi, Kerala, India

J. Yesodharan
Department of Pathology, Amrita Institute of Medical Sciences, Kochi, Kerala, India

E. Dhamija, S. V. S. Deo (eds.), *Imaging in Management of Breast Diseases*,
https://doi.org/10.1007/978-981-96-4998-3_12

able morbidity and psychological distress in relatively young females.

The common queries that a clinician faces while evaluating a patient with mastitis is how to decide on the etiology, any specific biomarkers that could indicate autoimmune etiology, when to change treatment and long-term follow-up of established mastitis. It is essential for the radiologists to know the clinical features and imaging appearance of varying stages of mastitis so that the patient can be directed to appropriate management. Once diagnosis is suspected, following a certain algorithm helps in early medical management of mastitis by obtaining optimal image-guided tissue biopsy for histopathological and microbial assessment, thereby avoiding indolent disease progression and inevitable breast tissue scarring. A thorough clinical history helps in approaching the differential diagnosis and timely identification of underlying malignancy.

12.2 Classification of Mastitis

There are several classifications of mastitis available in literature. Mastitis is most commonly classified based on its etiology as lactational (puerperal) or nonlactational (nonpuerperal). Based on the pathogenesis, mastitis is further classified as infectious or noninfectious. The presentation of mastitis can be either acute or chronic. The inflammatory process based on histopathology is seen either within the ducts or surrounding the ducts, that is, periductal in location. Based on serological tests, further immunological classification shows mastitis to be either autoimmune or nonautoimmune. From a clinical point of view, it is better to classify mastitis as either lactational or nonlactational.

Kamal et al. in 2009 classified mastitis into three groups: infectious, noninfectious, and malignant [1]. The classification was fairly comprehensive with subdivisions of each component:

- Infectious mastitis was further classified into simple mastitis (lactational and nonlactational), complicated mastitis (complications like abscess, draining sinus tracts, infected cysts, infected galactocele, and infected postinterventional collections), and specific mastitis (tubercular, fungal).
- Noninfectious mastitis was further classified into periductal mastitis/duct ectasia, plasma cell mastitis, granulomatous mastitis, diabetic mastopathy, postirradiation mastitis, and secondary mastitis (secondary to vascular diseases, collagen disorders, traumatic fat necrosis and foreign bodies).
- Malignant mastitis was subdivided into inflammatory carcinoma and malignant abscess.

12.3 Etiopathogenesis of Mastitis

Mastitis defined as inflammation of the breast can affect patients of any age group and may or may not be associated with infection. While infectious mastitis and breast abscesses are predominantly caused by bacteria that colonize the skin, causes of noninfectious mastitis range from the commoner duct ectasia/periductal mastitis to less frequent conditions including idiopathic granulomatous mastitis, diabetic mastopathy, vasculitis, and postirradiation/augmentation procedure-related mastitis [2]. The term malignant mastitis should be used in the context of inflammatory breast carcinoma or the rare but well-described presentation of malignancy as breast abscess [1]. Biopsy is not indicated in all cases of mastitis. It is resorted to in situations like unusual presentation, uncertainty of diagnosis, recurrent infections, or failure to respond to treatment. Fine-needle aspiration or tissue biopsies provide material for pathological and microbiological evaluation to look for evidence of infections and inflammation including granulomas and malignancy [3]. Discharges from nipple or draining sinuses could also be subjected to cytopathological examination. Though mastitis is most common among women in childbearing age group, all inflammations cannot be attributed to infectious cause. Mastitis is also seen in pediatric age group and in adult males, and its recognition is essential for prompt treatment. Mastitis classified broadly as infectious and noninfectious groups have distinctive clinical presentation, etiopathogenesis, imaging features, and clinical management which has been discussed in detail in the following sections.

12.4 Infectious Mastitis

Infectious mastitis is an acute inflammation of the breasts from which causative organism can be isolated. This is found more commonly in puerperal status (up to 33%) and less commonly in nonpuerperal status (less than 10%) [1]. It can be further subdivided into simple mastitis, complicated mastitis, and specific mastitis.

12.4.1 Simple Mastitis-Lactational Mastitis

Also known as puerperal mastitis, it is less common during pregnancy and occurs anytime during lactation. It is most common within initial six weeks and subsides within three months postpartum having a peak incidence within first three weeks of delivery. The incidence of lactational mastitis in breastfeeding women worldwide is 2–30% and occurs secondary to problems in breastfeeding resulting from prolonged engorgement or obstruction of drainage [3, 4].

Clinical Presentation: In a lactating lady with recent history of childbirth who presents with symptoms of focal pain, redness, malaise, and fever, clinical diagnosis of acute mastitis can be made. Subacute mastitis has subtle symptoms like sharp needling pain with burning sensation. This leads to a lower rate of diagnosis attributed to clinical misdiagnosis or lack of symptom understanding by the woman. There may be associated history of mastitis in prior pregnancy, nipple fissures or cracks, inadequate milk drainage, ill-fitted nursing bra, maternal stress, and topical antifungal creams [5].

Etiopathogenesis: Human milk was traditionally considered to be sterile and any contamination occurs from the mother's skin or infant's mouth. The process of bacterial transition from commensal to infective is still unclear. The most common bacteria isolated from cultures include *Staphylococcus aureus* (MRSA) in acute mastitis and *S. epidermidis* in subacute mastitis. However, they can be polymicrobial and aerobes like *Streptococcus* and *Enterobacteriaceae*, and anaerobes including *Peptostreptococcus* and *Propionibacterium* may be isolated [5].

Role of Imaging in Diagnosis and Management: Most forms of acute mastitis resolve on their own with symptomatic relief like hot fomentation and antibiotics. If the symptoms persist despite antibiotics, referral to specialist center is suggested where ultrasound can be performed to confirm collection before further intervention [1, 3].

Preventive measures include predelivery counseling and examination of nipple abnormalities by pediatricians and lactation experts with education on correct technique of latching [6].

Bacteria in breast milk can grow and proliferate if there is incomplete emptying, so constant emptying with avoidance of stasis is encouraged. In view of predominance of staphylococcus, appropriate antibiotics can be started without waiting for the microbial culture reports. They have to be given for duration of 7–14 days. In the event of recurrent episodes, material for microbiological cultures should be submitted from mother and the baby to determine their staphylococcal carrier status.

Biopsy is not routinely done in acute mastitis as it is often effectively managed nonsurgically. Unattended or incompletely treated mastitis can lead to breast abscess formation. Traditional treatment option was open surgical incision and drainage [3]. This is performed when the abscess at presentation has a size of maximum diameter of 5 cm size or other minimally invasive interventions fail. Incision is taken over the point of maximum fluctuation, pus drained, and loculi broken and wound is packed with gauze. The disadvantages include general anesthesia with interruption of breastfeeding, scarring to the breast, longer hospitalization, and increased financial implications. The recurrence rate of lactational mastitis in subsequent pregnancy is 8–30% [7].

When the abscess is less than 3 cm in maximum diameter at presentation, needle aspiration is the method of choice. Under local anesthesia with a 20 ml syringe attached to a 14–18 G needle, the pus is aspirated as completely as possible. The procedure can be repeated daily or every alternate day subject to a maximum of five times. Studies have shown 86–90% of women have symptomatic relief within a mean of 8.6 days (range 5–12 days) as against 10 days (range 6–15 days) with I&D. Ultrasound-guided vacuum-assisted biopsy can also be tried for the abscess with locules which has shown results similar as needle aspiration [8] (Fig. 12.1).

Infection can also occur within the sebaceous cysts in nipple areolar complex like *Montgomery tubercles*. They can present as an abscess that on ultrasound seems to arise within the skin in subcutaneous tissue plane. Majority of these infections resolve with oral antibiotics with surgical drainage reserved for nonresponsive cases [9] (Fig. 12.2).

Simple Mastitis—Nonlactational Infectious Mastitis (NLIM): Infectious mastitis in nonlactating women is rare but is significant as it is difficult to diagnose and the delay causes significant morbidity.

Clinical Presentation: This is commonly seen in female patients of reproductive age group though it has been reported in males of any age.

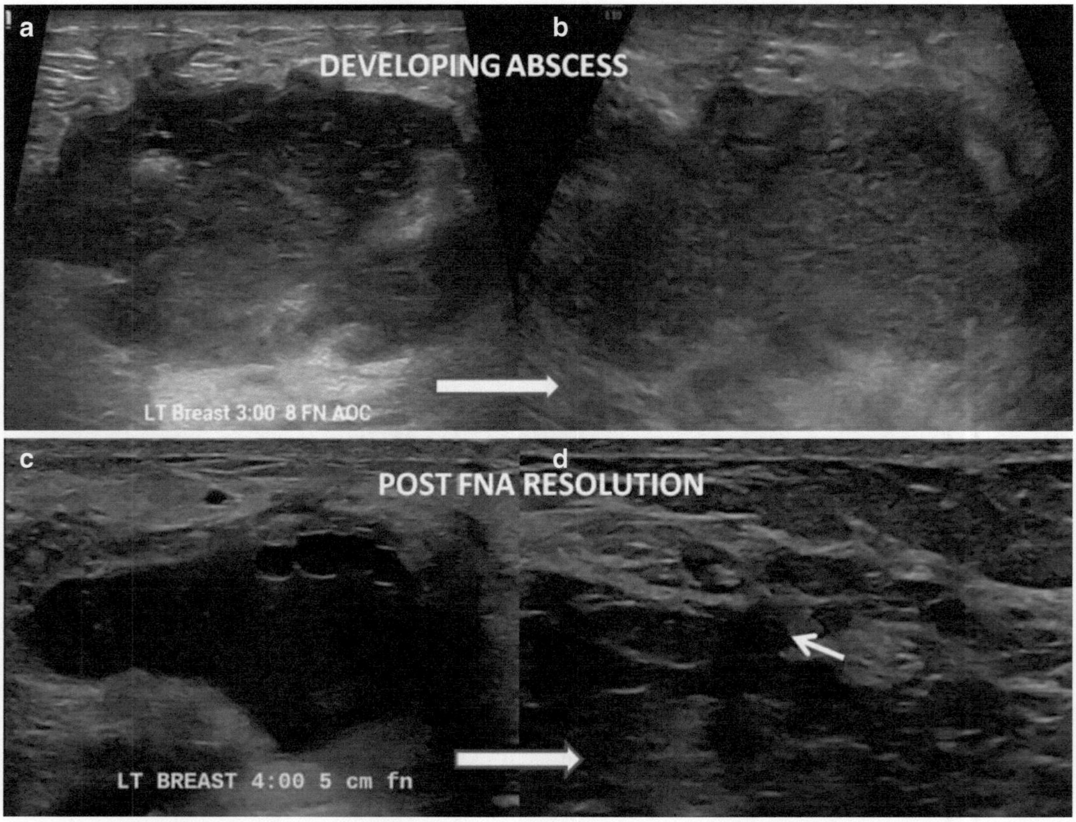

Fig. 12.1 A 28-year-old female, delivered 1 month ago with left breast acute-onset tender lump and fever. (**a**) US showed evolving collection of 50 cc. Treated with antibiotics; (**b**) follow-up after two weeks of antibiotics showed palpable organized abscess of 44 cc. Guided near complete aspiration with 18 G. Culture grew Staphylococcus aureus. (**c**) Follow-up after a month of FNA showed a hypoechoic collection of 13 ml with fat globules in nondependent part. (**d**) Five months after initial aspiration showed residual scar

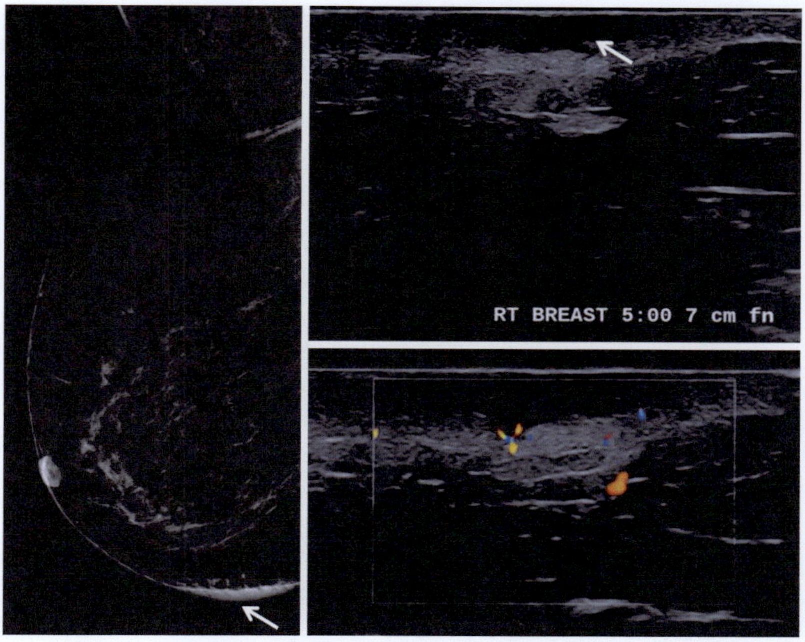

Fig. 12.2 A 52-year-old female with recent onset tender nodule in right breast lower inner quadrant. Diagnosis is infected sebaceous cyst that responded to oral antibiotics. MLO view (arrow) shows focal skin thickening. US shows a dermal-based hypoechoic collection with irregular margins (arrow). Marginal vascularity is seen

Varying clinical presentations and variable time for definitive diagnosis are noted in different parts of the world. In North American and European population, it usually presents with local inflammatory symptoms or a unilateral mass. Abscess is the most common presentation in Latin American countries. In a study from India, periductal mastitis was noted in elderly women with associated ductal dilatation. They presented with lump in periareolar region. There can be associated nipple abnormalities like congenital retraction or exposure to chronic smoking [10, 11].

Etiopathogenesis: The most commonly isolated organism belonged to *Staphylococcus* genus. However it was polymicrobial in about 30% of cases consisting of other types of bacteria like *Enterobacteriaceae*, *Peptostreptococcus*, *Propionibacterium*, *Bacteroides*, and occasionally *Klebsiella* and *Pseudomonas* [10].

Role of Imaging: Mammography may be normal or show focal asymmetry. Tubular tortuous structures can be seen in retroareolar region on tomosynthesis. Ultrasound features include a dilated duct with ill-defined hypoechoic area near the periareolar region. MRI breast has limited role in initial stages. Documentation of initial collection volume is essential for follow-up assessment when conservative approach is planned [11].

Management: The length of treatment is dictated by the underlying cause. It can be a combination of incision and drainage with antibiotics or long-term antibiotics alone with a close response monitoring [10]. Follow-up in conservative cases is done by clinical and ultrasound response assessment till complete clinical resolution. A bimonthly clinical follow-up is recommended for at least six months if symptoms remain stable or regress [11] (Fig. 12.3).

Complicated mastitis includes breast abscess, draining sinus tracts, infection of preexisting cysts, galactoceles, and postinterventional collection.

Clinical Presentation: The common presentation is a palpable tender painful mass with associated axillary lymphadenopathy in 25% of patients. There is abscess formation with breakdown that usually occurs as a complication of

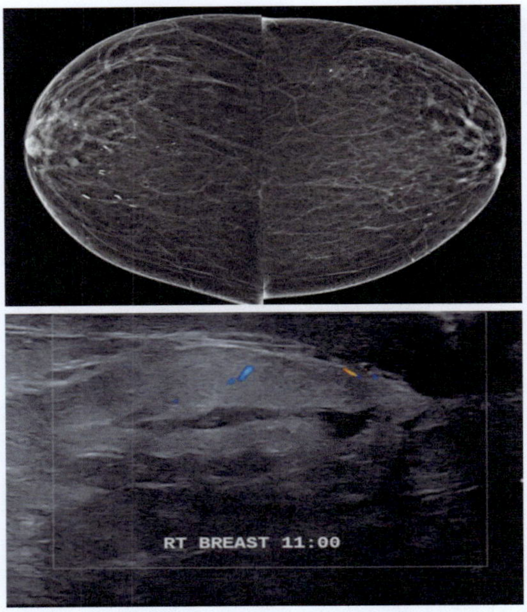

Fig. 12.3 A 61-year-old female with right breast tender mass in upper outer quadrant periareolar region. She had a single episode of yellowish nipple discharge on expression. There is history of type 1 diabetes mellitus of an eight-year duration. Treated with antibiotics. Partial resolution was documented at one month. Mammography shows focal asymmetry in right breast outer quadrant. Ultrasound shows a prominent duct with surrounding echogenic subcutaneous tissue with vascularity

untreated or delay in treatment of acute mastitis. Superadded infection of preexisting collection like a cyst, galactocele, or postoperative seroma can also lead to complicated mastitis.

Etiopathogenesis: Even though staphylococci and streptococci are the most common organism, rarer bacteria like *Nocardia*, *Pseudomonas*, and fungi can also be isolated.

Imaging Features: Mammography has limited role when complicated abscess is suspected. Adequate compression cannot be given in extremely tender breasts which are already dense due to inflammatory process. In addition to skin thickening and focal asymmetry on MG (if performed), abscess formation may appear as irregular mass or architectural distortion [12]. Ultrasound shows multiple round or oval collections with homogenous internal echoes and posterior enhancement. There is increased vascularity and surrounding echogenic subcutaneous tissue suggestive of edematous changes. Secondary infected cyst and infected galactocele appear as thick-walled cavities on ultrasound containing low levels and fluid levels [1, 12] (Fig. 12.4).

Management: Majority of the complicated abscesses initially respond to oral antibiotics. However incision and drainage may be required in nonresponding cases. Some surgeons prefer to remove adjacent ducts while draining abscess to prevent the possibility of fistula formation [1, 9].

12.4.2 Specific Mastitis

Whenever breast abscess culture yields growth of atypical organisms like *Mycobacterium* (tuberculosis, nontuberculous mycobacteria (NTM), and *Corynebacterium* spp.), fungal (*Histoplasma*, *Cryptococcus*, *Aspergillus*), hydatid, or parasites like *Wuchereria bancrofti* causing filariasis, it is termed as specific mastitis [1]. Indolent nature of the abscess formation, lack of acute symptoms, absence of specific imaging features, and lack of awareness of the condition among the physicians leads to misdiagnosis or delayed diagnosis of specific mastitis. On microscopic examination, inflamed and eventually fibrotic breast parenchyma is noted surrounding a central cavity with secretion and neutrophils along with obliteration of the lobular architecture. These may be complicated by the development of fistulous tracts resulting in discharging skin sinuses [13].

Tuberculous Mastitis (TM): The rare condition can involve both lactating and nonlactating females and is common in endemic areas as well as in patients originating from these areas. In primary TM where the breast is the only source of infection, introduction of bacilli can occur from direct inoculation into lactiferous duct from the mouth of a suckling infant harboring TB in faucial tonsils. In secondary TM, the spread from

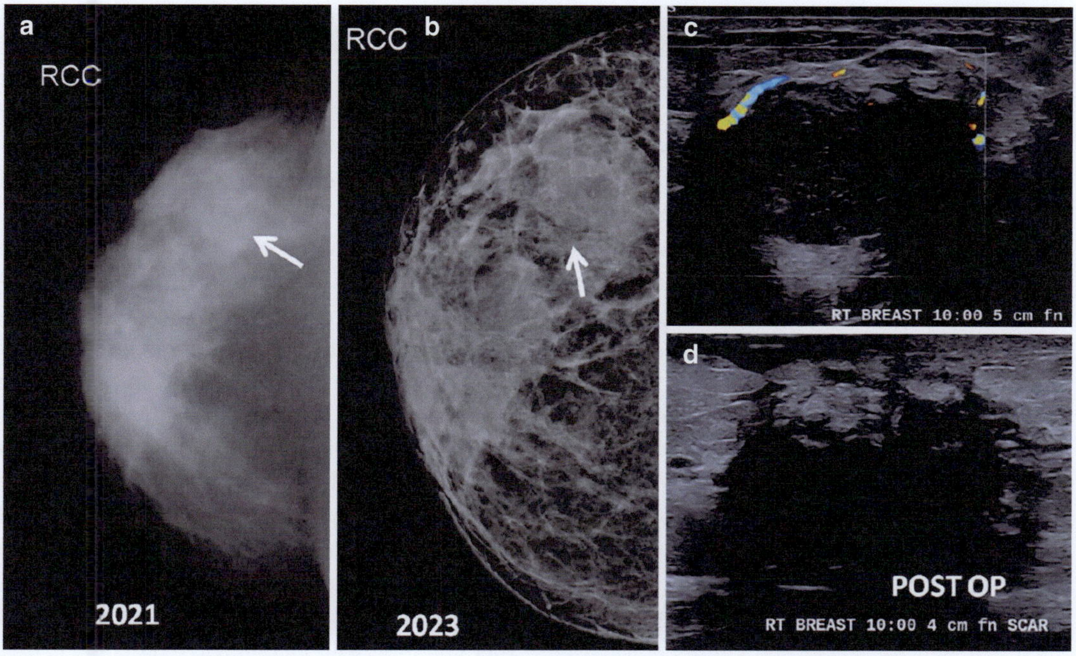

Fig. 12.4 A 49-year-old female with history of multiple bilateral simple cysts now presents with recent onset tender right breast lump of two-week duration: (**a**) MG right CC view in 2021 showed mass in outer quadrant, (**b**) MG in 2023 showed progression of the mass, and (**c**) US showed multiple simple cysts. Palpable concern at 10 o'clock position about 5 cm from nipple showed a deeply located irregular thick-walled collection with marginal vascularity. US aspiration with 18 G needle yielded 4 ml of brownish pus that grew Klebsiella pneumonia sensitive to most antibiotics. Progression of symptoms noted while on oral antibiotics leading to incision and drainage. (**d**) Postoperative changes with no residual collection

infection can occur from other site in body or directly from underlying chest wall involvement. It has been rarely reported in men too constituting about 3% of the reported cases [14].

Clinical Presentation: The most common presentation is a unifocal or multifocal palpable mass with or without sinus tract formation. Skin changes include thickening, discoloration, or ulcer. Nipple discharge with retraction is also noted. Axillary lymphadenopathy is seen in almost a quarter of the patients. There can be mastalgia and accompanying constitutional symptoms like fever, night sweat, and weight loss. The most common site of involvement is right breast upper outer quadrant followed by left retroareolar region [14].

Etiopathogenesis: Abscess can be positive for acid fast bacilli (AFB). Histologically, finding of a granulomatous lesion with Langhans' giant cells is indicative of tuberculosis even when AFB cannot be demonstrated. ESR is usually elevated in all patients.

Imaging Features: Mammography findings are usually abnormal and depend on early or late clinical presentation. The masses when present can be single or multiple; asymmetry is either global or focal. There can be associated findings like skin thickening, nipple retraction, and axillary lymphadenopathy. Ultrasound of palpable masses have solid, cystic, or complex solid cystic appearance. Inflammatory changes like subcutaneous tissue edema, subareolar duct dilatation, and skin thickening can be present alone or with associated features. Axillary lymphadenopathy with abnormal features is also noted. The nodular type presenting as masses can mimic benign fibroepithelial masses in initial stages. In later stages, healing with cicatrization sets in and is indistinguishable from breast carcinoma. Diffuse involvement is seen in patients with low immunity or virulent organisms, and multiple pockets of abscess with edematous changes are frequent. Cross-sectional imaging like the CT chest and MRI breast are useful to determine the extent of involvement and extramammary spread like pulmonary or rib involvement [14] (Fig. 12.5).

Management: History of pulmonary tuberculosis was found in only about 28% of the patients in one study. In case of abscess formation, it is aspirated and sent for smear and culture sensitivity. Core biopsy should be performed for diffuse breast involvement or when single or multiple masses are present. Biopsy is preferred from the periphery of the mass when tissue sample has to be sent for rapid tuberculous PCR tests.

Treatment is similar to that for pulmonary tuberculosis. However, demonstration of TM does not exclude the possibility of concomitant malignancy, and thorough clinical and imaging follow-up is warranted [14].

Nontuberculous mycobacteria mastitis: NTM can cause acute, subacute, or chronic mastitis. The main causative organisms include *Mycobacterium fortuitum*, *M. avium*, *M. abscessus*, and less commonly *M. chelonae*. It is difficult to differentiate clinically from other forms of mastitis; however, bilateral involvement is more common. There is also association with prior breast interventions or infections. Antimicrobials should be started empirically while waiting for culture sensitivity. Once growth is obtained and confirmed, further treatment and duration will be based on antibiotic sensitivity. Long-term targeted antibiotics are essential as recurrence is very common with incomplete treatment [15].

Cystic Neutrophilic Granulomatous Mastitis (CNGM): CNGN is a rare subtype characterized by the presence of suppurative lipogranulomas caused by *Corynebacterium* species. It is

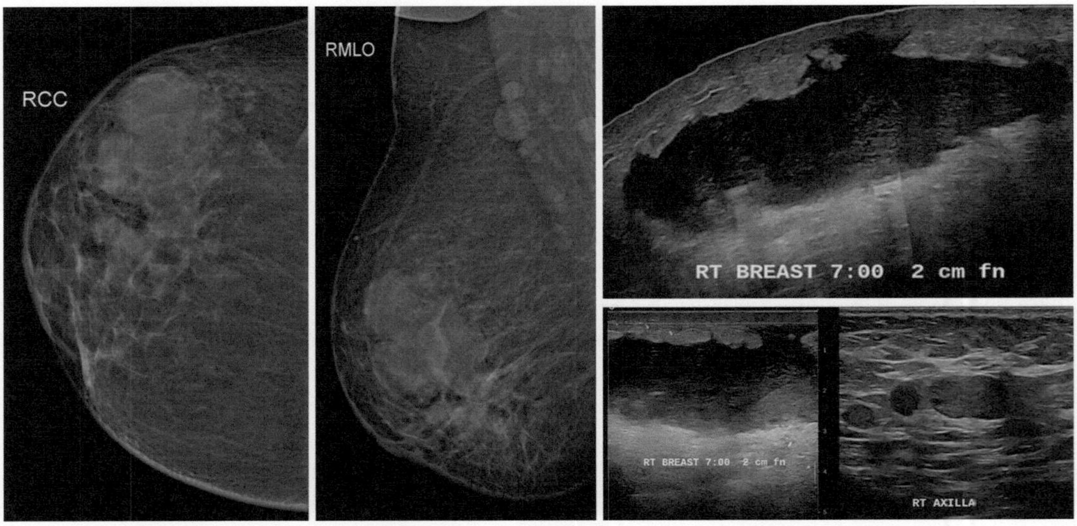

Fig. 12.5 A 49-year-old female with history of right breast recurrent abscess in different quadrant with sinus formation. Right mammography showed postoperative changes in medal quadrant. In lateral quadrant, there is a newly appeared equal density mass with lobulated margins. Overlying skin thickening noted. Multiple round dense axillary lymph nodes are also seen. In lower outer quadrant, there is a large collection with tracking pattern into the hypodermis on US. Surrounding vascularity noted. Multiple round hypoechoic lymph nodes are seen at axillary level I. FNAC of the lymph node showed reactive changes. Biopsy from the abscess wall showed granuloma. Pus aspirate grew AFB, though smear was negative. AKT started

common among women of reproductive age group. Clinically it is indistinguishable from other forms of infectious mastitis and breast neoplasm.

Clinical Features: The most common presentation is breast mass, nipple inversion, and sinus formation. It can be associated with pain, erythema, nipple discharge, and abscess formation.

Etiopathogenesis: Histological features of lipogranulomas consist of central lipid cells surrounded by rim of neutrophils that are surrounded by epithelioid histiocytes. There may be gram-positive bacillus (GPB) in the central lipid vacuole. These features should prompt for further microbiological tests to identify corynebacteria (Fig. 12.6).

Imaging Features: Mammography features include mass and asymmetry. Ultrasound features include mass, dilated ducts, subcutaneous tissue edema, fluid collection, and abscess formation.

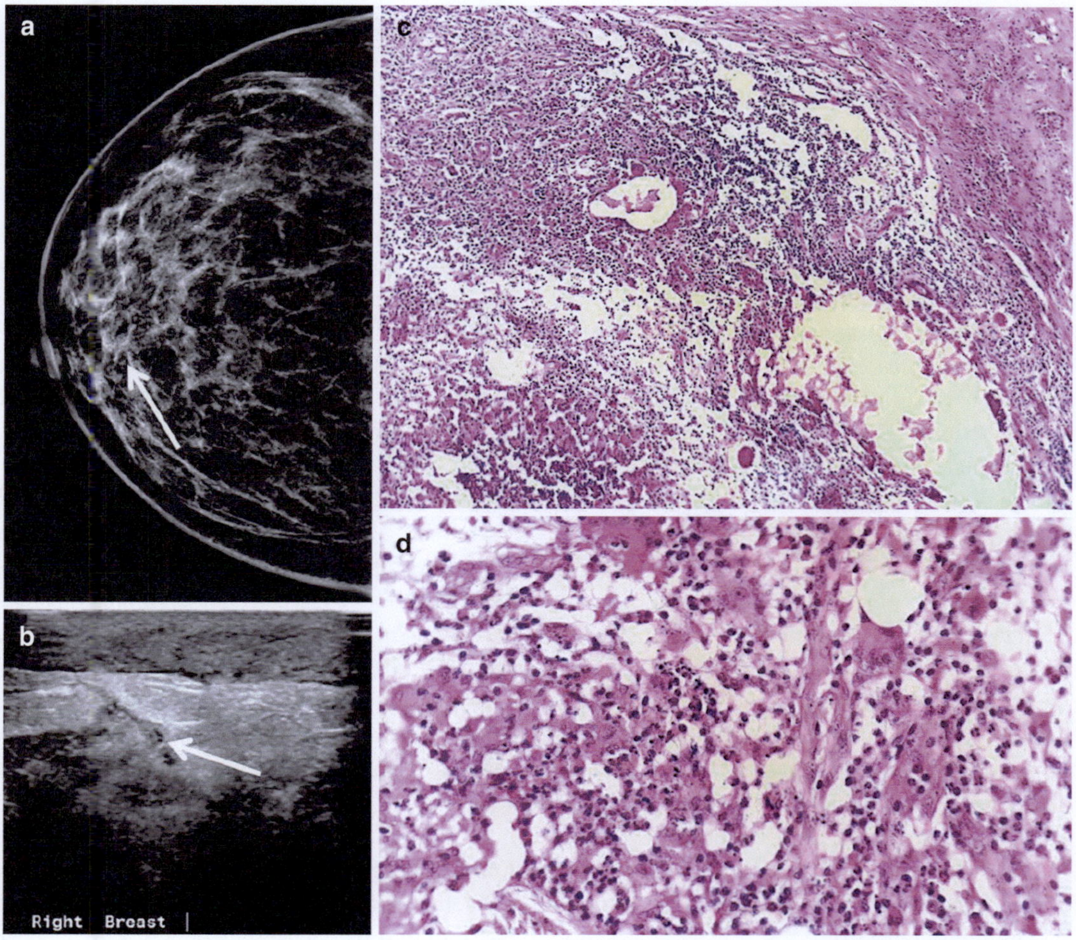

Fig. 12.6 A 36-year-old lady, nonlactating parous with right breast tender lump. Recent incision and drainage was performed elsewhere: (**a**) MG showed global asymmetry of the parenchyma with no suspicious calcifications; (**b**) US showed echogenic collection with multiple dilated ducts and reactive axillary lymph nodes; (c and d) (HPE high power), Pus was aspirated under guidance and microbiological culture showed gram-positive bacilli? diphtheroids. Biopsy of the abscess cavity yielded granulomatous inflammation with cystic spaces rimmed by neutrophils, as seen in cystic neutrophilic granulomatous mastitis (CNGM)

Management: The optimal treatment is yet to be standardized due to rarity of the disease. It ranges from surgical drainage of abscess to conservative management with steroids and aspiration. Targeted antimicrobial therapy for long term can be introduced after culture of *Corynebacteria* [16].

Hydatid Disease: Hydatid disease involving the breast is extremely rare consisting of 0.27% of all known hydatid cases, affecting women between the ages of 30 and 50 years. They present with a painless progressive palpable breast lump.

Mammography shows a high-density homogenous mass with circumscribed margins. Overpenetrated view may show ring-shaped opacities within that represents mother and daughter cysts. Ultrasound is the modality of choice and has imaging features ranging from solid to complex solid cystic or completely cystic mass depending on the evolution of the cyst. Internal echoes represent hydatid sand. MRI shows daughter cysts paralleling water intensity on all sequences. On postcontrast sequences, pericyst wall enhancement signifies sterile inflammation.

Complete surgical excision is the treatment of choice with care being taken to avoid rupture or spillage to prevent potential anaphylaxis or recurrence [17].

Filariasis: In endemic areas, breast swelling can occur as sequelae to chronic obstruction of the axillary lymphatics by the microfilariae. It can also present as painless mass located in the upper outer quadrant. There can be associated skin thickening and axillary lymphadenopathy. Ultrasound showing a cystic lesion with vigorous internal movements of the filarial larvae termed "filarial dance" is pathognomonic. Treatment is by antimicrobials [17].

Cysticercosis: Usually the muscles are affected in cysticercosis. Hardly a few cases of breast involvement are reported worldwide. Patients present with nontender breast lumps located far posteriorly. Ultrasound shows a cystic lesion with eccentric echogenic nidus. There are four types of appearance based on the internal cyst and scolex location ranging from a cyst within the collection to a calcified cyst. FNAC is the modality of choice for diagnosis. If inconclusive for cyst fragments and eosinophilic infiltrates, excision biopsy is indicated for diagnosis. Treatment is by appropriate anthelminthic and follow-up is recommended till complete resolution [17].

12.5 Noninfectious Mastitis

12.5.1 Periductal Mastitis

This commonest form of noninfectious mastitis is of two types based on etiopathogenesis and age at presentation: squamous metaplasia of lactiferous ducts (SMOLD) which is related to tobacco smoking and common in younger women and mammary duct ectasia which is not related to smoking and is common in older women [9, 12].

Squamous Metaplasia of Lactiferous Ducts: It is also known as periductal mastitis, recurrent subareolar mastitis, or Zuska's disease.

Clinical Presentation: Younger women and men of any age with history of tobacco smoking present with pain and discomfort around the nipple region. There is associated erythematous tender lump or nipple discharge in initial stages. Progression leads to abscess formation with fistulous track in periareolar region. Recurrence and persistence of the symptoms have led to many patients being diagnosed as Munchausen's syndrome.

Etiopathogenesis: The keratinizing squamous epithelium normally extends for a distance of 1–2 mm into the lactiferous duct orifice. Deeper extension of keratin leads to blocking of lactiferous sinus orifice due to accumulated keratin plug. Subsequent dilatation of the duct and rupture can lead to keratin debris inciting inflammatory response. Secondary infection of inflamed ducts can occur, leading to duct damage and possible rupture with abscess formation and subsequent draining periareolar fistula [12]. They are mostly peripheral in lactating and subareolar in nonlactating women. They are usually single, of average size 1–2 cm, unilocular and well localized. There is an association with tobacco use [7].

Imaging Features: Due to the presence of exquisite pain in periareolar region, mammography with compression is challenging. When performed, there can be an irregular mass or focal asymmetry in retroareolar region. However, the fistulous tract is not visible. MRI is helpful to identify deep-seated abscess cavity and fistula formation [12] (Figs. 12.7 and 12.8).

Pathologic Features: The most common I&D specimen has shown mixed acute and chronic periductal or stromal inflammatory infiltrate and foreign body giant cells associated with keratinaceous debris. There can be abscess formation with secondary bacterial infection. Infectious process must be excluded by performing both aerobic and anaerobic cultures. SMOLD can be diagnosed in only 1% of core biopsy samples. A high degree of clinical suspicion and history is a must to avoid delay in optimal treatment.

Management: Initial treatment is with incision and drainage with antibiotics that are useful in secondary infection. In case of recurrent symptoms, excision of the affected duct with wedge resection of the nipple is performed for definitive treatment. Cessation of smoking if history present is also a must [12].

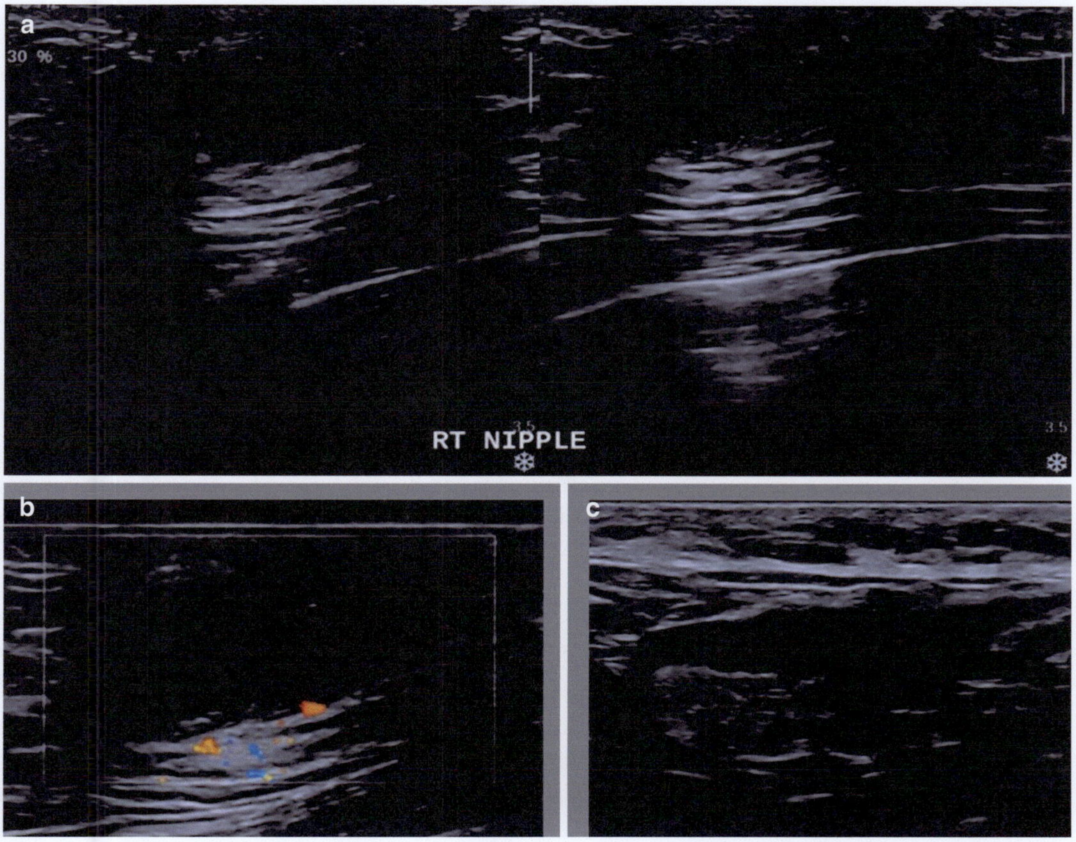

Fig. 12.7 22 F, recurrent right breast tender retroareolar lumps not responding to antibiotics. History of incision and drainage multiple times in recent past. US showed right retroareolar residual collection with two reactive lymph nodes at axillary level I. Treated with excision biopsy. Acute on chronic inflammation with dilated ducts. Diagnosis was subareolar chronic abscess with secondary infection that responded to antibiotics

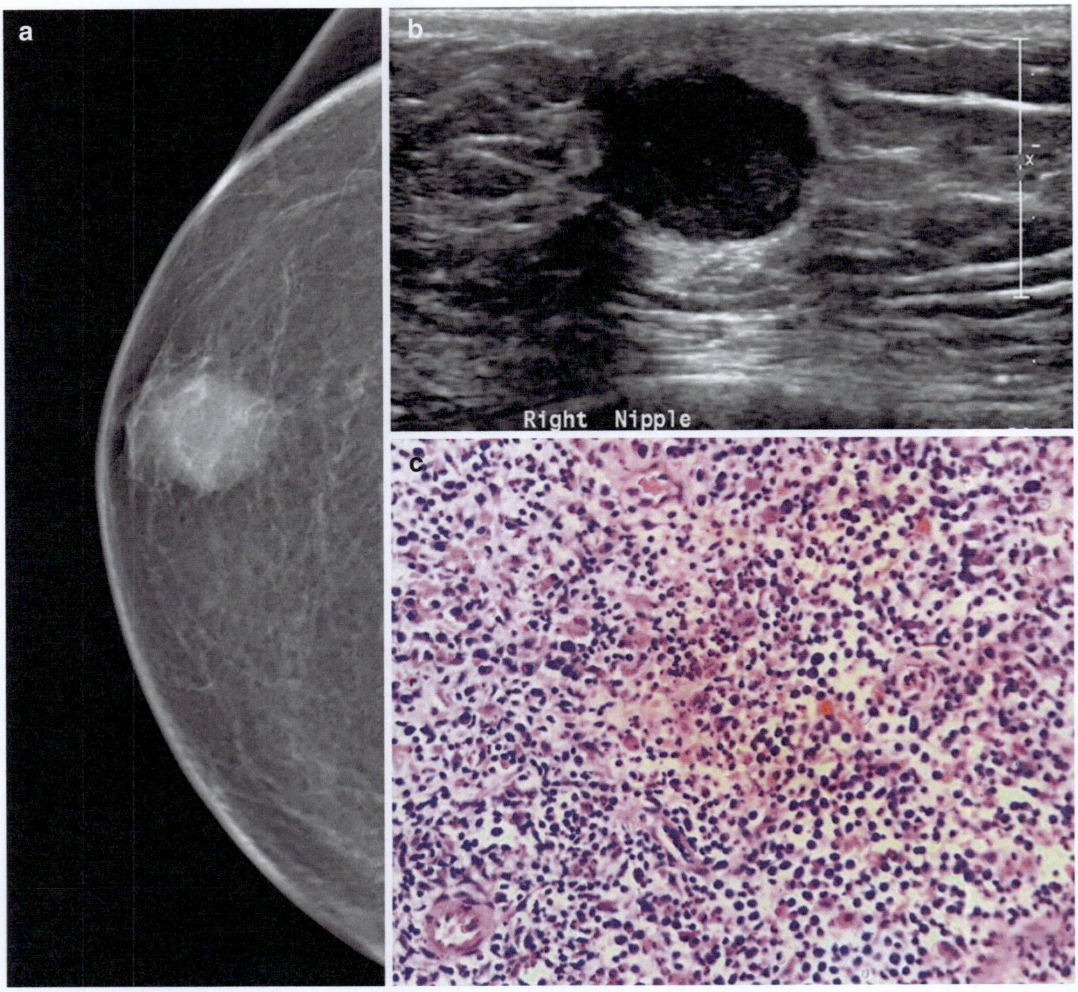

Fig. 12.8 A 61-year-old gentleman with right breast lump and spontaneous serous nipple discharge. There is no accompanying pain or fever. History of chronic smoking present. (**a**) MG showed a high-density round mass in retroareolar region with circumscribed margins. (**b**) US showed a complex cystic solid mass with indeterminate lymph nodes. c. HPE high power of core biopsy. US-guided initial aspirate yielded pus. Culture grew gram-positive bacilli. Biopsy from the collapsed wall showed fibrocollagenous tissue along with granulation tissue with collections of predominantly plasma cells along with lymphocytes, macrophages, and multinucleated giant cells

Mammary Duct Ectasia: Large multiple dilated lactiferous ducts in subareolar region are seen in perimenopausal and postmenopausal women. There is associated periductal inflammation and fibrosis and presents as a painless irregular subareolar mass. Duct ectasia seen in older females is not associated with tobacco use or fistula formation [9].

Plasma cell mastitis refers to an extreme form of aseptic periductal mastitis characterized by prominent plasma cell reaction to retained secretions in ducts. Accompanying atypical epithelial hyperplasia in these cases may be mistaken for carcinoma especially in small biopsies. The rare possibility of a plasma cell dyscrasia also needs exclusion in cases of overwhelming plasma cell infiltration.

Clinical Symptoms: Unilateral or bilateral thick nipple discharge of varying color is noted. Painless subareolar mass is seen with or without skin retraction and can mimic breast carcinoma.

Pathogenesis: Secretory stasis due to weakening of elastic fibers of contractile myoepithelial cells leads to ductal dilatation. The intraluminal contents include eosinophilic proteinaceous material, lipid/ceroid pigment-laden histiocytes, desquamated epithelial cells, cholesterol crystals, and calcific debris. These ducts may rupture with discharge of stasis material inciting periductal inflammation composed of neutrophils, foamy histiocytes, lymphocytes, and plasma cells along with stromal fibrosis and hyperelastosis. Subsequent healing with periductal fibrosis leads to formation of a mass with skin retraction [2, 12, 18].

Imaging Features: Mammography shows multiple dilated tubular structures, irregular mass with or without calcifications. The calcifications with benign features are large and rod like. When they are linear and branching, they can mimic DCIS. Ultrasound demonstrates multiple subareolar anechoic dilated ducts. When filled with echogenic nonmobile secretions, they can mimic intraductal malignancy. Real-time imaging showing movement of particulate matter is diagnostic [12] (Fig. 12.9).

Rarely ductal carcinoma in situ (DCIS) presents as a noninflammatory mastitis or noninflammatory breast cancer. This unusual form of DCIS is palpable and does not show calcification. Noninflammatory mastitis is presumed to be a risk factor for DCIS even though the mechanism is unclear. It is also unclear if DCIS precedes mastitis. Damiani S et al. have suggested that high-grade DCIS damages the myoepithelial and basement layer leading to chronic irritation of the lumen, thereby inciting inflammatory response. Imaging features are helpful in differentiating malignant inflammatory breast cancer from simple infectious mastitis. However, there are no specific imaging features pathognomonic to noninfectious mastitis, and biopsy is a must for definitive diagnosis especially in recurrent cases [19].

Management: Duct ectasia is self-limiting and does not require treatment.

12.5.2 Idiopathic Granulomatous Mastitis (IGM)

IGM is a rare disease of women of childbearing age that mimics breast carcinoma clinically and radiologically. IGM is characterized by noncaseating granuloma and microbscess formation centered on breast lobules. It constitutes about

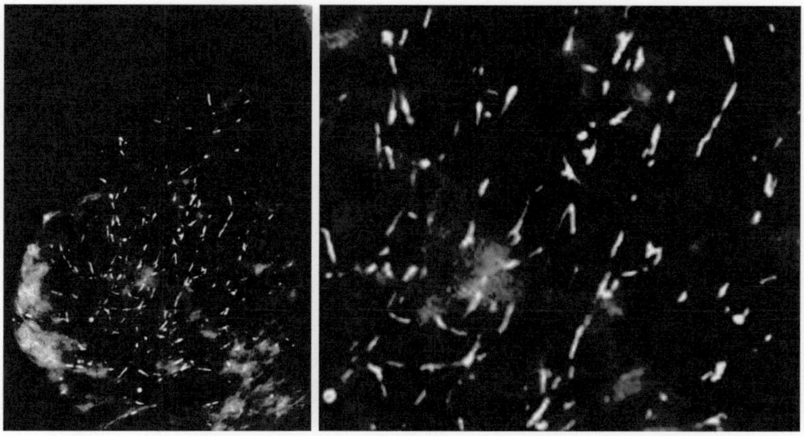

Fig. 12.9 MG right MLO view and digitally zoomed images show linear smooth calcifications without a smooth center. Smooth and regular edges are noted. Plasma cell mastitis is incidentally detected and usually bilateral

0.4–1.6% of breast biopsies [20]. The etiology of idiopathic granulomatous mastitis is still not certain. It is commonly seen in ladies between the age of 30–40 years within 5 years of pregnancy or on oral contraceptives.

Etiopathogenesis: Theories include localized autoimmune reactions to extravasated materials from the milk ducts, manifestation of a generalized autoimmune disease, impact of hormone treatment, and specific bacterial infections or fungal infestations [12]. There is a possibility of focal autoimmune reaction induced by an unknown insult. A few studies noted large T-cell population on immunostaining [21–23] while one study noted the presence of predominant CD3 positive T-cell population in the lesion distributed in and around the inflamed lobule [11]. Though it is thought to be a cell-mediated reaction to substances in mammary secretions or in lobular epithelial cells, the exact inciting antigen is not known. The primary histopathologic finding is granulomatous lobulitis [2] comprising multiple granulomatous abscesses composed of epithelioid histiocytes, Langhans giant cells, neutrophils, lymphocytes, plasma cells, and fat necrosis with a lobulocentric pattern [24].

Ogura et al. categorized granulomatous lobular mastitis into IgG4-related and non-IgG4-related. As we know, IgG4-related disease refers to a syndrome characterized by mass-forming lesions in various organs composed of dense lymphoplasmacytic infiltrates with increased tissue IgG4 plasma cells, stromal sclerosis, and elevated serum IgG4 levels [25].

However, like any other site, granulomatous inflammation in the breast could be attributed to a variety of other infectious and noninfectious etiologies which need exclusion before zeroing in on a diagnosis of idiopathic granulomatous lobular mastitis. Infections include tuberculosis, brucellosis, leprosy, and certain bacterial infections, fungal and parasitic infestations which need confirmation or exclusion with careful morphological evaluation, histochemical stains, microbiology cultures, polymerase chain reaction, or other relevant investigations. Noninfectious causes include sarcoidosis, rheumatoid arthritis and vasculitides like localized polyarteritis nodosa, giant cell arteritis, and granulomatosis with polyangiitis involving different types and sizes of vessels with varied nature of inflammatory cell infiltrates, with or without accompanying necrosis.

Rarely, duct ectasia or leakage of foreign filler substances in mammary implants may incite foreign body giant cell granulomatous reaction. Occasionally, sarcoid-like inflammatory response may be seen with breast carcinomas in the peritumoral tissue and draining axillary lymph nodes [2]. A histologic variant of breast carcinoma with osteoclastic giant cells is also well described.

Clinical Features: The most common symptom is mass followed by tenderness. There can be associated erythema, skin sinus or nipple discharge, and abscess formation at presentation. Unilateral involvement predominantly on right side or bilateral breast involvement can occur with different stages of disease progression. Definitive diagnosis is by core biopsy. Most of the patients would have already taken a course of systemic antibiotics at the time of presentation [26].

Imaging Features: Mammography shows the following features in the order of frequency: asymmetry, mass, and architectural distortion. Calcifications are usually not seen. Associated skin thickening with nipple retraction is also noted infrequently. In about 20–24% of cases, mammography will be normal. Ultrasound showed irregular-shaped hypoechoic mass, either single or multiple contiguous. Abscess when formed follows a tracking pattern along the subcutaneous tissue with subsequent skin fistula. There may be surrounding inflammatory changes in subcutaneous tissue. Associated ipsilateral axillary lymphadenopathy is noted in 15–25% of the cases. MRI breast features are variable and depend on the severity of disease. It is indicated in nonresponsive mass to know the exact disease extent. The appearance is of an irregular mass with heterogeneous enhancement or nonmass enhancement depending on the inflammatory changes. Fazzio et al. have described T2 bright peripherally enhancing masses with central non-areas typical of an abscess in advanced cases [26, 27] (Figs. 12.10 and 12.11).

Management: Since mastitis is the presenting symptom, most of the patients get initial empirical antibiotic therapy though response is not present. Confirmation of granulomatous mastitis and exclusion of neoplasm on core biopsy is mandatory before initiating the treatment. There are two treatment options once GM is confirmed. The first and favored is conservative management with high-dose steroids, tapering over 2–6 months. A response of 66–72% can be obtained with a recurrence rate of 15% [27]. When steroid treatment fails, the second option of excision and debridement of the granulomatous cavity becomes mandatory with a recurrence rate of 6.8% [28]. When abscess is the initial presenting symptom, depending on the size, it is aspirated, drained, or incised. Aspiration can be difficult due to the presence of necrotic tissue in the center. Recent studies have shown promising results for the residual abscess after oral steroids using ultrasound-guided triamcinolone injection into the abscess cavity directly after aspirating the abscess [27, 28].

12.5.3 Diabetic Mastopathy (DMP)

Diabetic mastopathy or lymphocytic mastopathy is a rare benign fibroinflammatory disease of the breast associated with hard painless breast lumps in premenopausal women mostly with type I diabetes mellitus. There may be other diabetes-related complications at presentation. It has to be

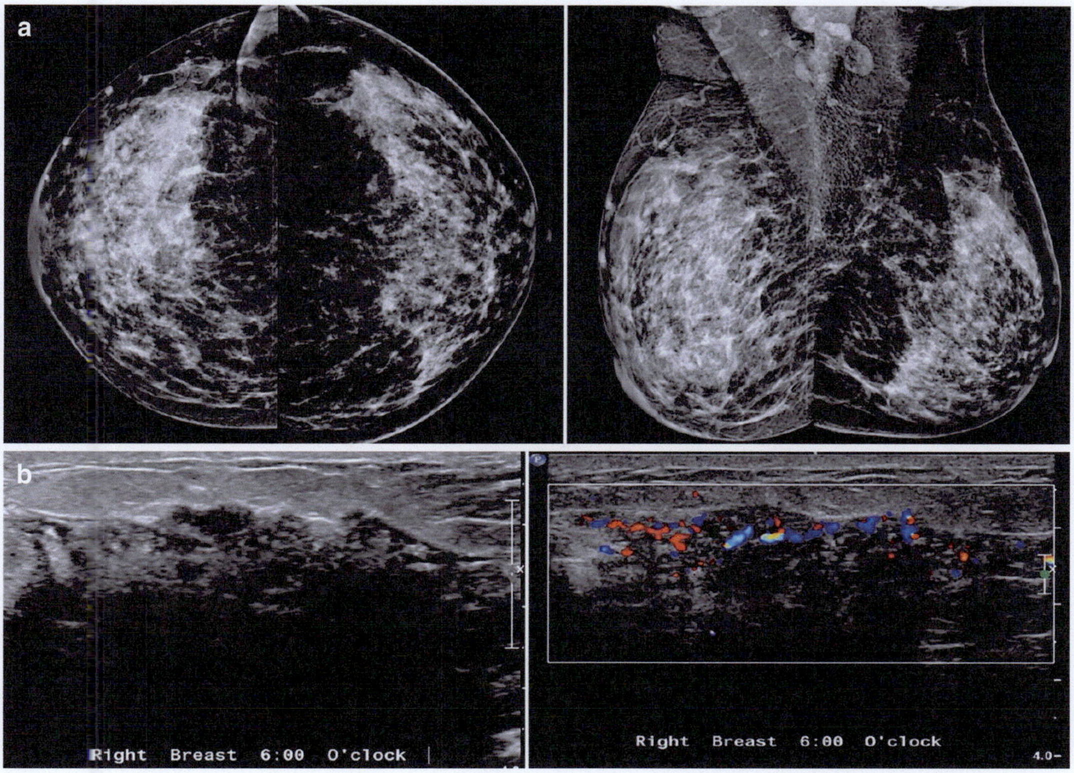

Fig. 12.10 A 41-year-old lady with recent onset right breast tender lump. She is not lactating and her last child birth was four years ago: (**a**) Right breast shows global asymmetry with periareolar skin thickening and nipple retraction. (**b**) US showed nonmass area with marginal vascularity. No collections at that time. US-guided core biopsy confirmed idiopathic granulomatous mastitis. Oral steroids were started with good initial response

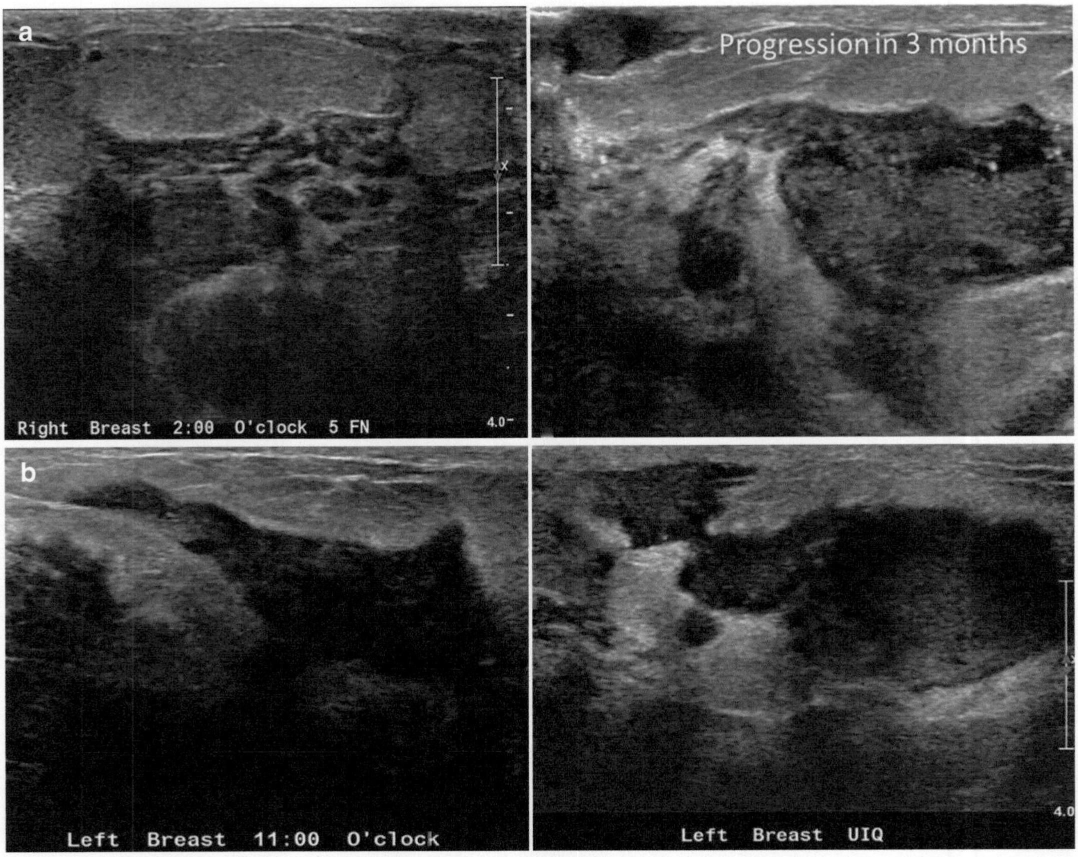

Fig. 12.11 A 29-year-old lady with bilateral concurrent biopsy-proven idiopathic granulomatous mastitis with abscess formation despite oral steroids necessitating incision and drainage. Her last child birth was three years before the symptom onset. (**a**) Right breast nonmass area progresses into an abscess with sinus formation. (**b**) Left breast abscess shows progression into a larger collection while on steroids

distinguished from breast malignancy. The prevalence is up to 13% of all type I DM [29]. Association with type II DM and other autoimmune diseases are also noted less frequently.

Pathophysiology: Histopathological features include keloid-like dense fibrosis with epithelioid myofibroblasts in the stroma and B-cell-rich lymphocytic infiltrates in perilobular, periductal, and perivascular locations with lobular atrophy. Though the terms lymphocytic mastitis and diabetic mastopathy are often considered synonymous, the latter term must be used only when there is a palpable mass and established association with diabetes mellitus. Similar histological changes may also be seen in other autoimmune conditions including Hashimoto thyroiditis. The term "sclerosing lymphocytic mastitis" can be applied in cases with marked sclerosis [29].

Clinical Presentation: There is often a palpable hard, painless, and irregular mass either in one breast or bilateral breasts.

Imaging Features: Mammography shows dense glandular tissue with focal asymmetry or mass with no associated suspicious calcifications. Ultrasound shows a mixed echogenic mass with posterior partial shadowing and poor vascularity. There is no associated axillary lymphadenopathy. Ultrasound-guided core biopsy is mandatory for diagnosis (Fig. 12.12).

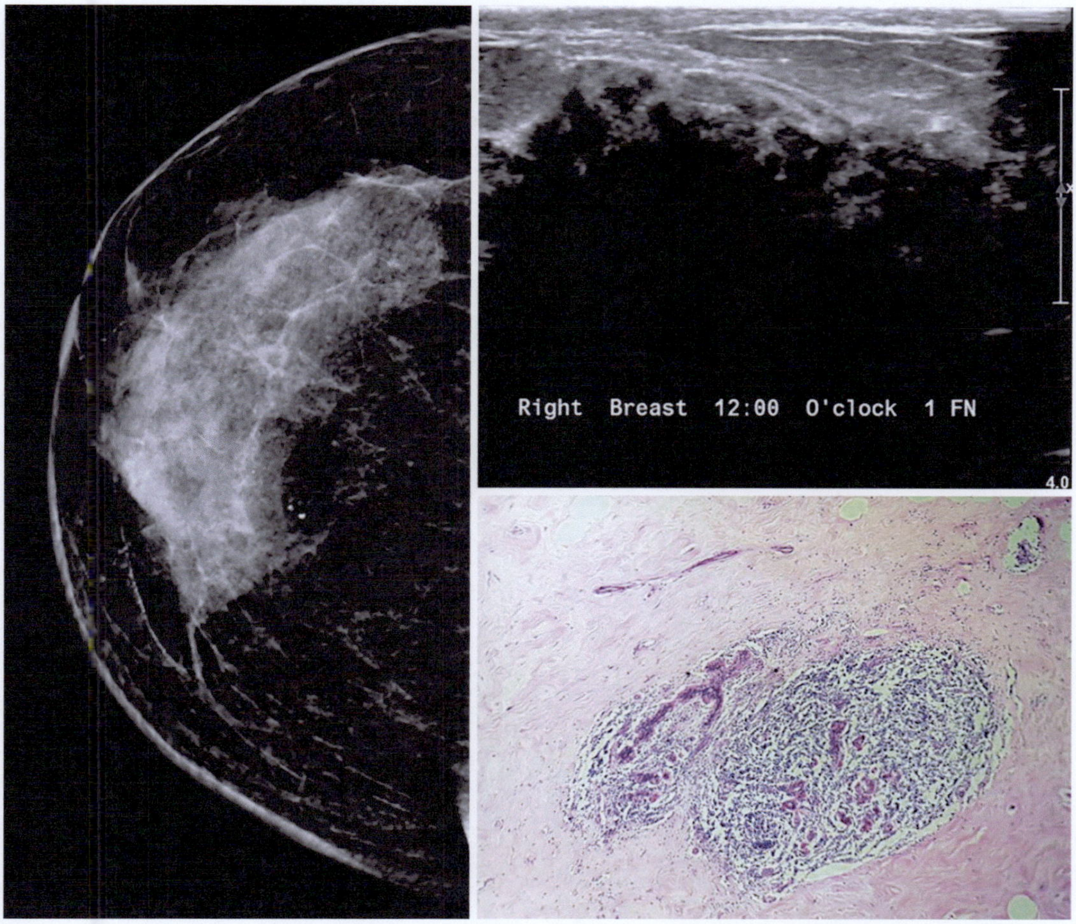

Fig. 12.12 A 56-year-old lady with right breast lump of one-year duration associated with occasional throbbing pain. History of type II DM on oral treatment since past ten years. (**a**) MG showed dense breast tissue with a focal asymmetry at 12 o'clock position periareolar region. There were no suspicious calcifications. (**b**) US showed an oval mixed echogenic mass with indistinct margins measuring maximum of 3.8 cm. The mass was poorly vascular and had posterior shadowing. Axillary lymph nodes were normal. (**c**) US-guided core biopsy showed hyalinized core showing interconnecting spaces lined by fibroblasts. Excision biopsy after persistent symptoms was performed. Final pathology was reported as fibrosing mastopathy—in keeping with diabetic mastopathy

Management: The clinical and imaging findings are inconclusive, and these lesions are often misdiagnosed as breast carcinomas. The recognition of this rare but benign disease is crucial to avoid surgical biopsies. There is an increased risk of recurrence after attempted surgical excision. There is no increased risk of development of breast carcinoma [30].

12.5.4 Eosinophilic Mastitis

Eosinophilic mastitis is a rare inflammatory condition of the breast resulting from infiltration of the eosinophils around ducts and lobules with admixed lymphocytes and plasma cells. It can clinically present with features similar to a breast malignancy.

Pathophysiology: Eosinophils constitute the main infiltrate in the sampled tissue. Though it is often attributed to an immune response to ductal secretions, these can also be associated with other allergic conditions, peripheral eosinophilia, eosinophilic granulomatosis with polyangiitis (Churg-Strauss syndrome), or hypereosinophilic syndrome. The activated eosinophils degranulate with release of cytotoxic inflammatory mediators which result in tenderness, erythema, and mass formation (Fig. 12.13a–c).

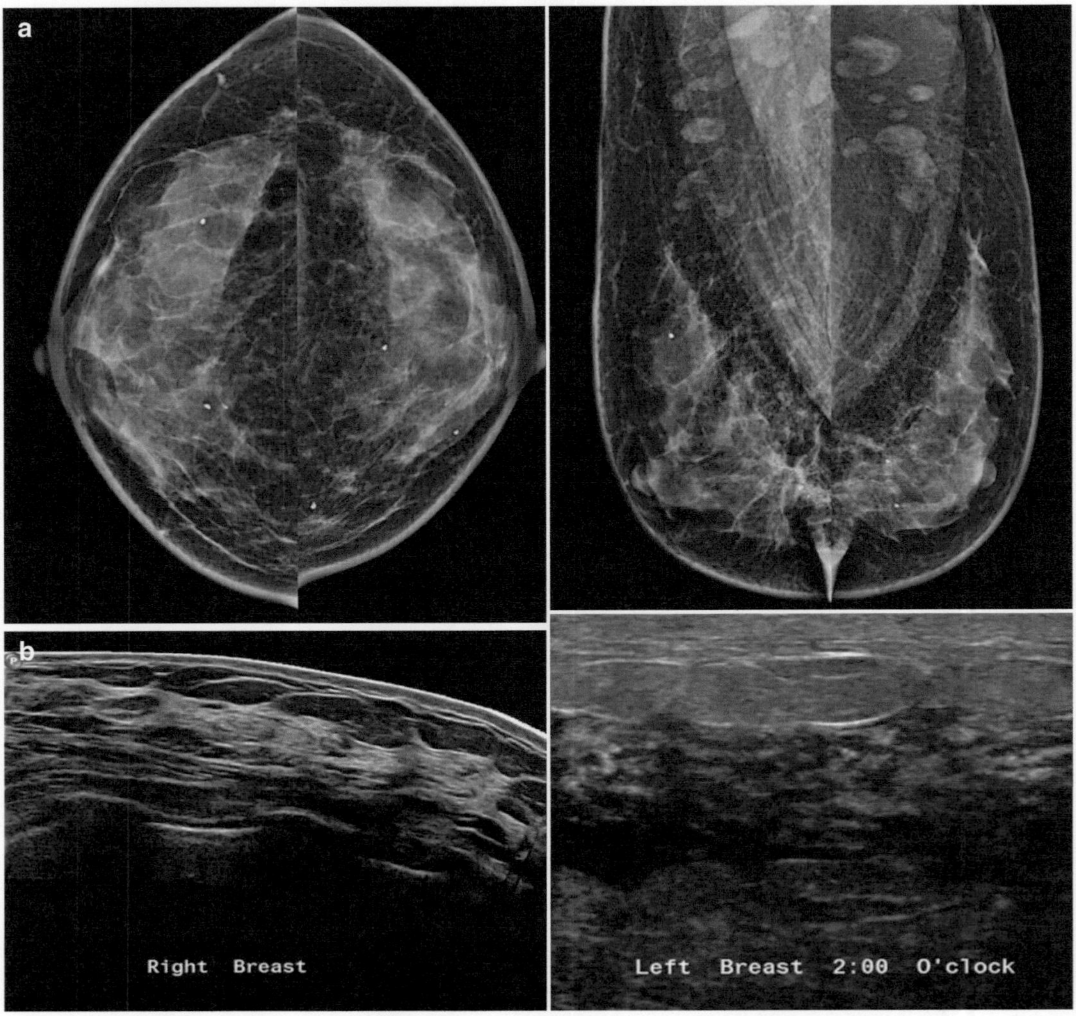

Fig. 12.13 A 41-year-old lady with recent onset left breast tender lumpiness. History of DM. Clinically ill-defined lump with skin erythema and enlarged axillary lymph node: (**a**) MG showed dense breasts. No suspicious features. US showed normal right breast. Left breast showed diffuse skin thickening, subcutaneous tissue edema, and thickened and hypoechoic parenchyma with an enlarged lymph node; (**b**) MRI breast was performed to assess the extent of lesion. Inflammatory changes with regional nonmass enhancement was noted with no significant restriction on DWI. US core biopsy showed inflammatory lesion. Stromal edema with periductal and interstitial infiltrates predominantly eosinophils. Negative for DCIS/malignancy. FNAC of left axillary lymph node was reactive. Diagnosis of eosinophilic mastitis was confirmed with hematological parameters. (**c**) A course of antibiotics and anthelmintic was given. US follow-up after two weeks of antibiotics showed complete response

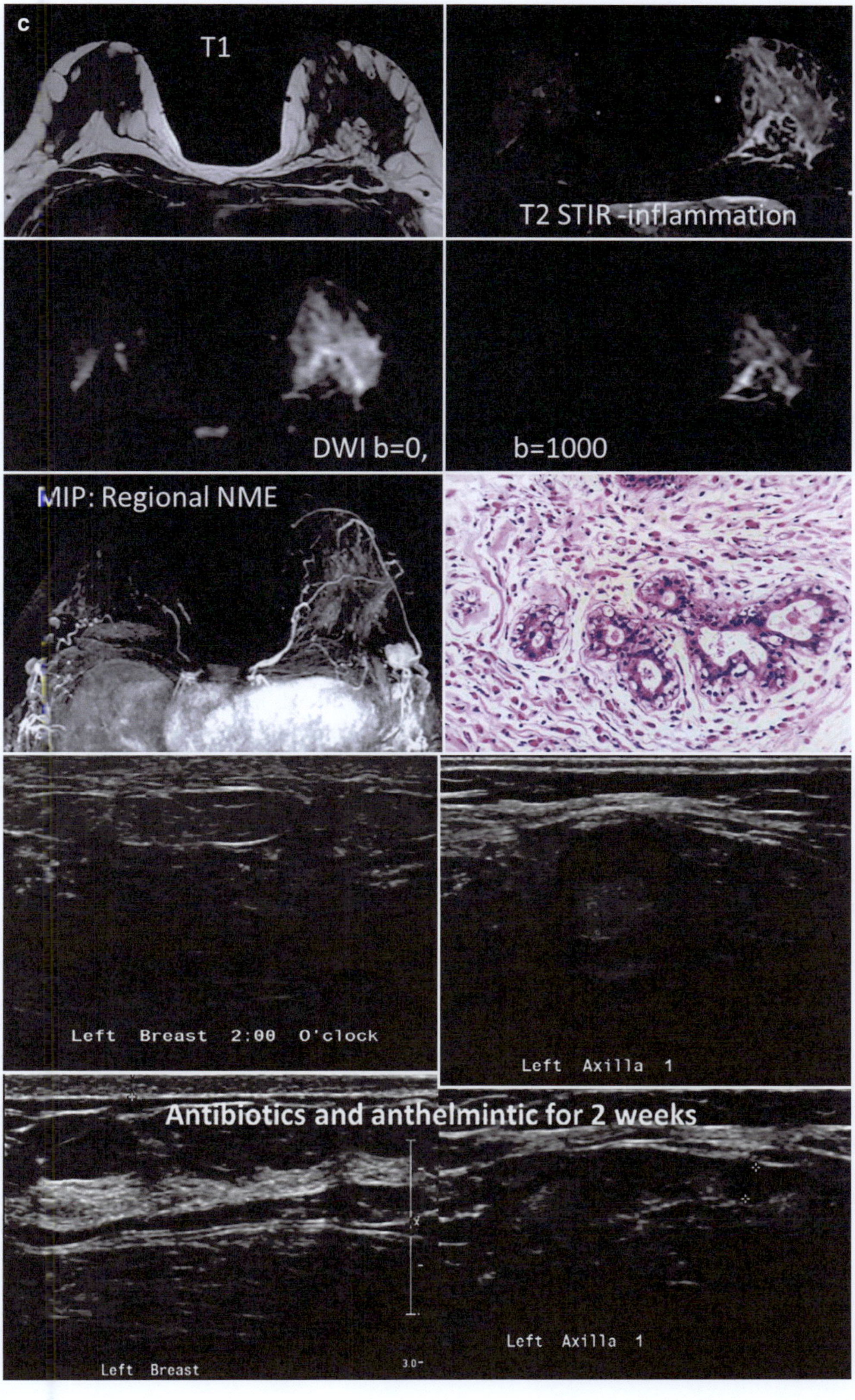

Fig. 12.13 (continued)

Clinical Presentation Unilateral breast mass, with or without edema and breast pain. There may be associated skin thickening or nipple discharge rarely.

Imaging Features Mammography shows focal or global asymmetry. Ultrasound shows mass or heterogeneous area, skin thickening, and dilated duct with thickened walls. MRI shows edematous changes and dilated ducts.

Management Medical management with serial imaging is the mainstay. If infective cause could be identified, appropriate therapy with anthelmintic should be given. If not, treatment with steroids and antihistaminic is effective. There is no role for surgical intervention [31].

12.5.5 Miscellaneous Causes of Mastitis/Rarer Forms of Mastitis

Postbiopsy Changes: Benign excision biopsy changes are among the commonest reactive conditions in the breast. Obtaining history of the surgical procedure and duration elapsed since treatment is mandatory to correlate with evolving changes.

Pathophysiology: These include a variety of morphological alterations like hemorrhage, inflammation with infiltration of foreign body giant cells, granulation tissue formation, fat necrosis, and scarring. Squamous metaplasia of adjacent ducts, infarction of lesional tissue, and reaction to marking devices placed during imaging may all confound pathological interpretation of subsequent excision biopsy specimens [29].

Imaging Features: Mammography signs of postoperative changes include skin thickening, increased trabecular markings, postoperative fluid collection, scar, fat necrosis, and dystrophic calcifications. These changes are marked up to six months after surgery. Skin thickening more than 2 mm is abnormal. It is seen in 90% of postoperative patients. It stabilizes or returns to normal in 2–3 years postsurgery. Postoperative collection consisting of fluid alone or mixed with blood presents as a mass in half of the patients after one month. In some patients, it is seen to persist after years. However, there is gradual regression in size on serial studies. Seroma retracts and is replaced with fibrous tissue. Fat necrosis is tissue necrosis resulting from damage to intima of vessels during surgery or during radiation can manifest as curvilinear calcifications in 3–6 months [32] (Fig. 12.14).

Radiation Mastitis: During the acute period after irradiation, inflammatory markers are induced, and the expression of these proteins contributes to increased vascular permeability of breast tissue. Breast edema that manifests as skin and trabecular thickening appears generally in the first week but persists several weeks after completion of radiation therapy. Initially, there is engorgement of the dermal as well as of the intramammary lymphatics (trabecular thickening). This edema usually resolves over a period of weeks, months, or sometimes years.

Radiographically, an irradiated breast with skin and trabecular thickening appears denser as compared to the contralateral normal breast. Postirradiation mastitis is characterized by diffuse edema, coarsened breast trabeculae, and skin thickening on mammography of the irradiated breast. These findings should be interpreted with caution as they may mask underlying residual or recurrent malignancies [1].

Baseline mammography posttherapy is obtained 6 months after completion of radiation and thereafter after 12 months annually. Skin

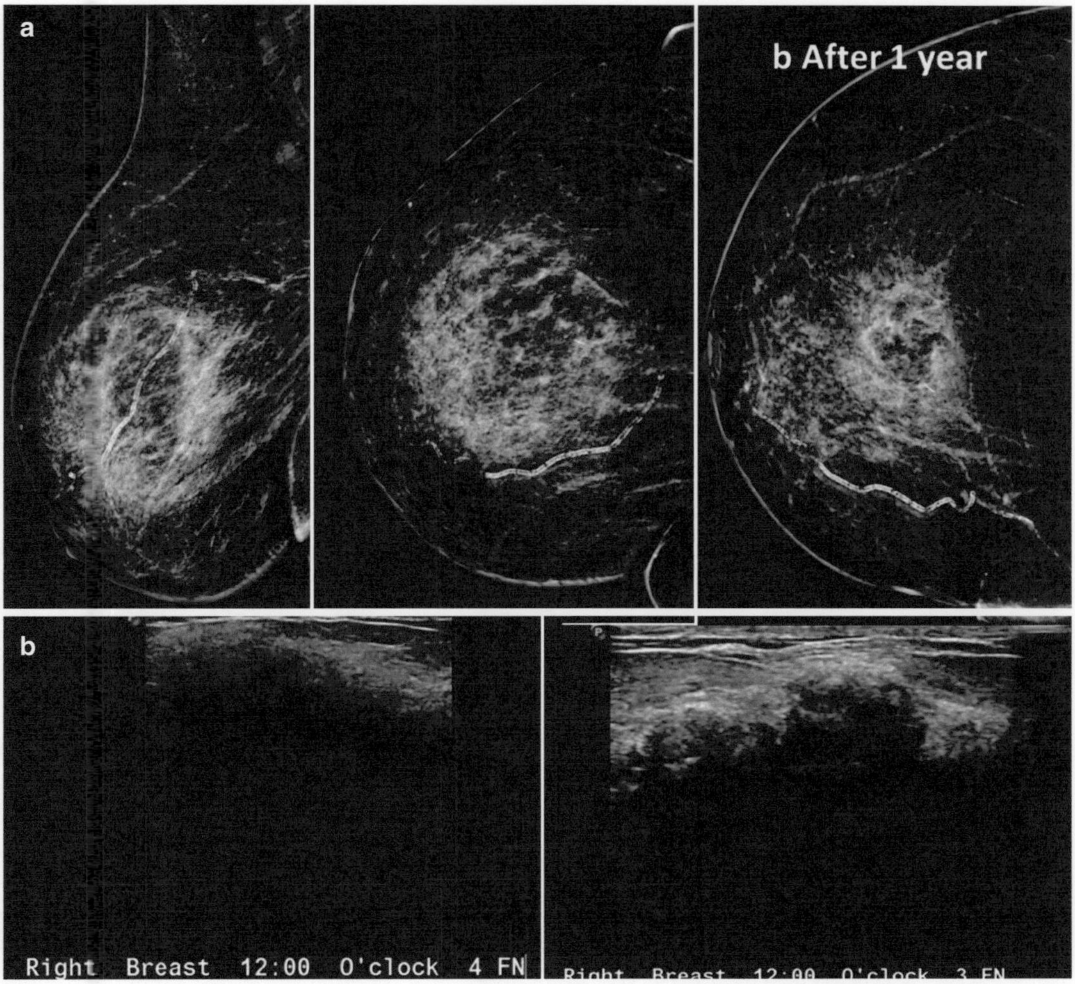

Fig. 12.14 A 60-year-old lady with multiple chest wall debridements following angioplasty presents with right breast lump. (**a**) MG showed a mixed density fat containing mass with no calcifications. US showed an echogenic mass with shadowing. US-guided core biopsy showed fat necrosis that was benign concordant. (**b**) Follow-up MG and US after one year show significant interval regression of the findings

changes and increased trabecular markings should subside or stabilize in 2–3 years. The changes take longer to regress for intracavitary beam radiation as compared to external beam radiation. Features suggestive of recurrent disease on mammography include interval appearance of mass near scar site, suspicious calcifications, skin thickening after stabilization, and axillary lymphadenopathy (Fig. 12.15).

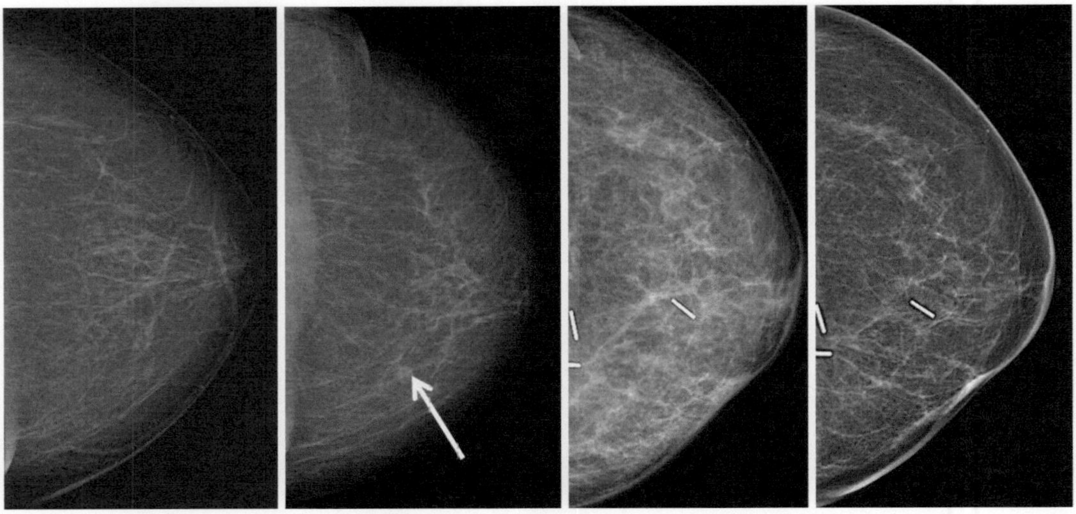

Fig. 12.15 A 64-year-old lady on screening detected left breast neoplastic mass (arrow) underwent breast conservation surgery and radiotherapy. Postradiation changes in the form of skin thickening and increased trabecular markings show regression in two years

12.6 Malignant Mastitis

Whenever a nonlactating female patient presents with inflammatory breast symptoms that do not respond to antibiotics, exclusion of malignancy is of utmost importance with appropriate imaging modalities and biopsy/aspiration as when required, as inflammatory breast cancer has poor prognosis and diagnosis should not be delayed. The rare presentation of malignancy as breast abscess should also be borne in mind in atypical cases.

Inflammatory Breast Cancer: Inflammatory breast cancer (IBC) is a rare form of locally advanced breast neoplasm with atypical presentation simulating common condition like mastitis, thereby leading to delay in diagnosis and treatment.

Clinical Presentation: The diagnosis of IBC is based upon the presence of all of the following clinical criteria: rapid onset of breast erythema occupying at least one-third of the breast, edema, and/or peau d'orange and/or warm breast, duration of history of no more than six months, and dominant mass may not be present. Presence of fever and leukocytosis would suggest infectious mastitis.

Imaging Features: Routine screening rarely helps in diagnosis of IBC. Mammographic features include enlarged breast, skin thickening, increased trabecular markings, and axillary lymphadenopathy; dominant mass and calcification may or may not be present. Ultrasound shows diffuse skin thickening with subdermal lymphatic channels and diffuse subcutaneous tissue edema. Hypoechoic nonmass areas are seen with enlarged multiple lymph nodes involving all three axillary levels. MRI breast shows diffuse enlargement with abnormal enhancement helping one to optimize targeting the biopsy under ultrasound guidance.

Pathology: Neoplastic cells should be demonstrated in the core biopsy samples. There is also pathological infiltration of the dermal lymphatics by tumor emboli. Lobular histology cases are less commonly seen in IBC. The punch biopsy samples of skin showing tumor are also considered confirmatory for IBC (Fig. 12.16).

Management: The threefold approach of neoadjuvant chemotherapy, surgery in the form of modified radical mastectomy, and radiation to chest wall and axilla for the mainstay of treatment. A potential underlying IBC necessitates follow-up of all cases of mastitis to complete regression. In the event of persistence of symptoms after 7–10 days of antibiotic course, core biopsy sample should be obtained for definitive diagnosis [33].

Malignant Abscess: Presentation of malignancy as breast abscess is well documented. There can be thickened wall with pathological nodes. Tissue biopsy should be attempted from the periphery of the abscess cavity as central portion may be necrotic [1] (Fig. 12.17).

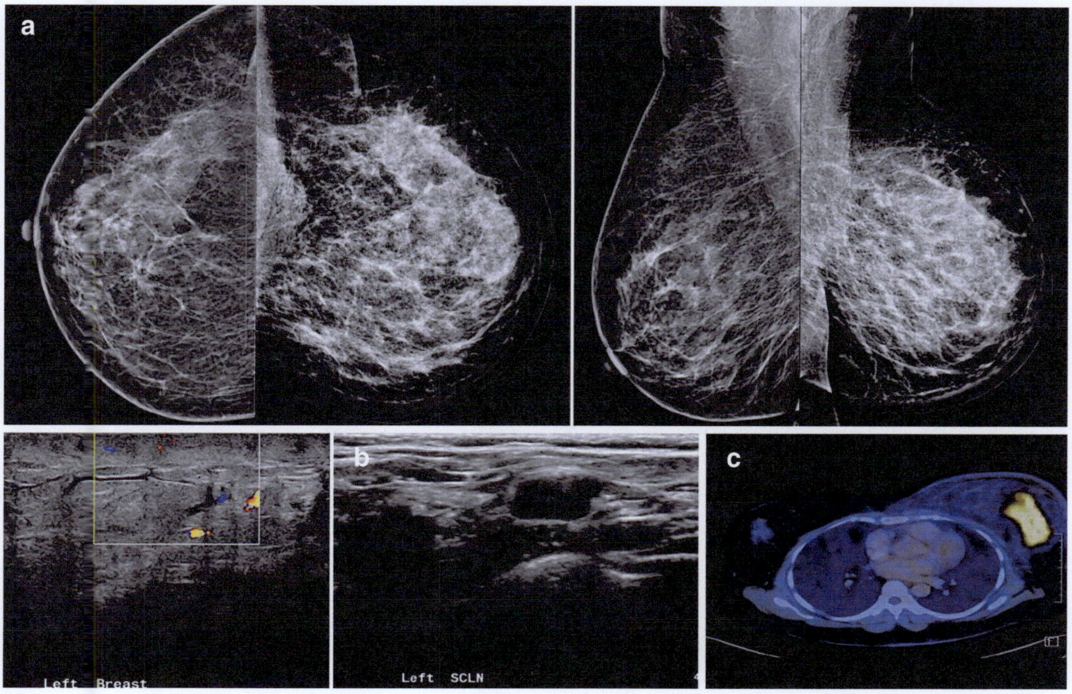

Fig. 12.15 A 38-year-old lady with left breast enlargement of three-month duration. There is no history of trauma or fever. (**a**) MG showed left breast significant enlargement with diffuse skin thickening and increased trabecular markings. There were no discrete masses or suspicious calcifications. (**b**) US images show skin thickening with prominent subdermal lymphatic channels. Diffuse hypoechoic parenchyma with no discrete solid masses. Lymph nodes at all levels including left supraclavicular region were suspicious. US-guided core biopsy of the most suspicious area showed invasive neoplasm grade III with DCIS. Her 2neu-enriched and supraclavicular lymph node FNAC was positive for malignancy. (**c**) PET-CT confirmed the left breast enlargement with skin involvement and underlying extensive mass. Diagnosis of inflammatory breast neoplasm was made

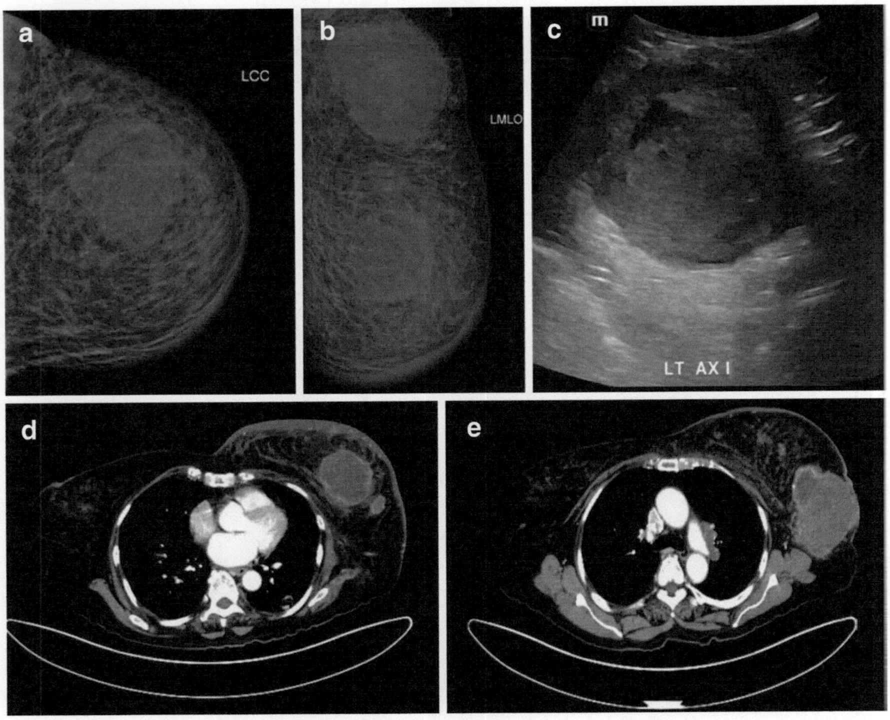

Fig. 12.17 A 56-year-old lady with recent onset left breast and axillary masses. Core biopsy from the mass and lymph node confirmed triple-negative invasive breast cancer with necrosis and high proliferative index. (**a**) CC view shows left breast round mass with circumscribed margins. (**b**) MLO view shows a larger similar mass in axilla. (**c**) Ultrasound of the large axillary mass with convex probe shows necrotic nature. (**d**) CECT thorax section through the mass in lateral quadrant. € CECT thorax through the axillary regions shows necrotic malignant mass

12.7 Conclusion

Recognition of the type of mastitis based on relevant clinical history, history of smoking exposure, lactational status, and associated autoimmune disorders help to direct appropriate investigations and the mode of intervention. Once mastitis is diagnosed, it must be followed to complete regression as there is always a rare chance of missing an underlying or coexisting breast neoplasm (Fig. 12.18).

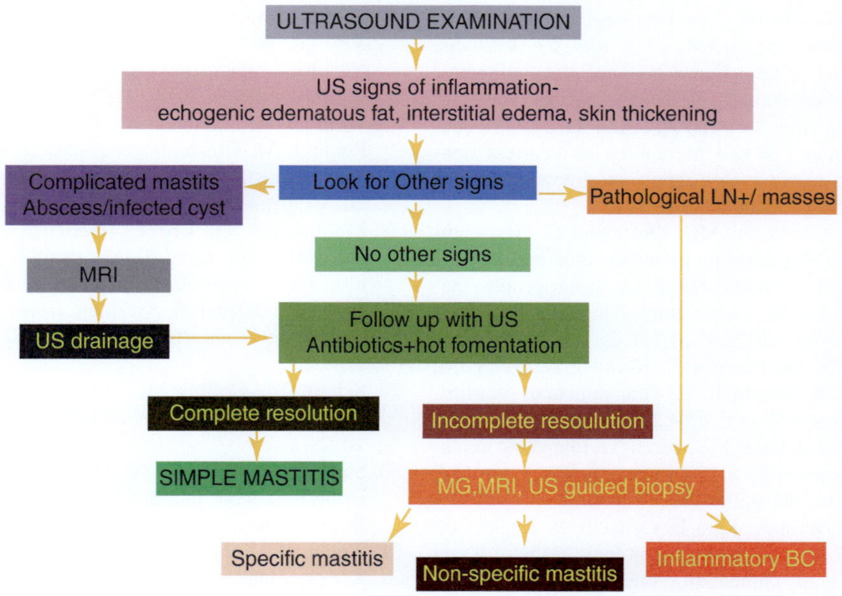

Fig. 12.18 Algorithmic approach to mastitis

References

1. Kamal RM, Hamed ST, Salem DS. Classification of inflammatory breast disorders and step by step diagnosis. Breast J. 2009;15(4):367–80.
2. Hoda SA, Brogi E, Koerner FC, Rosen PP. Rosen's breast pathology. 4th ed; 2014. 1 p.
3. Boakes E, Woods A, Johnson N, Kadoglou N. Breast infection: a review of diagnosis and management practices. Eur J Breast Health. 2018;14(3):136–43. https://doi.org/10.5152/ejbh.2018.3871.
4. Blackmon MM, Nguyen H, Mukherji P. Acute mastitis. In: StatPearls [Internet]. Treasure Island: StatPearls Publishing; 2023. Available from: http://www.ncbi.nlm.nih.gov/books/NBK557782/.
5. Angelopoulou A, Field D, Ryan CA, Stanton C, Hill C, Ross RP. The microbiology and treatment of human mastitis. Med Microbiol Immunol (Berl). 2018;207(2):83–94.
6. Giri A, Basu S, Ghosh A. Impact of lactational training and nipple evaluation during pregnancy in reducing lactational mastitis and breast abscess. Asian J Clin Pediatr Neonatol. 2023;11(2):1–3.
7. Almasad JK. Mammary duct fistulae: classification and management. ANZ J Surg. 2006;76(3):149–52.
8. Ghunaim H. Percutaneous ultrasound-guided needle aspiration for management of breast abscesses – a review. J Med Radiat Sci. 2023;70(3):327–37.
9. Febery A, Bennett I. Sonographic features of inflammatory conditions of the breast. Australas J Ultrasound Med. 2019;22(3):165–73.
10. Costa Morais Oliveira V, Cubas-Vega N, López Del-Tejo P, Baía-da-Silva DC, Araújo Tavares M, Picinin Safe I, et al. Non-lactational infectious mastitis in the Americas: a systematic review. Front Med. 2021;8:672513.
11. Gopalakrishnan Nair C, Null H, Jacob P, Menon RR, Null M. Inflammatory diseases of the non-lactating female breasts. Int J Surg Lond Engl. 2015;13:8–11.
12. Turashvili G, Li X. Inflammatory lesions of the breast. Arch Pathol Lab Med. 2023;147(10):1133–47.
13. Dixon JM. Periductal mastitis/duct ectasia. Br J Surg. 1982;69(7):423–5.
14. Farrokh D, Alamdaran A, Laeen AF, Rastegar YF, Abbasi B. Tuberculous mastitis: a review of 32 cases. Int J Infect Dis. 2019;87:135–42.
15. Yoo H, Choi SH, Kim YJ, Kim SJ, Cho YU, Choi SJ. Recurrent bilateral breast abscess due to nontuberculous mycobacterial infection. J Breast Cancer. 2014;17(3):295–8.
16. Wu JM, Turashvili G. Cystic neutrophilic granulomatous mastitis: an update. J Clin Pathol. 2020;73(8):445–53.
17. Dhamija E, Gulati S, Hari S. Imaging spectrum in tropical breast infections. Br J Radiol. 2024;97(1154):315–23.

18. Periductal Mastitis – an overview | ScienceDirect Topics [Internet]. [cited 2024 Mar 3]. Available from: https://www.sciencedirect.com/topics/medicine-and-dentistry/periductal-mastitis
19. Liong YV, Hong GS, Teo JGC, Lim GH. Breast ductal carcinoma in situ presenting as recurrent non-puerperal mastitis: case report and literature review. World J Surg Oncol. 2013;11:179.
20. Barra F, Centurioni MG, Gustavino C, Alessandri F, Ferrero S. Idiopathic granulomatous mastitis: the importance of summarizing the heterogenous evidence of the current literature. J Investig Surg Off J Acad Surg Res. 2022;35(3):721–2.
21. Diesing D, Axt-Fliedner R, Hornung D, Weiss JM, Diedrich K, Friedrich M. Granulomatous mastitis. Arch Gynecol Obstet. 2004;269(4):233–6.
22. Al-Khaffaf B, Knox F, Bundred NJ. Idiopathic granulomatous mastitis: a 25-year experience. J Am Coll Surg. 2008;206(2):269–73.
23. Erhan Y, Veral A, Kara E, Ozdemir N, Kapkac M, Ozdedeli E, et al. A clinicopthologic study of a rare clinical entity mimicking breast carcinoma: idiopathic granulomatous mastitis. Breast Edinb Scotl. 2000;9(1):52–6.
24. Dabbs DJ. Breast pathology. 2nd ed. Philadelphia: Elsevier; 2017.
25. Ogura K, Matsumoto T, Aoki Y, Matsumoto T, Aoki Y, et al. IgG4-related tumour-forming mastitis with histological appearances of granulomatous lobular mastitis: comparison with other types of tumour-forming mastitis. Histopathology. 2010;57:39–45. Mastitis: Clinical features, classification and management
26. Barreto DS, Sedgwick EL, Nagi CS, Benveniste AP. Granulomatous mastitis: etiology, imaging, pathology, treatment, and clinical findings. Breast Cancer Res Treat. 2018;171(3):527–34.
27. Wolfrum A, Kümmel S, Theuerkauf I, Pelz E, Reinisch M. Granulomatous mastitis: a therapeutic and diagnostic challenge. Breast Care Basel Switz. 2018;13(6):413–8.
28. Moldoveanu D, Lee C, Hesley G. Framework and guide for intralesional steroid injections in idiopathic granulomatous mastitis. Eur J Radiol [Internet]. 2023;168. Available from: https://www.ejradiology.com/article/S0720-048X(23)00432-1/fulltext
29. Schnitt SJ, Collins LC. Biopsy interpretation of the breast. 2nd ed. Lippincott Williams & Wilkins; 2012.
30. Shrikrishnapalasuriyar N, Atkinson M, Kalhan A, Evans P. Diabetic mastopathy: a diagnostic challenge. Br J Diabetes. 2018;18(1):32–4.
31. Arnott W, Leong G, Davis A, Diab J, Clement Z. Eosinophilic mastitis: a rare benign inflammatory condition and review of the literature. J Surg Case Rep. 2022;2022(10):rjac456.
32. Ramani SK, Rastogi A, Mahajan A, Nair N, Shet T, Thakur MH. Imaging of the treated breast post breast conservation surgery/oncoplasty: pictorial review. World J Radiol. 2017;9(8):321–9.
33. Hester RH, Hortobagyi GN, Lim B. Inflammatory breast cancer: early recognition and diagnosis is critical. Am J Obstet Gynecol. 2021;225(4):392–6.

Unusual Breast Cancers

13

Bhawna Dev and Leena Joseph Dennis

Abstract

Unusual breast masses present a diagnostic challenge due to their unusual presentation or mixed imaging features, often requiring a comprehensive triple approach for accurate diagnosis and evaluation. Imaging plays a pivotal role in the assessment and management of breast masses. While clinical examination remains a fundamental diagnostic tool, imaging techniques provide crucial insights into the nature, location, and characteristics of unusual breast masses, aiding in differential diagnosis. Histopathology and immunohistochemistry definitely lead to the closest or definitive diagnosis helping accurate treatment planning. These masses encompass a gamut of breast diseases. Among malignancies, the most common type is invasive ductal carcinoma, no special type/not otherwise specified. These tumours originate from the terminal duct lobular unit. They can also feature some special subtypes like apocrine change, neuroendocrine differentiation, lobular carcinoma, etc. There are some rare variants like mucinous carcinoma, metaplastic carcinomas, and sarcomas that can also develop in the breast. This chapter mentions the unusual manifestations and imaging features of such rare neoplasms in the breast.

Keywords

Unusual breast cancer · Mucinous carcinoma Medullary carcinoma · Granular cell tumour Metaplastic breast tumour · Sarcomas of the breast

13.1 Introduction

This chapter deals with not so common malignancies found in the breast. Most of the times, these masses have overlapping clinical and imaging features; hence histopathology and immunohistochemistry are mandatory for final diagnosis. Certain specific imaging features may raise suspicion of the underlying variability; therefore diligent radiological evaluation becomes essential. Appropriate and judicial role of various imaging modalities, such as mammography, ultrasound, magnetic resonance imaging (MRI), and modern techniques like contrast-enhanced digital mammogram (CEDM), and contrast-

B. Dev (✉)
Department of Radiology, Sri Ramachandra Institute of Higher Education and Research, Chennai, India
e-mail: bhawnadev@sriramachandra.edu.in

L. J. Dennis
Department of Pathology, Sri Ramachandra Institute of Higher Education and Research, Chennai, India
e-mail: leenadennisj@sriramachandra.edu.in

E. Dhamija, S. V. S. Deo (eds.), *Imaging in Management of Breast Diseases*,
https://doi.org/10.1007/978-981-96-4998-3_13

enhanced ultrasound (CEUS), helps in narrowing the differential diagnosis and assessment of unusual breast masses.

The incidence of these rare tumours is very less. Most often, we come across benign neoplasms like fibroadenomas, and malignant lesions include invasive mammary or ductal carcinoma (IMC/IDC)-NOS (not otherwise specified). The presence of mucin in malignancies to the extent of more than 90% qualifies it as mucinous carcinoma. IMC with medullary features is yet another type, with a characteristic syncytial pattern of tumour cells and presence of infiltrating lymphocytes. The gross appearance is very deceptive, due to its fairly well-circumscribed margins. Another benign tumour which can clinically resemble malignancy is the granular cell tumour (GCT). This lesion arises from intralobular breast stroma and occurs within the distribution of the cutaneous branches of the supraclavicular nerve. The light microscopic appearance is quite classic, with the presence of abundant granular cytoplasm. On the other hand, differentiation of glandular epithelium into a nonglandular mesenchymal tissue is called metaplasia. These metaplastic changes include squamous cell, spindle cell, and heterogeneous mesenchymal changes. Sarcomas of the breast, primary or secondary, is yet another class of rare tumours in the breast. Their histology resembles the soft tissue sarcomas at other sites.

Understanding the clinical signs and examination, imaging characteristics, and histopathology of unusual breast masses is essential to achieve accurate diagnoses and for guiding appropriate management strategies, ultimately optimizing patient outcomes.

13.2 Mucinous Carcinoma

Mucinous carcinoma (MC) is also called colloid carcinoma or gelatinous carcinoma of the breast and is a relatively rare subtype of breast cancer, accounting for about 2% of all invasive breast carcinomas [1]. Postmenopausal women, mean age, are more affected.

These are breast neoplasms with mucinous component that comprises >90% of tumour and usually have a favourable prognosis. Based on the cellularity of the tumour, mucinous carcinomas can be divided into two subtypes: (a) the pure type consists of tumour tissue with extracellular mucin production in more than 90% of the tumour and (b) the mixed type or invasive carcinoma with mucinous features containing infiltrating ductal epithelial component without any mucin or mucin less than 90%.

It usually presents as a palpable, soft mass, or as a nonpalpable mammogram detected mass.

13.2.1 Imaging Features

MC can present as equal or low density round or oval mass with circumscribed or microlobulated/partially obscured margins on mammogram (MG) (Fig. 13.1a, b). Tumours with high mucin content can appear as circumscribed or lobulated mass, whereas spiculated or irregular margins may indicate mixed type of tumour [2]. Rarely it can present as isolated architectural distortion. Calcifications can be seen in both forms of MC or when there is an adjacent ductal carcinoma in situ.

Ultrasound (USG) often shows a round or microlobulated mass with complex mixed echogenicity containing solid and cystic components (Fig. 13.1c). The mass can have posterior enhancement with minimal vascularity (Fig. 13.1d). Pure mucinous cancers can be homogenous and isoechoic to the mammary fat. Mixed form is usually heterogenous in echotexture (Fig. 13.1e).

Mucinous cancers show bright, high signal intensity on fat saturated T2WI (Fig. 13.2f) due to the water content in mucin. Variable signal intensity is seen on fat saturated T1WI (Fig. 13.2g) depending upon the protein content and composition. DWI shows lower signal intensity due to plenteous mucin and ADC values are high. DWI can also show high signal intensity (Fig. 13.2h) likely due to the increase in cell density with corresponding ADC showing no signal drop (Fig. 13.2i). After the administration of gadolinium-based contrast agent, MC may show

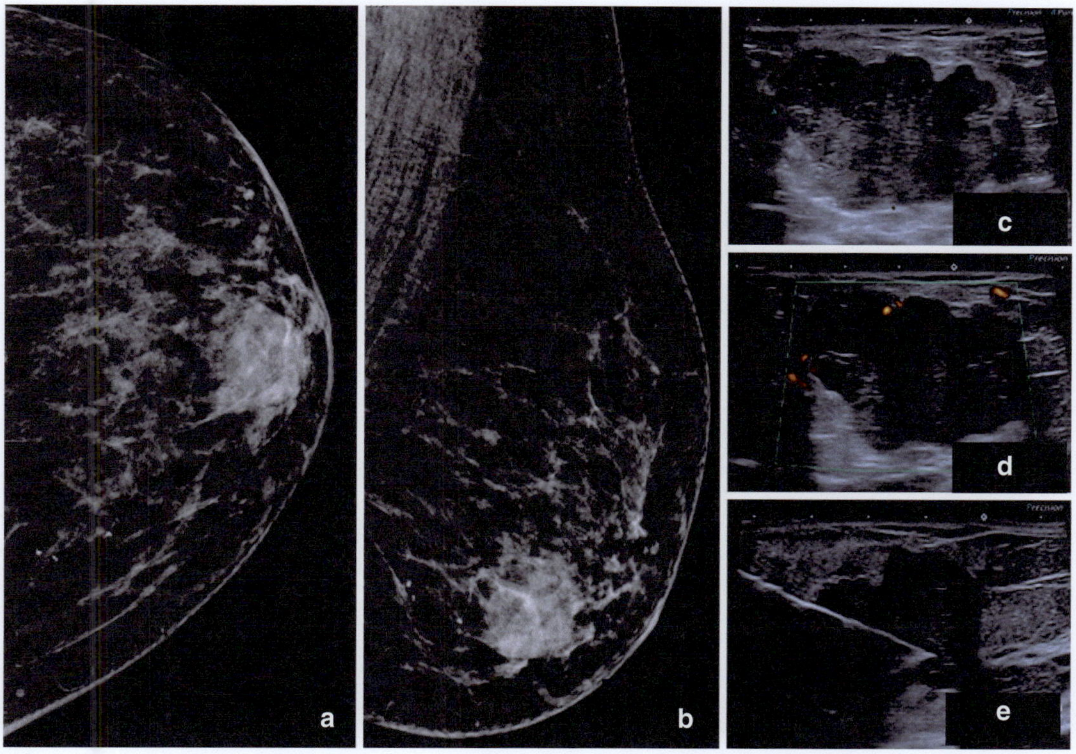

Fig. 13.1 (**a** and **b**) Mammogram: CC & MLO view of the left breast showing an irregular high density mass with partially obscured margins in central lower quadrant. (**c** and **d**) Ultrasound: showing irregular circumscribed mass with macrolobulations and mixed echogenicity, minimal vascularity is seen on colour flow imaging. (**e**) Core biopsy needle in situ Biopsy confirmed it as mixed type mucinous carcinoma

any of the three different enhancement patterns depending upon the mucin content. Pattern one has no evident enhancement when mucin is predominant in tumour; second pattern is seen as a heterogenous enhancement corresponding to island of neoplastic epithelial cells in a puddle of mucin; and the third pattern is seen as rim enhancement (Fig. 13.2j, k) mapping presence of peripheral distribution of tumour cells and central location of mucin [3]. Time-signal intensity curves obtained usually show a gradually enhancing pattern or plateau-type pattern after the initial rise.

13.2.2 Pathology Findings

Gross: Mucinous carcinoma of the breast shows a soft glistening gelatinous mass with pushing margins (Fig. 13.3l). The tumours range in size from less than 1 cm to more than 20 cm (mean = 3 cm).

Histopathology: Mucinous carcinoma is composed of at least 90% of abundant extracellular mucin admixed with invasive neoplastic epithelial cells (Fig. 13.3m).

The mucinous component of a mixed MC will be less than 90% of the tumour. Extensive sampling may be needed to detect the neoplastic epithelium, when there is predominantly mucin. The carcinoma cells of MC are arranged in a variety of patterns, including strands, alveolar nests, papillary and micropapillary clusters, and large cribriform sheets. Most of the MC are well to moderately differentiated. Calcifications associated with MC tend to be coarse and irregular.

Histological subtypes of MC have been classified by Capella et al. [4] into three subtypes: type

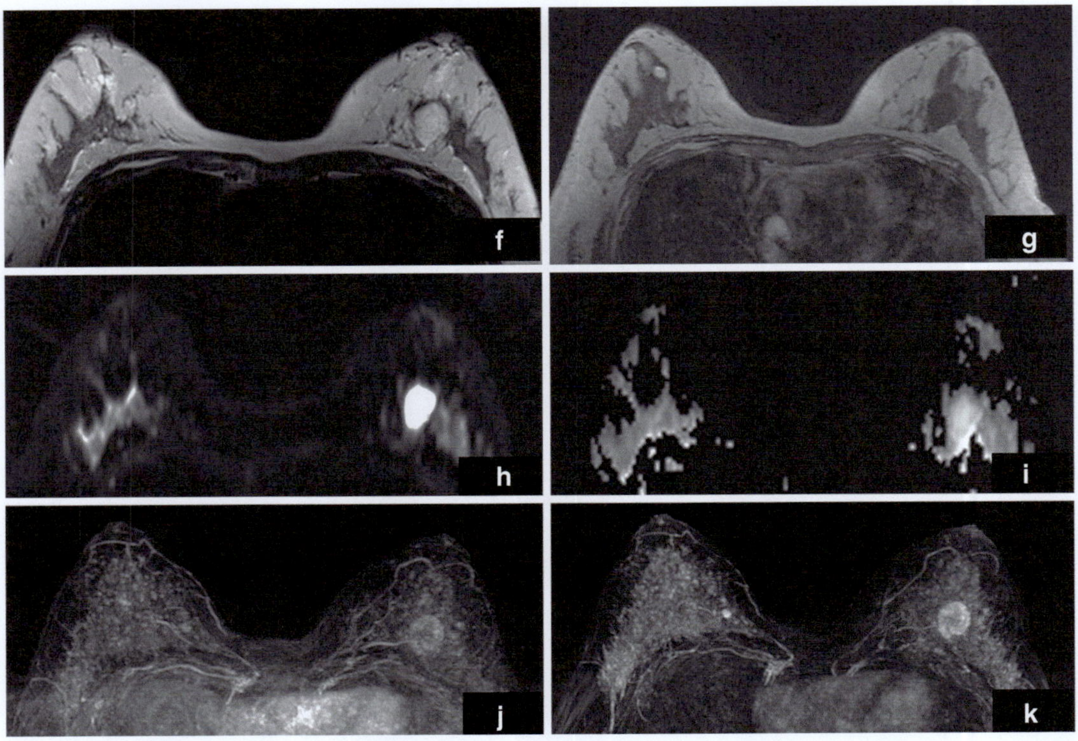

Fig. 13.2 MRI features of mucinous carcinoma of the breast T2W (**f**), T1W (**g**), DWI (**h**), ADC (**i**), MIP Early (**j**), and MIP late postcontrast (**k**) images showing an irregular T2W hyperintense mass and hypo- to isointense on T1W images, with facilitated diffusion and slow filling in contrast from the periphery to the centre of the mass, suggestive of a mucinous tumour

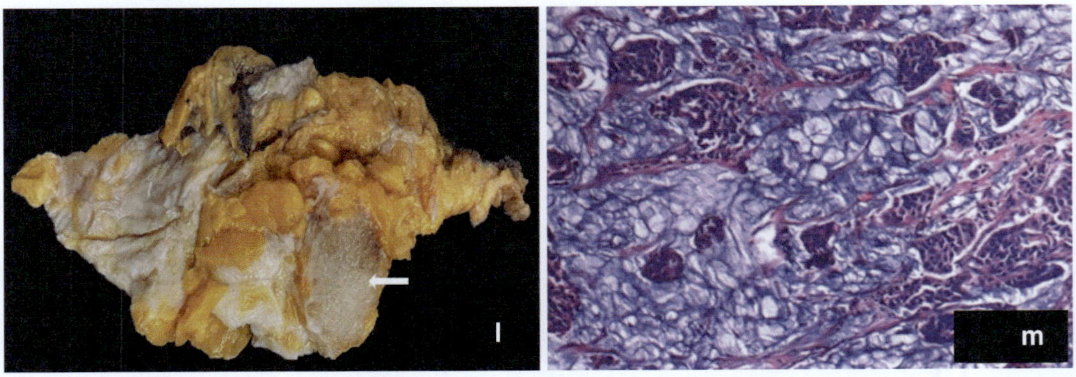

Fig. 13.3 (**l**) Cut surface of the excision biopsy specimen showing glistening and gelatinous appearance of the tumour. (**m**) H&E stain (x200) show tumou cells floating in pools of mucin

A is characterized by abundant extracellular mucin with epithelium seen in trabeculae and ribbons or festoons; type B has less-abundant extracellular mucin and consists of "clumps" of cells with intracytoplasmic mucin and often granular cytoplasm; and type AB shows indeterminate features. Some authors consider type B to be having endocrine differentiation.

There may be some rare variants like micropapillary variant, which shows tumour cells arranged in small clusters, and may have psammomatous calcifications. At times the cells may have a signet ring morphology. The MC may also be seen associated with solid papillary carcinoma,which are usually type B.

Immunohistochemistry: Typically, MC shows positive expression for oestrogen and progesterone receptors, while androgen receptors are expressed at a low level, and HER 2 is not amplified.

Microscopic differential diagnosis includes mucocele-like lesion, nodular mucinosis, and metastatic mucinous carcinoma.

13.2.3 Management and Prognosis

Surgery followed by hormone therapy in hormone-responsive (ER/PR) tumours is often the management approach for MC along with axillary staging by sentinel lymph node biopsy and administration of adjuvant radiotherapy and hormone therapy after breast conservation [5].

Since most mucinous carcinomas are negative for the protein HER2/neu, they are not treated with trastuzumab [6]. Mucinous breast cancer carries a favourable prognosis with a low recurrence rate and a low incidence of lymph node metastasis. Pure mucinous carcinoma has a relatively good prognosis and lower incidence of axillary nodal metastasis [7].

13.3 Invasive Breast Carcinoma of no Special Type with Medullary Pattern

This is another rare type of breast carcinoma constituting less than 5% of all invasive breast carcinomas [8]. The mean age ranges between 45 and 54 years [9]. They rarely affect the male breast. To diagnose a mass lesion as this histological variant, unique stern criteria have been set which includes complete circumscription, the syncytial growth pattern of at least 75% of the tumour, intermediate to high nuclear grade, an associated diffuse lymphocytic infiltrate, and a lack of intraductal components or glandular differentiation. WHO updated the classification of medullary carcinoma under an umbrella term of "carcinomas with medullary features," in 2012. These also include atypical medullary carcinoma and invasive carcinoma of no special type with medullary features [10].

Invasive ductal carcinoma with medullary features are known to be associated with BRCA1 gene mutation [11]. However, not all BRCA 1 mutated cancers are likely to be medullary cancers. Among BRCA1-associated breast cancers, 7.8–19% are medullary carcinomas, and 35–60% show the presence of medullary features [12].

They typically present as a soft palpable rapidly growing mass which mimic fibroadenoma on physical examination.

13.3.1 Imaging Features

These cancers are seen as circumscribed round, oval or macro lobulated, and equal or high density masses (Fig. 13.4a, b) on MG, just like fibroadenomas. Calcifications are usually not found in these well-defined masses [13].

On USG, the features are similar to mammogram—round or lobulated well-circumscribed hypoechoic mass with posterior enhancement [14] (Fig. 13.4c). Internal vascularity on colour doppler may be noted [15]. Posterior enhancement is more likely seen in medullary carcinoma then fibroadenomas; however, biopsy is mandatory for final diagnosis and for management decision. MRI reveals round, oval, or lobular mass with smooth margin showing rim enhancement with or without enhancing internal septation as a common feature [16]. Homogeneous or heterogeneous internal enhancement with delayed peripheral enhancement after contrast administration can also be seen [14, 16]. These features are present consistently, yet they are not specific for medullary cancer and can be noted in benign as well as other types of cancers [14, 16]. Dynamic contrast-enhanced MRI may show a rapid initial rise with a plateau or washout.

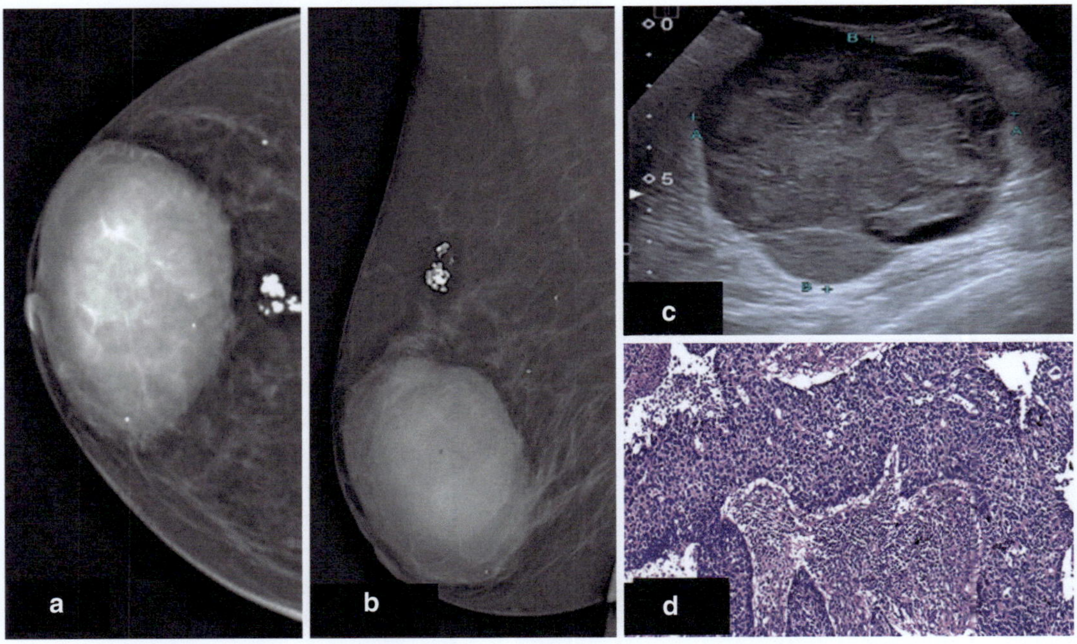

Fig. 13.4 (**a** and **b**) Mammogram: CC and MLO view showing an oval high density mass with circumscribed margins in subareolar region of the right breast. Two focal microcalcifications are seen within the mass. Coarse popcorn calcification seen adjacent to mass. (**c**) Ultrasound shows an oval circumscribed parallelly oriented heterogeneously hypoechoic mass with posterior acoustic enhancement in the subareolar region of the right breast. (**d**) Light microscopy shows sheets of tumour cells with a lymphoplasmacytic infiltrate (H&Ex200)

13.3.2 Pathology

Gross: This variant is a moderately firm and discrete tumour, which resembles a fibroadenoma. A distinct margin can be made out at the edge of the tumour. The cut surface of the tumour has a lobulated or nodular architecture, sometimes with haemorrhage and necrosis.

Histopathology: For microscopic features, criteria set by Ridolfi et al. [17] are important for a diagnosis and all the criteria should fit in. These criteria include prominent lymphoplasmacytic infiltrate, noninvasive microscopic circumscription, and growth in sheets—syncytial pattern (Fig. 13.4d), poorly defined nuclear grade, and a high mitotic rate. If some of these features are not seen, it is termed as infiltrating ductal carcinoma with medullary features.

A syncytial growth pattern refers to the formation of broad, irregular sheets, or islands of tumour cells, with indistinct cell borders. It may give the appearance of a poorly differentiated squamous cell carcinoma.

At least 75% of the tumour should show a syncytial pattern, for fitting in this category.

The lymphoplasmacytic reaction usually is seen at the periphery and also should be present diffusely in the substance of the tumour. At times, there is also an admixture of neutrophils, eosinophils, and monocytes, especially when there is a presence of necrosis or cystic degeneration.

Immunohistochemistry: These tumours are most often negative for oestrogen and progesterone receptors and HER 2neu with variable expression of keratins 5/6 and 14, smooth muscle actin, EGFR, P-cadherin, p53, and caveolin-1. They have a high Ki-67 proliferation index.

Microscopic differential diagnosis includes lymphoma in the breast, Epstein-Barr virus (EBV)-associated lymphoepithelial like carcinoma and undifferentiated ductal carcinoma.

13.3.3 Management and Prognosis

The treatment of typical or atypical medullary breast carcinoma is identical to invasive ductal carcinoma which includes modified or radical mastectomy along with radiation or chemotherapy, depending on the stage of the cancer [18]. Tumours of size 3 cm or smaller are treated by breast conservative surgery followed by adjuvant radiation.

Despite its histopathologically highly malignant characteristics, these tumours carry a favourable prognosis and lower risk of nodal involvement as compared with the more common IDC-NOS. The extensive presence of a dense lymphoplasmacytic response may prevent it from growing and spreading quickly.

Patients whose tumours are larger than 3 cm or who have four or more involved lymph nodes have high recurrence rates that are not appreciably different from the recurrence rates of patients with usual IDC.

13.4 Granular Cell Tumour of the Breast

Granular cell tumour (GCT) is a soft tissue tumour with neuroectodermal differentiation [19]. GCT was originally named granular cell myoblastoma, but currently, it is considered to be neural in origin according to immunohistochemical studies [20]. Granular cell tumour accounts for 0.5% of all soft tissue tumours [21] which commonly affects peripheral soft tissues (38%), trunk (36%), upper limbs, head, and neck. Tongue is the most common location in the head and neck region. In around 5–6% of cases, GCT is observed in the breast, where it can be clinically and radiologically confused with a malignant breast tumour [19]. GCT of the breast arises from intralobular breast stroma and occurs within the distribution of the cutaneous branches of the supraclavicular nerve. It usually presents as a solitary nontender nodule but not uncommonly is multifocal and may present as a part of a multicentric disease.

It is an uncommon tumour of the breast in premenopausal women presenting as a painless lump. The tumour is often found in the upper inner quadrant unlike breast cancer that is found in the upper outer quadrant.

13.4.1 Imaging Features

Mammogram may present with features simulating malignancy like irregular iso- to hyperdense mass showing noncircumscribed spiculated margins. Rarely focal skin thickening and local invasion into pectoralis muscle can be seen [22, 23]. Sometimes the mass/nodule may appear well defined or solid circumscribed.

Ultrasound is usually nonspecific with features more inclined toward malignancy, like heterogenic irregular mass with ill-defined margins. Vascularity and posterior acoustic shadowing may or may not be present. It may present as a solid well-circumscribed mass/nodule (Fig. 13.5a) with the presence of anisotropy, a very specific feature. This is present due to the of fibrillary composition and varies according to the angle of ultrasound used to image the mass [24]. Contrast-enhanced ultrasound (CEUS) can prove helpful in exhibiting benign features in GCT [25].

It is almost invisible on T2-weighted sequences, showing low to intermediate signals on T1 weighted images. After the administration of gadolinium, variable enhancement patterns are noted. Rim enhancement and irregular margins may be noted. Either type 1 or type 3 dynamic time kinetic curves can be seen. Benign and malignant GCT can be differentiated on PET. Hoess et al. stated in their series that a benign GCT shows an uptake value of 1.8 which is less than the cut-off value of 2.5 of malignant masses [26].

13.4.2 Pathology

Histopathology: It shows the presence of characteristic large polygonal cells with abundant eosinophilic cytoplasm (Fig. 13.6b). There are

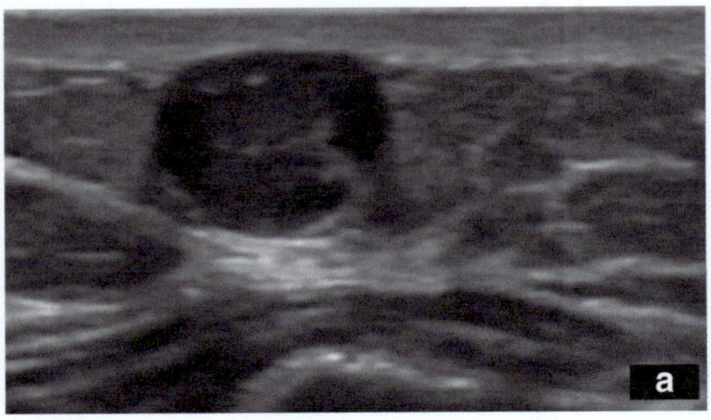

Fig. 13.5 (**a**) Ultrasound features of granular cell tumour: Round circumscribed hypoechoic parallelly oriented mass with no obvious posterior features seen in the upper inner quadrant of the right breast

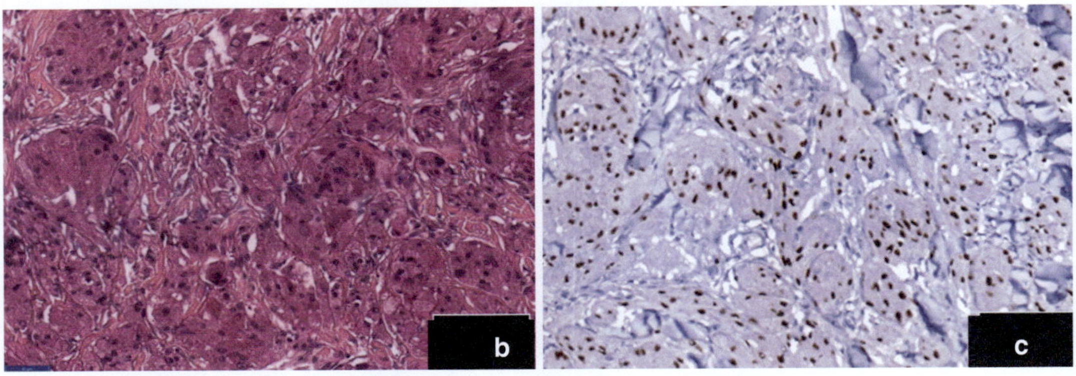

Fig. 13.6 (**b**) Light microscopy showing the tumour cells with abundant eosinophilic granular cells (H&Ex200). (**c**) Immunohistochemical stain showing SOX 10 nuclear positivity in the tumour cells (IHCx200)

six histological parameters to distinguish benign from malignant granular cell tumours. This includes the presence of necrosis, spindling of the nuclei, vesicular nuclei with large nucleoli, increased mitotic activity (>2mitosis/10 high power field), high nuclear to cytoplasmic ratio, and nuclear pleomorphism [27, 28].

Immunohistochemistry: Multiple granular cell tumours may be seen in the context of LEOPARD syndrome, due to a mutation in the PTPN11 gene. Immunohistochemical staining for S100, SOX 10 (Fig. 13.6c), and CD 68 are known to be 100% positive.

13.4.3 Management and Prognosis

Surgical excision with a clean margin is the best treatment for this tumour and patient recovers and responds well to the surgery. Poor prognostic factors associated with malignant granular cell tumour (MGCT) include large tumour size, older patient age, increased mitotic activity, and Ki-67 labelling index greater than 10% [29].

13.5 Metaplastic Carcinoma of the Breast

Most benign and malignant tumours of the breast arise from glandular epithelium. However, in some cases, glandular epithelium differentiates into a nonglandular mesenchymal tissue, and this process is called metaplasia [30]. Metaplastic changes include squamous cell, spindle cell, and heterogeneous mesenchymal changes which occur in less than 5% of breast carcinomas [31, 32].

13.5.1 Imaging Features

The mammogram, ultrasound, and MRI imaging characteristics of metaplastic breast carcinomas can be similar to invasive ductal carcinoma as

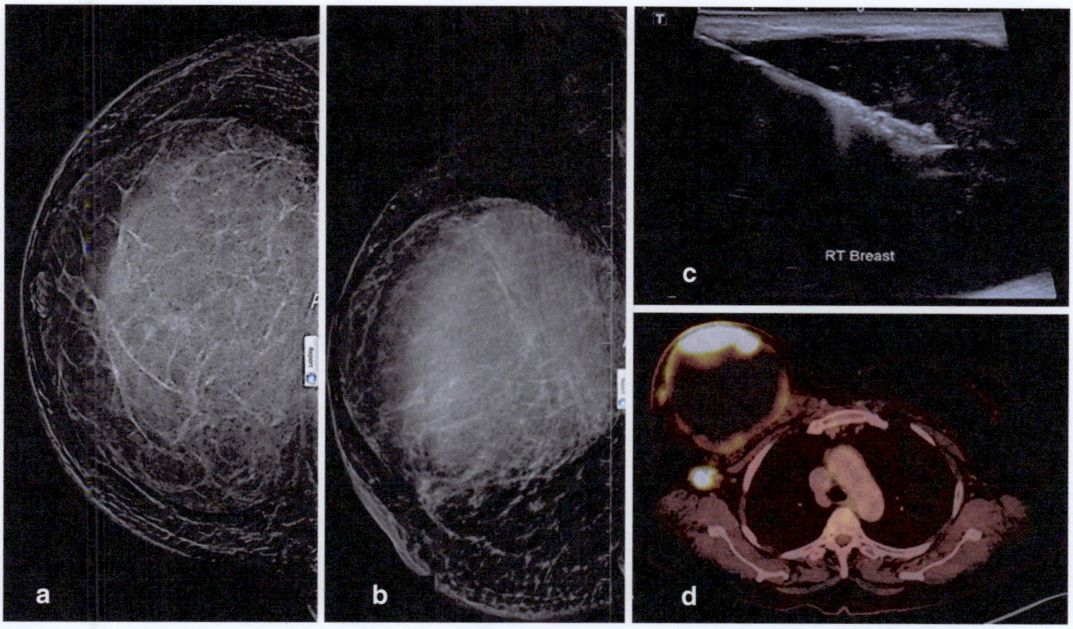

Fig. 13.7 (**a** and **b**) Mammogram: CC and MLO view showing a large round high density mass with circumscribed margins occupying almost the entire right breast. (**c**) Ultrasound shows an oval well-circumscribed solid cystic mass with posterior acoustic enhancement, core biopsy needle seen in situ. (**d**) PET CT: showing the increased uptake in the solid part of the tumour with an uptake in the ipsilateral enlarge axillary lymph node

well as benign masses, leading to misinterpretation [32].

On mammogram, these tumours usually present as circumscribed dense masses (Fig. 13.7a, b). Microcalcifications can be observed in 25% of the cases, with greater frequency in the carcinoma with chondroid metaplasia [33]. These may appear as complex cystic solid masses (Fig. 13.7c) on USG, some showing gentle lobulations. Posterior acoustic enhancement is seen commonly due to cystic component caused due to necrosis [34].

These can present as a round or lobular mass with smooth margins on MRI, which commonly shows high signal intensity on T2-weighted images due to necrotic component and cystic degeneration [35]. The reported enhancement patterns of these lesions include heterogeneous, rim-like, or as nonenhancing internal components. The commonly seen kinetic pattern is early enhancement and a delayed washout.

Differential diagnosis of high T2 signal are mucinous carcinoma, invasive ductal carcinoma with infarction or necrosis, intracystic papillary carcinoma, and invasive papillary carcinoma, in addition to metaplastic breast carcinoma.

PET CT shows increased uptake in the solid part of the tumour (Fig. 13.7d).

13.5.2 Pathology

Gross: These tumours are often firm, well circumscribed, and solid. The cut surface has a pearly, white to greyish, and glistening surface in areas of squamous and chondroid differentiation. The mean size is 3.9 cm, ranging from 2 cm to >10 cm.

Histopathology: The diagnosis is mainly by histopathological examination and morphology is usually heterogenous. These can be purely epithelial-only carcinomas, pure (monophasic) sarcomatoid carcinomas, and biphasic epithelial and sarcomatoid carcinomas (Fig. 13.8e, f). The epithelial-only carcinomas include low-grade adenosquamous carcinoma, high-grade adenosquamous carcinoma, and pure squamous cell

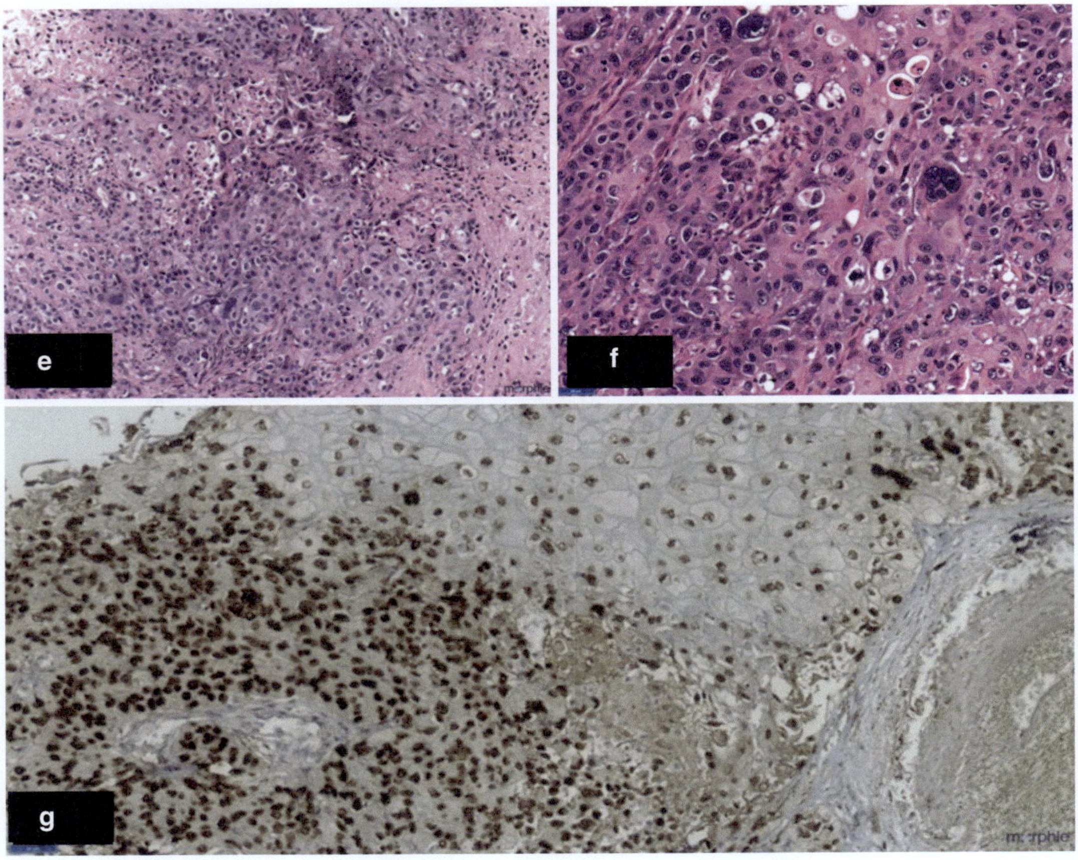

Fig. 13.8 (**e**) Metaplastic carcinoma with tumour showing marked pleomorphism and squamoid areas (H&E x200). (**f**) Tumour cells showing squamoid morphology with marked nuclear pleomorphism and bizarre giant cells (H&Ex400). (**g**) Tumour cells showing nuclear positivity for P63 (IHCx400)

carcinoma. The pure (monophasic) sarcomatoid carcinomas include fibromatosis like metaplastic carcinoma and spindle cell carcinoma.

Heterologous mesenchymal components may be included like chondroid, osseous, rhabdomyosarcomatous, angiosarcomatous, liposarcomatous, and neuroglial differentiation or in combination. Mesenchymal component can show a wide spectrum of atypia, ranging from minimal atypia to frankly malignant.

Immunohistochemistry: In difficult situations where the epithelial component cannot be demonstrated, immunohistochemical stains like broad-spectrum keratins like AE1/AE 3, CAM 5.2, 34 beta E12, and high molecular weight keratin like CK5/CK6 and CK 14 may be useful. P63 is another marker which is positive in 77% cases (Fig. 13.8g). ER, PR, HER 2, CD 34, Desmin, and SMA is usually negative.

The differential diagnosis includes phyllodes tumour, primary breast sarcoma, metastatic sarcoma, and adenomyoepithelioma.

13.5.3 Management and Prognosis

It is of utmost importance to differentiate metaplastic breast cancer from invasive ductal carcinoma and primary breast sarcoma to decide the correct treatment and management [36].

Preoperative diagnosis of metaplastic breast carcinoma is quite difficult by core needle biopsy as in most cases, transition foci of metaplastic element usually is found after excision biopsy. Hence excision biopsy is preferred to avoid misleading diagnosis from core biopsy sample [37].

The biological behaviour of this tumour varies from low to high grade. These tend to have large tumour size, less nodal involvement, and higher American Joint Committee on Cancer (AJCC) stage. There is a poor response to neoadjuvant systemic therapy with pathology complete response (pCR) rate of ~10–17%.

13.6 Sarcomas of the Breast

These are heterogenous group of malignant tumours of mesenchymal origin accounting for 1% of malignant breast tumours and <5% of all sarcomas [38]. They can be either *primary sarcomas* (spontaneous) occurring sporadically or *secondary sarcomas*, which occur as a sequalae to breast cancer treatments like external beam radiation and chronic lymphedema.

Angiosarcomas are the most common subtype of sarcomas, estimated at 20–30% of primary breast sarcomas and 50–70% of secondary breast sarcomas [39].

Other common subtypes include *malignant fibrous histiocytoma* and *fibrosarcoma*. These are aggressive tumours with poor prognosis because of local recurrence and early development of hematogenous distant metastasis.

Primary and secondary breast sarcomas usually present as a solitary, rapidly enlarging breast lump, with pain in 7–21% patients [40]. Associated skin thickening and nipple retraction can be seen, especially with angiosarcomas, which are more infiltrative. Sarcomas tend to grow larger than primary carcinomas with a median size of approximately 5 cm [41].

Primary angiosarcoma of the breast (PAB) is a much rarer variant that occurs sporadically among young women in their third and fourth decade with no known risk factors [42]. Secondary angiosarcomas of the breast on the contrary occur frequently in elderly women in their sixth and seventh decade, associated with the risk factor of radiation therapy postbreast conservation surgery. An average latency period of about 7–10 years has been observed between the radiation therapy and the development of secondary angiosarcoma [42].

13.6.1 Imaging Features

Imaging findings in sarcoma vary and may depend on histologic subtype. Mammogram may show equal to hyperdense mass with well-defined or ill-defined margins (Fig. 13.9a) or architectural distortion without associated calcifications. Mass may rarely give soap bubble appearance on mammogram. About 19% of the angiosarcomas have negative mammogram [41]. These are seen as hypoechoic to heteroechoic, round, oval, or irregular (Fig. 13.9b) mass with indistinct margins, internal vascularity (Fig. 13.9c), and variable posterior features on USG. Tumour can also present as a complex solid cystic mass [43] surrounded by adjacent tubular structures—vessels [44] on ultrasound. Diffuse oedema and overlying skin thickening may also be present. Large vessels with turbulent flow may be seen within the mass.

Lymph nodes are not involved as the tumour tends to metastasize hematogenously rather than through lymphatics.

MRI features include heterogeneous mass which is usually hypointense on T1-weighted and hyperintense on T2-weighted images. Large anastomotic vascular spaces containing slow flowing blood give high signal intensity on T2-weighted images. T1-weighted images may show hyperintense foci due to intratumoural haematoma or haemorrhagic nature of tumour. High-grade tumours show more rapid enhancement (Fig. 13.10d, e) with washout kinetics (Fig. 13.10f) in dynamic contrast-enhanced MRI. Most frequently type 1 kinetic curve is noted [45].

13.6.2 Pathology

Gross: Most of the sarcomas range in size from 1 to 20 cm with majority being more than 2 cm; average size is 5 cm. Central portion of tumour

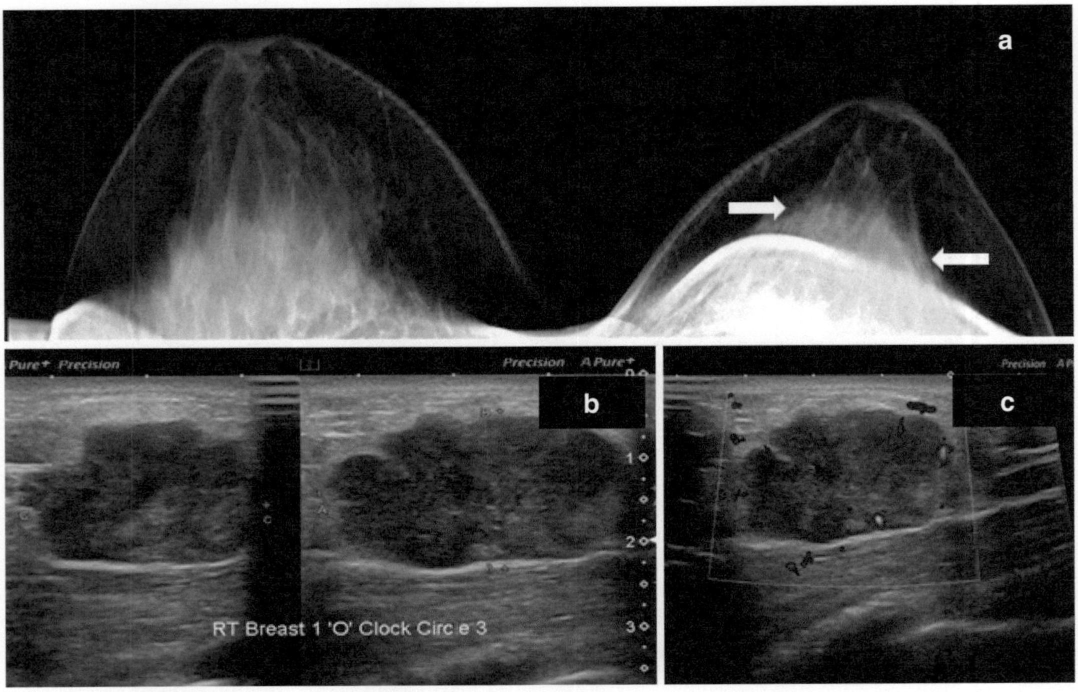

Fig. 13.9 (**a**) Mammogram: Cleavage view showing a high density irregular mass (white arrows), posterior border of the mass is not seen clearly. (**b** and **c**) Ultrasound: showing irregular circumscribed mass with internal vascularity, seen abutting the pectoralis major muscle

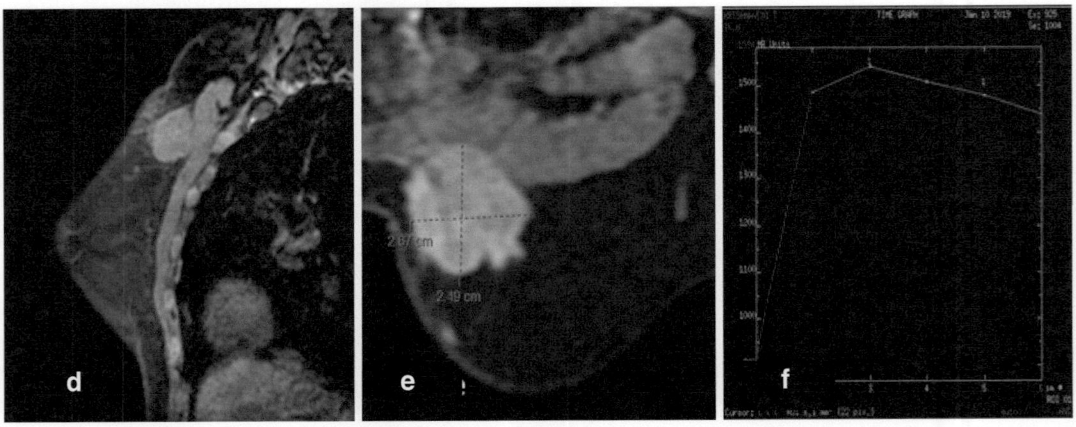

Fig. 13.10 (**d** and **e**) Contrast-enhanced MRI shows intensely enhancing mass abutting the pectoralis. (**f**) Postcontrast time kinetic curve showing rapid enhancement with type 3 curve

may be haemorrhagic, myxoid, or calcified or may show lipomatous changes with firm to hard areas on palpation. Infiltrative periphery of tumour can blend into surrounding tissue and may not be visible. Necrosis may or may not be present depending on the pathological type of sarcoma.

Histopathology: Angiosarcoma: This is characterized by abnormal, anastomosing vascular channels (Fig. 13.11a) with infiltrative borders and is usually not well circumscribed. In poorly differentiated tumours, solid areas without evident vessel formation may be present. Blood lakes due to massive extravasation from tumour

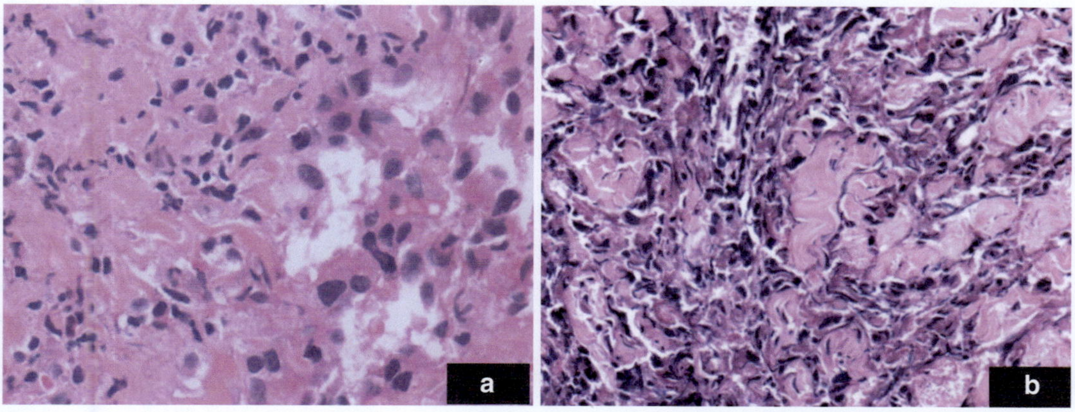

Fig. 13.11 (**a**) Tumour cells forming vascular channels with atypical mitoses H&E X200. (**b**) Highly pleomorphic tumour cells with lumen formation H&E X200

vessels are helpful diagnostic features. Tumour cells are abnormal in appearance with pleomorphic nuclei and frequent mitotic figures (Fig. 13.11b).

Liposarcoma: All grades of liposarcomas reported arising in breast have been primary tumour. Low-grade tumours and myxoid variants are commoner than pleomorphic variant in most series, and the low-grade tumours have more favourable outcome compared with pleomorphic variants. The tumour cells include lipoblasts and other atypical appearing adipocytic cells. Liposarcomatous heterologous differentiation can be seen more often in phyllodes tumour rather than in primary sarcomas. Diagnosis of primary liposarcoma of breast is one of exclusion and must be distinguished from lipomas.

Leiomyosarcoma (LMS) [5]: These tumours show intersecting bundles of spindle cells with eosinophilic cytoplasm and elongated nuclei with blunt ends and varying degrees of pleomorphism with mitotic activity. Morphologic and immunohistochemical findings are similar to LMS arising in other sites. Immunohistochemistry shows positivity for keratin in some tumours.

Extraskeletal osteogenic sarcoma (OGS): Extraskeletal OGS rarely arises in the breast. All histologic variants, including fibroblastic, osteoblastic, chondroblastic, and telangiectatic, have been reported. It is a high-grade, mitotically active tumour which tends to have worse outcome. Extraskeletal OGS of the breast is diagnosis of exclusion. Osteogenic differentiation can be seen in metaplastic carcinoma or phyllodes tumour and may be prominent.

Pleomorphic spindle cell sarcoma: Some tumours in this category have been classified as fibrosarcomas or malignant fibrous histiocytoma. It is a malignant spindle cell proliferation arranged in herringbone or storiform pattern. These tumours tend to be high grade with frequent mitotic activity and areas of necrosis. These may arise at sites of prior breast radiation. It is important to exclude metaplastic carcinoma and malignant phyllode tumour. Tumour cells should be cytokeratin negative (including high molecular weight keratins) and p63 negative.

Sarcomas in adolescents and children: Rarely rhabdomyosarcomas and synovial sarcomas can involve the breast in younger patients. This may represent primary or metastatic disease. Primary tumours are usually alveolar rhabdomyosarcoma on histopathology.

Immunohistochemistry:

Lineage-specific markers are helpful to identify the specific types of sarcoma. For angiosarcoma, the vascular markers are positive; for leiomyosarcoma, the smooth muscle markers (smooth muscle actin, desmin, caldesmon); for rhabdomyosarcoma, the skeletal muscle markers (desmin, myogenin, myoglobin); and S100 in malignant peripheral nerve sheath tumours. Keratins are used to exclude carcinomas.

Differential Diagnosis on Pathology: Metaplastic carcinoma: Subsets of these carcinomas show feature characteristic of myoepithelial cells. Most of them show spindle cell morphology with or without a squamous differentiation with matrix (basement membrane) formation. The matrix can resemble cartilage or osteoid. Extensive sampling to detect areas of epithelial differentiation and/or DCIS can help exclude sarcoma. Panel of immune stains for cytokeratin (particularly high molecular weight) and P 63 are important to help in confirming the diagnosis.

Phyllode tumour: High-grade phyllode tumours can have areas of heterologous differentiation like liposarcoma, rhabdomyosarcoma, or osteogenic sarcoma. Extensive sampling looking for biphasic pattern can help to identify phyllode tumour.

Fibromatosis occurs more commonly in the breast than sarcomas. This can invade into normal tissue, into skeletal muscle, and around nerves. Minimal nuclear pleomorphism and absence of mitoses distinguish fibromatosis from sarcoma.

Nodular fasciitis: These are usually seen in superficial location or in muscle fascia. Cells have haphazard arrangement whereas malignant spindle cell tumours usually grow in organized fascicular patterns. Minimal to no nuclear pleomorphism with fine chromatin and atypical mitotic figures should not be seen.

Dermatofibrosarcoma protuberans: These are spindle cell neoplasms arising in dermis and infiltrating into subcutaneous tissue. Dermal-based lesions can invade into the breast. Spindle cells are arranged in storiform pattern with minimal pleomorphism and rare mitoses.

Myofibroblastoma: Benign neoplastic proliferation of myofibroblasts with minimal nuclear pleomorphism does not infiltrate around normal breast epithelium.

Secondary sarcoma arising after radiation: The most common is angiosarcoma and undifferentiated sarcomas. Postradiation angiosarcomas usually occur on an average of six years following radiation to breast or and chest wall as skin lesions with ecchymosis, with or without ulcers [46]. The criteria for defining post-radiation sarcoma is histological confirmation of sarcoma and prior history of radiotherapy.
Secondary sarcoma arising in setting of chronic lymphedema: Chronic oedema increases risk of sarcoma at multiple sites. In Stewart-Treves syndrome, one of the components is angiosarcoma of edematous arm. Lymphedema-associated lymphangiosarcoma very rarely can also occur.

13.7 Inflammatory Breast Cancer

Inflammatory breast cancer (IBC) is an unusual and aggressive clinicopathologic variety of breast cancer. This form of invasive breast cancer presents clinically as a sudden localized increase in warmth, erythema, and breast oedema. This condition can be extremely painful and have a protracted morbidity [47]. A wide range of additional nonspecific symptoms may also be present, which might result in a delayed diagnosis and unsuccessful treatment [48]. Clinical characteristics include induration and increased volume of the affected breast with a palpable ridge at the borders of induration, elevated warmth, discomfort, pain, and peau d'orange, or cutaneous oedema [49]. The nonspecific findings often lacking an underlying palpable or image detected mass, with the biopsy diagnosis of invasive cancer, are considered in the diagnostic criteria set forth by the American Joint Committee on Cancer [50]. A previously normal breast developing cancer is referred to as primary inflammatory breast cancer. The development of inflammatory skin alterations in a breast affected by invasive cancer or following noninflammatory breast cancer surgery is known as secondary inflammatory breast cancer [51].

13.7.1 Imaging Features

Mammogram may show diffusely increased breast density, with or without a mass, calcifications, and/or parenchymal deformation, diffuse oedema, widespread skin, and trabecular thickening (Fig. 13.12a, b). Suboptimal tissue compression can cause masses and other features seem unclear on mammography [52].

On ultrasound, the increase in the breast parenchyma's echogenicity resulting from tissue oedema, ill-defined masses or areas of parenchymal distortion, and thickened Coopers ligaments can be seen (Fig. 13.12c, d). An additional important indicator of inflammation is breast hyperaemia or increased vascularization of the breast tissues [53].

The difficulty of locating the main breast lesion using ultrasound in order to enable core needle biopsy may increase in cases with diffuse tissue oedema and parenchymal architectural distortion. Sonography is useful for assessing the regional nodes and for planning biopsy (Fig. 13.12e) in patients with detectable masses [54]. The best imaging method for identifying primary breast parenchymal lesions in IBC patients is magnetic resonance imaging (MRI). Skin thickening and parenchymal abnormalities are better visualized on MRI. Thicker skin and parenchyma on MRI may provide helpful details for the diagnosis of inflammatory breast cancer [55]. The MRI characteristics of inflammatory breast cancer include several tiny, confluent, heterogeneously enhancing masses and global skin thickening in the affected breast [56]. In complex circumstances, skin punch biopsies may be guided by MRI. An early assessment with fluorodeoxyglucose PET/CT scan can be helpful as it offers more information on distant metastases or lymph nodes [57].

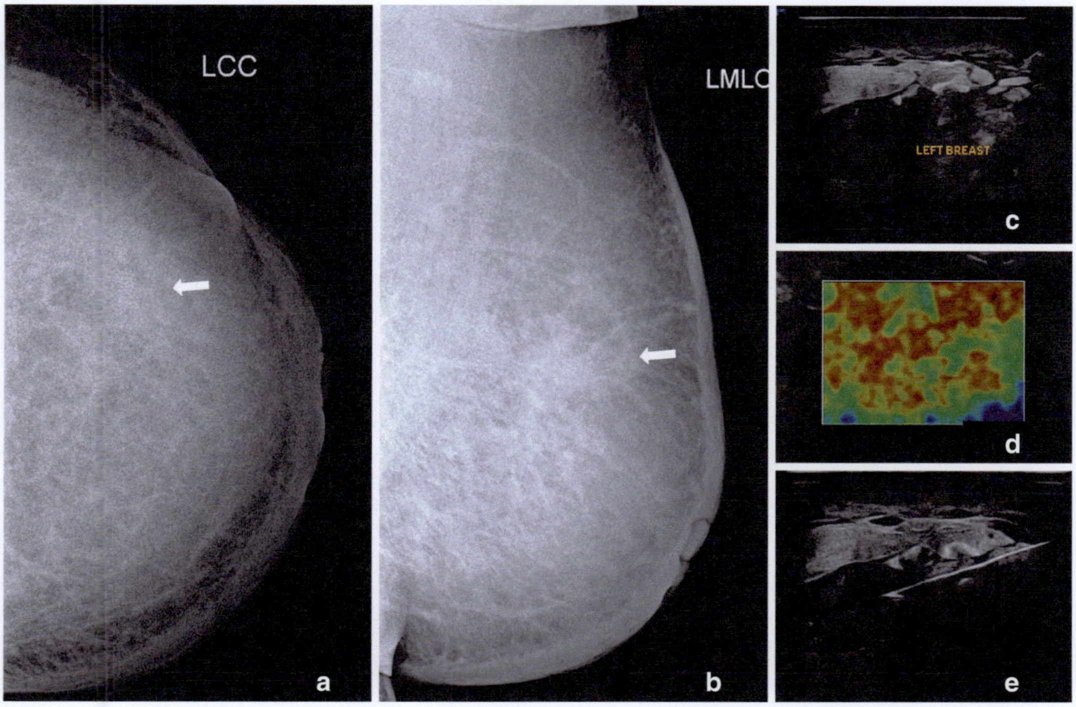

Fig. 13.12 (**a** and **b**) Mammogram: CC and MLO views of the left breast showing diffuse skin thickening with an irregular ill-defined equal density mass with surrounding architectural distortion (white arrows). (**c** and **d**) Ultrasound imaging shows diffuse skin thickening with skin and subcutaneous oedema. Irregular noncircumscribed heterogeneous mass which is hard on elastography. (**e**) Core biopsy needle in situ

13.7.2 Pathology

Histopathology: The first step in diagnosing invasive cancer is obtaining a core needle biopsy. Tumour cell invasion of dermal lymphatics is a characteristic histologic finding in inflammatory breast cancer discovered after skin biopsy [58]. Hormone receptors are often negative and indicate worse prognosis and shorter disease-free lifetime [51].

13.7.3 Management and Prognosis

Neoadjuvant chemotherapy, a mastectomy, and postmastectomy radiation comprise the course of treatment. Using a trimodality strategy (1) systemic treatment, (2) surgery, and (3) radiation therapy, recommended internationally by expert guidelines, should be followed by patients with primary inflammatory breast cancer in order to obtain the greatest local control and survival outcome [58].

Nonmetastatic noninflammatory locally advanced breast cancer (LABC) and nonmetastatic inflammatory breast cancer are treated similarly. Neoadjuvant chemotherapy, axillary dissection, modified radical mastectomy, and postmastectomy radiation treatment are the components of conventional therapy. Neoadjuvant treatment frequently involves chemotherapy regimens based on anthracycline and taxane [51].

Stage IV illness is present in around one-third of individuals with inflammatory breast cancer at the time of diagnosis. Although there is a risk of local advancement, the aim of systemic therapy is to enhance quality of life, improve signs and symptoms, maintain survival, and prolong survival [51].

The prognosis for inflammatory breast cancer is quite poor, and there is a significant chance of an early recurrence. Negative receptor status, the presence of four or more lymph nodes at the time of presentation, and the inability to respond to neoadjuvant treatment are indicators that signify a poor prognosis. Trimodality therapy has resulted in an overall five-year survival rate which currently ranges from 30% to 70% [51].

13.8 Summary

The chapter aimed at highlighting the imaging features of unusual breast cancers which could facilitate planning of further steps like need of biopsy, short-term follow-up or an extra investigation needed. Role of histopathology and immunohistochemistry forms a crucial component of patient management. Rad-path correlation assists in further management of the patient.

Acknowledgement We would like to thank and acknowledge Dr. Seema Sud, Professor, Sr. Consultant, Department of CT & MRI, and Sir Ganga Ram Hospital, New Delhi, for her contribution in the form of images to this chapter.

References

1. Kaoku S, Konishi E, Fujimoto Y, Tohno E, Shiina T, Kondo K, Yamazaki S, Kajihara M, Shinkura N, Yanagisawa A. Sonographic and pathologic image analysis of pure mucinous carcinoma of the breast. Ultrasound Med Biol. 2013;39(7):1158–67.
2. Memis A, Ozdemir N, Parildar M, Ustun EE, Erhan Y. Mucinous (colloid) breast cancer: mammographic and US features with histologic correlation. Eur J Radiol. 2000;35:39–43.
3. Linda A, Zuiani C, Girometti R, et al. Unusual malignant tumors of the breast: MRI features and pathologic correlation. Eur J Radiol. 2010;75:178–84.
4. Capella C, Eusebi V, Mann B, et al. Endocrine differentiation in mucoid carcinoma of the breast. Histopathology. 1980;4:613–30.
5. Barkley CR, Ligibel JA, Wong JS, Lipsitz S, Smith BL, Golshan M. Mucinous breast carcinoma: a large contemporary series. Am J Surg. 2008;196(4):549–51.
6. Garcia Hernandez I, Canavati Marcos M, Garza Montemayor M, Lopez Sotomayor D, Pineda Ochoa D, Gomez Macias GS. Her-2 positive mucinous carcinoma breast cancer, case report. Int J Surg Case Rep. 2018;42:242–6.
7. Zhang L, Jia N, Han L, Yang L, Xu W, Chen W. Comparative analysis of imaging and pathology features of mucinous carcinoma of the breast. Clin Breast Cancer. 2015;15(2):e147–54.
8. Foulkes WD, Smith IE, Reis-Filho JS. Triple-negative breast cancer. N Engl J Med. 2010;363:1938.
9. Foschini MP, Eusebi V. Rare (new) entities of the breast and medullary carcinoma. Pathology. 2009;41:48.
10. Chu Z, Lin H, Liang X, Huang R, Zhan Q, Jiang J, Zhou X. Clinicopathologic characteristics of typical medullary breast carcinoma: a retrospective study of 117 cases. PLoS One. 2014;9:e111493.

11. Jacquemier J, Padovani L, Rabayrol L, Lakhani SR, Penault-Llorca F, Denoux Y, Fiche M, Figueiro P, Maisongrosse V, Ledoussal V, Martinez Penuela J, Udvarhely N, El Makdissi G, Ginestier C, Geneix J, Charafe-Jauffret E, Xerri L, Eisinger F, Birnbaum D, Sobol H. Typical medullary breast carcinomas have a basal/myoepithelial phenotype. J Pathol. 2005;207:260.
12. Pathology of familial breast cancer. Differences between breast cancers in carriers of BRCA1 or BRCA2 mutations and sporadic cases. Breast Cancer Linkage Consortium Lancet. 1997;349(9064):1505–10.
13. Meyer JE, Amin E, Lindfors KK, Lipman JC, Stomper PC, Genest D. Medullary carcinoma of the breast: mammographic and US appearance. Radiology. 1989;170:79.
14. Yoo JL, Woo OH, Kim YK, Cho KR, Yong HS, Seo BK, Kim A, Kang EY. Can MR imaging contribute in characterizing well-circumscribed breast carcinomas? Radiographics: a review publication of the Radiological Society of North America. Inc. 2010;30:1689.
15. Selvi R. Breast diseases: imaging & clinical management. Springer; 2015. https://doi.org/10.1007/978-81-322-2077-0_33.
16. Tominaga J, Hama H, Kimura N, Takahashi S. MR imaging of medullary carcinoma of the breast. Eur J Radiol. 2009;70:525.
17. Ridolfi RL, Rosen PP, Port A, et al. Medullary carcinoma of the breast: a clinicopathologic study with 10 year follow-up. Cancer. 1977;40:1365–85.
18. Eichhorn JH. Medullary carcinoma, provocative now as then. Semin Diagn Pathol. 2004;21:65.
19. Adeniran A, Al-Ahmadie H, Mahoney MC, Robinson-Smith TM. Granular cell tumor of the breast: a series of 17 cases and review of the literature. Breast J. 2004;10(6):528–31. https://doi.org/10.1111/j.1075-122X.2004.21525.x.
20. Abrikossoff AI. Weitere untersuchungen uber myoblastenmyome. Virchows Arch Pathol Anat Physiol Klin Med. 1931;280:723–40.
21. Rose B, Tamvakopoulos GS, Yeung E, Pollock R, Skinner J, Briggs T, et al. Granular cell tumours: a rare entity in the musculoskeletal system. Sarcoma. 2009;2009:765927.
22. Leo C, Briest S, Pilch H, Schütz A, Horn LC, Leinung S. Granular cell tumor of the breast mimicking breast cancer. Eur J Obstet Gynecol Reprod Biol. 2006;127:268–70.
23. Gavriilidis P, Michalopoulou I, Baliaka A, Nikolaidou A. Granular cell breast tumour mimicking infiltrating carcinoma. BMJ Case Rep. 2013;18:2013.
24. Stavros AT. Breast ultrasound. 1st ed. Lippincott Williams & Wilkins; 2004.
25. Wang H, Feng D, Zou T, Liu Y, Wu X, Zou J, Huang R. Contrast-enhanced ultrasound of granular cell tumor in breast: a case report with review of the literature. Front Oncol. 2022;12:894261. https://doi.org/10.3389/fonc.2022.894261.
26. Hoess C, Freitag K, Kolben M, et al. FDG PET evaluation of granular cell tumor of the breast. J Nucl Med. 1998;39:1398–401.
27. Fanburg-Smith JC, Meis-Kindblom JM, Fante R, Kindblom LG. Malignant granular cell tumor of soft tissue: diagnostic criteria and clinicopathologic correlation. Am J Surg Pathol. 1998;22:779–94.
28. Battistella M, Cribier B, Feugeas JP, Roux J, Pelletier F, Pinquier L, et al. Vascular invasion and other invasive features in granular cell tumours of the skin: a multicentre study of 119 cases. J Clin Pathol. 2014;67:19–25.
29. Soukup J, Hadzi-Nikolov D, Ryska A. Dermatofibroma-like granular cell tumour: a potential diagnostic pitfall. Pol J Pathol. 2016;67(3):291–4.
30. Brenner RJ, Turner RR, Schiller V, Arndt RD, Giuliano A. Metaplastic carcinoma of the breast: report of three cases. Cancer. 1998;82:1082–7.
31. Pitts WC, Rojas VA, Gaffey MJ, et al. Carcinomas with metaplasia and sarcomas of the breast. Am J Clin Pathol. 1991;95:623–32.
32. Wargotz ES, Norris HJ. Metaplastic carcinoma of the breast. IV. Squamous cell carcinoma of ductal origin. Cancer. 1990;65:272–6.
33. Oberman HA. Metaplastic carcinoma of the breast. Am J Surg Pathol. 1987;11:918–29.
34. Park JM, Han BK, Moon WK, Choe YH, Ahn SH, Gong G. Metaplastic carcinoma of the breast: mammographic and sonographic findings. J Clin Ultrasound. 2000;28:179–86.
35. Tashjian J, Kuni CC, Bohn LE. Primary squamous cell carcinoma of the breast: mammographic findings. Can Assoc Radiol J. 1989;40:228–9.
36. Evans HA, Shaughnessy EA, Nikiforov YE. Infiltrating ductal carcinoma of the breast with osseous metaplasia: imaging findings with pathologic correlation. AJR. 1999;172:1420–2.
37. Wargotz ES, Deos PH, Norris HJ. Metaplastic carcinoma of the breast. II. Spindle cell carcinoma. Hum Pathol. 1989;20:732–40.
38. Smith TB, Gilcrease MZ, Santiago L, Hunt KK, Yang WT. Imaging features of primary breast sarcoma. Am J Roentgenol. 2012;198(4):W386–93.
39. Yin M, Wang W, Drabick JJ, Harold HA. Prognosis and treatment of non-metastatic primary and secondary breast angiosarcoma: a comparative study. BMC Cancer. 2017;17(1):295.
40. Yang WT, Hennessy BTJ, Dryden MJ, Valero V, Hunt KK, Krishnamurthy S. Mammary angiosarcomas: imaging findings in 24 patients. Radiology. 2007;242(3):725–34.
41. Wienbeck S, Meyer HJ, Herzog A, Nemat S, Teifke A, Heindel W, et al. Imaging findings of primary breast sarcoma: results of a first multicenter study. Eur J Radiol. 2017;88:1–7.
42. Arora TK, Terracina KP, Soong J, Idowu MO, Takabe K. Primary and secondary angiosarcoma of the breast. Gland Surg. 2014;3(1):28–34.
43. Marchant LK, Orel SG, Perez-Jaffe LA, Reynolds C, Schnall MD. Bilateral angiosarcoma of the

breast on MR imaging. AJR Am J Roentgenol. 1997;169:1009–10.
44. Liberman L, Dershaw DD, Kaufman RJ, Rosen PP. Angiosarcoma of the breast. Radiology. 1992;183:649–54.
45. Lee K, Seo KJ, Whang Y. Primary angiosarcoma of the breast: MRI findings. iMRI Investigative Magnetic Resonance Imaging. 2018;22:194–9.
46. Abdou Y, Elkhanany A, Attwood K, et al. Primary and secondary breast angiosarcoma: single center report and a meta-analysis. Breast Cancer Res Treat. 2019;178:523–33. https://doi.org/10.1007/s10549-019-05432-4.
47. Kushwaha AC, Whitman GJ, Stelling CB, Cristofanilli MC, Buzdar AU. Primary inflammatory carcinoma of the breast: retrospective review of mammographic findings. AJR Am J Roentgenol. 2000;174:535–8.
48. Kasales CJ, Han B, Smith JS Jr, Chetlen AL, Kaneda HJ, Shereef S. Nonpuerperal mastitis and subareolar abscess of the breast. AJR Am J Roentgenol. 2014;202:W133–9.
49. Haagensen CD. Diseases of the breast. 2nd ed. Philadelphia: Saunders; 1971. p. 576–84.
50. Green FL, Page DL, Fleming ID, et al. Breast. In: Green FL, Page DL, Fleming ID, et al., editors. AJCC cancer staging manual. 6th ed. New York: Springer; 2003. p. 223–40.
51. Chippa V, Barazi H. Inflammatory breast cancer. In: StatPearls [Internet]. Treasure Island: StatPearls Publishing. p. 2024. Available from: https://www.ncbi.nlm.nih.gov/books/NBK564324/.
52. Yang WT, Le-Petross HT, Macapinlac H, Carkaci S, Gonzalez-Angulo AM, Dawood S, Resetkova E, Hortobagyi GN, Cristofanilli M. Inflammatory breast cancer: PET/CT, MRI, mammography, and sonography findings. Breast Cancer Res Treat. 2008;109:417–26. https://doi.org/10.1007/s10549-007-9671-z.
53. Leong PW, Chotai NC, Kulkarni S. Imaging features of inflammatory breast disorders: a pictorial essay. Korean J Radiol. 2018;19(1):5–14.
54. Barkana BD, El-Sayed A, Khaled RH, Helal M, Khaled H, Deeb R, Pitcher M, Pfeiffer R, Roubidoux M, Schairer C, Soliman AS. Imaging modalities in inflammatory breast cancer (IBC) diagnosis: a computer-aided diagnosis system using bilateral mammography images. Sensors (Basel). 2022;23(1):64. https://doi.org/10.3390/s23010064.
55. Lee KW, Chung SY, Yang I, Kim HD, Shin SJ, Kim JE, Chung BW, Choi JA. Inflammatory breast cancer: imaging findings. Clin Imaging. 2005;29:22–5.
56. Le-Petross HT, Cristofanilli M, Carkaci S, Krishnamurthy S, Jackson EF, Harrell RK, Reed BJ, Yang WT. MRI features of inflammatory breast cancer. AJR Am J Roentgenol. 2011;197(4):W769–76.
57. Sager S, Asa S, Doner RK, Leblebici C, Halac M. Initial evaluation of inflammatory breast cancer with fluorodeoxyglucose positron emission tomography. Indian J Nucl Med. 2012;27(1):33–4.
58. Dawood S, Merajver SD, Viens P, Vermeulen PB, Swain SM, Buchholz TA, Dirix LY, Levine PH, Lucci A, Krishnamurthy S, Robertson FM, Woodward WA, Yang WT, Ueno NT, Cristofanilli M. International expert panel on inflammatory breast cancer: consensus statement for standardized diagnosis and treatment. Ann Oncol. 2011;22(3):515–23.

Imaging in Special Clinical Scenarios

14

Palak Thakkar Popat, Soujanya Mynalli, and Aparna Katdare

Abstract

Breast cancer detection is often challenging in certain clinical scenarios such as young age, pregnancy, lactation, and high-risk genetic profile. Not only the risk is higher, some of these cohorts are associated with more aggressive disease warranting early detection and intervention. Special care needs to be given to detection, appropriate locoregional and distant staging, treatment, and posttreatment surveillance.

Keywords

Young · Pregnancy · Bilateral · Synchronous Metachronous breast cancer

14.1 Introduction

Breast cancer (BC) encompasses a spectrum of malignancies with distinct entities which have variable demographics and histopathology. Its ease in diagnosis in middle age and elderly women with spiculated masses and pleomorphic microcalcifications contradicts the increasing complexities in special scenarios such as morphologic misinterpretation of triple-negative cancers from fibroepithelial lesions and added challenges of breast density masking detection of malignancies in young, pregnant, and lactating women. In this chapter, we shall encompass these special scenarios to enhance understanding and skills in early detection of breast cancer and its management in such cases.

14.2 Breast Cancer in Young Females

Among women with BC, 'young women' is defined as those diagnosed with BC at an age under 40 years [1]. They are underrepresented in recent research focusing on risk-stratification models as well as molecular tools. This cohort comprises an important subgroup to address in terms of biologically more aggressive BC, often diagnosed in advanced stages of outside screening, and have a higher societal impact.

Young women with breast cancer (YWBC) account for 7–12% of diagnosed BC with increased occurrence of highly proliferative, poorly differentiated cancers, greater association with lymphovascular invasion, and increased relapse and mortality rates regardless of stage at diagnosis [2]. Even though the incidence of YWBC is 4% in the United States, it is elevated

P. Thakkar Popat (✉)
Department of Radiodiagnosis, Officer in Charge, Breast Imaging and Interventions, Tata Memorial Hospital, Mumbai, India

S. Mynalli · A. Katdare
Department of Radiology, Tata Memorial Hospital, Homibhabha National Institute, Mumbai, India

E. Dhamija, S. V. S. Deo (eds.), *Imaging in Management of Breast Diseases*,
https://doi.org/10.1007/978-981-96-4998-3_14

in low- and middle-income nations [2]. One of the factors attributed is breast density, an independent moderate risk factor for BC. BC in young women are linked with tumours having aggressive biology like triple-negative (TN) and human epidermal growth factor 2 (HER2)-positive tumours, but increasing incidence of luminal cancer is also revealed, particularly in developing nations [3]. Tumour biology may differ in this age group, and the vast BC survival gap indeed is with the less-aggressive luminal BCs. The rate of distant-stage BC has been growing by 4.6% annually in women aged 20–39 years according to Surveillance, Epidemiology, and End Results (SEER) database [4], emphasising on need of research to understand differences in behaviour of luminal BCs in young women.

Noninclusion of this cohort in existing screening programmes reduces rates of early detection as they usually enrol women from 40 to 50 years depending on country-specific guidelines, with the American College of Radiology and Society of Breast Imaging, recommending annual screening from age 40 [5]. While screening guidelines are well established for individuals with BRCA1 or BRCA2 gene mutations, they represent only a small proportion of YWBC, as approximately 90% of early-onset BCs occur in noncarriers [6]. Survivors of childhood cancer having undergone radiotherapy are also at elevated risk, and early screening is advised, beginning either 8 years posttreatment or at age 25, whichever occurs later [7].

Young women from certain racial and ethnic backgrounds face a disproportionately high burden of disease. African American women under the age of 35 have three times the BC-specific mortality rate and twice the incidence of invasive BC [3]. Numerous factors, including low socioeconomic position, restricted access to care, and treatment delays further contribute to poorer outcomes, creating a vicious cycle that not only impacts individual health but also undermines socioeconomic productivity and disrupt family life.

The treatment of young women with BC is complex and calls for specialised, committed multidisciplinary care, including counselling on sexual health, fertility, genetic susceptibility, and socioeconomic repercussions as well as mental support. The Breast Health Global Initiative (BHGI) and the National Comprehensive Cancer Network (NCCN) in Oncology have created resource-stratified guidelines with ways to address the poor outcomes for YWBC in low-income countries [8]. Prioritising fertility preservation, choosing measures to preserve ovarian function, and addressing psychological and quality of life (QoL) concern upon diagnosis are all part of the care. Above all, raising awareness towards early detection is the key to better outcomes.

14.2.1 Diagnostic Imaging for Screening, Staging, and Follow-Up

There is no evidence for regular screening with any imaging technique in average risk, healthy young women. Annual surveillance with MG and MRI has been suggested for high-risk women. Identifying higher-risk individuals with targeted focus on clinical breast examination and screening imaging may be more viable in low middle-income countries.

Choice of Imaging Imaging is challenging in the subset of YWBC because of higher density of breast parenchyma, higher frequency of benign pathologies, and misleading features of malignancy that may miss a positive diagnoses. High-grade tumours in this group and TNBC can simulate benign lesions since they are known to exhibit increased cellularity and necrosis, leading to internal heterogeneity, circumscribed margins, posterior enhancement, and T2W hyperintensity, contrary to stromal reaction and desmoplasia leading to spiculated margins in low-grade tumours [9].

Young women, with self or clinically detected palpable mass in breast or axilla, usually undergo a USG examination first, followed by MG or MRI for an equivocal or suspicious finding [5].

MG in young: It has a compromised diagnostic accuracy and detection due to the higher density and asymmetric parenchyma, often masking even clinically palpable masses. This can lead to both false-positive and false-negative results. The masses detected on MG require USG correlation for characterisation. Cysts, abscesses, papillary neoplasms, fibroepithelial lesions, and malignancies may share similar appearance. Masses may present with spiculated or microlobulated margins with secondary features of skin and nipple changes. Of the suspicious microcalcifications, amorphous pattern may be difficult to be seen amidst dense parenchyma. These architectural distortion and margins may be better appreciated with digital breast tomosynthesis (DBT), an adjunct to routine mammography (MG), improving diagnostic accuracy particularly in young women and dense breast tissue [10]. A synthesised projected two-dimensional view from acquired tomographic views seems promising especially in this population due to reduced radiation exposure.

Functional imaging may be performed by contrast-enhanced MG (CEM), which improves detection of occult index and satellite lesions despite possibility of background parenchymal enhancement (BPE) in this cohort which may pose a challenge (Fig. 14.1). CEM is called a poor woman's MRI and has proven to have sensitivity and specificity close to MRI because of similar principle of neoangiogenesis. CEM does not provide temporal information on enhancement pattern as of MRI but focuses on detecting abnormal enhancing lesions and guides triaging multiple lesions for biopsy.

USG in young: It is used to detect and characterise masses, as solid or cystic, provide appropriate access for biopsy, and assess ductal and nonmass findings, additional lesions, and nodal assessment. It has a distinct advantage over MG to detect masses occult on MG and DBT in background of dense parenchyma. Certain interpretation challenges are encountered such as dense parenchyma with Cooper's ligaments causing posterior shadowing that may mask posterior lesions and misinterpret posteriorly located cysts as solid mass due to improper sound attenuation, or shadowing may be misinterpreted as malignancy. Mastopathy and sclerosing changes also cause diffuse posterior shadowing limiting optimal evaluation. Characterisation of ductal pathologies is limited in background of fibrocystic changes. USG has high false-negative biopsy rates because of high incidence of benign lesions in the young like mastitis, fibroepithelial lesions, and hormonal parenchymal changes. Handheld or automated breast ultrasonography may help in wider population access for early detection in this cohort versus screening MG in resource-

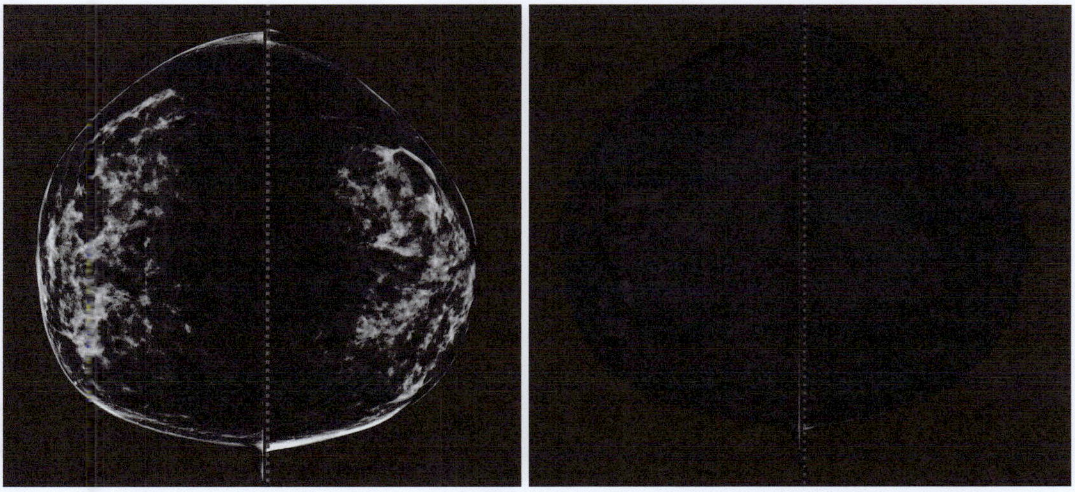

Fig. 14.1 Bilateral CC view showing dense breast parenchyma. CEM shows nonmass enhancement in the inner and central region of the right breast. Histopathology suggestive of ductal carcinoma in situ

constrained settings. Contrast-enhanced USG has its limited role in vascular solitary lesions; however it is not widely practised despite being modality without using ionising radiations.

Preoperative MRI is a superior functional diagnostic modality for better assessment in dense breasts and especially helps in delineating ductal disease, masses, detection of occult-enhancing findings, and characterisation of the detected findings. It has the most superior true-negative predictive value but poorer specificity causing increased rates of ipsilateral mastectomy and contralateral biopsy of abnormal findings; nonetheless, the importance of additional malignancies detected by MRI cannot be negated. Preoperative breast MRI is not mandatory for all cases but should be reserved for select cases as a personalised management protocol, such as in dense and asymmetric breasts, histopathologies such as lobular carcinomas, and high-risk genetic status. MRI is not identified as a significant prognostic factor for recurrence-free survival in women aged 35 years and YWBC [11]. Abbreviated MRI, which involves acquiring only two sequences—before and immediately after contrast administration—demonstrates equivalent performance to standard MRI protocols in diagnostic settings [12]. Hence, it may be considered to ease resources and subject more women to undergo an MRI. DCE-MRI has its advantages to assess the enhancement and washout pattern of abnormal enhancing lesions that can be mapped on kinetic curve and compared with normal breast parenchymal enhancement and with index mass. Kinetics may help in triaging the most suspicious and most distant lesion from the index mass to diagnose multifocality and multicentricity to guide surgical planning.

Newer developments such as ultrafast technique acquires images at a high temporal resolution immediately after contrast administration. Ultrafast MRI is used in screening high-risk patients that saves time as well as prevents misjudgements by BPE as observed in DCE-MRI. It is also proven to be as sensitive as that of DCE-MRI in detection of enhancing lesions (Fig. 14.2). It compromises on the spatial resolution, and hence detection of significant findings is superior on the subtracted ultrafast sequences while characterisation is superior on the routine-subtracted DCE sequences. Papillomas and intramammary nodes show false-positive functional characteristics on MRI and hence always need to be confirmed with a second-look USG.

14.2.2 Molecular Subtypes of Cancer in Young Females

Triple-Negative Cancers TNBC represents up to 24.9% of YWBC [9]. Of these, 70–80% are basal-like subtypes [13], which are commonly linked to BRCA1 mutations and are typically characterised by larger size, high nuclear grade (>80% high grade), and poor survival rates. Since they may appear benign on ultrasound, radiologists must carefully evaluate its morphology to distinguish from fibroepithelial tumours. MRI remains the most sensitive imaging tool for detecting TNBC, often revealing round masses with rim enhancement. When in doubt, it is rather recommended to biopsy for any atypical features.

Fig. 14.2 Extremely dense breast with heterogenous parenchyma. She has a personal history of earlier lumpectomy for a benign pathology in the left breast. Follow-up MG with a circle shows an asymmetric new density in the inner aspect of the left breast. USG showed irregular indeterminate masses. Ultrafast sequence of MRI shows small enhancing masses and additional areas of nonmass enhancement in the inner aspect of left breast corresponding to the MG detected asymmetric density. Histopathology suggestive of lobular carcinoma

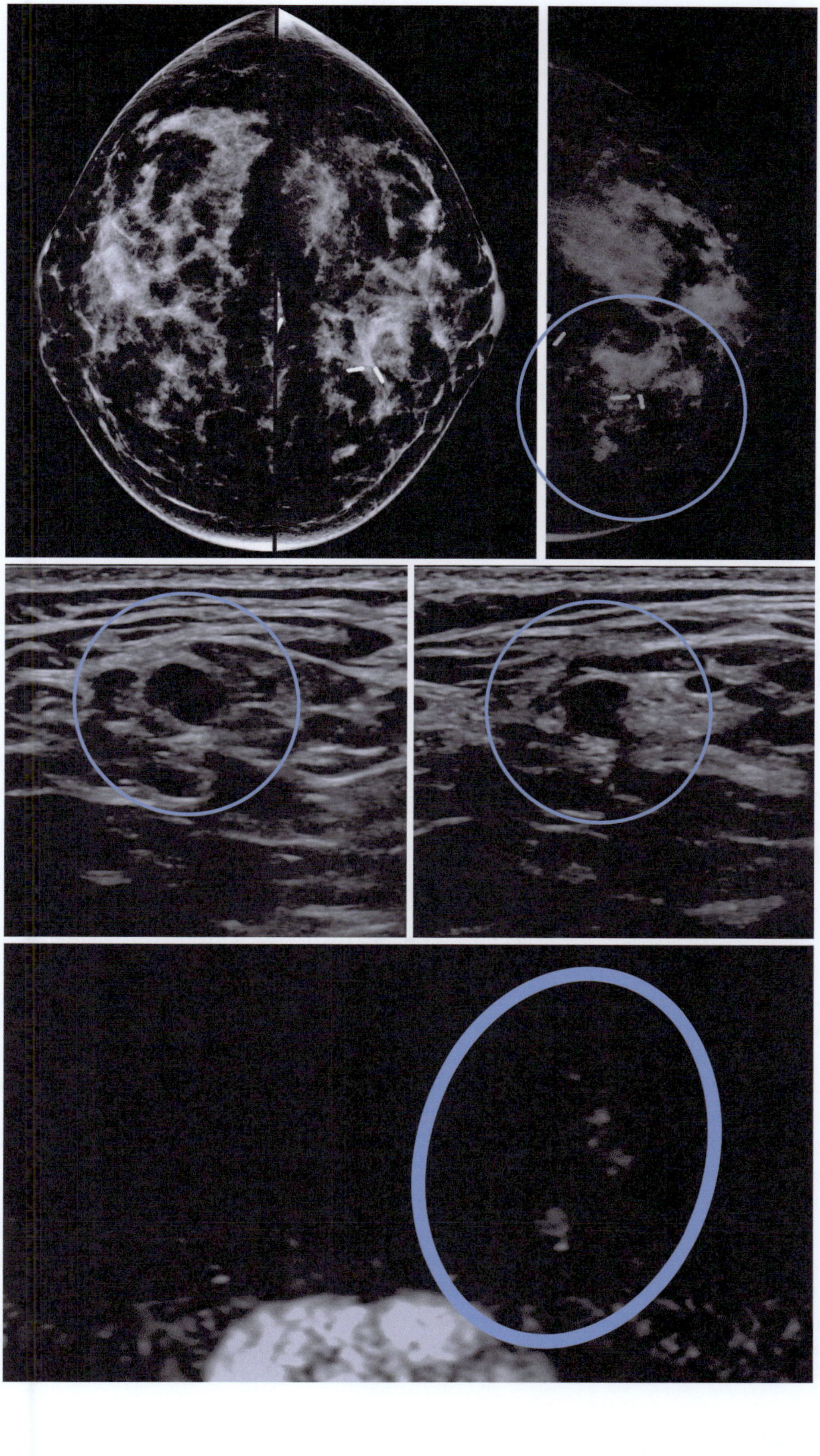

TNBCs especially the basal-like subtype tend to respond well to neoadjuvant chemotherapy, leading to better long-term outcomes, but there is also a significantly increased risk for early recurrence and mortality, particularly within the first 1–3 years following treatment [10] highlighting importance of close and continuous follow-up. TNBCs also follow a unique metastatic pattern, frequently spreading to the lungs and brain rather than the bones and liver, further contributing to poor prognosis in advanced stages [10].

HER2-Enriched Tumours HER2-enriched tumours account for up to 25% of YWBC [1]. These tumours are characterised by overexpression of the HER2 receptor on the surface of tumour cells, leading to increased cellular proliferation, indicated by high Ki-67 levels, and aggressive clinical profile. They are often associated with multifocal or multicentric disease, lymph node involvement, and higher recurrence rates, all contributing to poorer disease-specific and overall survival. Notably, HER2-positive nonluminal cancers tend to have a lower disease-free survival compared to their luminal counterparts.

On mammography, HER2-positive tumours are commonly linked to microcalcifications in over 60% of cases, due to their frequent association with high-grade ductal carcinoma in situ (DCIS). They also carry a higher likelihood of being multifocal, multicentric, or bilaterallity [9]. Digital breast tomosynthesis (DBT) and ultrasound (USG) can enhance lesion detection and visualisation, particularly in patients with dense breast tissue [14]. Despite their aggressive nature, HER2-positive tumours—especially when locally advanced—tend to respond well to targeted chemotherapy, which has been associated with improved survival outcomes.

Stage I–III luminal cancers: In YWBCs with stage I–III luminal type, both five-year breast cancer-specific and disease-free survival rates tend to be poorer, despite the use of adjuvant endocrine therapy aimed at reducing recurrence. Interestingly, this survival disadvantage is primarily seen in those with luminal A subtypes [9], reflecting distinct tumour biology and potentially different oncogenic pathways involved in younger patients.

Unfortunately, radiologists often encounter these patients only after the disease has progressed, limiting opportunities for early intervention. Even short delays in initiating treatment—particularly in cases of metastatic breast cancer—can negatively impact survival. Therefore, thorough staging is crucial for early identification of metastases.

14.2.3 Genetic Counselling and Testing

Genetic counselling and testing should be offered to all YWBC, regardless of tumour subtype or family history. Traditional testing criteria based on personal or family history alone can miss nearly 50% of germline mutations [6]. BRCA1 mutation carriers are more likely to develop TNBC, whereas BRCA2 carriers typically present with oestrogen receptor (ER)-positive tumours, which are more frequently associated with ductal carcinoma in situ (DCIS), and hence mammographic screening is especially beneficial in BRCA2 carriers, by detecting DCIS-associated microcalcifications [15]. Risk of developing a second breast cancer within 10 years of the initial diagnosis is significantly higher in BRCA mutation carriers, ranging from 7% to 17%, increasing to 21% in BRCA1 carriers diagnosed before the age of 40 [10]. As a result, continued close imaging surveillance is essential for early detection unless a risk-reducing mastectomy was performed after the initial diagnosis. Additionally, BRCA mutation carriers are at greater risk for central nervous system (CNS) involvement, entailing need of comprehensive local and systemic follow-up imaging. Preventive strategies such as risk-reducing salpingo-oophorectomy (RRSO) and gynaecologic surveillance are also strongly recommended. A common misconception is that the absence of a BRCA1 or BRCA2 mutation significantly lowers the risk of breast cancer in young. Other moderate- to high-penetrance genes such as ATM, CHEK2, and

PALB2 should be considered through multigene panel testing in YWBC [16]. Identifying genetic mutation impacts treatment plans such as considering risk-reducing surgery, using specific medications like platinum derivatives or PARP inhibitors [16], and personalising surveillance strategies such as annual screening MRI brain and whole body imaging in individuals with a TP53 mutation (Li-Fraumeni syndrome) due to increased risk of secondary radiation-induced malignancies [6].

14.2.4 Management of Young Females with BC

Young age is an independent risk factor for increased locoregional recurrence especially in HER2-positive and TNBC irrespective of type of surgery performed. No improvement in long-term survival is seen despite growing trend toward bilateral mastectomies among young women. Hence, breast-conserving surgery (BCS) with careful assessment of surgical margins remains an acceptable and effective standard of care. Oncoplastic surgical techniques can be offered to patients undergoing BCS when postoperative breast asymmetry is expected. In cases where mastectomy is necessary, skin- and nipple-sparing procedures with immediate breast reconstruction (IBR) may be offered except in inflammatory breast cancers where reconstruction is delayed due to the need for extensive radiation therapy and the recommendation to wait until the highest risk of recurrence has passed. Similarly, patients with locally advanced disease poorly responding to initial systemic therapy may be offered delayed reconstruction [13].

Postoperative radiotherapy (RT) recommendations do not differ with age or genetic status [17]. Postmastectomy RT following implant-based reconstruction is associated with increased risks of reconstructive failure (over 15%) and capsular contracture (over 30%) and should be discussed, especially in high-risk patients such as those with TP53 mutations [17].

Prophylactic radiation to the contralateral, unaffected breast is not recommended for BRCA mutation carriers who do not undergo contralateral mastectomy [17].

Adjuvant systemic treatment for invasive breast cancer in young women should be determined by disease extent and tumour biology—including tumour size, nodal involvement, hormone receptor status, HER2 expression/amplification, Ki-67 levels, tumour grade, comorbidities, and patient preferences.

Genomic assays like Oncotype DX, MammaPrint, Prosigna, EndoPredict, and Breast Cancer Index estimate recurrence risk and can help guide adjuvant chemotherapy decisions [16]. In select women aged 35 or younger with favourable clinical, genomic, and pathological features, it may be appropriate to omit chemotherapy [18].

Tamoxifen, at a standard dose of 20 mg daily for five years, has been shown to reduce breast cancer risk by 35–40% and is recommended for chemoprevention in women at elevated risk. For women with breast intraepithelial neoplasia who are at lower risk of recurrence, a low-dose tamoxifen regimen (5 mg daily for three years) may offer a well-tolerated alternative with fewer side effects while still providing effective risk reduction [19]. Postchemotherapy OFS (ovarian function suppression) is seen in 22–61% of women <40 years with greater improvement in <35 years age [20]. Endocrine therapy (ET) is recommended for high-risk patients as per USPSTF but with limited data available in Asian population.

In young women (under 40) undergoing chemotherapy, adding gonadotropin-releasing hormone agonists can help protect ovarian function [21]. However, the method of ovarian suppression (medical or surgical) requires balancing fertility preservation, treatment adherence, and cost. Younger patients often struggle with adherence to hormone therapy.

The timing of these agonists does not seem to impact their effectiveness in preserving ovarian reserve, but coordination with fertility teams is crucial to avoid complications. Anti-HER2 therapies, like trastuzumab and chemotherapy regimens, such as taxane- and anthracycline-based treatments, are effective across age groups. However, anthracyclines carry long-term risks like heart failure and leukaemia. Nonanthracycline regimens are considered for certain tumour types. Immune-related endocrine issues can impact fertility, and their long-term effects are under study [22]. Zoledronic acid for osteoporosis prevention requires counselling for potential risks to fertility and pregnancy outcomes [23].

Psychosocial Issues YWBC face a heightened risk of psychosocial challenges, during and after treatment. Common sources of distress include concerns about body image, sexuality, and sexual dysfunction, often linked to premature menopause, treatment-induced amenorrhea, weight gain, hair loss, and the physical impact of breast surgery. It is important to involve spouses and family members early in the care process, to provide meaningful benefits throughout the various stages of treatment. Comprehensive care for YWBC should also include guidance and support regarding fertility preservation, contraception, management of premature menopause, sexual health, pregnancy after breast cancer, bone health, cognitive changes, and recommended lifestyle modifications. Additionally, care considerations for women diagnosed with breast cancer during pregnancy must be incorporated into the treatment planning.

Overview and Path Forward A multidisciplinary approach is essential to address the unique concerns among YWBC. Early breast cancer awareness is crucial, particularly given the rising incidence of advanced disease and increased mortality rates among women aged 20–39 [24]. Timely referral for diagnostic workup is vital for young women with significant breast symptoms. Clinical breast exams are recommended every 1–3 years for women aged 25–39 and annually for those over 40 [25]. Population-based genetic testing may be a more efficient and cost-effective approach to identifying high-risk individuals, as most carriers of germline mutations remain unidentified [25]. Liquid biopsy, which detects circulating tumour DNA, shows promise in monitoring treatment response and relapse, offering potential benefits for patients with early-onset breast cancer [4].

14.3 Bilateral Breast Cancers

The overall incidence of bilateral breast cancer ranges from 1.4% to 12% with only 1–2% of cases being pathologically distinct. Invasive ductal carcinoma (IDC) of no special type (NST), previously referred to as IDC not otherwise specified (NOS), is the most common form of invasive BBC, comprising 50–75% of all cases [1]. Contralateral breast cancer may develop as a metastatic lesion or as a second primary tumour, either synchronously (at the same time) or metachronously (at a different time). Incidental detection of contralateral malignancy on radiological workup for diseased breast is the most common form of presentation. Occasionally they present as bilateral palpable masses. Bilateral histopathological and molecular receptor evaluation is recommended as different tumour biology may be encountered.

14.3.1 Bilateral Synchronous Breast Cancers

This is defined as the diagnosis of invasive or in situ BC in both breasts within a six-month interval. The incidence ranges from 0.7% to 3.0% with worse survival rates because of early distant metastasis and limited treatment options [26].

Diagnosing bilateral BC can be challenging, as the disease may present at different stages with varied clinical features and histopathological profiles, leading to differences in prognosis and treatment approaches.

The detection of asymptomatic contralateral BC at the time of initial diagnosis of ipsilateral disease particularly through MG and USG offers improved survival outcomes [27]. Additionally, routine MRI screening of the contralateral breast shows survival benefit, particularly in larger primary histologic grade 3 tumours [28] (Fig. 14.3).

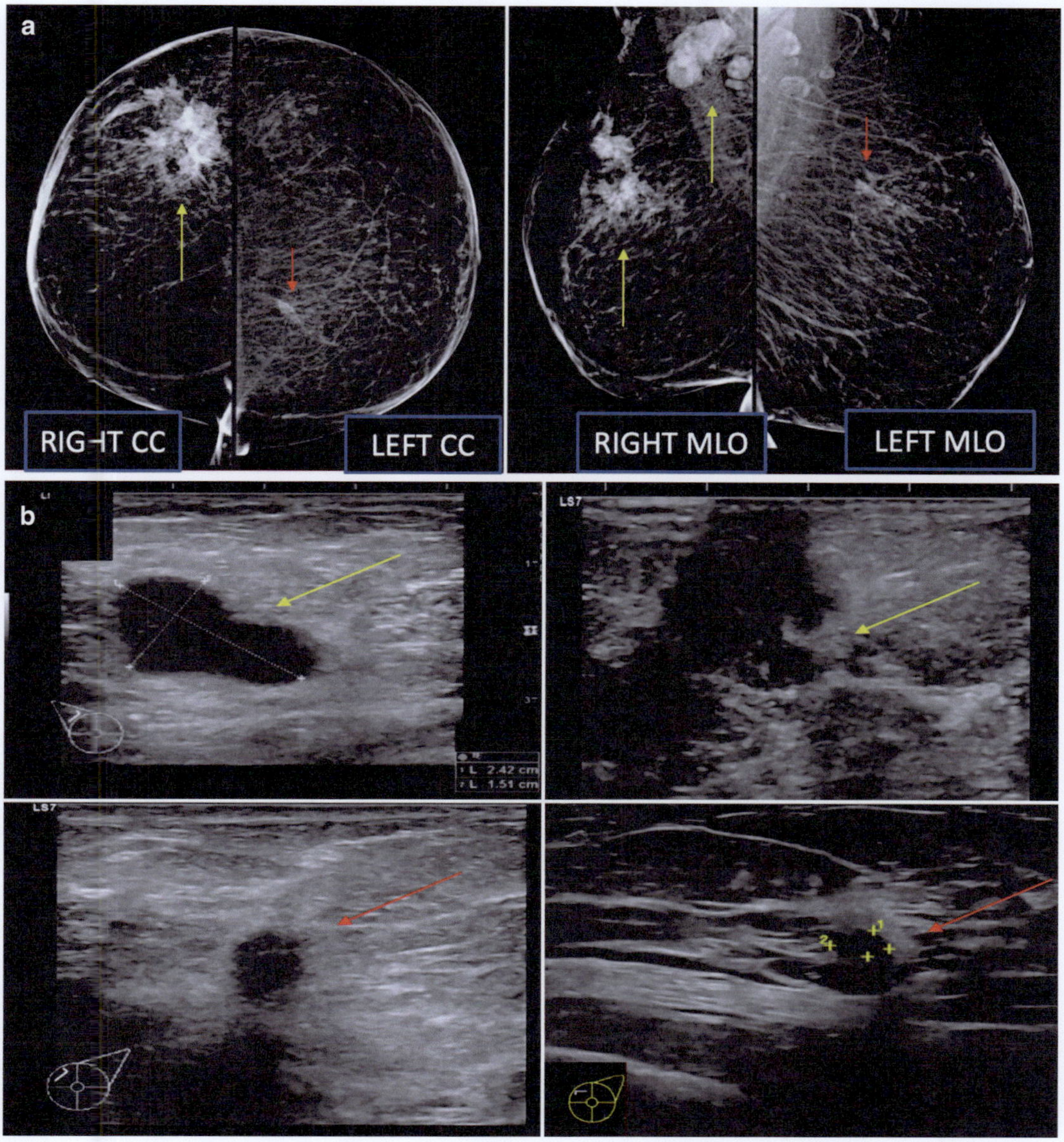

Fig. 14.3 Bilateral BC: Locally advanced right breast cancer (IBC NST, grade 3 with DCIS) seen as spiculated mass (yellow arrow) on MG in upper outer quadrant reaching up to the skin along with metastatic right axillary nodes (yellow arrow), confirming above findings on USG (hypoechoic solid) as well as on PET (FDG avid). Incidentally detected, left breast upper inner quadrant focal asymmetry (red arrow) and hypoechoic and round solid lesion showing posterior acoustic shadowing (red arrow) on USG with no uptake on FDG-PET (red arrow)—HPR: invasive lobular carcinoma, grade 2

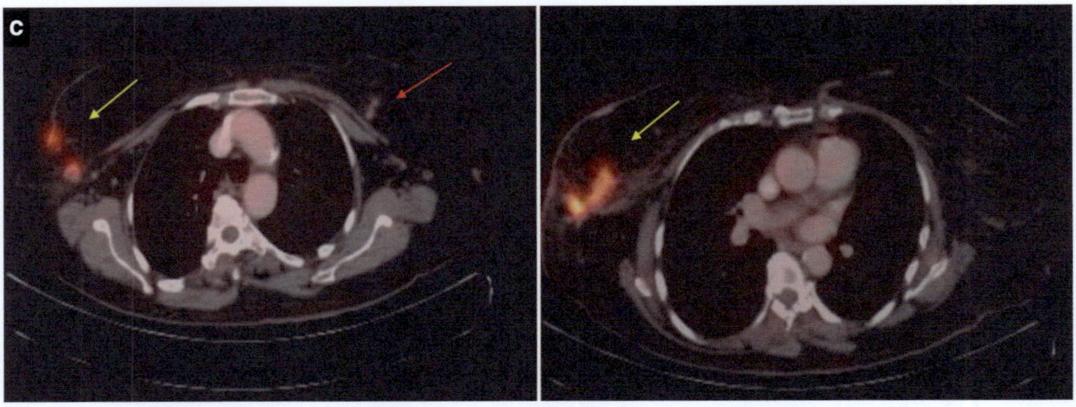

Fig. 14.3 (continued)

Bilateral BC risk is increased by factors such as invasive lobular carcinoma in the index breast, family history, young age at diagnosis, and BRCA mutations. High-risk patients should undergo genetic counselling, broad-panel germline testing, and next-generation sequencing. Treatment depends on disease stage, tumour characteristics, patient health, age, and comorbidities and may include breast-conserving surgery, mastectomy, radiation therapy, chemotherapy, endocrine therapy, or targeted therapy. Bilateral breast irradiation can be complex due to differing tumour aggressiveness, but hypofractionated schedules are feasible, minimise acute side effects, and do not increase the risk of late effects like secondary malignancies like angiosarcoma [29].

14.3.2 Multiple Ipsilateral Synchronous Breast Cancer

The incidence of multiple ipsilateral synchronous BC has risen, largely due to advancements in imaging techniques and the increased use of breast MRI for screening and staging purposes. This condition is defined by the presence of synchronous tumours within the same breast, occurring either within the same quadrant (multifocal) or across different quadrants (multicentric) [30].

Breast MRI is the most sensitive imaging modality for identifying additional satellite lesions in the ipsilateral breast that may be occult on conventional imaging. Given the overlap in imaging features, accurate interpretation requires consideration of both morphological and functional characteristics. Restricted diffusion with low ADC values has sensitivity and specificity of 62.5% to 92.8% and 45.8% to 96.7%, respectively [31], with superior yield led by contrast kinetics. A second-look ultrasound (USG) is often useful for evaluating MRI-detected lesions followed by USG-guided biopsy. One of the primary limitations of breast MRI is its relatively low specificity ranging from 40–80% [31]. As a result, any new MRI-detected significant finding with no USG correlate must be subject to MRI-guided biopsies or wire localized excision, if it potentially alters management.

CEM, another supplemental tool to MG for dense and asymmetric breast parenchyma, may incidentally detect additional occult cancers in the ipsilateral and/or contralateral breasts. Its benefit outweighs poorer accuracy in the presence pf background parenchymal enhancement. CEM detected lesions may be biopsied or wire localised under CEM guidance in the absence of a correlate on USG.

14.3.3 Bilateral Metachronous Breast Cancer (Fig. 14.4)

It refers to a second primary BC detected in the contralateral breast more than six months after the initial diagnosis, with an incidence rate of approximately 2.2% [29].

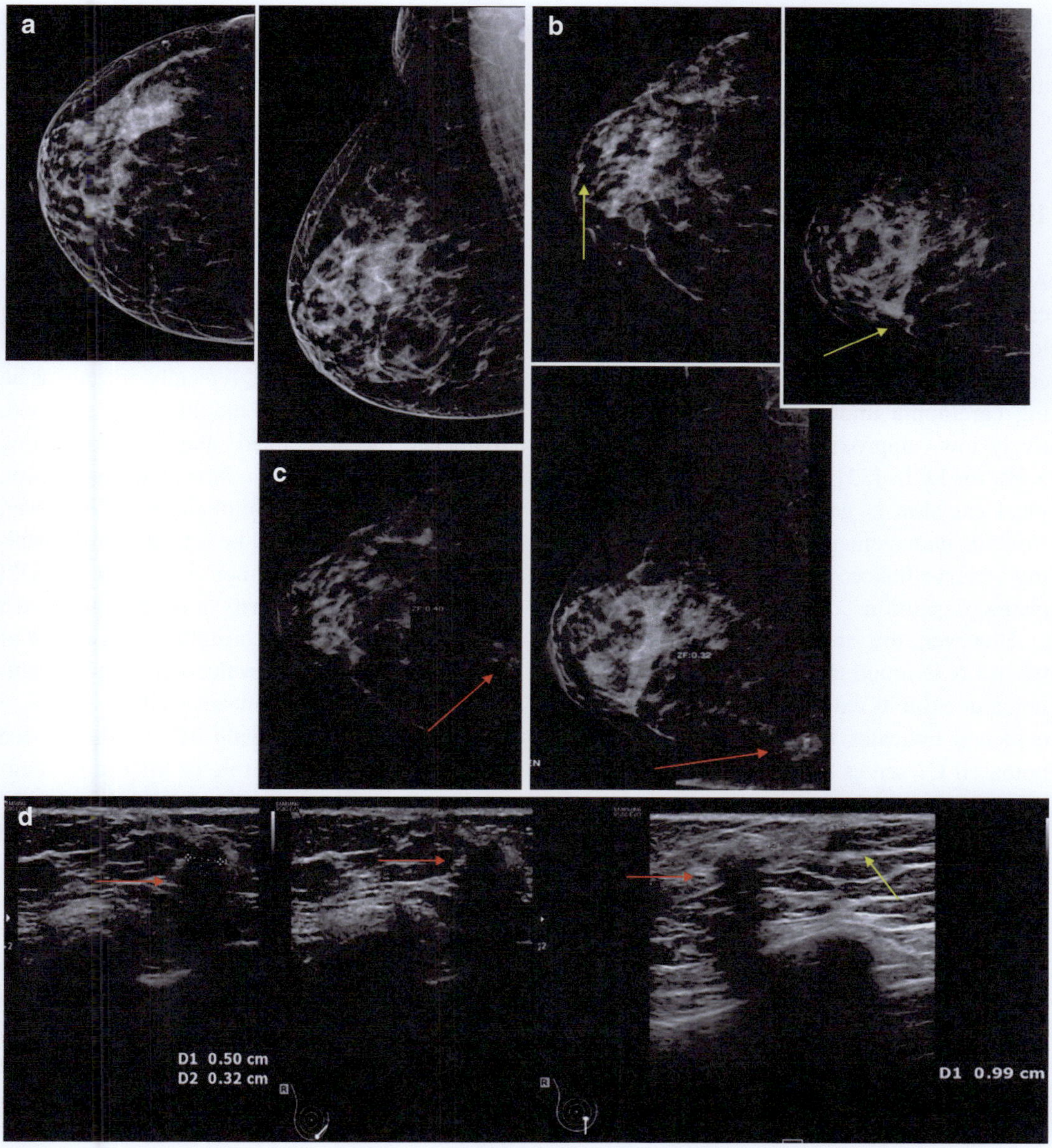

Fig. 14.4 Metachronous breast cancer—Post left mastectomy for locally advanced left breast cancer (IDC NOS, grade 3), with normal contralateral MG (**a**). Right mastopexy changes seen in lower inner quadrant of the right breast (yellow arrow) on follow-up MG (**b**). A new onset mass with spiculated margins and pleomorphic microcalcifications within (red arrow) was detected on further follow-up MG (**c**) in lower inner quadrant away from scar site. The suspicious mass (red arrow), away from scar changes (yellow arrow), was confirmed on USG. USG-guided biopsy revealed IDC with intermediate-grade DCIS

Dynamic study of the level of serum tumour markers like CA-125, CA-15-3, and CA-27-29 in BC patients may be a screening tool for early diagnosis of the development of metachronous tumours and monitor treatment response, of which CA-15-3 is widely used. The most unfavourable factor is germline mutations in the BRCA1/BRCA2 genes [16].

Routine follow-up protocols are based on MG, which has a higher sensitivity to detect DCIS and masses. But for all asymmetries, a correlating MRI improves sensitivity in detecting occult, noncalcific DCIS and invasive cancers with sensitivity ranging from 94% to 100% for invasive carcinoma and 40–100% for ductal carcinoma in situ (DCIS) [32].

14.3.4 Lobular Neoplasia Spectrum

Atypical lobular hyperplasia (ALH) and lobular carcinoma in situ (LCIS) fall in spectrum of lobular neoplasia (LN). When identified through core needle biopsy, the likelihood of discovering carcinoma upon surgical excision is relatively low—approximately 2.5% for ALH and 5.8% for LCIS [33]. Consequently, routine surgical excision is generally not recommended. Instead, management typically includes imaging surveillance and consideration of chemoprevention.

However, the approach becomes less clear when LN is found alongside synchronous carcinoma or exhibits extensive involvement. Current evidence indicates that invasive lobular carcinoma (ILC) serves as a risk marker for future breast cancer, whereas LCIS is considered a nonobligate precursor to invasive disease [34]. On the other hand, ductal carcinoma in situ (DCIS)—which represents 20–25% of breast cancer cases—is frequently detected via mammographic calcifications and is associated with a favourable prognosis [35]. Importantly, nonsurgical management strategies for LN are not appropriate when there is concurrent invasive carcinoma or DCIS.

14.3.5 Bilateral Breast Cancer in Males

Male breast cancer is an uncommon condition, accounting for approximately 1% of all BC with large hormone expression [36]. Among the various subtypes, invasive ductal carcinoma is by far the most prevalent in men. A bilateral synchronous presentation—where cancer is found in both breasts at the same time—is extremely rare, occurring in only about 1.5–2% of male BCs [37].

Clinically, male BC often presents as a painless, firm mass located near the nipple (subareolar region in eccentric location). Other common signs and symptoms include nipple retraction, spontaneous bloody nipple discharge, skin ulceration over the lesion, and palpable axillary lymphadenopathy.

On imaging, male BC typically appears as an irregular mass centred in the subareolar area with spiculated or ill-defined margins, suggesting malignancies. Unlike in female breast cancer, calcifications are not commonly seen. However, if identified, they should be regarded with suspicion and warrant further investigation [37] (Fig. 14.5). Due to its rarity, it is often diagnosed at a later stage, underscoring the importance of awareness and timely evaluation of any suspicious breast changes in means well.

Given the rarity of male BC and the limited literature available, the role of MRI in its diagnosis and management is not clearly established. However, MRI has demonstrated superiority over ultrasound and mammography in certain contexts, primarily in detecting additional disease. It can identify occult lesions in the ipsilateral breast in approximately 15% of cases and in the contralateral breast in about 10% of cases [38]. Despite this, the use of MRI in male breast cancer is typically reserved for highly selected cases where conventional imaging is inconclusive or further assessment is clinically necessary.

Risk factors for bilateral involvement in males include positive family history, increasing age, black race, BRCA2 mutations, radiation exposure, hyperoestrogenic conditions (liver diseases, obesity, alcoholism, and oestrogen treatment), hypoandrogenic and testicular conditions (Klinefelter's syndrome, undescended testis, orchitis, orchiectomy), and hyperprolactinemia [16].

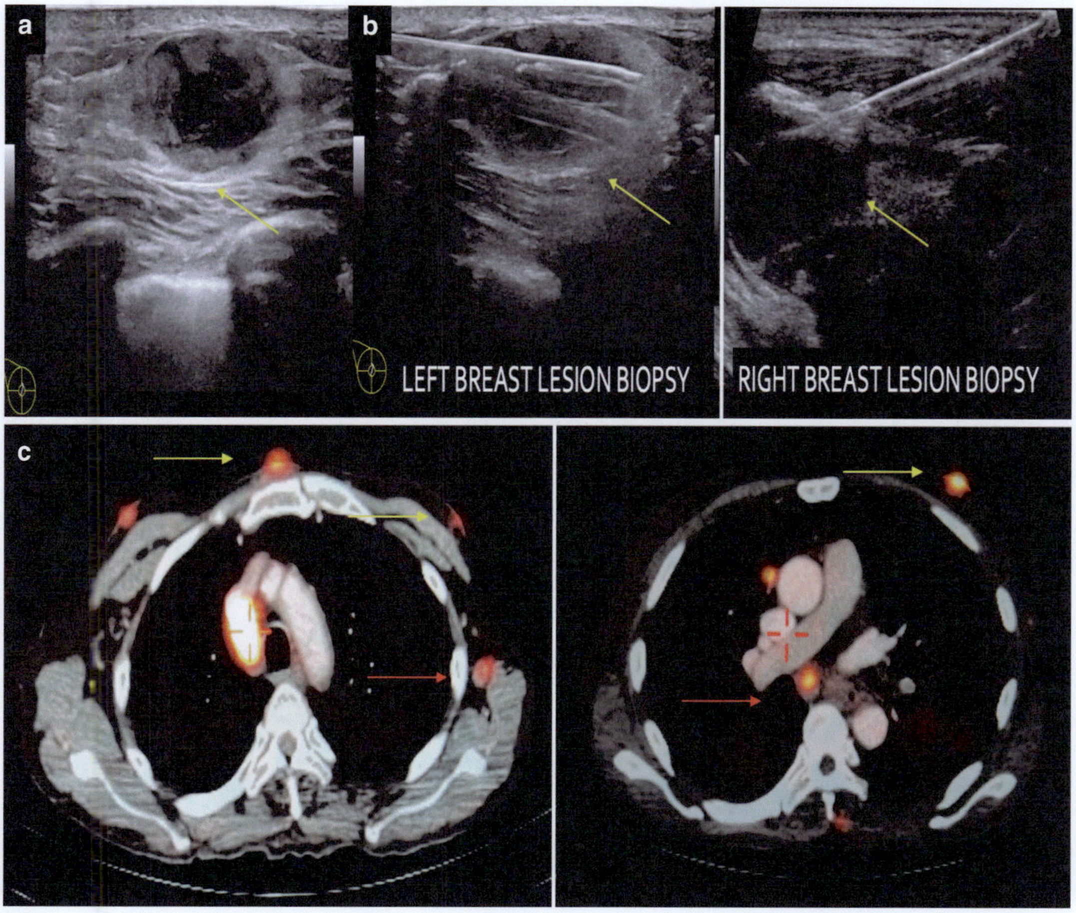

Fig. 14.5 Elderly male with palpable breast masses showing round heteroechoic vascular masses in bilateral breasts (yellow arrow) that show FDG avidity on PET (yellow arrow). USG-guided biopsy (yellow arrow in 'b') revealed high-grade lymphoma. PET also revealed FDG avid suspicious left axillary and mediastinal lymph nodes (red arrow)

14.3.6 Ipsilateral Breast Tumour Recurrence (Fig. 14.6)

Ipsilateral breast tumour recurrence (IBTR) is defined as the reappearance of in situ or invasive carcinoma within the skin or parenchyma of the same breast following breast-conserving surgery (BCS), in the absence of clinical or radiologic evidence of regional or distant metastasis. Early detection of IBTR, which has an incidence of 5% to 10%, is associated with significantly improved survival outcomes.

The most common site of recurrence is within the original tumour quadrant or along the chest wall scar following radical surgery, accounting for approximately 60–95% of cases [14]. Recurrences identified through routine surveillance imaging—both clinically and radiologically—tend to have a better prognosis than those detected by the patient, as delays in diagnosis increase the risk of distant metastases and negatively affect overall outcomes. Several risk factors are associated with earlier onset and higher rates of IBTR. These include young age, BRCA

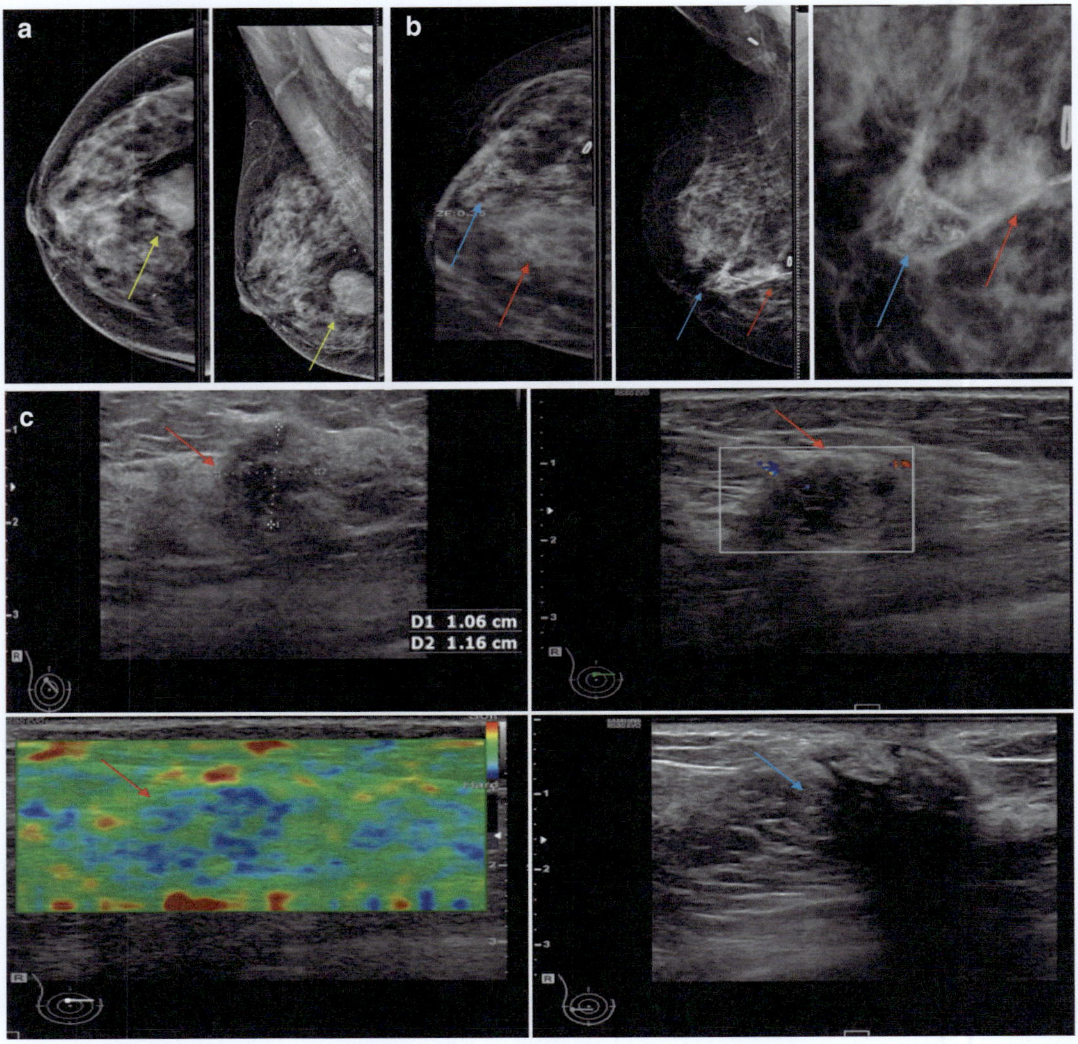

Fig. 14.6 Case of ipsilateral breast tumour recurrence: Significant family history of BC in a woman with baseline MG (**a**) right lower central region prepectoral microlobulated mass (yellow arrow), post-BCT status. Follow-up MG after two years showed scar site dystrophic calcifications (blue arrow) with new-onset pleomorphic microcalcifications in inner central region (red arrow) with associated density (**b**). USG (**c**) confirmed the 2 o clock hypoechoic suspicious mass (red arrow), HPR revealed IDC NOS, along with fat necrosis at 8 o clock (blue arrow)

gene mutations, TNBC subtype, advanced nodal involvement (N2), and a positive family history. Additionally, treatment-related factors such as positive surgical margins, inadequate radiotherapy, or noncompliance with treatment protocols contribute to recurrence risk [17].

The sensitivity of mammography (MG) for detecting IBTR in a previously treated breast is limited—ranging from 65% to 78% [14]—due to postsurgical and radiation-induced changes, which can obscure or mimic recurrent disease. Mammographic signs of recurrence often resemble those of the primary tumour and include suspicious calcifications (pleomorphic, indistinct, coarse heterogeneous, or linear) near or at the tumour bed in about 75% of cases. Other findings include architectural distortion (3%) and increasing skin oedema [39]. Calcifications caused by fat necrosis typically present with characteristic ring- or arc-shaped appearances appearing benign. Early dystrophic calcifications may appear indeterminate and require close follow-up to monitor their evolution or may necessitate MRI for better soft tissue characterisation.

USG has limited sensitivity in this context, and when findings on MG and/or USG are inconclusive, breast MRI becomes a valuable tool [14, 35]. When performed at least 12–18 months after completing breast-conserving therapy (BCT), MRI can reliably differentiate between postsurgical scar tissue and true recurrence, offering a sensitivity of 90–100% and specificity of 83–93% [12].

CEM is emerging as a promising alternative and may offer additional diagnostic value over conventional, noncontrast MG in the evaluation of suspected IBTR [14, 35].

To summarise, inherent risk factors are associated with development of bilateral BCs, be it contralateral metastasis or bilateral index masses at similar time point or delayed intervals. As per current national comprehensive cancer network (NCCN) guidelines (version 3.2023), an indication for testing for high penetrance cancer susceptibility genes (BRCA1/BRCA2, CDH1, PALB2, PTEN, and TP53) is indicated in women with multiple primary BCs, regardless of age, and this includes both types of bilateral BC [8]. Early detection using appropriate screening modalities according to risk assessment improves outcome and survival.

In cases of synchronous breast cancer, especially with similar histomorphologic features and receptor status, high grade or advanced stage, axillary lymph node involvement, and absence of in situ carcinoma (DCIS or LCIS) in the contralateral breast, metastatic spread to the contralateral breast is a greater possibility rather than two independent primary tumours.

Imaging modalities and diagnostic pathway are similar to unilateral BCs. Women with multiple ipsilateral synchronous malignancies undergoing breast-conserving therapy (BCT) experience similar rates of locoregional recurrence (LRR) as those with unifocal disease at an equivalent stage [40]. This is due to improvement in adjuvant therapies that make salvageable surgery successful, and this emphasises the critical role played by imaging in detecting accurate disease extent for appropriate surgical resection.

14.4 Pregnancy-Associated Breast Cancers

Pregnancy-associated breast cancer (PABC) refers to breast cancer that occurs during pregnancy, within one year of delivery or may encompass any phase of lactation. The incidence of PABC varies between 1 in 3000–10,000 women and increases with maternal age [41]. Incidence of PABC is 0.2–3.8% of all BC [42]. Lactational period varies among women, and close follow-up is recommended for six years postpartum; however, it is usually detected in the first 2–3 years [43].

PABC shows difference in behaviour and prognosis, with worse outcomes [44]. This is likely due to mammary gland involution (tissue remodelling) after pregnancy through wound healing and inflammation, supposedly creating a protumour microenvironment, apart from hormonal tissue stromal effect and immune tolerance. Particularly in the postpartum phase, PABC present with aggressive biology (higher tumour grade, nodal stage, and lymphovascular invasion) and usually hormone receptor (HR) negative. Delayed diagnosis leads to poor outcome in overall and disease-free survival [6].

Given the comparable oncologic and obstetric outcomes to non-PABC patients, it is important to promote awareness to ensure prompt diagnosis and effective treatment of PABC [45]. There are no specific pregnancy or lactating screening guidelines for high-risk (BRCA/CHEK2 germline mutants) women [46]. It is essential to be vigilant and employ a timely multimodality imaging evaluation for diagnosis and staging, maintaining a primary focus on the foetus and mother safety while planning a multidisciplinary management strategy [47].

Unique challenges of diagnosing PABC arise because many of the physiological changes of pregnancy (breast engorgement, hypertrophy,

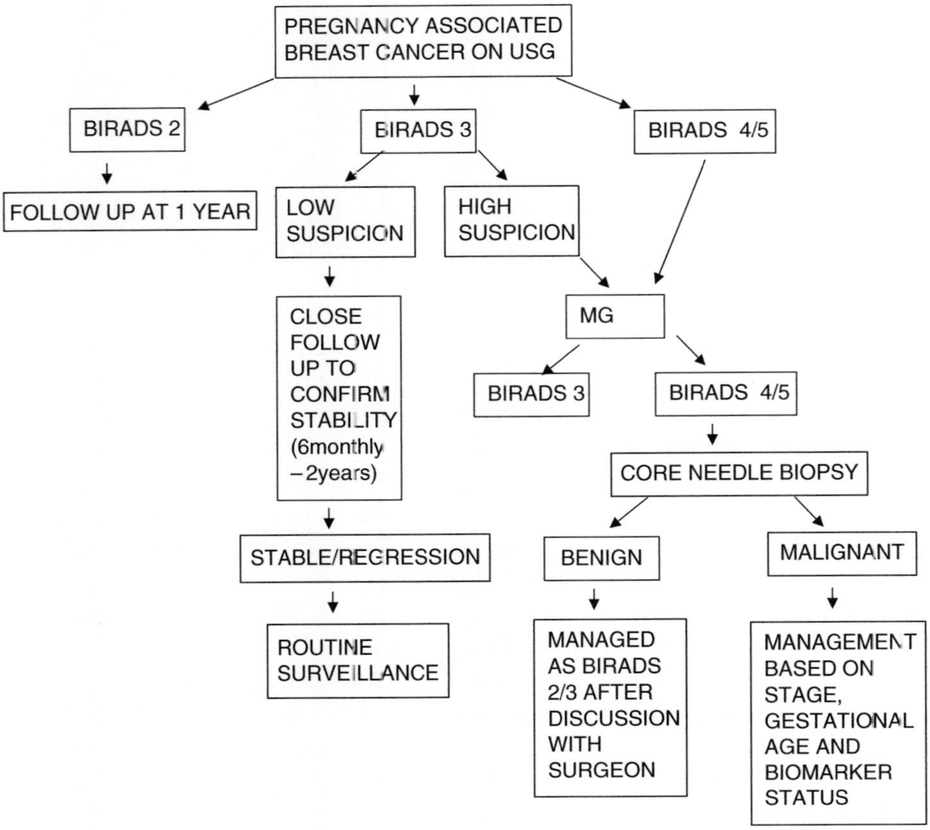

Fig. 14.7 Algorithm for imaging PABC

increased nodularity, and density) mask detection of malignant transformation both clinically and radiologically (Fig. 14.7).

14.4.1 Diagnostic and Prognostic Role of Imaging

Symptoms at presentation could range from a mass, ulcer, nipple discharge, diffuse breast oedema or pain. Any clinically palpable breast lump in pregnancy for two weeks or more should be evaluated promptly, despite higher occurrence of benign findings [48]. USG breast is the first investigation of choice during any trimester and shows almost 100% sensitivity and near 90% negative predictive value for detection of PABC [15]. During pregnancy and lactation, the physiological changes in the breast lead to progressive ductal and lobular hyperplasia along with ductal ectasia, which can cause large hypoechoic ducts and lobules to appear against a background of diffusely reduced breast echogenicity [16]. Multiparametric USG including Doppler and elastography can give additional information for lesion characterisation. Growing experience can reliably identify benign findings like complicated cysts, galactoceles, lactating adenomas, and breast abscesses to best avoid unnecessary biopsies [8], as a relatively higher incidence of complications including bleeding, pain, and rarely milk fistula is associated with biopsies during pregnancy. But for all suspicious palpable findings and BIRADS 4 or above category findings, supplemental mammography and USG-guided biopsy should be preferred. USG also helps evaluate axillary lymph nodes and in assessing disease response to neoadjuvant chemotherapy received during pregnancy (Fig. 14.8).

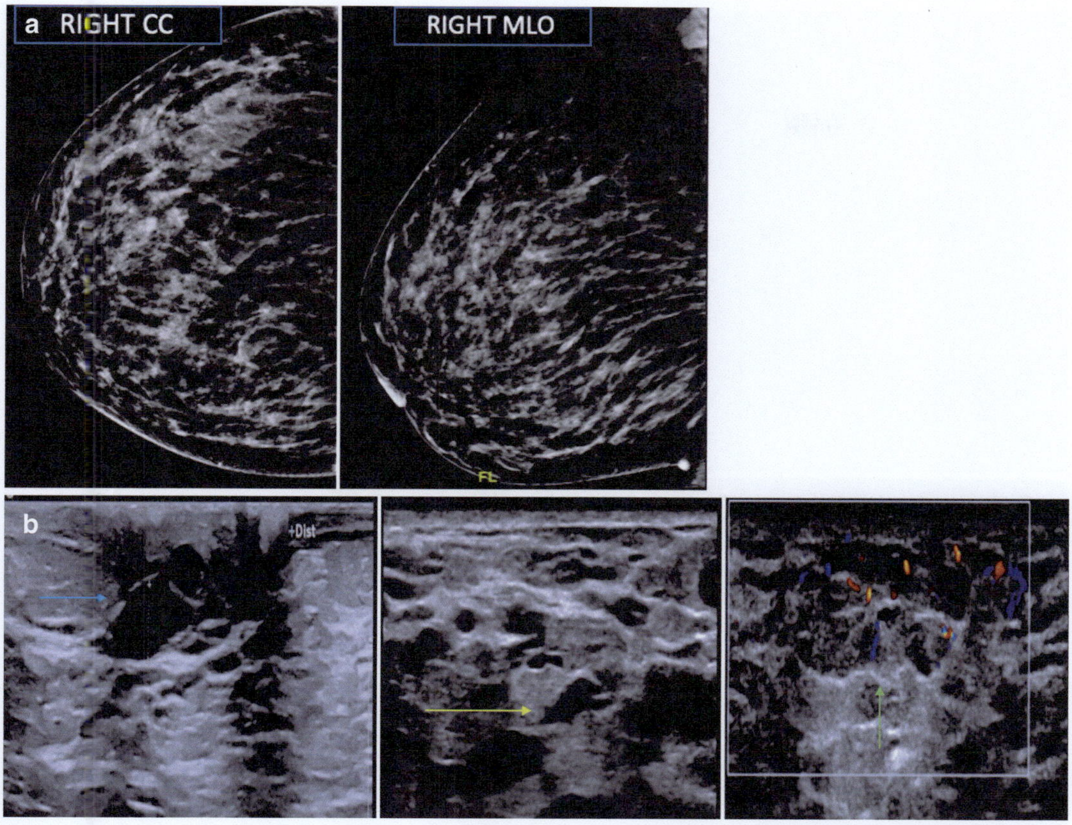

Fig. 14.8 Normal lactating breast with increased density and stromal glandular parenchyma seen on MG (**a**) as well as on USG (**b**) showing parenchyma heterogeneity (yellow arrow) with dilated ducts (blue arrow) and increased vascularity (green arrow)

There are limitations to MG screening in pregnancy due to increased breast density and pseudoconcerns with radiation exposure, although the total radiation dose of a bilateral two-dimensional MG is <3 mGy which is below the exposure limits for either stochastic or deterministic effects [49]. Lead apron shielding should be made available to pregnant patients undergoing diagnostic MG. For lactating women, MG can be performed after nursing to decrease the attenuation of x-rays by breast milk. The mammographic features of PABC include asymmetries or masses, architectural distortion, microcalcifications, skin thickening, and/or axillary lymphadenopathy. Additional MG views like spot compression or single view tomosynthesis can be used in ambiguous findings (Fig. 14.9).

Stereotactic-guided biopsy and MG-guided hookwire localisation may be considered for MG-only detected suspicious findings [48]. Routine annual mammography screening is not recommended during pregnancy and can resume 3 months after lactation for women greater than 40 as per ACR [5].

MRI without contrast would be the method of choice over ionising radiation-based imaging modalities [such as computed tomography (CT) and positron emission tomography (PET)] in the evaluation of pregnant females unless clinical benefits for the mother outweigh the potential risks to the foetus. Regardless, MRI techniques, such as T2-weighted image and diffusion-weighted image (DWI), have a diagnostic role in assessing PABC by exhibiting the low signal of

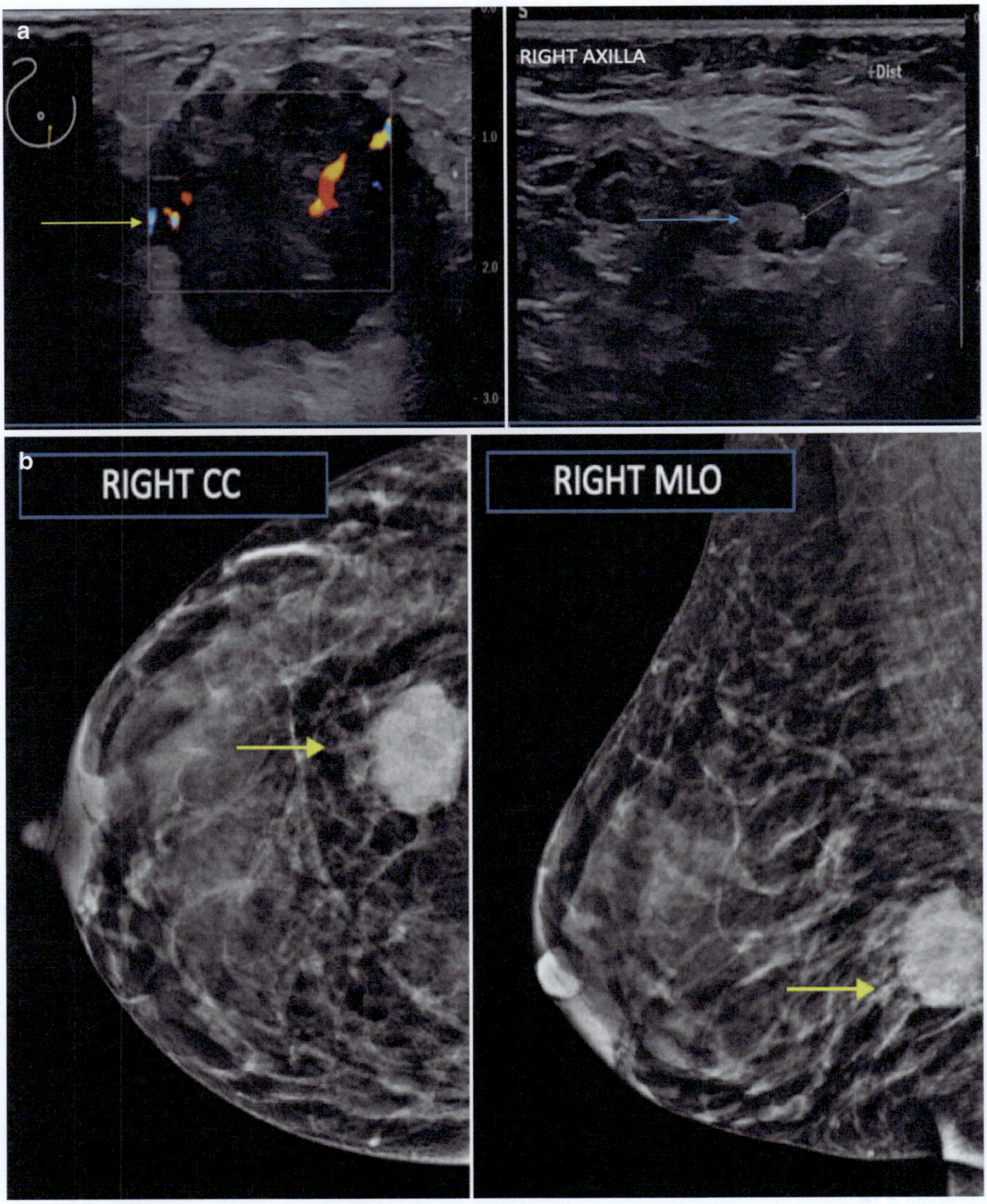

Fig. 14.9 Pregnant lady presenting with palpable right breast lump showed hypoechoic microlobulated mass with vascularity at 5 o'clock position (yellow arrow) as well as suspicious right axillary node (blue arrow) with eccentric cortical hypertrophy on USG (**a**). Diagnostic MG (**b**) confirmed solitary mass with no microcalcifications (yellow arrow). USG-guided biopsy revealed metaplastic carcinoma grade 3

disease against the background of high signal from the lactating breast parenchyma [50]. DCE-MRI, despite its diagnostic superiority, is contraindicated during pregnancy because of gadolinium-associated fetotoxic properties [18]. DCE-MRI can be considered after planned pregnancy termination or postdelivery. Extensive BPE limits sensitivity to detect cancer, and this normalises three months postcessation of breastfeeding [51]. Poorer accuracy in the presence of BPE can be overcome with ultrafast sequences which offer superior detection of suspicious findings (Fig. 14.10). A single DCE MIP image has an average sensitivity of 93.3% and a negative predictive value (NPV) of 96.2% to detect malignancy in lactational breast MRI. Limitations

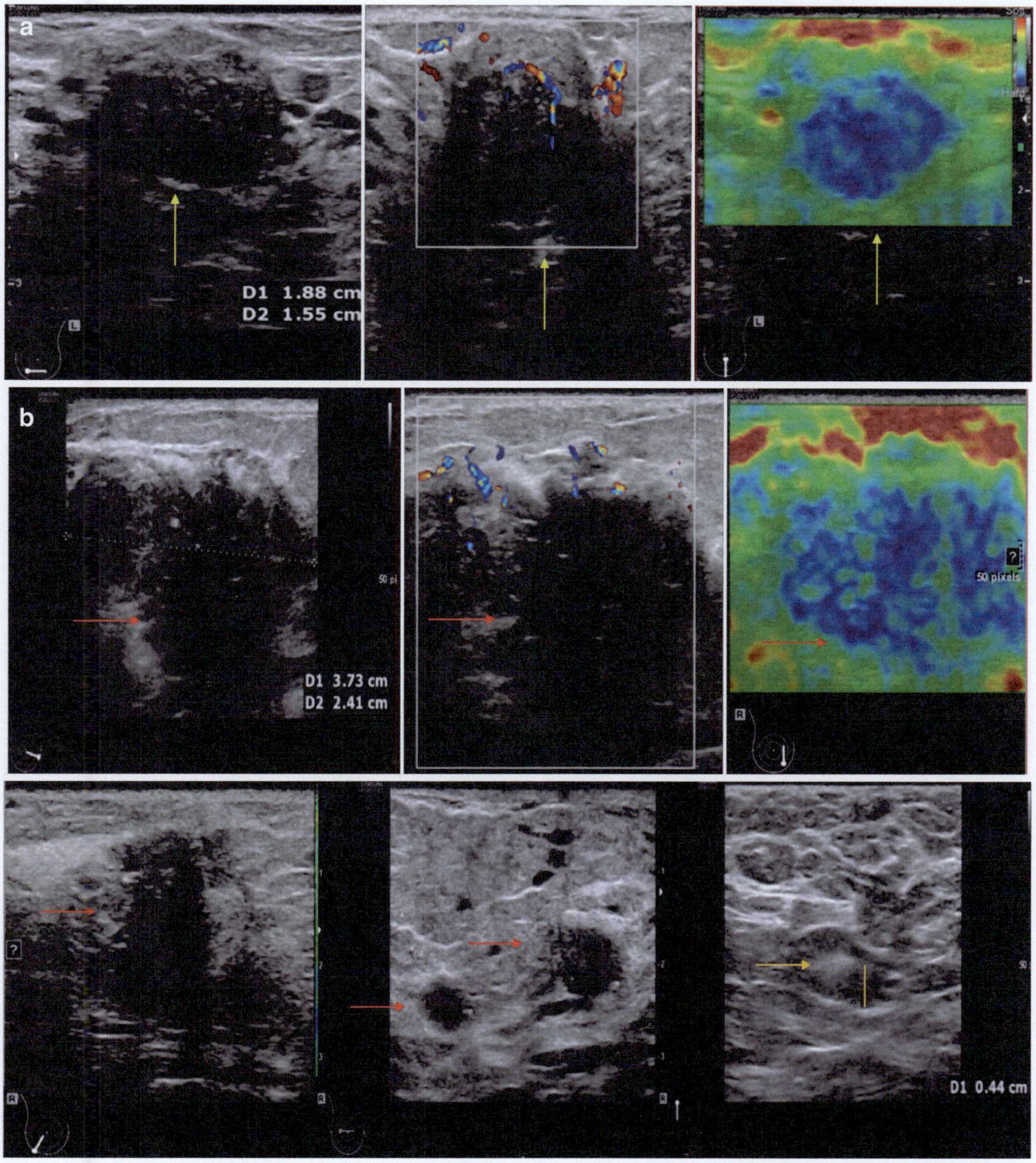

Fig. 14.10 Lactating mother since six months presented with bilateral breast lumps showed mixed echogenic mass (yellow arrow) with vascularity and hard on elastography at 6 o'clock left breast on USG (**a**). Right breast USG (**b**) showed 4 o'clock index spiculated mass and additional hypoechoic masses at 7 and 10 o'clock (all in red arrows). Right axillary node shows eccentric cortical hypertrophy—suspicious (orange arrow). HPR revealed IDC NOS CE-MRI (**c**) both breasts confirmed right breast multicentric T1 hypo-T2 intermediate enhancing masses with diffusion restriction (red arrows) along with intervening nonmass enhancement (blue arrow)—contemplating for conservative surgery. The left breast 6 o'clock lesion (yellow arrow) showed T1 iso-T2 hypointense enhancement with no diffusion restriction and categorised as BIRADS 4a—HPR revealed lactating adenoma

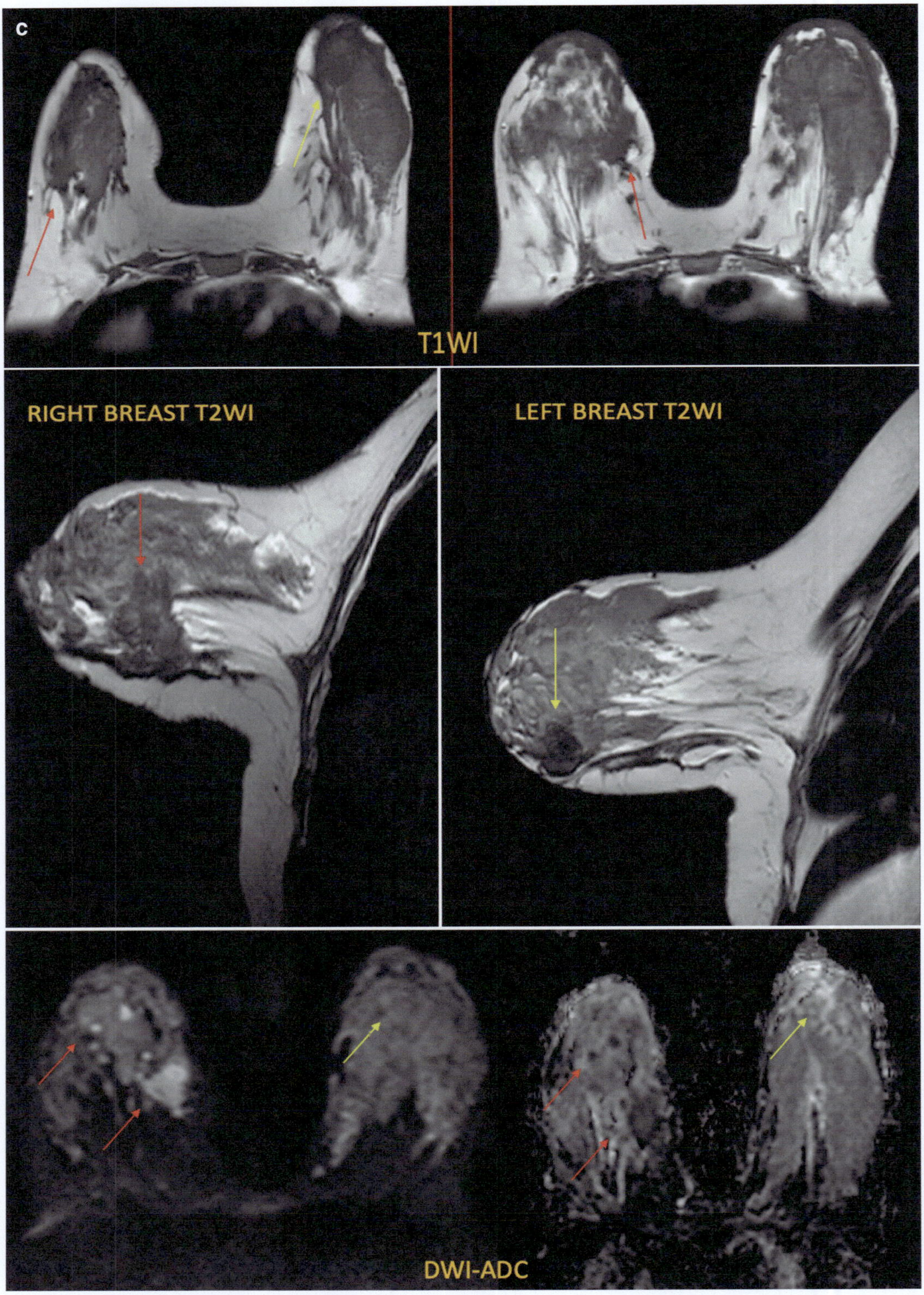

Fig. 14.10 (continued)

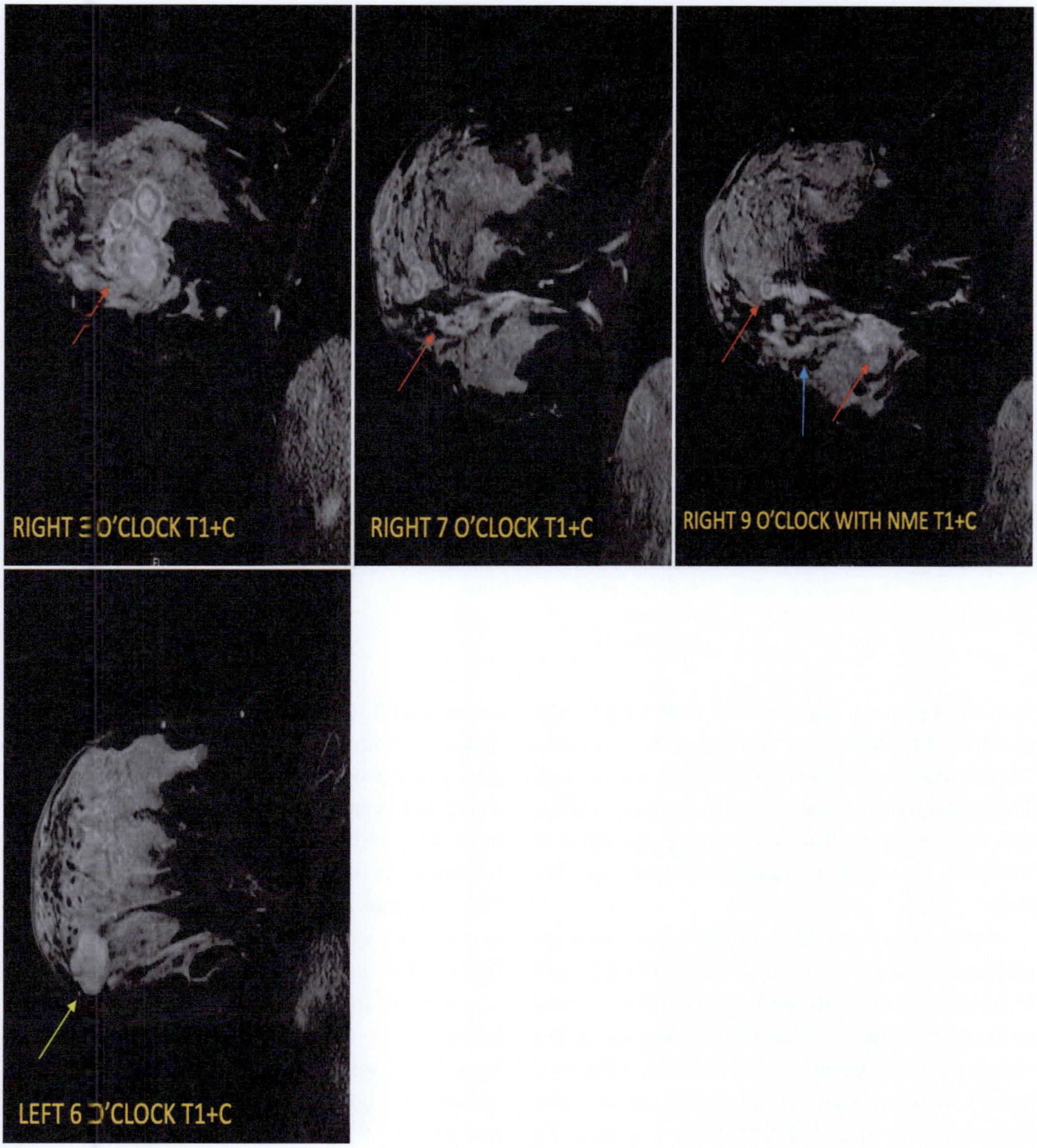

Fig. 14.10 (continued)

like artefacts, eddy currents, image distortions, and low sensitivity for nonmass enhancement preclude its use for screening [17]. DCE MRI and guided procedures are safe in lactating women. It is recommended to abstain from breastfeeding for at least 6 hours after MRI, in view of gadolinium-related effects. Annual screening MRI for high-risk patients is resumed within 6–8 weeks following cessation of lactation [5].

The various indications for imaging modalities have been enumerated in Table 14.1.

Recent advances on MRI techniques like diffusion tensor imaging (DTI) of the breast (increases tumour conspicuity in background of linear ductal tree skeleton), DWI whole body

Table 14.1 Imaging modalities for pregnancy-associated breast cancer

Modality	Pregnancy-associated breast cancer	Postpartum-related breast cancer	Use	Limitation
USG	First investigation of choice		Diagnose typical benign pathologies avoiding unnecessary biopsy. Detect suspicious findings and categorise level of suspicion and for need of biopsy.	Indeterminate USG features require supplemental imaging.
MMG	Adjuvant tool for diagnosis		Locoregional staging, detection of microcalcifications, and guided procedures in absence of USG correlate	Mammographic density and radiation exposure
MRI—Unenhanced	Recommended in selected cases	DWI, DTI, and T2WI may detect early cancers.	Annual MRI screening in genetically high-risk postpartum. Whole body DWI—an alternative for distant staging	Artefacts and challenges in interpretation
DCE MRI	Contraindicated	Diagnostic and prognostic role	Can be used in lactation	Gadolinium use is controversial.
Nuclear imaging	Last choice based on risk-benefit ratio	Strict guidelines pre- and postprocedure	Distant staging	Tracer toxicity and teratogenic effects

with background suppression (DWI-BS), MR spectroscopy (MRS) for choline peak, and intravoxel incoherent motion (IVIM) are under trial. These sequences have shown promising results and are being evaluated for being included in standard screening or diagnostic protocols for PABC [19].

When using nuclear imaging in pregnant patients, 18F-fluorodeoxyglucose (FDG) and technetium (Tc-99 m) can be safely administered with careful dose calculation and precautions like bladder catheterisation and hydration. However, hybrid imaging with CT increases foetal radiation exposure [52]. PET/MRI is a promising alternative, offering better detection of distant metastases than PET/CT [21]. For distant staging in pregnancy-associated breast cancer, whole body diffusion-weighted imaging (DWI-BS) is effective in detecting skeletal, liver, peritoneal, and nodal metastases [21].

14.4.2 Treatment

PABC patients and their families need comprehensive multidisciplinary treatment, and strong social support since decision-making after diagnosis and prognosis evaluation is intellectually, psychosocially, and physically demanding. There are many options for treatment, like any other BC, with the difference that in pregnancy, treatment is scheduled around gestational age [22]. Purpose of treatment as curative or palliative must be individualised on case-by-case basis. Initiation of cancer treatment in pregnancy tends to increase the risk of prematurity and early labour [43]. Prognosis influences decisions regarding continuation of pregnancy, but termination does not influence the overall survival of the patient. Surgery, chemotherapy, and radiotherapy along with targeted therapies are available options.

BC surgery is feasible at any gestational age with the assistance of nonteratogenic anaesthetics [14]. The timing of operation for PABC must be determined based on patient and tumour factors, gestational age, and patient preference. Elective operation is generally deferred until after pregnancy. For reconstruction of the breast, prosthetic implants can be considered, whereas autologous reconstruction is generally deferred until after delivery. Sentinel lymph node biopsy can be safely done during pregnancy, but blue dye must be avoided because of the risk of anaphylaxis [24]. Alternatively, Technetium-99 m with a one-day protocol is used.

Chemotherapy is the treatment of choice in metastatic PABC, and agents are anthracyclines, taxanes, and platinum derivates, particularly as dose-dense regimens that yield improved overall survival Chemotherapy may be started at 12 weeks of pregnancy as neoadjuvant or adjuvant therapy [25]. Preexposure prophylaxis before 12 weeks poses risks for congenital anomalies (21.7%) and foetal growth restriction [6]. For both maternal and foetal recoveries, the chemotherapy should be discontinued by the end of the third trimester, with an optimal gap of three weeks between termination and delivery to avoid peripartum complications [23].

Lesser evidence is available for targeted therapies regarding teratogenic effects. Trastuzumab and Pertuzumab, which are large molecules, need active transport by the placenta, whereas tyrosine kinase inhibitors are transplacental. Targeted therapies consequently impact foetal growth and development [50] by decreasing the volume of amniotic fluid and hence contraindicated during pregnancy. This also adds to foetal renal and pulmonary anomalies and thus is administered following delivery only [24].

Hormonal therapy is contraindicated during pregnancy and must be delayed until after delivery. Pregnancy with tamoxifen has been associated with a higher risk of foetal malformations and spontaneous abortions, although current evidence is still sparse [32]. Likewise, immunotherapy is not indicated during pregnancy, since PD-1/PD-L1 interactions potentially increase the risk of foetal endocrinopathies [26].

In pregnant women, the risks and benefits of radiation therapy should be weighed carefully with regard to the potential risk to the foetus. Foetal tissues are sensitive to radiation and its toxicities, and the sensitivity depends on the pregnancy stage. The foetal dose depends on the distance from the target, the target volume size and location, and the technical aspects of the radiation therapy [19]. For oligometastatic disease, metastasis-directed radiation therapy is the usual approach, with a preference for ultrahypofractionated courses over one week [3]. If the target lesion is away from foetus like brain metastases, targeted radiotherapy can be an option. Good coordination between the medical physics and radioprotection groups should be maintained to minimise risk to both foetus and patient.

In BC-treated offspring, careful assessment of the offspring must be done with echocardiogram and ECG in those who were exposed to in utero anthracyclines [4].

In utero-exposed infants to platinum derivatives need vigilant monitoring for hearing loss.

Poorer outcome of pregnancy-associated breast cancer (PABC) than non-PABC seems to be a result of delayed diagnosis rather than pregnancy. This emphasises the importance of more stringent screening measures in high-risk groups and better imaging modalities for the detection of the disease at an early stage. Radiologists need to have a high index of suspicion, use appropriate imaging modalities, and perform a biopsy in cases of any doubt. Treatment needs to be planned through proper multidisciplinary channel, following standardised protocols while taking extra care regarding foetal protection.

14.5 Summary

Breast cancer is the leading cause of cancer-related deaths among women under 40, as they are more likely to develop aggressive subtypes such as triple-negative and HER2-enriched cancers, which tend to progress to advanced stages rapidly. A multidisciplinary approach is essential for ensuring the best possible outcomes for young women with breast cancer, especially considering the void of routine screening protocols for this population. Clinical breast examination is the base to screening in young population; however, inherent risk factors must be borne in mind to begin early imaging.

MG with USG, MRI, and CNB are the pillars of evaluation of BCs with accurate and early detection. Other modalities like tomosynthesis, elastography, and contrast-enhanced MG show promising adjunct role in decision-making.

Bilateral BC must be foreseen in high-risk target patients based on biomarker and grade of tumour. It emphasises need of a close follow-up and prognostication in such patients, not to forget the simultaneous rapid advancement of targeted therapy to improve outcome and survival.

PABC is BC during pregnancy or lactation. Postpartum BC is associated with poor prognosis and aggressive behaviour, attributing to delay in diagnosis and also protumour microenvironment. Locoregional staging is done by USG and MG and unenhanced MRI techniques if required (DWI, T2WI, DTI). DCE MRI retains significant value in breast imaging during lactation, particularly with emerging ultrafast sequences that enhance early detection of malignant lesions while minimising background parenchymal enhancement. The use of DWI-BS versus nuclear imaging for distant staging requires further validation to determine the optimal risk-benefit balance. Additionally, pregnant women with breast cancer should be referred for genetic counselling to address potential hereditary factors.

References

1. Ramirez SA, Menegaz BA, Roark A, Bonefas E, Sepulveda KA, Thompson AM, et al. Abstract P1-05-08: assessment and diagnosis of breast pathology in young women: what can we learn? Cancer Res. 2023;83(5_Supplement)
2. Hendrick RE, Helvie MA, Monticciolo DL. Breast cancer mortality rates have stopped declining in U.S. women younger than 40 years. Radiology. 2021;299(1):143.
3. Leung JWT. Invited commentary: learning about breast cancer outcomes in Asian women to close the health equity gap. Radiographics. 2022;42:E203.
4. Davey MG, Brennan M, Ryan ÉJ, Corbett M, Abd Elwahab S, Walsh S, et al. Defining clinicopathological and radiological features of breast cancer in women under the age of 35: an epidemiological study. Ir J Med Sci. 2020;189(4):1195.
5. diFlorio-Alexander RM, Slanetz PJ, Moy L, Baron P, Didwania AD, Heller SL, et al. ACR appropriateness criteria® breast imaging of pregnant and lactating women. J Am Coll Radiol. 2018;15(11):S263.
6. Gao Y, Samreen N, Heller SL. Non-BRCA early-onset breast cancer in young women. Radiographics. 2022;42(1):5.
7. Heller SL, Lourenco AP, Niell BL, Ajkay N, Brown A, Dibble EH, et al. ACR appropriateness criteria® imaging after mastectomy and breast reconstruction. J Am Coll Radiol. 2020;17(11):S403.
8. Gradishar WJ, Moran MS, Abraham J, Aft R, Agnese D, Allison KH, et al. NCCN guidelines® insights: breast cancer, version 4.2021. J Natl Compr Cancer Netw. 2021;19(5):484.
9. Castro Reyes B. Breast cancer characteristics in young women. Rev Senol Patol Mamar. 2021;34(2):209–17.
10. Durhan G, Azizova A, Önder Ö, Kösemehmetoğlu K, Karakaya J, Akpınar MG, et al. Imaging findings and clinicopathological correlation of breast cancer in women under 40 years old. Eur J Breast Health. 2019;15(3):147–52.
11. Park AR, Chae EY, Cha JH, Shin HJ, Choi WJ, Kim HH. Preoperative breast MRI in women 35 years of age and younger with breast cancer: benefits in surgical outcomes by using propensity score analysis. Radiology. 2021;300(1):39.
12. Taourel P. MRI to detect contralateral breast cancer in patients with newly diagnosed breast cancer: an increase in overall survival to be confirmed. Radiology. 2022;304:308.
13. Di Nubila B, Cassano E, Urban LABD, Fedele P, Abbate F, Maisonneuve P, et al. Radiological features and pathological-biological correlations in 348 women with breast cancer under 35 years old. Breast. 2006;15(6):744.
14. Cheun JH, Kim HK, Lee HB, Han W, Moon HG. Abstract P2-11-07: mammographic density is associated with increased risk of contralateral breast cancers but not of ipsilateral breast tumour recurrences. Cancer Res. 2022;82(4_Supplement):P2-11-07.
15. Monticciolo DL. Invited commentary: the challenges of early-onset breast cancer. Radiographics. 2022;42:E16.
16. Kamishov SV, Izrailbekova KS, Balenkov OY. Study of the level of tumour markers and mutations in the BRCA1/2 genes in breast cancer patients with metachronous tumours. J Clin Oncol. 2022;40(16_suppl):e12563.
17. Tsujino K, Hirota S, Takahara K, Takada Y, Konishi M, Kono N, et al. Breast conservation therapy for early breast cancer: comparison of breast conserving surgery with or without radiotherapy. J JASTRO. 2000;12(1)
18. Prihantono, Faruk M. Breast cancer resistance to chemotherapy: when should we suspect it and how can we prevent it? Ann Med Surg. 2021;70:102793.
19. Hruska CB, Hunt KN, Conners AL, Geske JR, Brandt KR, Degnim AC, et al. Impact of short-term low-dose tamoxifen on molecular breast imaging background parenchymal uptake: a pilot study. Breast Cancer Res. 2019;21(1):38.
20. Chavarri-Guerra Y, Higgins MJ, Szymonifka J, Cigler T, Liedke P, Partridge A, et al. Drug withdrawal in women with progressive metastatic breast cancer while on aromatase inhibitor therapy. Br J Cancer. 2014;111(11):2046.
21. Huang J, Lin Q, Cui C, Fei J, Su X, Li L, et al. Correlation between imaging features and molecular

subtypes of breast cancer in young women (≤30 years old). Jpn J Radiol. 2020;38(11):1062.
22. Bullier B, MacGrogan G, Bonnefoi H, Hurtevent-Labrot G, Lhomme E, Brouste V, et al. Imaging features of sporadic breast cancer in women under 40 years old: 97 cases. Eur Radiol. 2013;23(12):3237.
23. Greally M, Kielty J, Watson GA, Das G, Malouf C, McSorley L, et al. Where youth matters—clinicopathologic characteristics and emerging trends in treatment and outcomes in young Irish women with breast cancer. Ir J Med Sci. 2019;188(1):59.
24. Gao Y, Perez CA, Chhor C, Heller SL. Breast cancer screening in survivors of childhood cancer. Radiographic. 2023;43(4):e220155.
25. Paluch-Shimon S, Cardoso F, Partridge AH, Abulkhair O, Azim HA, Bianchi-Micheli G, et al. ESO–ESMO fifth international consensus guidelines for breast cancer in young women (BCY5). Ann Oncol. 2022;33(11):1097.
26. Agarwal S, Singhal V. Bilateral invasive synchronous breast cancer: Atypical presentation. Clin Radiol [Internet]. 2022 Nov 1 [cited 2023 May 27];77:e24. Available from: http://www.clinicalradiologyonline.net/article/S0009926022005931/fulltext
27. Copur MS, Ramaekers R, Gauchan D, Crockett D, Clark D. Synchronous bilateral breast cancer with different histology. Radiol Case Rep. 2023;18(7):2491–7.
28. Freitas V, Li X, Amitai Y, Au F, Kulkarni S, Ghai S, et al. Contralateral breast screening with preoperative MRI: long-term outcomes for newly diagnosed breast cancer. Radiology [Internet] 2022 [cited 2023 May 27];304(2):297–307. Available from: https://pubs.rsna.org/doi/10.1148/radiol.212361
29. Megaro G, Rossi L, Ceddia S, Sinjari M, Mannino A, Gozzi E, et al. Synchronous and metachronous metastatic breast cancer, with different histology and opposite immunophenotype, treated with combination of chemotherapy, anti-Her2, and endocrine therapy: a case report. Case Rep Oncol. 2020;13(2)
30. Linshaw D, Tonneson J, Rosenkranz K. Surgical therapy for women with multiple synchronous ipsilateral breast cancer (MIBC): current evidence to guide clinical practice. Curr Breast Cancer Rep. 2019;11:67.
31. Rehman S, Rehman B, Rehman AU, Din IU, Iftikhar A, Javaid A, et al. MRI features of synchronous masses in known breast cancer patients in predicting benign versus malignant lesions: a case based review at tertiary care cancer hospital. South Asian J Cancer. 2023;12(1):068.
32. Clauser P. Clinical value of contralateral breast cancers detected by pre-operative MRI in patients diagnosed with DCIS: a population-based cohort study-commentary. Eur Radiol [Internet]. 1:3. Available from: https://doi.org/10.1007/s00330-023-09396-4
33. Crary IL, Parker EU, Lowry KP, Patwardhan PP, Soong TR, Javid SH, et al. Risk of lobular neoplasia upgrade with synchronous carcinoma. Ann Surg Oncol. 2022;29(10)
34. Hu J, Lanitis S, Dimopoulos N, Bright-Thomas R, Cunningham D, Faissola B, et al. Invasive lobular carcinoma: imaging characteristics, size at presentation and bilaterality. Cancer Res. 2009;69(24_Supplement):4015.
35. Roubidoux MA, Lai NE, Paramagul C, Joynt LK, Helvie MA. Mammographic appearance of cancer in the opposite breast: comparison with the first cancer. Am J Roentgenol. 1996;166(1):29–31.
36. Sharma S, Fischer A, Hatch P, Sharma S. A case of bilateral male breast cancer- what does it teach us? Radiol Case Rep. 2023;18(4):1592.
37. Özgür C, Sunal BS, Tunçbilek N. A rare case of bilateral synchronous male breast cancer: a multimodality approach. Eur J Breast Health. 2022;18(2):199.
38. Amornsiripanitch N, Nguyen VT, Rahbar H, Hippe DS, Gadi VK, Rendi MH, et al. Diffusion-weighted MRI characteristics associated with prognostic pathological factors and recurrence risk in invasive ER+/HER2– breast cancers. J Magn Reson Imaging. 2018;48(1):226.
39. Heine JJ, Malhotra P. Mammographic tissue, breast cancer risk, serial image analysis, and digital mammography: part 2. Serial breast tissue change and related temporal influences. Acad Radiol. 2002;9(3):317–35.
40. Mishra A, Oberoi AS, Deo S, Sharma J, Gogia A, Sharma DN, Mathur S, Dhamija E. Bilateral breast cancer: clinical profile and management. Indian J Surg Oncol. 2023;14(3):651–8.
41. Kaur D, Jain R, Rai S, Mangal KS. Incidence of breast carcinoma in pregnant and lactating women. Int J Sci Res. 2021:46.
42. Jin YC, Du JX, Fu SM, Chen Q, Qiu YR, Pei A, et al. A retrospective clinical study of patients with pregnancy-associated breast cancer among multiple centers in China (CSBrS-008). Chin Med J. 2021;134(18):2186.
43. Shao C, Yu Z, Xiao J, Liu L, Hong F, Zhang Y, et al. Prognosis of pregnancy-associated breast cancer: a meta-analysis. BMC Cancer. 2020;20(1):746.
44. Jo H, Park S, Kim HR, Kim H, Hong J, Lee JE, et al. Long-term breast cancer outcomes of pregnancy-associated breast cancer (PABC) in a prospective cohort. Cancers (Basel). 2022;14(19)
45. Tan QT, Alcantara VS, Sultana R, Loh KWJ, Go AL, Wong FY. Pregnancy-associated breast cancer: a multicenter study comparing clinicopathological factors, diagnosis and treatment outcomes with non-pregnant patients. Breast Cancer Res Treat. 2023;198(1):53.
46. Faermann R, Friedman E, Kaidar-Person O, Brodsky M, Neiman OH, Shalmon A, et al. Pregnancy associated breast cancer among Israeli BRCA1/BRCA2 carriers in a high-risk clinic. Acad Radiol. 2023;30(2):248–54.
47. Safi N, Saunders C, Anazodo A, Dickinson JE, Boyle F, Ives A, et al. Clinical decision making in the management of breast cancer diagnosed during preg-

nancy: a review and case series analysis. J Adolesc Young Adult Oncol. 2022;11:245–51.
48. Parokonnaya AA, Petrovskiy AV, Avtomonov DE, Sergeev YS. Errors in the diagnosis of breast cancer during pregnancy and lactation based on clinical cases. Онкогинекология. 2021;3
49. Kieturakis AJ, Wahab RA, Vijapura C, Mahoney MC. Current recommendations for breast imaging of the pregnant and lactating patient. Am J Roentgenol. 2021;216:1462–75.
50. Nissan N, Massasa EEM, Bauer E, Halshtck-Neiman O, Shalmon A, Gotlieb M, et al. MRI can accurately diagnose breast cancer during lactation. Eur Radiol. 2022;33:2935.
51. Fruchtman-Brot H, Mango VL. Pregnancy-associated breast cancer in BRCA1/2 carriers: is intensified breast ultrasound surveillance warranted? Acad Radiol. 2023;30:255.
52. Despierres M, Boudy AS et al. Feasibility, safety and impact of (18 F) FDG PET CT in patients with pregnancy associated cancers: French CALG network. Acte Oncol. 2022;61(3).

Imaging and Approach in Male Breast Diseases

15

Upasna Sinha, Ruchi Sinha, and Ekta Dhamija

Abstract

The male breast is a rudimentary structure composed predominantly of adipose tissue and atrophic ductal tissue in the subareolar region, as compared to developed terminal ductal-lobular units and the ductal system in female breast. The male breast diseases are rarer and different from the female breast and therefore need understanding of basic anatomy and pathologies separately. The majority of male breast pathologies are benign, the most common being gynecomastia. Male breast cancer is very rare, and invasive ductal carcinoma is the most commonly seen histologic subtype. The incidence of lobular diseases such as fibroadenomas, phyllodes, sclerosing adenoses, fibrocystic disease, and lobular carcinoma is very low in men compared with women because men do not have terminal ductal-lobular unit differentiation. Diseases arising from the skin and subcutaneous tissue are also common in the male breast. There is no standardized imaging algorithm or screening protocol, so all imaging assessment in men are mostly diagnostic in nature. Mammography and ultrasound are the two main imaging modalities used to evaluate the male breast. Although male breast disease is uncommon, it is imperative to understand the differences between male and female breast anatomy and pathologies for making an accurate diagnosis and avoiding unnecessary investigations.

Keywords

Male breast · Gynecomastia
Pseudogynecomastia · Male breast cancer
Epidermal inclusion cyst

15.1 Introduction

Despite its rudimentary structure, the male breast can suffer from a spectrum of benign and malignant diseases, although incidence is low. The common clinical symptoms are unilateral or bilateral breast enlargement, breast pain, and palpable lump. The majority of male breast lesions are benign, with gynecomastia being the most common. Male breast cancer is rare, often present with advanced stages, and has worse prognosis than female breast cancer. Therefore, it is important to differentiate cancer from the more

U. Sinha (✉)
Department of Radiodiagnosis, AIIMS, Patna, India
e-mail: drupasnasinha@aiimspatna.org

R. Sinha
Department of Pathology/Laboratory Medicine, AIIMS, Patna, India

E. Dhamija
Department of Diagnostic and Interventional Onco-Radiology, IRCH, AIIMS, New Delhi, India

E. Dhamija, S. V. S. Deo (eds.), *Imaging in Management of Breast Diseases*,
https://doi.org/10.1007/978-981-96-4998-3_15

common benign breast lesions. Since there is no standardised algorithm and no screening protocol for early cancer detection, male breast undergoes gamut of imaging evaluation with diagnostic indication and purpose. This chapter attempts to discuss the basic differences and describe various pathologies in male breasts.

15.2 Development and Anatomy

At birth and until the prepubescent stage, the male and female breasts have similar histological anatomy. Male and female breasts develop differently during adolescence due to distinct hormonal environments. Peripubertal oestrogen and progesterone promote ductal system proliferation and branching in females, as well as stromal and terminal duct lobular unit (TDLU) development [1]. A mature female breast is thus composed primarily of fibroglandular tissue, which comprises ducts, stroma, and lobular tissue, as well as a well-developed nipple-areolar complex.

The initial surge of oestrogen that occurs in males during the peripubertal period results in a transient proliferation of the stroma and ductal system. However, the concomitant sharp increase in testosterone antagonises the effect of oestrogen and leads to significant involution and atrophy of the ductal system [2]. In addition, the TDLU does not develop because of the absence of progesterone. Therefore, the typical adult male breast is a rudimentary structure with a small nipple-areolar complex. It consists of skin, subcutaneous fat (which accounts for most of the breast volume), and an atrophic ductal system with little stromal tissue in the retroareolar region [3]. Cooper's ligaments are absent, and the underlying pectoralis muscle is prominent [4]. Histology shows predominantly adipose tissue with few scattered ducts in the dense collagenised stroma, with sparse and underdeveloped lobules (Fig. 15.1a).

On digital mammography (MG), male breast shows homogeneously radiolucent subcutaneous fat with subareolar few high-density strands of connective tissue, indicating an atrophic ductal system and stroma (Fig. 15.2a, b). The pectoralis muscle appears prominent. In contrast, the mature female breast is larger and shows predominantly high-density fibroglandular tissue with a less prominent pectoralis muscle (Fig. 15.2c, d).

Similarly, male breast ultrasound (US) shows subcutaneous isoechoic fat with a small hypoechoic area in the retroareolar region representing ductal remnants (Fig. 15.3a), whereas female breast shows a variable amount of heterogeneous echotexture representing fibroglandular parenchyma (Fig. 15.3b and Table 15.1).

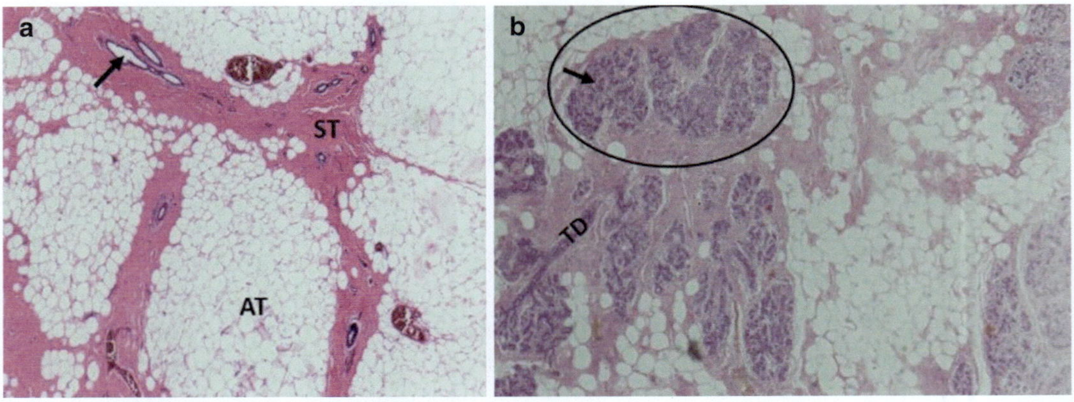

Fig. 15.1 Normal histopathological image—photomicrograph of male breast parenchyma (hematoxylin and eosin, 40×) (**a**) shows few scattered ducts (arrow) in dense collagenised stroma (ST) and extensive adipose tissue (AT). There is absence of acini and terminal ductal lobular unit as compared to female breast (**b**) which shows multiple TDLU consisting of terminal duct (TD) and lobules (circle) of acini (arrow)

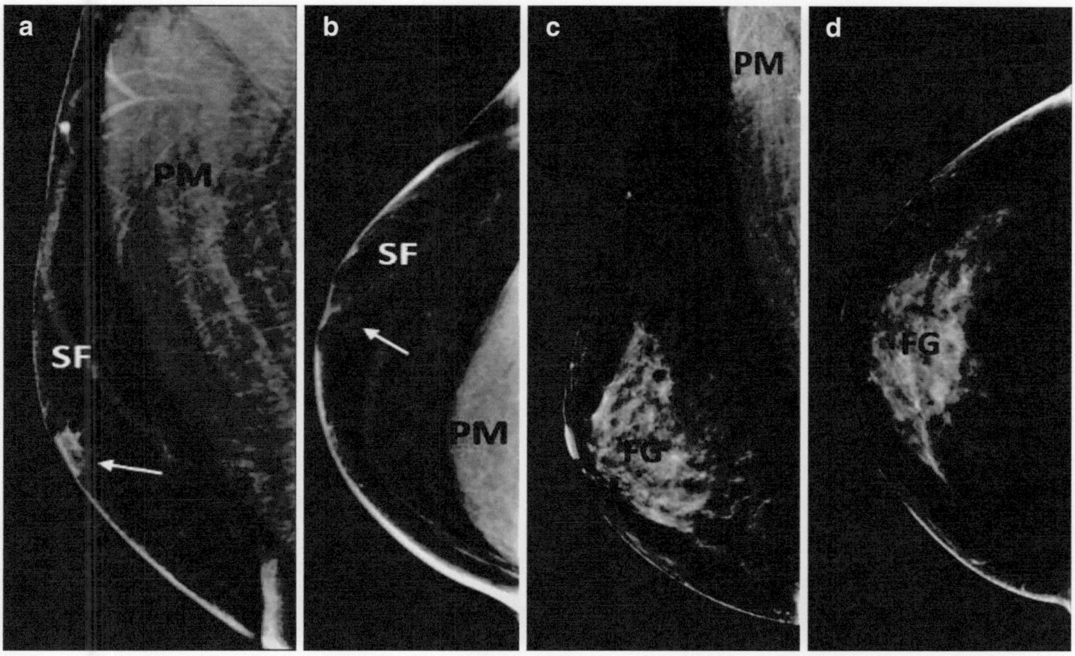

Fig. 15.2 Normal imaging anatomy on digital mammogram—mediolateral oblique (**a**) and craniocaudal views (**b**) of normal male breast show homogenous radiolucent subcutaneous fat (SF) with prominent pectoralis muscle (PM) and remnant ductal tissue in subareolar region (arrow) as compared to female breast (**c**, **d**) which show predominant high-density fibroglandular tissue (FG) with less prominent pectoralis muscle

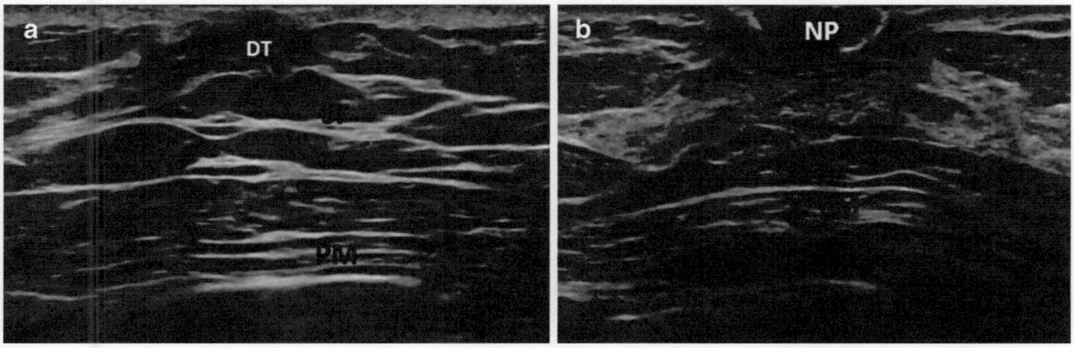

Fig. 15.3 Normal imaging anatomy of the breast on ultrasound: Transverse ultrasound of male breast (**a**) shows predominant isoechoic subcutaneous fat (SF) with hypoechoic remnant ductal tissue (DT) in subareolar region whereas female breast (**b**) shows heterogenous echotexture of fibroglandular tissue (FG) at the level of nipple (NP). Pectoralis muscle (PM) is also seen posteriorly

Table 15.1 Anatomy of male and female breast

	Male breast	Female breast
Predominant component	Subcutaneous fat	Fibroglandular tissues
Ductal system	Atrophic	Well developed
Terminal ductal-lobular unit	Development rare	Well developed
Stromal tissue	Minimal subareolar stromal tissue	More stromal tissue scattered in the breast
Cooper's ligament	Absent	Present
Pectoralis muscle	Prominent	Less prominent
Nipple areolar complex	Small	Large
Mammogram	Homogenous radiolucent fat with small retroareolar density of remnant ductal system	Variable densities depending upon the amount of fibroglandular tissue

15.3 Clinical Presentation and Assessment

The clinical presentation is often with symptomatic breast as either unilateral or bilateral breast enlargement, pain, or palpable lump [4, 5]. The onset-progress-duration and age group are important factors while approaching any symptomatic male breast. For instance, the history of bilateral breast enlargement/lump with or without associated pain is almost always due to gynecomastia, and evaluation consists of ruling out any underlying cause for the condition. On the other end, an elderly male with painless mass should be evaluated with suspicion of malignancy because the incidence of breast cancer in young males (less than 40 years) is up to 1.6% and the lumps are predominantly benign in nature for this age group.

Several studies demonstrated that physical examination has a high sensitivity of 85–100% and a high NPV of 95–99.5% but low PPV in detecting malignancy [4, 6, 7]. Hence, no additional imaging is needed if the physical examination is normal or benign. However, if it is suspicious or indeterminate, the man should undergo imaging evaluation prior to tissue sampling or biopsy.

The main imaging modalities include digital MG with or without digital breast tomosynthesis (DBT) and breast US. Just like in female patients, MG involves acquisition of two standard views: mediolateral oblique (MLO) and craniocaudal (CC) view. The small size of the breast can make MG a technical challenge and may need an expert radiographer and use of small compression paddles.

At times, the enlarged pectoralis muscle opacity may obscure posteriorly located lesions, which can be dealt with acquisition of the pectoralis-displaced view—in which the technician pushes the pectoralis muscle posteriorly and instructs the patient to contract the pectoralis muscle while pulling the breast anteriorly onto the detector [3]. Most of the times, male breast needs comprehensive assessment using MG as the primary modality and US as adjunct modality, for detection and characterization of the underlying pathology.

The MG has been reported to have a high sensitivity of 95–100%, specificity of 90–95%, and NPV of 99–100% for cancer detection [6–9]. In a study by Taylor et al. on efficacy of triple assessment in male breast diseases, the combined NPV of clinical examination and mammography was 100% in ruling out cancers in men above 40 years of age [10]. US has a sensitivity of 80–100%, a specificity of 74–99.5%, and an NPV of 99–100% for the detection of cancer [5–7, 11]. Thus ultrasound is the most specific imaging modality and mammography has a high sensitivity; no further assessment is necessary if the results of both imaging modalities are benign [7].

US is particularly helpful in determining the relationship between a mass and the nipple because gynecomastia tends to be concentric with the nipple, whereas malignant masses tend to be eccentric. US is also preferable for the assessment of axillary nodes. Few studies have also attempted to study the added value of elastography to differentiate benign and malignant masses of the male breast; however, it is not routinely recommended [12].

According to American College of Radiology (ACR) appropriateness criteria, targeted breast US should be the first imaging modality in men younger than 25 years of age who have a palpable mass. If ultrasound findings are suspicious, diagnostic MG should be performed. In patients above 25 years, evaluation should begin with MG, and if it is indeterminate, a targeted ultrasound should be performed as a complementary tool. Regardless of the patient's age, a MG should be the first imaging modality when there is a clinical suspicion of cancer [13].

MRI is not routinely recommended and there are no established indications or guidelines for the male breast. According to Shin et al.'s analysis of MRI breast in men over a ten-year period, breast MRI may be useful to evaluate skin involvement, posteriorly located masses (for chest wall invasion), occult breast cancer, inflammatory breast cancer, and postoperative residual disease, and it may occasionally be used to assess response to neoadjuvant chemotherapy [14].

Imaging findings are described according to the ACR Breast Imaging Reporting and Data System (BIRADS) lexicon, similar to the female breast, and each breast is assigned BIRADS categories 0–6 [15]. However, the readers should note that the ACR categories for breast composition do not apply to the male breast because it lacks normal fibroglandular tissue.

If imaging findings are indeterminate or suspicious, US-guided biopsy is usually preferred to establish pathological diagnosis.

15.4 Benign Breast Diseases

There is a wide spectrum of benign and malignant lesions described in literature which affect male breasts. Ductal and stromal proliferative diseases such as gynecomastia, myofibroblastoma, ductal carcinoma, etc. are more common than lobular pathologies because of the lack of lobular development in men [2]. Therefore, pathologies arising in lobular units like fibroepithelial lesions (fibroadenomas and phyllodes), cysts, sclerosing adenosis, lobular carcinoma in situ, and invasive lobular carcinoma are extremely rare in males, in contrast to females in whom some of these pathologies are very common [16]. Dermal and subcutaneous lesions are also common in the male breast.

Gynecomastia Gynecomastia is the most common pathology of the male breast. It refers to benign proliferation of glandular tissues. It is caused by an oestrogen-androgen imbalance, that is, androgen deficiency and/or oestrogen excess [17]. Depending on the aetiology, gynecomastia can be physiological in 25% of cases, idiopathic in 25% (where no abnormality can be seen), and pathological in the remaining cases (where an underlying cause can be identified) [18, 19].

Physiologic gynecomastia occurs in neonates due to transplacental transfer of estradiol, pubescent boys due to a hormonal surge in which the initial rise in oestrogen causes proliferation of breast tissue, and in senescence due to decreased testosterone levels. Pubertal gynecomastia occurs in 65% of male adolescents and spontaneously regresses in 90% of them. Pathological gynecomastia can have underlying endocrinological, metabolic, neoplastic, and pharmacological causes [1] (Table 15.2). Clinically, it manifests as

Table 15.2 Causes of gynecomastia

Physiological
Neonatal
Pubertal
Senescence
Idiopathic
Pathological
Endocrinological—Klinefelter syndrome, hypogonadism, and hyperthyroidism
Systemic/metabolic—Cirrhosis, chronic renal failure, obesity, and malnutrition
Neoplastic—Adrenal cortical carcinoma, testicular tumour, pituitary adenoma, hepatocellular carcinoma, lung carcinoma, and renal carcinoma
Pharmacological/drug induced
Hormonal-androgen inhibitor, exogenous oestrogen, and anabolic steroids
Cardiovascular-ACE inhibitor, amiodarone, spironolactone, and thiazide diuretics
CNS—Diazepam, haloperidol, and tricyclic antidepressant
Antiulcer—Cimetidine, ranitidine, and omeprazole
Marijuana

unilateral, bilateral symmetric, or bilateral asymmetric breast enlargement with or without soft, mobile, subareolar lump or thickening, with or without associated breast pain. It is the most common cause of palpable lumps in men.

According to the ACR Appropriateness Criteria, imaging is not indicated if a man has classic clinical signs and symptoms of gynecomastia or pseudogynecomastia [13].

Appelbaum has described three mammographic patterns of gynecomastia-nodular, dendritic, and diffuse-depending on the degree and stage of ductal and stromal proliferation [20].

Nodular gynecomastia (acute and reversible)—It is the most common type (72%) of gynecomastia and correlates with the florid histologic phase characterised by florid ductal epithelial hyperplasia with micropapillary architecture, periductal inflammation, and cellular, edematous stroma (Fig. 15.4). It may present with a tender lump and is reversible with treatment of underlying cause. MG shows a subareolar nodular or disk-shaped density or a fan-shaped density that gradually merges with the surrounding parenchymal fat (Fig. 15.5). US shows a

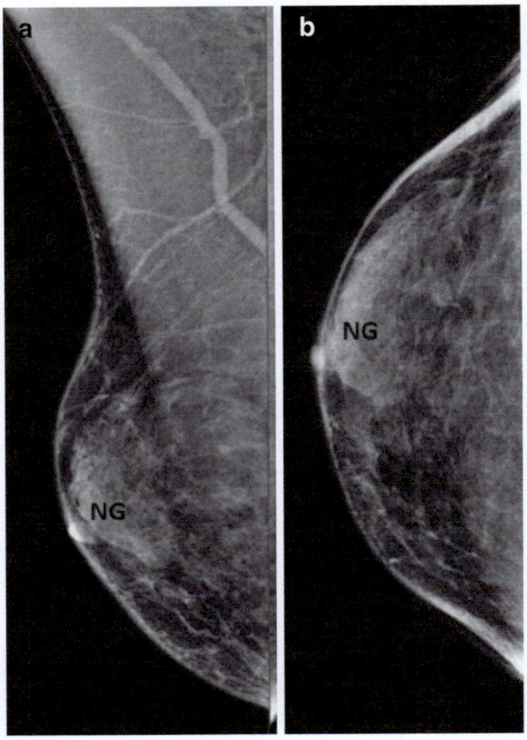

Fig. 15.5 Nodular gynecomastia: Mediolateral oblique (MLO) (**a**) and craniocaudal (CC) (**b**) mammogram of the right breast shows fan-shaped subareolar density (NG)

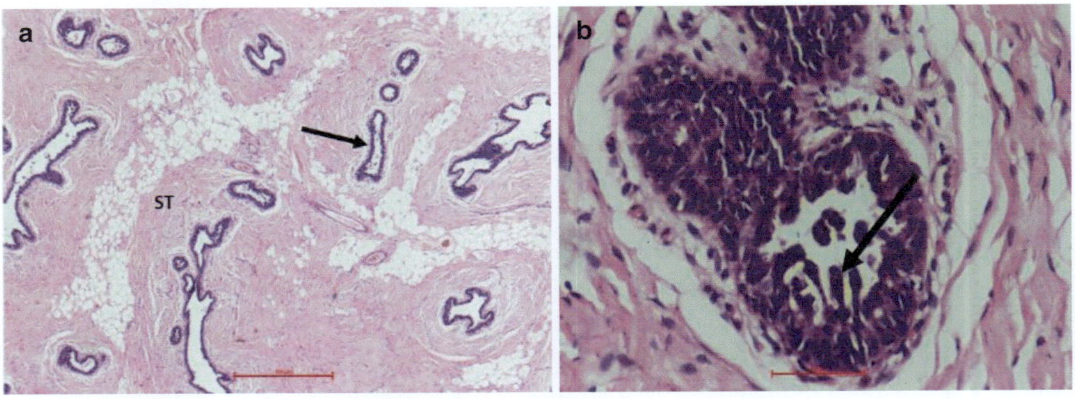

Fig. 15.4 Gynecomastia. (**a**) Photomicrograph (Hematoxylin & eosin; 40×) shows benign ducts (thin arrow) surrounded by cellular stroma (ST). (**b**) Photomicrograph (Hematoxylin & eosin; 400×) shows micropapillary hyperplasia (thick arrow) of ductal lining epithelium

well-circumscribed oval/-disk-shaped or fan-shaped hypoechoic area enclosed by surrounding normal adipose tissue, just beneath the nipple [4, 16]. Hypervascularity can be demonstrated due to stromal proliferation.

Dendritic gynecomastia (chronic and irreversible)—It accounts for 20% of gynecomastia and occurs after one year of duration of onset. It corresponds to the late inactive or fibrous stage of histology which shows dilated ducts with minimal epithelial proliferation surrounded by a dense collagenous hypocellular stroma representing periductal fibrosis [21, 22]. MG shows a flame- or star-shaped irregular retroareolar density originating from the nipple-areolar complex with prominent extensions in the surrounding fat that may extend into the upper outer quadrant (Fig. 15.6). US shows an irregular, heterogeneous, hypoechoic lesion with an irregular, star-shaped posterior margin that has the appearance of spider legs or finger-like projections radiating into the surrounding echogenic fibrous tissue [1, 4, 16].

Diffuse glandular gynecomastia—It accounts for only 3% of cases and has components of both a nodular and dendritic pattern. It occurs due to excessive exogenous oestrogen administration as in the treatment of prostate cancer or in transgender individuals. Imaging shows diffuse proliferation of fibroglandular tissue mimicking a female breast. MG and US show an enlarged breast with features similar to a heterogeneous dense female breast [23] (Fig. 15.7).

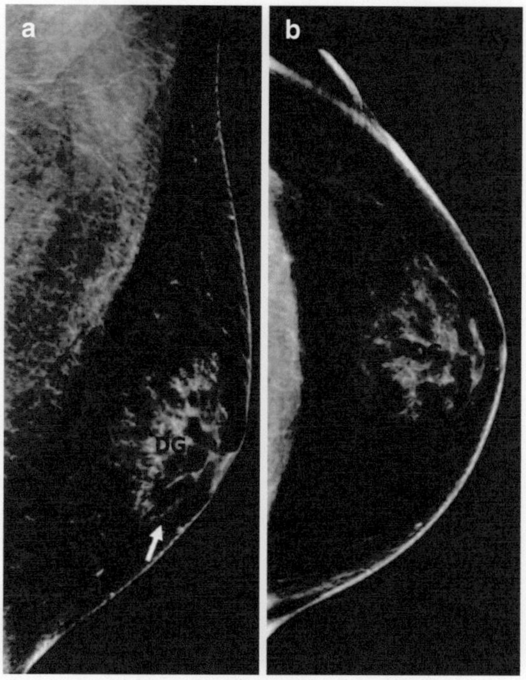

Fig. 15.6 Dendritic gynecomastia: MLO and CC mammogram of the left breast shows flame-shaped subareolar opacity (DG) arising from posterior border of nipple, with dendritic extensions (arrow) posteriorly

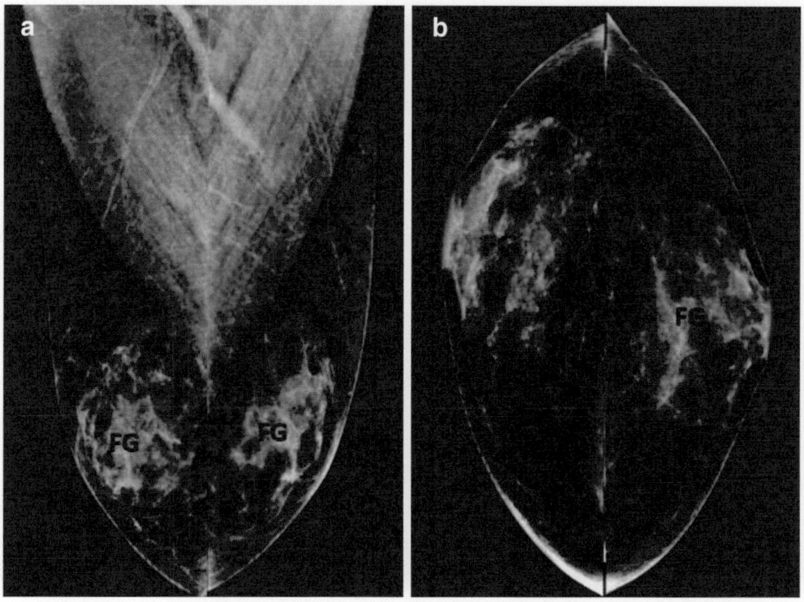

Fig. 15.7 Diffuse gynecomastia: MLO and CC mammogram of male breast shows bilateral enlarged breast with diffuse fibroglandular density (FG) resembling heterogeneously dense female breast

Table 15.3 Clinicoradiological characteristics of gynecomastia and male breast cancer

	Gynecomastia	Male breast cancer
Family and genetic risk factors	Absent	Present
Age of presentation	Any age	Usually above 60 years
Physical examination	Soft, mobile, and usually tender lump	Soft to hard, mobile or fixed, painless lump
Laterality	Can be unilateral or bilateral	Usually unilateral
Relation to the nipple	Subareolar and central to nipple	Subareolar, eccentric to nipple, or in periphery
Mammogram	Fan- or flame-shaped subareolar opacity with posterior margins merging with the surrounding fat. No discrete mass	Usually discrete mass with noncircumscribed (indistinct, spiculated, microlobulated) margin
Ultrasound	Subareolar disc- or fan-shaped or irregular hypoechoic area, with posterior finger-like projections. No cystic component	Usually discrete hypoechoic solid mass with noncircumscribed margin and may have cystic component
Secondary signs of skin and nipple involvement and axillary adenopathy	Absent	Usually present

Gynecomastia may mask the presence of early breast cancer clinically and radiologically. Although gynecomastia and cancer can occur concurrently, there is no documented association between the two. The majority of physiological gynecomastia and idiopathic gynecomastia show spontaneous regression. During the reversible phase, pathological gynecomastia can be treated by stopping the offending drugs and treating the underlying systemic or endocrine problems. Hormonal therapies and other medications like aromatase inhibitors and oestrogen receptor modulators can also be helpful if it has not reached the chronic fibrotic phase. There are surgical options including liposuction and reduction mammoplasty for refractory cases or for cosmetic purposes [17].

The two main differential diagnoses are pseudogynecomastia and cancer. Certain clinicoradiological characteristics may aid in differentiating between cancer and gynecomastia, albeit they may not always rule out malignancy in cases of gynecomastia (Table 15.3).

Pseudogynecomastia (Adipomastia) It is a unilateral or bilateral enlargement of the breast due to excessive deposition of adipose tissue without glandular proliferation [24]. Unlike lipoma, which is a well-circumscribed, encapsulated lesion, pseudogynecomastia is a diffuse lesion. The symptoms are similar to those of gynecomastia, but pseudogynecomastia is nontender and has no palpable lump. It usually occurs in overweight and obese individuals. MG shows only fatty tissues but no subareolar density as in gynecomastia.

Lipoma It is the second most common benign lesion of the male breast after gynecomastia. Clinically, it presents as a subcutaneous, palpable, nonpainful, soft mass. On MG, it may be indistinguishable from adjacent fat tissue or show a typical circumscribed, low-density mass with thin isodense capsule. US shows a circumscribed, oval, parallel oriented, homogeneous, isoechoic to mildly hyperechoic mass with a thin echogenic capsule and no internal vascularity. Pathologically, it is a well-circumscribed, encapsulated subcutaneous lesion composed of mature adipose tissue [21]. Because it remains predominantly asymptomatic, excision is not required. However, surgical excision may be performed for cosmetic reasons.

Epidermal Inclusion Cyst It is the third most common benign breast lesion in men. It is a benign dermal lesion arising due to the occlusion of hair follicles or from sites of previous skin trauma. Patients present with smooth, palpable, usually painless mass and may have a visible opening on the skin as a blackhead and give the history of whitish discharge. MG shows a well-circumscribed, oval-shaped, equal to high-density superficial mass. US shows a well-circumscribed mass with variable echotexture ranging from anechoic (cystic) to hypoechoic to heterogenous, depending upon the internal content in the dermal and/or in the subcutaneous region. No internal vascularity is seen on colour Doppler. US may demonstrate an onion skin-like appearance of mass due to concentric alternating hypo- and hyperechoic rings of lamellated keratin [25]. If the cyst is completely intradermal, the claw sign may be seen on US, in which the posterior margin of the echogenic dermis is seen beneath the lesion. US may reveal a hypoechoic tract extending from the mass to the skin which is diagnostic [26]. The cyst may rupture and cause inflammation when the margin becomes indistinct/irregular on US and shows peripheral vascularity that may mimic malignancy. On histology, the cyst wall is lined by stratified squamous epithelium with the presence of laminated keratin debris in the cyst lumen [4].

Sebaceous cyst is another benign dermal cyst that is indistinguishable from epidermal inclusion cyst both clinically and on imaging. It results from occlusion of a sebaceous gland and is usually smaller than an epidermal inclusion cyst.

FNAC or biopsy should be avoided because rupture of the cyst can induce surrounding inflammatory reaction [26]. Treatment is conservative, and if symptomatic, surgical excision may be attempted.

Intraductal/Intracystic Papilloma It is a rare benign neoplastic lesion of the ductal epithelium. It may present as a nipple discharge or as a solitary, painless subareolar mass. It may also be associated with gynecomastia.

MG may show a well-circumscribed subareolar mass of equal to high density. US illustrates a single or multiple, oval, circumscribed, hypoechoic mass in a cystic dilated duct with a stalk of internal vascularity on colour Doppler. Imaging cannot distinguish it from papillary carcinoma, and biopsy may miss the malignant component due to undersampling. Grossly, it is a cystic lesion with a mural nodule/papilloma protruding into the cyst lumen. The cavity may contain clear fluid, blood, or clots. Microscopy shows a broad fibrovascular core lined by proliferating ductal epithelial as well as myoepithelial cells. Apocrine metaplasia may be focally present [21]. Because of the possibility of underlying atypia/malignancy, surgical excision is the treatment of choice.

Pseudoangiomatous Stromal Hyperplasia (PASH) It is a rare benign mesenchymal tumor of male breast. Clinically it may be asymptomatic and detected incidentally on imaging and on pathology for other lesions. In male it is frequently a component of gynecomastia supporting its postulated hormonal etiology. It may present as a palpable mass referred to as a tumoral PASH. It often has non-specific benign imaging features where MG shows a circumscribed or partially circumscribed noncalcified mass and the US shows a solid, circumscribed, usually hypoechoic and less frequently heterogenous mass. Microscopy shows benign stromal myofibroblastic proliferation resembling a vascular lesion [27]. It has anastomosing spaces in a dense collagenous stroma. Some of the spaces are lined by spindle- shaped myofibroblasts and a few of these spaces may contain red blood cells. Thus pathologically it may mimic low-grade angiosarcoma but PASH lacks malignant cytologic features such as atypia, mitosis, and necrosis [28]. Routine surgical excision is not recommended when diagnosed on biopsy with no suspicious features on imaging, however local excision may be required for symptomatic masses.

Myofibroblastomas It is the only pathology more common in males than females. It is a rare benign stromal tumour of the breast that frequently affects middle-aged males. It resembles a fibroadenoma on clinical examination and seen as a firm, palpable, mobile lump. On MG, it appears as a circumscribed, noncalcified mass, and on US, it is seen as a well-circumscribed, mixed echotexture mass with variable internal vascularity that can have posterior acoustic shadowing, likely due to an incorporated fat component. Biopsy is required for nonspecific imaging findings and microscopy shows the proliferation of bland spindle cells within hyalinised collagen [22]. It is treated by wide surgical excision.

Pilomatrixoma It is a rare benign cutaneous mass arising from the hair follicle matrix cell and is also known as calcifying epithelioma of Malherbe. It commonly occurs in children and adolescents and presents as a small, painless skin nodule. The overlying skin may get discoloured and rarely ulcerate due to inflammatory changes. MG shows a circumscribed mass with pleomorphic and coarse calcifications. US examination would show a circumscribed, heterogeneous, iso- to mildly hyperechoic mass with internal calcification and posterior acoustic shadowing. Thus imaging findings are a mimicker of breast cancer and biopsy is recommended. Pathology shows dermal-based lesion composed of nests of basaloid cells with abrupt keratinisation. Eosinophilic epithelial cells called Ghost or shadow cells are present in the centre. Foreign body giant cells and foci of calcification may be present. Complete surgical excision is the treatment of choice.

Angiolipoma The extremely rare male breast mass is a type of vascular tumour composed of mature adipocytes and a variable amount of angiomatous tissue [29]. Clinically, it presents as a painless, mobile, firm, palpable mass. MG shows variable findings such as asymmetry or a circumscribed mass with variable density depending on the amount of fat component, and US may demonstrate a well-circumscribed, iso- to hyperechoic homogeneous mass with internal vascularity. Imaging findings may mimic malignancy, and in such cases, biopsy is indicated.

Granular Cell Tumour It is a rare benign tumour of neural origin that can present as a unilateral palpable lump and often misdiagnosed as breast cancer [30]. Because of the sensory distribution of the supraclavicular nerve, it tends to occur in the upper inner quadrant. Imaging findings are variable, ranging from a round, circumscribed mass to an irregular, spiculated mass with occasional calcification on MG. USG findings range from visualization of benign circumscribed mass to an irregular mass with spiculated or angulated margin and posterior acoustic shadowing [28]. Biopsy is often performed for suspicious findings. Grossly, granular cell tumour of the breast (GCTB) is a firm to hard mass with well-circumscribed to infiltrative borders [21]. Microscopically, the tumour cells are seen in sheets and nests with intervening collagenous stroma. Tumour cells are seen infiltrating into lobules, adjacent fat, and dermis of the skin, mimicking invasive carcinoma [21]. However, GCTB lacks the component of in situ carcinoma. Sometimes, morphological distinction of GCTB from invasive carcinoma, histiocytic lesions, and metastatic carcinoma can be difficult, requiring IHC examination for differentiation. The lesion is treated with wide local excision to reduce recurrence which is reported in 2–8% of cases.

Cysts Simple cysts are the most common lesion of the female breast. However, they are extremely rare in the male breast because of the absence of lobular tissue, but few cases have been reported in literature. Breast cysts are often associated with gynecomastia. It is advised that all complicated and complex cysts and even simple cysts in men should be considered suspicious and should undergo a detailed evaluation including biopsy. However, Maimone et al. reviewed 19 cysts in the male breast and concluded that in the absence of suspicious findings (irregular shape, noncircumscribed margin, thickened wall, septation, solid component, and internal vascularity), cysts can be considered benign, and biopsy can be avoided [31].

Inflammatory Diseases Chronic periductal mastitis with duct ectasia may rarely occur in the male breast, with only a few cases reported in the literature [32]. It is characterised by dilated ducts with periductal chronic inflammation and fibrosis.

Nonpuerperal subareolar mastitis or abscess, also known as Zuska's disease, can also occur in men [33]. It is caused by squamous metaplasia and proliferation of the epithelium in the lactiferous ducts, resulting in obstruction and secretory stasis leading to abscess formation [34]. Histologically, the lactiferous ducts show squamous metaplasia with duct spaces filled with keratinous debris and periductal mixed stromal inflammation along with multinucleated foreign body-like type giant cells if the lactiferous duct ruptures [21].

Both these entities may present with nipple discharge, a subareolar lump, and nipple retraction that mimic malignancy. It might get complicated by recurrent abscess formation and mammary fistulae. MG might show an ill-defined retroareolar mass or asymmetry with signs of inflammation such as skin and trabecular thickening. US examination shows a complex cystic mass or heterogeneous hypoechoic mass and sometimes might show vascularity in solid inflammatory area. In chronic ductal ectasia, dilated ducts with intraductal debris are seen which needs to be differentiated from intraductal papillary lesions. Colour Doppler can be used to show the vascularity of the papillary lesions. Antibiotics and pus drainage are the standard treatment for abscesses, and surgical excision of the fistulous tract is an effective treatment to prevent recurrence [33].

Idiopathic and specific granulomatous mastitis may also affect the male breast, with clinical and imaging features similar to those of the female breast.

Diabetic Mastopathy It is a rare fibroinflammatory disease that typically occurs with longstanding type 1 diabetes that can be seen as regional asymmetry or a mass with indistinct margins on MG and irregular, hypoechoic, avascular mass with posterior acoustic shadowing on US. It appears suspicious both clinically and on imaging, so a biopsy is often performed.

Posttraumatic Fat Necrosis It can occur following trauma, breast surgery, or radiotherapy. Fat necrosis is an aseptic inflammation of adipose tissue. A palpable, painless lump is the most common presenting feature. The mass can be hard in consistency with retraction of the nipple or skin—features mimicking malignancy. Imaging findings depend on the stage of development, extent of fat liquefaction, fibrosis, and calcification. In the acute stage, fat necrosis shows asymmetry or an indistinct mass, with adjacent trabecular and skin thickening due to inflammatory changes that appears suspicious on MG. However, US examination can be helpful as it shows absence of definite mass but an area of increased echogenicity with a central hypoechoic area surrounded by edematous parenchyma and subcutaneous tissue. This area gradually becomes cystic due to liquefaction of fat and may form an oil cyst. The oil cyst is pathognomonic of fat necrosis on mammography and appears as a circumscribed radiolucent lesion with or without a thin peripheral curvilinear calcification and may have a fat-fluid level. The US shows a cystic lesion that may be completely anechoic or show internal debris or fat-fluid levels and may even form a complex sold cystic mass [35]. The chronic stage is characterised by the appearance of dystrophic calcifications and varying degrees of fibrosis. When extensive fibrosis replaces all adipose tissue, the mass appears as either indistinct or spiculated area on imaging that mimics malignancy and requires biopsy. The clinical history and evidence of fat on imaging may clinch the diagnosis. Histologically it is characterised by necrotic adipocytes, lipid-laden foamy macrophages, lymphocytes, plasma cells, and foreign body-multinucleated giant cells.

Many other benign lesions may also occasionally occur in the male breast, such as hematoma, seroma, fibromatosis, fibroadenoma, nodular fasciitis, nerve cell tumour (such as schwannoma, neurofibroma), and vascular lesions such as haemangioma and venous or lymphatic malformation.

Table 15.4 Risk factors for male breast cancer

Age
Race
Family history *Genetic syndrome*—Klinefelter syndrome, lynch syndrome, and Cowden syndrome
Germline mutation—BRCA1, BRCA2, PALB2, CHEK2, ATM, and NF1
Hyperestrogenism Endogenous source—Obesity, alcohol dependence, liver cirrhosis, and testicular dysfunction (due to undescended testes, orchitis, epididymitis, and congenital) Exogenous source—Prostate cancer therapy and transgender patients
Environmental exposure Ionic and electromagnetic radiation Hot working environment Exposure to chemical compounds like combustion products

15.5 Malignant Breast Diseases

Breast cancer is the most common cause of cancer in females. Male breast cancer, on the other hand, is a rare entity, accounting for approximately 1% of all breast cancers worldwide and less than 1% of all malignancies in male [36, 37]. However, over the past two decades, there has been an increase in diagnosed cancer cases in men. The lifetime risk of developing cancer is 1 in 1000 in males, compared with 1 in 8 in females [38]. The average age for diagnosis of breast cancer in male is about 67 years, at least 5–10 years later than in female [39], and only about 15% of patients are diagnosed at below 50 years of age [40]. The diagnosis is often made at an advanced stage due to lack of awareness among males and there are no screening guidelines, so 50% of them have axillary adenopathy at the time of diagnosis [41]. Therefore, men have a worse prognosis than their female counterparts.

Risk Factors (Table 15.4) Increasing age, race, and a history of cancer in the family, especially first-degree relatives, increase the risk of cancer in men. Similar to women, genetic syndromes also increase the risk of developing breast cancer in men. For example, Klinefelter syndrome increases the risk 50-fold; the cause is thought to be androgen deficiency due to hypogonadism. Several germline mutations of BRCA1, BRCA2, CHEK2, PLAB2, ATM, and NF1 [42, 43] are also associated with increased risk; BRCA2 mutations in particular are associated with younger age and poor prognosis and survival [44]. Hyperestrogenism, which may be due to an endogenous source (such as cirrhosis, testicular dysfunction, alcohol dependence, and obesity) or an exogenous source (such as in transgender patients and in prostate cancer therapy), also increases cancer risk.

There is no dedicated screening programme for asymptomatic male breast cancer because the incidence of male cancer is extremely low and therefore all male breast imaging is diagnostic. However, considering the factors of increasing number of male breast cancer cases and its presentation or detection at later stages with associated poor survival outcomes, screening of the male breast may be useful in men at high risk. Gao et al. reviewed breast imaging examinations over a 12-year period and concluded that screening mammography in high-risk men resulted in a cancer detection rate of 18 per 1000 examinations, which is higher than the cancer detection rate of 3–5 per 1000 for screening MGs in average-risk women [45]. They also stated that all occult malignancies detected on screening were stages 0–1 and node-negative, favouring a better prognosis. The NCCN also recommends that men with germline mutations should have breast self-examination and physical examination twice a year starting at age 35 for early detection of breast cancer [46]. The American Society of Clinical Oncology recommends annual ipsilateral mammography in men treated with lumpectomy, regardless of genetic predisposition, and annual contralateral mammography in men with a history of breast cancer with genetic predisposing mutation [38].

Clinical Symptoms The most common presenting complaint is a unilateral, painless, firm, palpable lump, usually in the subareolar region, often eccentric to the nipple. The mass may be fixed to the skin or underlying pectoral muscle. Bloody discharge from the nipple is noted in 25% of cases [28]. Because male breast is small, secondary signs such as thickening/ulceration/retraction of the skin, erosion/retraction of the nipple, and palpable axillary nodes occur earlier. The presence of bilateral cancer has been reported in 1.5–2% of patients [47].

On MG, cancers are usually high density, noncalcified mass in the subareolar region, often eccentric to the nipple. Less commonly, a mass with calcifications is seen, followed by presence of only calcifications [48]. The mass is usually irregularly shaped with indistinct or microlobulated or spiculated margins (Fig. 15.8). However, a round to oval mass with a well-circumscribed margin resembling a benign mass may also occur (Fig. 15.9). Microcalcifications are rare and occur in only 13–30% of cases. Calcifications, unlike cancers in women, are generally few and coarse and usually punctate rather than linear and widely scattered. Secondary signs of malignancy such as skin thickening, skin retraction, nipple retraction, thickened trabeculations, and axillary adenopathy may also be seen.

On US, they usually appear as an irregularly shaped, hypoechoic solid mass in the subareolar region, usually eccentric to the nipple. With US, the eccentric relationship of the mass to the nipple can be better visualised. The mass usually has a noncircumscribed margin (Fig. 15.10), and it may be a solid, cystic, or solid cystic mass with variable vascularity. Well-circumscribed masses on MG that show a cystic component on US should be biopsied because such complex cystic solid lesions have a high probability of malignancy in men [49].

MRI is not commonly used in male breast cancer. However, MRI features are similar to those of female breast cancer. Axillary adenopathy, skin, chest, and nipple involvement can also be better identified on MRI.

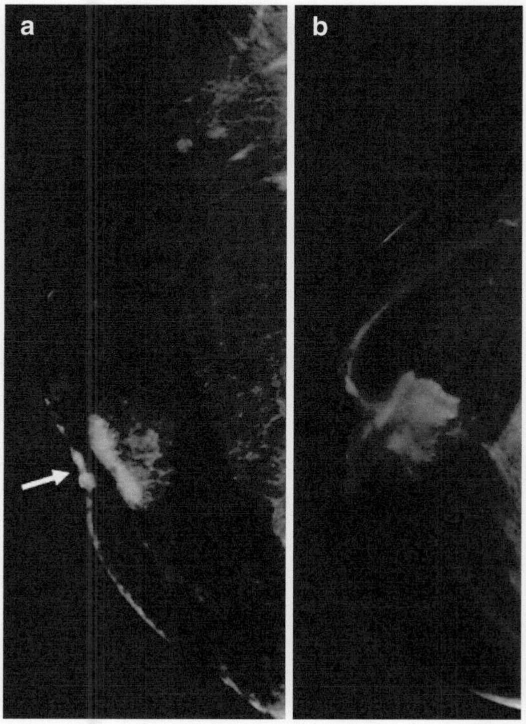

Fig. 15.8 Invasive ductal carcinoma. MLO mammogram (**a**) and tomosynthesis image of CC view (**b**) shows a high-density, irregular-shaped mass with spiculated margin (black arrow) in subareolar region associated with nipple retraction (white arrow)

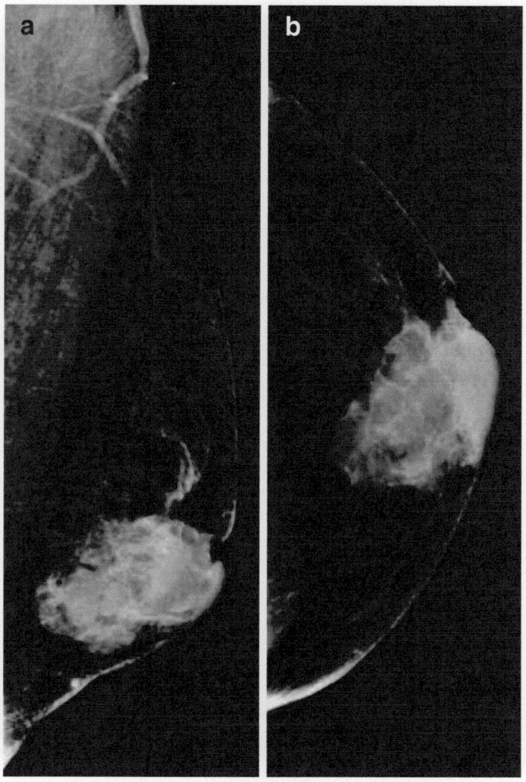

Fig. 15.9 Invasive lobular carcinoma: MLO (**a**) and CC (**b**) mammogram of the left breast shows a high-density irregular-shaped mass with circumscribed margin in subareolar region, eccentric to the nipple

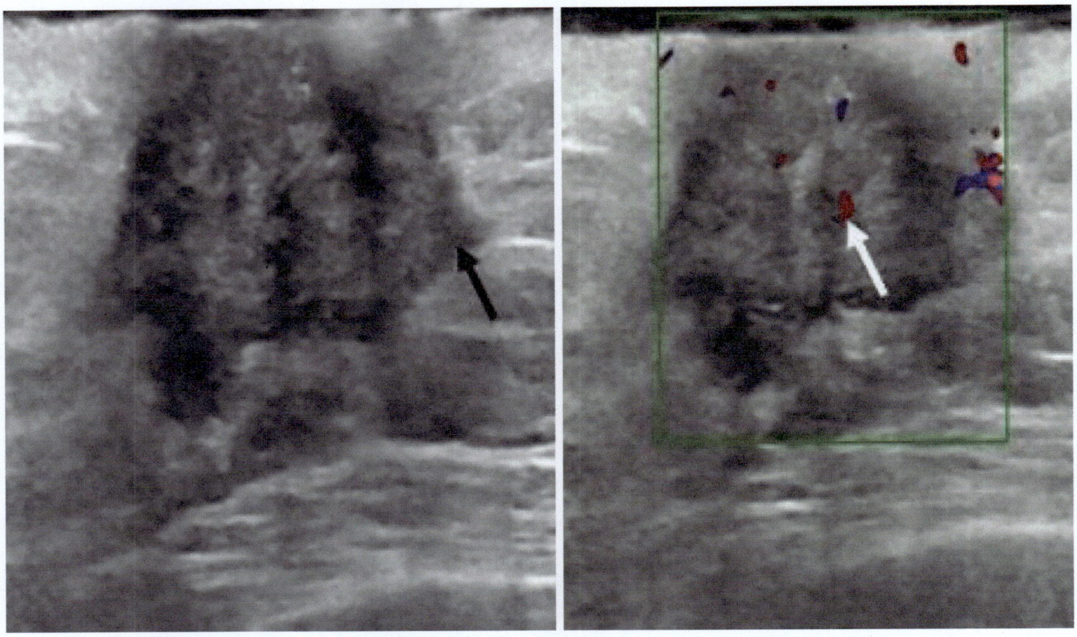

Fig. 15.10 Invasive ductal carcinoma. Transverse ultrasound shows an irregular-shaped, heterogeneously hypoechoic mass with angulated margin (black arrow) and minimal vascularity (white arrow) on colour Doppler

Invasive ductal carcinoma (IDC) is the most common histologic type, accounting for 85% of all cancers [50]. Histologically, the malignant cells forming glands, in solid nests and singly, are seen invading the desmoplastic stroma [21] (Fig. 15.11). IDC in males tend to be of higher (moderately to poorly differentiated) grade and pathologically advanced stage. Most common subtype of IDC is infiltrating ductal carcinomas, not otherwise specified, followed by papillary and mucinous carcinomas.

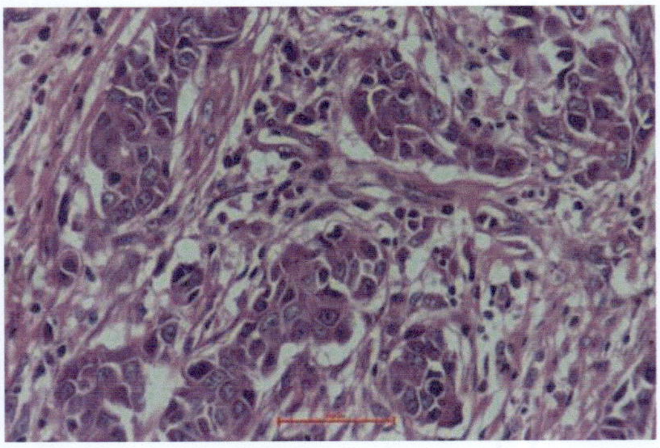

Fig. 15.11 Invasive ductal carcinoma. Photomicrograph (Hematoxylin & eosin; 400×) shows malignant ductal epithelial cells in solid nests invading the desmoplastic stroma

Ductal carcinoma in situ (DCIS) accounts for only 10% of male breast cancer cases. It is associated with 50% of invasive carcinomas, while pure DCIS is rare. The microscopic patterns of male

DCIS are predominantly cribriform or papillary and less commonly comedo and solid [51]. Nicosia et al. studied cases of pure DCIS over an 18-year period and found that palpable nodules followed by bloody nipple discharge were the most common clinical findings [52]. The most common histologic subtype was intracystic papillary carcinoma, and 10% of cases showed a cystic nodule on imaging [52]. Microcalcifications were found in only 5% of cases, in contrast to DCIS in women, where microcalcifications are common.

Male breast cancer have higher positivity for hormone receptors and lower positivity for human epidermal growth factor receptors compared to female breast cancer. The majority (80–90%) are strongly positive for ER and PR, and only 8.7% are Her-2 positive. The most common histologic subtype is luminal B and triple-negative cases are rare (0.3%) [41].

Papillary carcinoma is the second most common histologic subtype. It accounts for 3–5% of male breast cancer [4]. It consists of a complex proliferation of malignant ductal epithelial cells lining thin fibrovascular cores, with absence of myoepithelial cells, and the lesion is surrounded by a thick fibrous capsule. In invasive papillary carcinoma, infiltration of tumour cells into the adjacent stroma is seen. Clinically, it presents as a subareolar palpable mass. It has been noted that invasive and in situ papillary carcinomas often have a complex cystic and solid composition on US [4].

Lobular carcinoma is very rare due to paucity of lobules in the male breast and accounts for only about 1% of all male breast cancer [24]. Lobular carcinoma in situ is extremely rare and usually occurs in association with invasive lobular carcinoma (ILC). Klinefelter syndrome and excess oestrogen increase the risk of lobular carcinoma. Lobular carcinoma may, in rare cases, show up only as architectural distortion or asymmetry on MG, rather than a typical malignant mass (Fig. 15.12). Histologically, ILC is characterised by discontinuously scattered tumour cells infiltrating in a single row, "Indian file pattern" through a fibrous stroma [28] (Fig. 15.13).

Paget's disease of the male breast is rare and accounts for only 2% of all cases of Paget's disease [53]. The Clinical and imaging features are similar to that in female counterparts.

Management and Prognosis Treatment is similar to female breast cancer and depends on the stage of the disease. A combination of surgery, hormone therapy, chemotherapy, and radiation therapy is used. In most cases, a mastectomy is performed due to the small size of the breast and central location of the tumour. In male breast cancer, the overall survival rate is lower and mortality is higher than in female patients [54] (Table 15.5).

Sarcomas Primary mesenchymal tumours are rare and account for <1% of all breast cancers [55]. Dermatofibrosarcoma, also known as spindle cell tumour, is more common in males than in females and is seen between the ages of 30 and 50 years [2]. There are few case reports of liposarcomas, fibrosarcomas, and leiomyosarcomas [23, 56, 57]. Sarcomas usually present with nonspecific clinical and imaging findings. Treatment consists of either surgical excision or mastectomy.

Metastasis Metastasis to the breast is extremely rare. It is usually due to hematogenous spread of disseminated malignancy. Common nonmammary malignancies that metastasise to the breast include lymphoma, melanoma, gastrointestinal tumours, lung cancer, gastric cancer, prostate cancer, and sarcoma. Hormonal therapy in prostate cancer predisposes male to breast metastasis [58]. Multiple bilateral breast masses in patients with known extramammary primary tumour should raise suspicion of metastases. MG shows solitary or multiple round, dense masses with well-circumscribed or microlobulated margins that are usually not calcified [59]. US shows these as hypoechoic, circumscribed masses that often have increased internal vascularity.

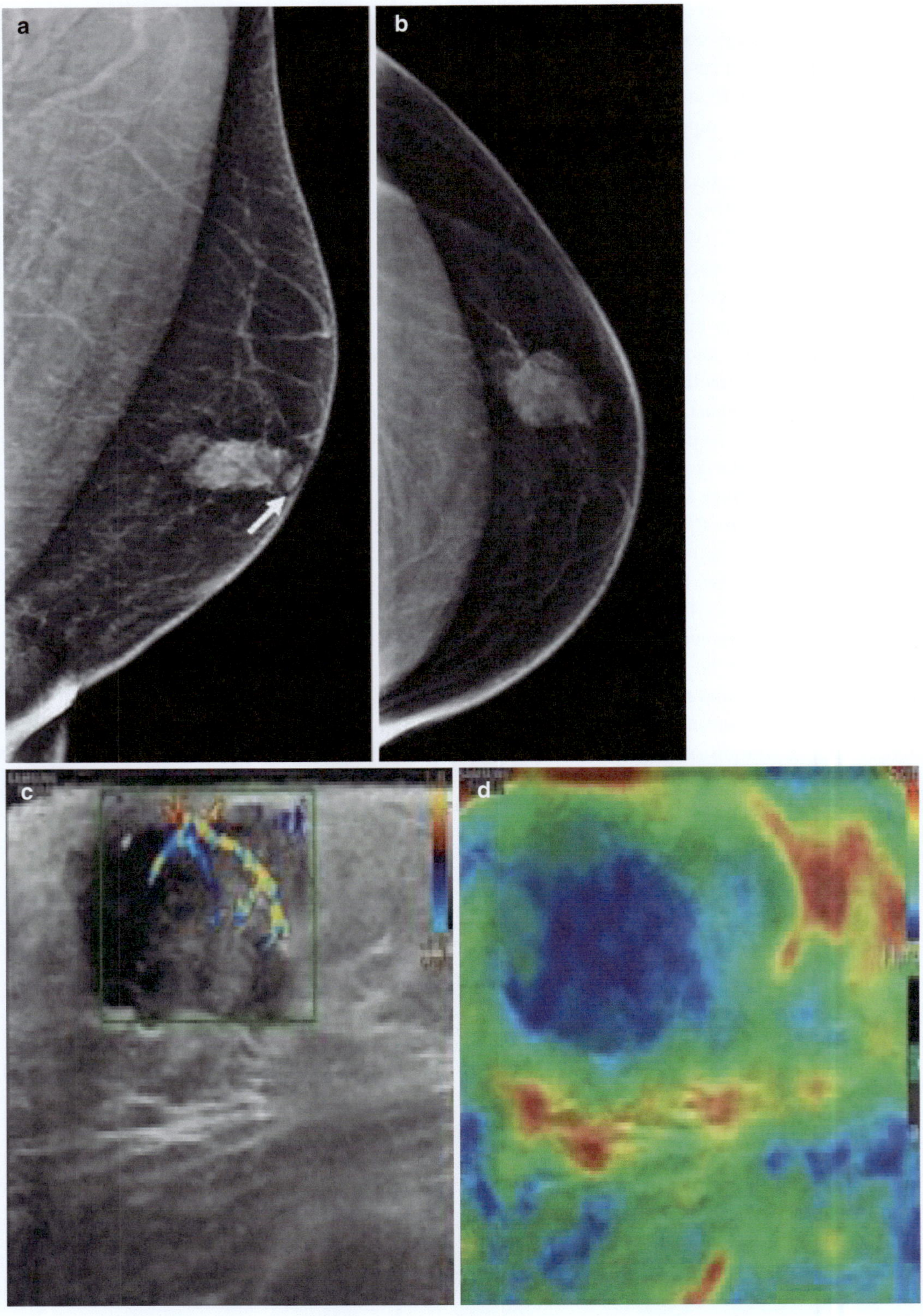

Fig. 15.12 Invasive lobular carcinoma. (**a**) MLO (**a**) and CC (**b**) mammogram of the left breast shows an irregular, high-density mass with a circumscribed margin in retroareolar region causing nipple retraction (arrow). Transverse ultrasound (**c**) of the same mass shows an irregular, heterogeneously hypoechoic mass with microlobulated and angular margins and increased internal vascularity. On strain elastography (**d**), the mass shows increased stiffness suggestive of hard consistency

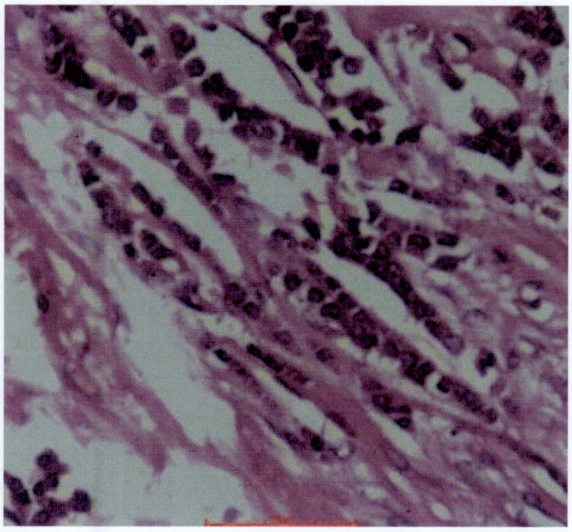

Fig. 15.13 Invasive lobular carcinoma. Photomicrograph (Hemotoxylin & eosin 400×) shows discohesive malignant cells invading the stroma in Indian file pattern

Table 15.5 Characteristics of male and female breast cancer

Characteristics	Male breast cancer (MBC)	Female breast cancer (FBC)
Mean age of diagnosis	67 years	62 years
Lifetime risk	1 in 1000	1 in 8
Common site	Subareolar	Upper outer quadrant
Anatomical site of origin of cancer	Central duct in subareolar region	Peripheral TDLU
Lobular carcinoma	Uncommon, 1.5% of all MBC	More common, 10–15% of all FBC
Intracystic papillary carcinoma	Relatively more common	Less common
DCIS	5% pure DCIS Papillary and cribriform subtype more common Low and intermediate grade	20% pure DCIS Solid subtype most common Usually high grade
Receptor positivity	High (80–90%) receptor positivity	Comparatively lower (60–70%) receptor positivity
Secondary signs of nipple/skin/chest wall involvement and axillary adenopathy at presentation	More common	Less common
Prognosis	Overall poor prognosis and survival rate as compared to female cancers	Better prognosis than male cancers
Malignant calcifications on mammogram	Less frequent, usually benign morphology—few coarse or punctate, scattered calcifications	More common, malignant morphology like pleomorphic, linear, or linear branching, and amorphous
Cystic lesions on ultrasound	Rarely seen Considered as suspicious	Complicated cysts without obvious solid components and simple cysts are usually benign lesions.

15.6 Conclusion

The male and female breasts have different histo-anatomy, so the spectrum and frequency of male and female breast lesions are different. The majority of male breast pathologies are benign with gynecomastia as the most common pathology. Male breast cancer is rare and often occurs in advanced stages with an overall poor prognosis. Therefore, any symptomatic male should be evaluated with the goal of confirming characteristic benign findings and ruling out underlying malignancy. Lobular pathologies such as cysts, fibroadenomas (benign lesions in female), and lobular carcinomas are extremely rare in men due to the absence of lobular tissue. All complex, and even simple cysts in the male breast, should be treated as a potentially malignant lesion. Therefore, knowledge of the clinic-radio-pathologic features of male breast lesions is extremely important for accurate diagnosis and management recommendations.

References

1. Nguyen C, Kettler MD, Swirsky ME, Miller VI, Scott C, Krause R, Hadro JA. Male breast disease: pictorial review with radiologic-pathologic correlation. Radiographics. 2013;33(3):763–79. https://doi.org/10.1148/rg.333125137. PMID: 23674773
2. Chen L, Chantra PK, Larsen LH, Barton P, Rohitopakarn M, Zhu EQ, Bassett LW. Imaging characteristics of malignant lesions of the male breast. Radiographics. 2006;26(4):993–1006. https://doi.org/10.1148/rg.264055116. PMID: 16844928
3. Iuanow E, Kettler M, Slanetz PJ. Spectrum of disease in the male breast. AJR Am J Roentgenol. 2011;196(3):W247–59. https://doi.org/10.2214/AJR.09.3994. PMID: 21343472
4. Chau A, Jafarian N, Rosa M. Male breast: clinical and imaging evaluations of benign and malignant entities with histologic correlation. Am J Med. 2016;129(8):776–91. https://doi.org/10.1016/j.amjmed.2016.01.009. Epub 2016 Feb 1. PMID: 26844632
5. Lapid O, Siebenga P, Zonderland HM. Overuse of imaging the male breast-findings in 557 patients. Breast J. 2015;21(3):219–23. https://doi.org/10.1111/tbj.12393. Epub 2015 Mar 13. PMID: 25772378
6. Patterson SK, Helvie MA, Aziz K, Nees AV. Outcome of men presenting with clinical breast problems: the role of mammography and ultrasound. Breast J. 2006;12(5):418–23. https://doi.org/10.1111/j.1075-122X.2006.00298.x. PMID: 16958958
7. Muñoz Carrasco R, Alvarez Benito M, Muñoz Gomariz E, Raya Povedano JL, Martínez Paredes M. Mammography and ultrasound in the evaluation of male breast disease. Eur Radiol. 2010;20(12):2797–805. https://doi.org/10.1007/s00330-010-1867-7. Epub 2010 Jun 23. PMID: 20571799
8. Woods RW, Salkowski LR, Elezaby M, Burnside ES, Strigel RM, Fowler AM. Image-based screening for men at high risk for breast cancer: benefits and drawbacks. Clin Imaging. 2020;60(1):84–9. https://doi.org/10.1016/j.clinimag.2019.11.005. Epub 2019 Nov 28. PMID: 31864206; PMCID: PMC7242122
9. Evans GF, Anthony T, Turnage RH, Schumpert TD, Levy KR, Amirkhan RH, Campbell TJ, Lopez J, Appelbaum AH. The diagnostic accuracy of mammography in the evaluation of male breast disease. Am J Surg. 2001;181(2):96–100. https://doi.org/10.1016/s0002-9610(00)00571-7. Erratum in: Am J Surg 2001 Jun;181(6):579. PMID: 11425067
10. Taylor K, Ames V, Wallis M. The diagnostic value of clinical examination and imaging used as part of an age-related protocol when diagnosing male breast disease: an audit of 1141 cases from a single centre. Breast. 2013;22(3):268–72. https://doi.org/10.1016/j.breast.2013.03.004. Epub 2013 Apr 6. PMID: 23570843
11. Rong X, Zhu Q, Jia W, Ma T, Wang X, Guo N, Ji H. Ultrasonographic assessment of male breast diseases. Breast J. 2018;24(4):599–605. https://doi.org/10.1111/tbj.12982. Epub 2018 Jan 8. PMID: 29316031
12. Crombé A, Hurtevent-Labrot G, Asad-Syed M, Palussière J, MacGrogan G, Kind M, Ferron S. Shear-wave elastography quantitative assessment of the male breast: added value to distinguish benign and malignant palpable masses. Br J Radiol. 2018;91(1082):20170676. https://doi.org/10.1259/bjr.20170676. Epub 2017 Dec 5. PMID: 29144159; PMCID: PMC5965781
13. Expert Panel on Breast Imaging, Niell BL, Lourenco AP, Moy L, Baron P, Didwania AD, diFlorio-Alexander RM, Heller SL, Holbrook AI, Le-Petross HT, Lewin AA, Mehta TS, Slanetz PJ, Stuckey AR, Tuscano DS, Ulaner GA, Vincoff NS, Weinstein SP, Newell MS. ACR appropriateness criteria® evaluation of the symptomatic male breast. J Am Coll Radiol. 2018;15(11S):S313–20. https://doi.org/10.1016/j.jacr.2018.09.017. PMID: 30392600
14. Shin K, Martaindale S, Whitman GJ. Male breast magnetic resonance imaging: when is it helpful? Our experience over the last decade. Curr Probl Diagn Radiol. 2019;48(3):196–203. https://doi.org/10.1067/j.cpradiol.2018.01.002. Epub 2018 Jan 10. PMID: 29454681
15. American College of Radiology. Breast imaging reporting and data system, breast imaging atlas. 5th ed. Reston: American College of Radiology; 2013.

16. Önder Ö, Azizova A, Durhan G, et al. Imaging findings and classification of the common and uncommon male breast diseases. Insights Imaging. 2020;11:27. https://doi.org/10.1186/s13244-019-0834-3.
17. Narula HS, Carlson HE. Gynaecomastia–pathophysiology, diagnosis and treatment. Nat Rev Endocrinol. 2014;10(11):684–98. https://doi.org/10.1038/nrendo.2014.139. Epub 2014 Aug 12. PMID: 2511223
18. Braunstein GD. Gynecomastia. N Engl J Med. 1993;328(7):490–5. https://doi.org/10.1056/NEJM199302183280708. PMID: 8421478
19. Derkacz M, Chmiel-Perzyńska I, Nowakowski A. Gynecomastia – a difficult diagnostic problem. Endokrynol Pol. 2011;62(2):190–202. PMID: 21528484
20. Appelbaum AH, Evans GF, Levy KR, Amirkhan RH, Schumpert TD. Mammographic appearances of male breast disease. Radiographics. 1999;19(3):559–68. https://doi.org/10.1148/radiographics.19.3.g99ma01559. PMID: 10336188
21. Rosen PP. Rosen's breast pathology. 3rd ed. Philadelphia: Wolters Kluwer/Lippincot Williams & Wilkins; 2009. p. 775–85. 787–801
22. Shaaban AM. Pathology of the male breast. Mini-symposium: breast pathology. Diagn Histopathol. 2019;25(4):138–42.
23. Chesebro AL, Rives AF, Shaffer K. Male breast disease: what the radiologist needs to know. Curr Probl Diagn Radiol. 2019;48(5):482–93. https://doi.org/10.1067/j.cpradiol.2018.07.003. Epub 2018 Jul 29. PMID: 30122313
24. Senger JL, Adams SJ, Kanthan R. Invasive lobular carcinoma of the male breast – a systematic review with an illustrative case study. Breast Cancer (Dove Med Press). 2017;9:337–45. https://doi.org/10.2147/BCTT.S126341. PMID: 28553141; PMCID: PMC5439541
25. Crystal P, Shaco-Levy R. Concentric rings within a breast mass on sonography: lamellated keratin in an epidermal inclusion cyst. AJR Am J Roentgenol. 2005;184(3 Suppl):S47–8. https://doi.org/10.2214/ajr.184.3_supplement.01840s47. PMID: 15728019
26. Giess CS, Raza S, Birdwell RL. Distinguishing breast skin lesions from superficial breast parenchymal lesions: diagnostic criteria, imaging characteristics, and pitfalls. Radiographics. 2011;31(7):1959–72. https://doi.org/10.1148/rg.317115116. PMID: 22084181
27. Seidman JD, Borkowski A, Aisner SC, Sun CC. Rapid growth of pseudoangiomatous hyperplasia of mammary stroma in axillary gynecomastia in an immunosuppressed patient. Arch Pathol Lab Med. 1993;117(7):736–8. PMID: 8323441
28. Lattin GE Jr, Jesinger RA, Mattu R, Glassman LM. From the radiologic pathology archives: diseases of the male breast: radiologic-pathologic correlation. Radiographics. 2013;33(2):461–89. https://doi.org/10.1148/rg.332125208. PMID: 23479708
29. Babiss E, et al. Radiologic and pathologic correlation for Angiolipomas of the breast. J Breast Imaging. 2022;4(2):177–82. https://doi.org/10.1093/jbi/wbac003.
30. Kim EY, Kang DK, Kim TH, Jung YS, Kim KS, Yim H. Granular cell tumor of the male breast: two case descriptions and brief review of the literature. J Ultrasound Med. 2011;30(9):1295–301. https://doi.org/10.7863/jum.2011.30.9.1295. PMID: 21876101
31. Maimone S, et al. Characteristics and management of male breast parenchymal cysts. J Breast Imaging. 2020;2(4):330–5. https://doi.org/10.1093/jbi/wbaa035.
32. Al-Masad JK. Mammary duct ectasia and periductal mastitis in males. Saudi Med J. 2001;22(11):1030–3. PMID: 11744981
33. Johnson SP, Kaoutzanis C, Schaub GA. Male Zuska's disease. BMJ Case Rep. 2014;2014:bcr2013201922. https://doi.org/10.1136/bcr-2013-201922. PMID: 24706699; PMCID: PMC3987215
34. Leong PW, Chotai NC, Kulkarni S. Imaging features of inflammatory breast disorders: a pictorial essay. Korean J Radiol. 2018;19(1):5–14. https://doi.org/10.3348/kjr.2018.19.1.5. Epub 2018 Jan 2. PMID: 29353994; PMCID: PMC5768507
35. Majithia J, Haria P, Popat P, Katdare A, Chouhan S, Gala KB, Kulkarni S, Thakur M. Fat necrosis: a consultant's conundrum. Front Oncol. 2023;(12):926396. https://doi.org/10.3389/fonc.2022.926396. PMID: 36873302; PMCID: PMC9978799
36. Weiss JR, Moysich KB, Swede H. Epidemiology of male breast cancer. Cancer Epidemiol Biomarkers Prev. 2005;14(1):20–6. PMID: 15668471
37. Centers for Disease Control and Prevention. Male breast cancer incidence and mortality, United States—2013–2017 No 19. Atlanta: Centers for Disease Control and Prevention, US Department of Health and Human Services; 2020.
38. Hassett MJ, Somerfield MR, Baker ER, Cardoso F, Kansal KJ, Kwait DC, Plichta JK, Ricker C, Roshal A, Ruddy KJ, Safer JD, Van Poznak C, Yung RL, Giordano SH. Management of male breast cancer: ASCO guideline. J Clin Oncol. 2020;38(16):1849–63. https://doi.org/10.1200/JCO.19.03120. Epub 2020 Feb 14. PMID: 32058842
39. Korde LA, Zujewski JA, Kamin L, Giordano S, Domchek S, Anderson WF, Bartlett JM, Gelmon K, Nahleh Z, Bergh J, Cutuli B, Pruneri G, McCaskill-Stevens W, Gralow J, Hortobagyi G, Cardoso F. Multidisciplinary meeting on male breast cancer: summary and research recommendations. J Clin Oncol. 2010;28(12):2114–22. https://doi.org/10.1200/JCO.2009.25.5729. Epub 2010 Mar 22. PMID: 20308661; PMCID: PMC2860409
40. Konduri S, Singh M, Bobustuc G, Rovin R, Kassam A. Epidemiology of male breast cancer. Breast. 2020;54:8–14. https://doi.org/10.1016/j.breast.2020.08.010. Epub 2020 Aug 22. PMID: 32866903; PMCID: PMC7476060
41. Cardoso F, Bartlett JMS, Slaets L, van Deurzen CHM, van Leeuwen-Stok E, Porter P, Linderholm B, Hedenfalk I, Schröder C, Martens J, Bayani J,

van Asperen C, Murray M, Hudis C, Middleton L, Vermeij J, Punie K, Fraser J, Nowaczyk M, Rubio IT, Aebi S, Kelly C, Ruddy KJ, Winer E, Nilsson C, Lago LD, Korde L, Benstead K, Bogler O, Goulioti T, Peric A, Litière S, Aalders KC, Poncet C, Tryfonidis K, Giordano SH. Characterization of male breast cancer: results of the EORTC 10085/TBCRC/BIG/NABCG International Male Breast Cancer Program. Ann Oncol. 2018;29(2):405–17. https://doi.org/10.1093/annonc/mdx651. PMID: 29092024; PMCID: PMC5834077
42. Pritzlaff M, Summerour P, McFarland R, Li S, Reineke P, Dolinsky JS, Goldgar DE, Shimelis H, Couch FJ, Chao EC, LaDuca H. Male breast cancer in a multi-gene panel testing cohort: insights and unexpected results. Breast Cancer Res Treat. 2017;161(3):575–86. https://doi.org/10.1007/s10549-016-4085-4. Epub 2016 Dec 22. PMID: 28008555; PMCID: PMC5241330
43. Zheng G, Leone JP. Male breast cancer: an updated review of epidemiology, Clinicopathology, and treatment. J Oncol. 2022;2022:1734049. https://doi.org/10.1155/2022/1734049. PMID: 35656339; PMCID: PMC9155932
44. Kwiatkowska E, Teresiak M, Filas V, Karczewska A, Breborowicz D, Mackiewicz A. BRCA2 mutations and androgen receptor expression as independent predictors of outcome of male breast cancer patients. Clin Cancer Res. 2003;9(12):4452–9. PMID: 14555518
45. Gao Y, Goldberg JE, Young TK, Babb JS, Moy L, Heller SL. Breast cancer screening in high-risk men: a 12-year longitudinal observational study of male breast imaging utilization and outcomes. Radiology. 2019;293(2):282–91. https://doi.org/10.1148/radiol.2019190971. Epub 2019 Sep 17. PMID: 31526252
46. Daly MB, Pal T, Berry MP, Buys SS, Dickson P, Domchek SM, Elkhanany A, Friedman S, Goggins M, Hutton ML, CGC, Karlan BY, Khan S, Klein C, Kohlmann W, CGC, Kurian AW, Laronga C, Litton JK, Mak JS, LCGC, Menendez CS, Merajver SD, Norquist BS, Offit K, Pederson HJ, Reiser G, CGC, Senter-Jamieson L, CGC, Shannon KM, Shatsky R, Visvanathan K, Weitzel JN, Wick MJ, Wisinski KB, Yurgelun MB, Darlow SD, Dwyer MA. Genetic/familial high-risk assessment: breast, ovarian, and pancreatic, Version 2.2021, NCCN clinical practice guidelines in oncology. J Natl Compr Canc Netw. 2021;19(1):77–102. https://doi.org/10.6004/jnccn.2021.0001. PMID: 33406487
47. Sun WY, Lee KH, Lee HC, Ryu DH, Park JW, Yun HY, Song YJ. Synchronous bilateral male breast cancer: a case report. J Breast Cancer. 2012;15(2):248–51. https://doi.org/10.4048/jbc.2012.15.2.248. Epub 2012 Jun 28. PMID: 22807945; PMCID: PMC3395751
48. Mathew J, Perkins GH, Stephens T, Middleton LP, Yang WT. Primary breast cancer in men: clinical, imaging, and pathologic findings in 57 patients. AJR Am J Roentgenol. 2008;191(6):1631–9. https://doi.org/10.2214/AJR.08.1076. PMID: 19020230
49. Yang WT, Whitman GJ, Yuen EH, Tse GM, Stelling CB. Sonographic features of primary breast cancer in men. AJR Am J Roentgenol. 2001;176(2):413–6. https://doi.org/10.2214/ajr.176.2.1760413. PMID: 11159083
50. Doebar SC, Slaets L, Cardoso F, Giordano SH, Bartlett JM, Tryfonidis K, Dijkstra NH, Schröder CP, van Asperen CJ, Linderholm B, Benstead K, Dinjens WN, van Marion R, van Diest PJ, Martens JW, van Deurzen CH. Male breast cancer precursor lesions: analysis of the EORTC 10085/TBCRC/BIG/NABCG International Male Breast Cancer Program. Mod Pathol. 2017;30(4):509–18. https://doi.org/10.1038/modpathol.2016.229. Epub 2017 Jan 13. PMID: 28084333
51. Hittmair AP, Lininger RA, Tavassoli FA. Ductal carcinoma in situ (DCIS) in the male breast: a morphologic study of 84 cases of pure DCIS and 30 cases of DCIS associated with invasive carcinoma–a preliminary report. Cancer. 1998;83(10):2139–49. https://doi.org/10.1002/(sici)1097-0142(19981115)83:10<2139::aid-cncr12>3.0.co;2-f. PMID: 9827718
52. Nicosia L, Lissidini G, Sargenti M, et al. Ductal carcinoma in situ of the male breast: clinical radiological features and management in a cancer referral center. Breast Cancer Res Treat. 2022;196:371–7. https://doi.org/10.1007/s10549-022-06689-y.
53. Sisti A, Huayllani MT, Restrepo DJ, Boczar D, Advani P, Lu X, Spaulding AC, Ball CT, McLaughlin SA, Forte AJ. Paget disease of the breast: a national retrospective analysis of the US population. Breast Dis. 2020;39(3–4):119–26. https://doi.org/10.3233/BD-200439. PMID: 32390594
54. Wang F, Shu X, Meszoely I, Pal T, Mayer IA, Yu Z, Zheng W, Bailey CE, Shu XO. Overall mortality after diagnosis of breast cancer in men vs women. JAMA Oncol. 2019;5(11):1589–96. https://doi.org/10.1001/jamaoncol.2019.2803. PMID: 31536134; PMCID: PMC6753503
55. Shukla S, Chauhan R, Jyotsna PL, Andley M. Primary fibrosarcoma of male breast: a rare entity. J Clin Diagn Res. 2014;8(4):FD11–2. https://doi.org/10.7860/JCDR/2014/7646.4296. Epub 2014 Apr 15. PMID: 24959458; PMCID: PMC4064845
56. Boehm D, Keller K, Schmidt M, Cotarelo C, Kern A, Lebrecht A, Koelbl H. Primary Leiomyosarcoma of the male breast. World J Oncol. 2010;1(5):210–2. https://doi.org/10.4021/wjon238w. Epub 2010 Nov 2. PMID: 29147209; PMCID: PMC5649800
57. Masannat Y, Sumrien H, Sharaiha Y. Primary leiomyosarcoma of the male breast: a case report. Case Rep Med. 2010;2010:534102. https://doi.org/10.1155/2010/534102. Epub 2010 Oct 27. PMID: 21048931; PMCID: PMC2965433
58. Mandaliya H, Sung J, Hill J, Samali R, George M. Prostate cancer: cases of rare presentation and rare

metastasis. Case Rep Oncol. 2015;8(3):526–9. https://doi.org/10.1159/000442045. PMID: 26668576; PMCID: PMC4677723
59. Sippo DA, Kulkarni K, Carlo PD, Lee B, Eisner D, Cimino-Mathews A, Harvey SC. Metastatic disease to the breast from Extramammary malignancies: a multimodality pictorial review. Curr Probl Diagn Radiol. 2016;45(3):225–32. https://doi.org/10.1067/j.cpradiol.2015.07.001. Epub 2015 Jul 4. PMID: 26293973

16

Staging and Management of Breast Carcinoma

Jyoti Sharma, Amitabha Mandal, and Anu Agrawal

Abstract

Breast cancer may be sporadic or familial. Familial breast cancer is associated with BRCA mutation. Most commonly, breast cancer presents with a lump. Triple assessment (clinical, radiological, and tissue diagnosis) is the main diagnostic modality. Breast cancer is staged as per eighth edition of the AJCC TNM staging system. The molecular classification is based on ER, PR, and Her 2 neu status. Broadly, breast cancers are categorized into early breast cancer (EBC), locally advanced breast cancer (LABC), and metastatic breast cancer (MBC). Surgery is the main treatment modality for EBC and LABC. In EBC, upfront surgery is preferred either MRM or BCS depending upon the various patient and tumor factors. For all BCS, postoperative radiotherapy is mandatory, whereas adjuvant chemotherapy is given in all patients with a tumor size more than 1 cm. For LABC, initial treatment of choice is systemic therapy, followed by BCS or MRM. PORT is given to all patients with LABC. All hormone receptor-positive patients should be treated with tamoxifen for 10 years irrespective of menopausal status. But aromatase inhibitors are given in hormone receptor-positive postmenopausal women. In any patients with TNBC subtype, initial treatment is NACT followed by surgery. Similarly for HER 2-positive patients, NACT is the preferred initial treatment modality, followed by surgery. After completion of treatment, every patient should be followed up 3 months for 2 years, then 6 months for next 3 years, and yearly thereafter. The follow-up should be lifelong. Evaluation of the treated breast (in case of BCS) and the opposite breast should be done with yearly mammogram.

Keywords

Breast cancer · Breast conservation surgery · Oncoplasty · Mastectomy

16.1 Introduction

Any woman diagnosed with breast cancer requires adequate staging of disease for appropriate management and prognostication. Currently, breast cancer is staged as per the eighth edition of the AJCC TNM staging system. This updated staging system is different from the previous seventh edition. In the new staging system, biomarker testing for ER, PR, and HER2 expression, tumor grade has been incorporated. In the case of

J. Sharma (✉) · A. Mandal
Department of Surgical Oncology, NCI-AIIMS, New Delhi, India

A. Agrawal
Department of Radiation Oncology, VMMC and Safdarjung Hospital, New Delhi, India

E. Dhamija, S. V. S. Deo (eds.), *Imaging in Management of Breast Diseases*,
https://doi.org/10.1007/978-981-96-4998-3_16

node-negative, ER-positive, and HER2-negative cancers, oncotype DX genomic assay has been included [1, 2]. Though recommended, the gene expression profile may not be available for all; therefore, the least expected is to classify breast cancer into morphological subtypes. Nevertheless, clinical breast examination remains the most important step in assigning stage and deciding treatment. Imaging and pathological evaluation plays a crucial role in treatment planning. Advancements in the surgical techniques, radiation treatment, and chemotherapeutic agents have led to improved survival and patient outcome. This chapter will provide an overview of the revised staging system and management strategies for breast cancer.

16.2 Staging of Breast Carcinoma

Similar to other cancers, breast cancer is also staged as per the TNM staging system. TNM includes three major criteria, tumor size (T), nodal status (N), and metastasis (M). The eighth edition of the TNM staging system has been effective from 1 January 2018, which incorporates the changes described in following section (Table 16.1). In the eighth edition, biologic prognostic factors like estrogen and progesterone receptor status (ER, PR), expression of human epidermal growth factor receptor (HER2) have been incorporated along with histologic grade and recurrence score.

Changes in T staging:

- Lobular carcinoma in situ (LCIS) is no longer classified as Tis. It is a benign entity as per eighth edition.
- Tumor size between 1 mm and 1.5 mm are not classified as microinvasive (T1mi); they are rounded to 2 mm.
- Small, microscopic, satellite tumor foci around a primary tumor should not be added to the maximum tumor size.
- When multiple synchronous tumors are present, the lesion with the largest size will be taken into the T staging. A suffix "m" should be mentioned in T stage.
- T4b lesion is defined as macroscopic satellite tumor nodule in the skin separate from the primary tumor.

Changes in N stage:

- The eighth edition clarified that the largest contiguous tumor deposit should define pN. Dimensions of satellite deposits are not added.
- Furthermore, clarification was added that cNX should only be used when a nodal basin has been removed and cannot be examined by imaging or clinical exam.
- cN0 is assigned to tumors in which nodal exam and imaging, if obtained, are negative.

Changes in metastases (M) classification:

- Pathological M0 should not be used.
- Cases are either cM0 or cM1 disease. If clinical M1 is confirmed by histopathology then use pM1.

Few commonly used terminologies have been tabulated in Table 16.2 for readers' convenience.

As per the AJCC staging system, stage 0, I—IIB are classified as early breast cancer (EBC). EBC would thus include DCIS, IA, T1N0; IB, T0N1mic/ T1N1mic; IIA, T0N1/T1N1/T2N0; IIB, T2N1/T3N0. In early breast cancer, staging assessment and evaluation are usually targeted at locoregional disease because distant or occult metastasis is unlikely, and, therefore, comprehensive metastatic workup is not recommended. On the other hand, large operable breast masses and locally advanced cancers would need metastatic work up. Metastatic workup includes CECT chest, abdomen, and pelvis along with bone scan or PET CT scan.

Table 16.1 TNM classification (eighth edition) of breast cancer [1]

Tx	Primary tumor cannot be assessed
T0	No evidence of primary tumor
Tis	Tis (DCIS)—Ductal carcinoma in situ Tis (Paget)—Paget disease of the nipple without any invasive carcinoma and/or DCIS in the underlying breast
T1 Tumor $\le$20 mm in greatest dimension	T1mi—Tumor $\le$1 mm in greatest dimension T1a—Tumor >1 mm but $\le$5 mm in greatest dimension T1b—Tumor >5 mm but $\le$10 mm in greatest dimension T1c—Tumor >10 mm but $\le$20 mm in greatest dimension
T2	Tumor >20 mm but $\le$50 mm in greatest dimension
T3	Tumor >50 mm in greatest dimension
T4 Tumor of any size with direct extension to the chest wall and/or the skin (ulceration or macroscopic skin nodules)[a]	T4a—Extension to the chest wall, not including only pectoralis muscle adherence/invasion T4b—Ulceration and/or ipsilateral satellite nodules and/or edema (including peau d'orange) of the skin, which do not meet the criteria for inflammatory carcinoma T4c—Both (T4a and T4b) T4d—Inflammatory carcinoma[b]
Clinical classification of regional lymph nodes	
cNX	Regional lymph nodes cannot be assessed (e.g., previously removed).
cN0	No regional lymph node metastases (neither by imaging nor clinical exam)
cN1	Metastasis to movable ipsilateral level I and II axillary lymph node(s). *cN1mi*[b]—Micrometastases (approximately 200 cells, larger than 0.2 mm, but none larger than 2.0 mm)
cN2	Metastasis to ipsilateral level I and II axillary lymph nodes that are clinically fixed or matted or in ipsilateral internal mammary nodes in the absence of clinically evident axillary node metastases *cN2a*—Metastasis to ipsilateral level I and II axillary lymph nodes fixed to one another (matted) or to other structures *cN2b*—Metastasis only in ipsilateral internal mammary nodes, and in the absence of clinically evident axillary node metastases
cN3	Metastases in ipsilateral infraclavicular (level III axillary) lymph node(s) with or without level I and II axillary lymph node involvement or in ipsilateral internal mammary lymph node(s) with clinically evident level I and II axillary lymph node metastases or metastases in ipsilateral supraclavicular lymph node(s) with or without axillary or internal mammary lymph node involvement *cN3a*—Metastasis to ipsilateral infraclavicular lymph node(s) *cN3b*—Metastasis to ipsilateral internal mammary lymph node(s) and axillary lymph nodes *cN3c*—Metastasis in ipsilateral supraclavicular lymph node(s)
Clinical classification of the metastatic disease	
M0	M0—No clinical or radiographic evidence of distant metastases (no pathologic M0; imaging studies are not required to assign the cM0 category) *cM0(i+)*—No clinical or radiographic evidence of distant metastases but deposits of molecularly or microscopically detected tumor cells that are no larger than 0.2 mm are present in circulating blood, bone marrow, or other nonregional nodal tissue in a patient without symptoms or signs of metastases
M1	Distant detectable metastases as determined by classic clinical and radiographic means and/or histologically proven metastases larger than 0.2 mm

[a] Invasion of the dermis alone does not qualify as T4

[b] Inflammatory carcinoma is restricted to cases with typical skin changes involving one-third or greater of the skin of the breast. While the histologic presence of invasive carcinoma invading dermal lymphatics is supportive of the diagnosis, it is not required, nor is dermal lymphatic invasion without typical clinical findings sufficient for a diagnosis of inflammatory breast cancer

Table 16.2 Commonly used terminology for breast cancer

Abbreviation	Terminology	Stage
EBC	Early breast cancer	Stage I, II
LOBC	Large operable breast cancer	Stage IIIA
LABC	Locally advanced breast cancer	Stage IIIB, IIIC
MBC	Metastatic breast cancer	Stage IV
OMBC	Oligometastatic breast cancer	
PMBC	Polymetastatic breast cancer	
YBC	Young breast cancer	Less than 40 years of age
PABC	Pregnancy-associated breast cancer	

16.3 Pretreatment Workup

Pretreatment workup includes bilateral mammogram/digital breast tomosynthesis and/or ultrasound breast for the primary breast tumor and ultrasound of bilateral axillae. Contrast enhanced MRI breast is advised in selected cases with age less than 35 and with clinical-imaging discordance. This is followed by core biopsy of primary tumor for confirming diagnosis of breast carcinoma and molecular subtyping. Genetic counseling and testing are advised in all patients with YBC, family history suggestive of pathogenic mutations, and those less than 60 years with TNBC. The routine investigations for anesthesia fitness include complete blood count (CBC), liver function test (LFT), kidney function test (KFT), prothrombin time, INR, chest X-ray, and 12 lead ECG. In authors' institute, viral markers are done routinely in all patients before surgery, including hepatitis B, hepatitis C, and HIV. The patients undergoing neo-adjuvant chemotherapy are advised for baseline and preoperative 2D-Echocardiogram.

The following parameters are recorded:

1. Complete history with details of the comorbid conditions
2. Physical examination
3. Imaging assessment
4. Tissue biopsy with diagnosis
5. Staging of the disease
6. Assessment of tumor-breast ratio, location of the tumor
7. Axilla evaluation
8. Plan of multidisciplinary team
9. Patient counseling and consent

16.4 Breast Conservation Treatment

Breast conservation treatment (BCT) consists of breast conservation surgery (BCS) followed by radiation therapy (RT) to the treated breast. Several randomized controlled trials had proved the efficacy of BCT, and it is equivalent to mastectomy [3, 4]. In Western countries, BCS is a well-established treatment modality, but in low-middle-income countries (LMIC) like India, the role of BCS is still evolving. The rate of BCS in India is still not touching the international benchmark. Several factors determine the choice of surgery like patient's preference, sociocultural background, age of the patient, availability of RT, stage of the disease, tumor-breast ratio, and other disease-related factors which have been discussed in subsequent sections. The goal of BCS is to provide a cosmetically acceptable breast without compromising oncological safety that is achieving a tumor-free margin.

Patient Selection for BCT Although BCS is an acceptable alternative to mastectomy, not all patients are suitable for BCS. Suitable patient selection is the main determinant for a successful BCS. The authors offer BCS to females with early-stage breast cancer (stage I and II) with a good tumor versus breast ratio, having no contraindication for RT, and patients motivated to complete the treatment course and having the required social and family support.

Absolute contraindications of BCT include the following:

1. Inflammatory breast carcinoma (IBC): Clinical diagnosis of IBC can be made by virtue of presence of extensive involvement of

the skin of the breast or the dermal lymphatic involvement. IBC is an absolute contraindication for BCS even after a complete response to neoadjuvant chemotherapy (NACT).
2. Presence of diffuse microcalcification in mammography.
3. Multicentric disease: When two or more tumors are present in the different quadrants of the breast and which cannot be resected by a single incision is called multicentric disease.
4. History of prior RT to the affected breast or chest wall [5].
5. Pregnancy: Although breast cancer developed in the later part of pregnancy can be considered for BCS where RT to the breast can be delivered after delivery, but in the first trimester, mastectomy is a suitable option.
6. Persistent positive margin after multiple excision [6].
7. Some connective tissue disorders like scleroderma and Sjogren syndrome tolerate RT poorly due to cutaneous fragility, and in those situations, BCT should not be considered as a treatment option [7]. Radiation toxicity is also increased in systemic lupus erythematosus and rheumatoid; hence, RT should be considered carefully [8].

Relative Contraindication of BCT The tumor-breast ratio is an important determinant of BCS. A large tumor in a small breast cannot provide a cosmetically acceptable breast, and so in such a situation, BCS can be individualized. Pendulous breast is not a contraindication to BCS, but homogenous delivery of RT is challenging in such cases. Although a large tumor is not a contraindication for BCT, it poses challenge in preservation of cosmesis. NACT can be offered to these patients in order to reduce the tumor size before considering BCS.

No longer considered as a contraindication for BCS

1. Age.
2. Local involvement of skin and nipple-areola complex (NAC) or retraction of the nipple: Excision of the NAC with a negative margin can provide an excellent cosmesis.
3. Lobular carcinoma.
4. Lymph node involvement.
5. Extensive intraductal component (EIC): Defined as the presence of more than 25 percent of ductal carcinoma in situ (DCIS) component in invasive ductal carcinoma. The presence of EIC indicates that the disease extends beyond the clinically apparent tumor. Studies have proven that EIC resected with a negative margin does not increase the rate of local recurrence as compared to EIC with a positive margin [9].
6. Tumor location.
7. Dense breast.
8. Inherited susceptibility: Patients with a strong family history of breast and ovarian cancer (BRCA1/BRCA2 mutation) can be offered BCS. Genetic counseling should be done in such a situation, and the patient should be explained about the pros and cons of bilateral prophylactic mastectomy. The patient should know that bilateral prophylactic mastectomy can reduce the risk of a second primary cancer but has no survival advantages of contralateral prophylactic mastectomy because it cannot eliminate the risk of metastasis or chest wall recurrence as the metastatic potential is determined by the primary tumor [10].

NACT Before BCS If the tumor size is large or the tumor-breast ratio is not optimum for BCS, NACT is a viable option for downstaging the disease in a nonmetastatic set up. Taking into account the possibility of a complete clinical response after NACT, a metallic tumor marker should be placed in the center of the tumor under the guidance of ultrasound before initiation of NACT. This marker can identify the site of tumor after complete response and can be localized using hookwire on the day of surgery.

Technique of BCS

1. *Skin incision*: Incision should be placed very carefully depending on the location of the tumor. A crescent incision is appropriate for the lesion of the upper outer and upper inner quadrant, whereas an inverted T-shaped incision can be used for the lower quadrant lesion.

For the central quadrant, an elliptical-shaped incision encompassing the NAC is appropriate. The incision plan should be discussed with radiologist at the time of hookwire placement for smooth retrieval of wire during surgery.
2. *The margin for BCS*: BCS with a negative margin has a lower rate of local recurrence than a positive margin [11]. For invasive carcinoma, "no ink on tumor" is the standard margin for BCS [12]. In the case of DCIS, a 2 mm margin is required [13]. Therefore, while excising, the index mass is removed three dimensionally along with surrounding 1 cm of normal breast tissue.
3. *Reconstruction of the breast*: Breast reconstruction depends on the volume of the breast tissue removed. Oncoplastic breast surgery is a potential option for the reconstruction of the breast. The goal of oncoplastic breast surgery is to resect the tumor with a negative margin and achieve acceptable cosmesis. Oncoplastic surgery (OPS) can be classified based on the amount of breast tissue removed. When <20% of the breast tissue is removed, it is called level I OPS, and when 20–50% of breast tissue is removed, it is level II OPS [14]. For level I defect, breast reconstruction is done by simple dermoglandular mobilization, and approximation of breast tissue using absorbable sutures. Complex reconstruction methods are required for level II defect. The commonly used complex oncoplastic techniques include lateral segmentectomy, batwing mastopexy, central breast-conserving surgery (BCS), reduction mammoplasty, vertical mastopexy, and donut mastopexy.

Complications of BCS

1. Seroma: Is the most common complication after BCS. Small seroma can be managed conservatively, but if the size is increasing, then aspiration can be done.
2. Hematoma: Hematoma is a common complication after BCS. It occurs due to primary or secondary hemorrhage, although most of the hematomas occur due to primary hemorrhage. Small hematoma can be managed conservatively, but expanding hematoma or large hematoma needs exploration and ligation of the bleeding vessels.
3. Wound infection: It can be superficial skin infection or deep-seated infection. Superficial infections can be managed with antibiotic, whereas deep skin infection requires wound exploration, pus evacuation, or sometimes debridement of the wound, along with the course of antibiotic.
4. Wound dehiscence: It may occur due to infected collection or mastectomy flap necrosis. This condition requires wound debridement and regular wound dressing with intravenous or oral antibiotic. At times, negative pressure dressing may be used to hasten healing and avoiding delay in postoperative radiotherapy. Secondary suturing should be attempted when the healthy granulation tissue is visible.

Postoperative RT Adjuvant whole breast irradiation (WBI) is essential for all patients after BCS. WBI decreases the incidence of locoregional recurrence and improves the overall survival [15–17]. The most commonly used conventional dose schedules consist of 45–50 Gray (Gy) at 1.8–2 Gy per fractions delivered daily to the whole breast, with an optional dose of 10–16 Gy tumor bed boost with or without lymph node irradiation over 4–5 weeks. However, hypofractionated dose schedule regimen (40 Gy in 15 fractions over 3 weeks duration) that is radiobiologically equivalent to conventional dose regimens with dose more than 2 Gy per fractions daily over 3–4 weeks has also been used [18].

The rationale for hypofractionation with a modest increase in fraction size accompanied by decrease in total dose results in similar local control, toxicity, and cosmesis along with better compliance and shorter duration of treatment time. Recently, ultrahypofractionation with dose regimens 27 Gy in 5 fractions over 1 week and 26 Gy in 5 fractions over 1-week duration has also been tried and compared with hypofractionation. It was noninferior to 40 Gy in 15 fractions over 3 weeks for tumor control and is safe in terms of normal tissue effects.

The acute toxicities reported are skin reactions, and late toxicities were breast shrinkage, arm edema, shoulder stiffness, telangiectasias, ischemic heart disease, symptomatic rib fractures, radiation pneumonitis, and radiation-induced brachial plexopathy which was similar as compared to conventional fractionation. Hence, a 1-week dose schedule has been adopted as a new standard for patients with early breast cancer requiring adjuvant radiation therapy to the whole breast in most of the centers globally [19].

Radiation Therapy After Neoadjuvant Chemotherapy Neoadjuvant chemotherapy (NACT) is being used in the treatment of breast cancer to downstage the tumor as already discussed. Along with downstaging the tumor, it has been increasingly used in patients with TNBC subtype, clinical stage III or above, and HER-2-positive tumors to decrease locoregional relapse [20]. Postoperative WBI is indicated after NACT and BCS irrespective of pathological response. In patients with clinical stage III disease and residual lymph node involvement, regional lymph node is irradiated irrespective of pathological response. However, in patients with clinical N1 disease with complete pathological response, approach to radiation therapy is a matter of controversy [21].

According to NCCN recommendations version 1.2024, considerations of radiation therapy in patients receiving NACT and BCS include the following [22]:

A. cN0 → ypN0 (SLNB) → WBI + tumor bed boost,
B. cN+ → ypN0 → WBI + tumor bed boost + comprehensive RNI (NSABP 51)
C. cN+ → ypN+ (SLNB) → WBI + tumor bed boost + ALND + comprehensive RNI

According to NCCN recommendations version 1.2024, considerations of radiation therapy in patients receiving NACT and mastectomy are the following:

A. cN0 → ypN0 (SLNB) → PMRT/observation
B. cN+ → ypN0 (SLNB) → PMRT + comprehensive RNI (NSABP 51)
C. cN+ → ypN+ → PMRT + ALND + comprehensive RNI

According to "Lucerne Toolbox," considerations of radiation therapy in patients receiving NACT have been mentioned below [23]. The presence of nonluminal A like grade 3, middle/high genomic risk, lymphovascular invasion, and extracapsular extension are considered as risk factors.

A. cN0 → ycN0 → SLNB → ypN0 → no local treatment
B. cN0 → ycN0 → SLNB → ypN+ → ALND or axillary RT → level III +/− IMN RT if risk factors +
C. cN+ → ycN0 → targeted axillary dissection → ypN0 → axillary RT → level III +/− IMN RT if risk factors +
D. cN+ → ycN0 → targeted axillary dissection → ypN+ → ALND or axillary RT → level III +/− IMN RT
E. cN0 → ycN+ → ALND→ ypN0 → no local treatment → level III +/− IMN RT if risk factors +
F. cN0 → ycN+ → ALND→ ypN+ → axillary RT + level III +/− IMN

16.5 Mastectomy

This includes modified radical mastectomy, simple mastectomy, skin-sparing or nipple-sparing mastectomy. Modified radical mastectomy involves resection of tumor, breast parenchyma, pectoral fascia, overlying skin, and level I and II axillary lymph nodes. In simple mastectomy, tumor with breast parenchyma and overlying skin are resected but the axilla is not addressed. In skin-sparing mastectomy, the skin envelope is preserved, while in nipple-sparing mastectomy, the nipple-areola complex is also preserved. In all these types except modified radical mastectomy, axilla can be addressed either through sentinel lymph node biopsy or through low axillary sampling. Whole breast reconstruction can be achieved after mastectomy also. In SSM and NSM, usually immediate reconstruction with silicone implant is done, while after MRM, delayed reconstruction with autologous tissue like pedicled or free myocutaneous flap is preferred.

16.6 Management of Early Breast Cancer (EBC)

Early breast cancers are tumors localized to the breast without involving the skin and chest wall and having limited spread to level I axillary lymph nodes. It includes AJCC stages cT1-T3, cN0 or cN1, and M0. There is controversy regarding stage cT3N1 whether it is EBC or LABC. Some consider it as large operable breast cancer (LOBC). All these patients are usually suitable for upfront surgery with adjuvant treatment. With the rapid evolution in local modalities (surgery and radiation) as well as advancements in systemic therapy, the treatment of EBC is becoming quite complex. The plan of management should be discussed by the multidisciplinary team and should have active involvement of the patient as per the algorithm (Fig. 16.1). Various factors need to be considered for planning treatment. These include the following:

1. *Tumor factors*—molecular subtype, gene profiling, multifocality/multicentricity, tumor size, and tumor location
2. *Patient factors*—age, performance status, desire, comorbidities, marital status, parity, menstruation, socioeconomic status, breast volume, history of prior radiation, and compliance
3. *Genetic factors*—hereditary breast cancer syndromes, pathogenic mutations, and familial breast cancer

Surgery BCS is usually the primary choice of treatment for early breast cancer [25]. Randomized trials did not show any difference in survival when mastectomy was compared with

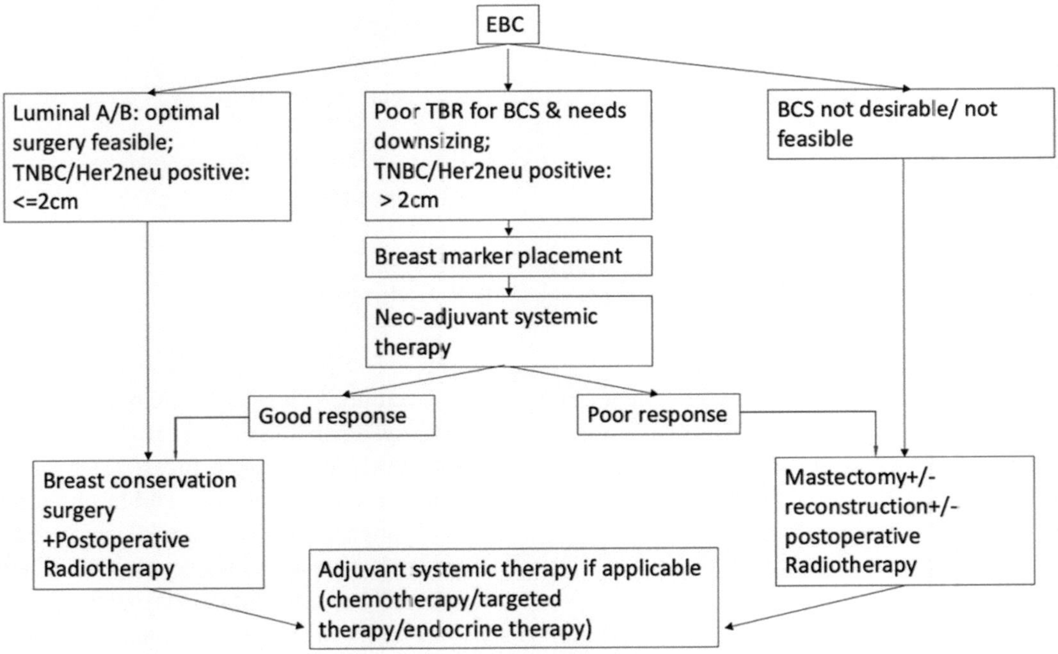

Fig. 16.1 Algorithm for management of early breast cancer [24] TBR tumor-breast ratio, BCS not feasible—multicentric tumors, prior scars, negative margins not achievable after lumpectomy

BCS plus radiation for stage I and stage II breast cancer [26, 27]. However, mastectomy may be indicated, depending on the factors described above. EBC with molecular subtypes Luminal A or B are considered as suitable candidates for upfront surgery. In triple-negative and Her-2-neu-positive breast cancers, upfront surgical excision is usually restricted to tumors up to 2 centimeters in diameter.

Upfront Breast Conversation Surgery BCS with radiation is the current global standard of care in EBC. It involves the excision of tumor along with surrounding normal breast tissue to ensure negative margins. This is combined with breast oncoplasty to maintain the breast aesthetics. The American Society of Breast Surgeons proposed a new consensus definition of oncoplastic surgery as "Breast conservation surgery incorporating an oncologic partial mastectomy with ipsilateral defect repair using volume displacement or volume replacement techniques with contralateral symmetry surgery as appropriate" [28].

Upfront BCS is preferred in patients with unifocal lesion, good tumor-breast ratio, luminal A molecular subtype, and no contraindication to radiation. The type of oncoplasty depends on the volume of resection, location of tumor, potential flap donor sites, and bilateral breast anthropometry. With refinement in oncoplastic techniques, better cosmesis can be achieved, even in large tumors or poor tumor-breast ratio [29].

For axillary staging, sentinel lymph node biopsy with dual-dye method is recommended in the absence of clinical axillary lymph nodes. However, in the presence of axillary lymph nodes, lymph node dissection should be performed.

Upfront Mastectomy In early breast cancer, mastectomy may be indicated in the presence of multifocal/multicentric lesions, diffuse microcalcifications, poor tumor-breast ratio, and inability to achieve negative margins after BCS. At times, age and frailty is a concern when mastectomy option is selected. Patient's or family's preference for mastectomy is another strong reason, especially in Indian population [30].

Mastectomy, usually skin sparing or nipple sparing, may be followed with immediate or delayed breast reconstruction. The reconstruction may be performed using autologous tissue (pedicled or free flaps) or silicone implants depending on the patient's age, surgical expertise, need for adjuvant radiotherapy, implant affordability, and availability of donor tissue sites. In case where radiotherapy is indicated, temporary tissue expander may be used during radiation followed by exchange with permanent implant.

In the West, there is a recent trend toward bilateral skin-sparing or nipple-sparing mastectomy with implant-based reconstruction even in patients suitable for BCS and in the absence of genetic predisposition [31]. However, in Indian patients, this is usually preferred in selected patients with pathogenic genetic mutations, where ipsilateral mastectomy and contralateral risk-reducing prophylactic mastectomy are performed [32].

Neoadjuvant Systemic Therapy Neoadjuvant systemic therapy refers to the administration of chemotherapy or endocrine therapy before definitive surgical treatment. Neoadjuvant chemotherapy (NACT) was introduced in the 1970s [33], with the aim to downstage locally advanced(inoperable) disease and make it operable. However, NACT was subsequently extended to operable (early) breast cancer, in order to perform breast-conserving surgery, and is now widely used, particularly for large tumors [34–36]. In the Early Breast Cancer Trialists' Collaborative Group (EBCTCG) meta-analysis, NACT led to more number of patients receiving breast-conservation therapy (65% vs. 49%) as compared to adjuvant chemotherapy; however, there was also an associated increased risk of local recurrence in patients (21.4% vs. 15.9%; RR 1.37, 1.17–1.61) [37]. Similarly, in the NSABP B-18 study, a higher rate of breast conservation was achieved in the preoperative chemotherapy group and the disease-free survival (DFS), distant disease-free survival, and overall survival were equivalent in patients receiving preoperative and postoperative chemotherapy (OS; $p = 0.99$, 0.70, and 0.83, respectively) [38]. In addition, response to NACT can be a prognostic factor and surrogate marker for survival outcomes in patients with triple-negative breast cancer and Her-2-neu gene amplification.

Therefore, in EBC patients who are eligible but not suitable for upfront breast conservation surgery in view of large tumor or poor tumor-breast ratio, NACT has a potential role in tumor downsizing and improving the breast conservation rate. Any patient planned for NACT should have adequate imaging and radiopaque marker placement in the index lesion before starting chemotherapy. Markers are used to guide the surgical excision because a residual tumor after chemotherapy may be clinically occult. Several techniques are in practice for breast tissue marking like wire-guided localization, metallic clip implantation, carbon tattooing, radioactive seed localization (RSL) using iodine-125 (125I) seeds, radiofrequency identification tags (RFIDs) and magnetic marker placement (Magseed/MaMaLoc) [39]. Metallic markers are made of 2- to 3-mm pieces of titanium or stainless steel and are the most commonly used markers today for wire-guided localization before surgery. These include clips in various shapes like ribbon, coil, oval, and heart [40].

Role of Radiation Therapy in EBC Accelerated partial breast irradiation (APBI), post BCS, in selected cases of EBC has been an alternative to whole breast irradiation involving treatment of limited and targeted breast tissue volume in much shorter duration of time. APBI is any scheme that delivers radiation to the tumor site and limited surrounding tissue over a short overall time. Improving quality of life, avoiding prolonged treatment regimens, reducing time cost and inconvenience, and potentially reducing acute and late toxicities are the advantages of APBI. Techniques used for APBI include multicatheter interstitial brachytherapy, balloon catheter intracavitary brachytherapy, external beam radiotherapy, and intraoperative radiation therapy [41] (Table 16.3).

Table 16.3 Dose schedules of various techniques of APBI

Techniques	Dose schedules
Multicatheter interstitial brachytherapy	34 Gy in 10 fractions BID
Balloon catheter intracavitary brachytherapy	MammoSite 34 Gy in 10 fractions BID
External beam radiotherapy (3DCRT)	38.5 Gy in 10 fractions BID
Intraoperative APBI	21 Gy—Electrons 20 Gy—50 KV photons

The American Brachytherapy Society (ABS) and American Society for Radiation Oncology (ASTRO) have different sets of selection criteria for patient eligibility for APBI in EBC [42, 43].

Patient eligibility selection criteria according to ABS are the following:

(a) Age >45 years
(b) All invasive subtypes and DCIS
(c) Tumor size <3 cm,unifocal and node negative
(d) ER +/−, Her 2 neu –
(e) Lymphovascular invasion absent

Patient eligibility selection criteria according to ASTRO are the following:

(a) Age >50 years
(b) All invasive subtypes
(c) Tumor size <3 cm and node negative
(d) ER +/−, Her 2 neu –
(e) Limited lymphovascular invasion and intraductal extension <3 cm

One of the questions faced by oncologists in daily clinical practice is the clinical indications of omitting adjuvant radiation in low-risk patients following BCS. Oncotype DX, PAM50, and ARCTIC are some of the techniques to better identify such patients by evaluating tumor biology and genetics. CALGB 9343 and PRIME II found that adjuvant breast irradiation has benefit in locoregional recurrence but had no impact on overall survival, distant disease-free survival, or breast preservation in EBC patients above the age of 70 years. Hence in patients >70 years of age with ER-positive early-stage breast cancer, adjuvant hormonal therapy remains a reasonable option by omitting adjuvant radiation [44, 45].

The GEC-ESTRO Breast Cancer Working Group classifies the patients into three groups for recommendation of APBI as low risk of ipsilateral breast tumor recurrence (IBTR)—suitable for APBI; intermediate risk of IBTR—suitable only in the context of trial; and high risk of IBTR—APBI is contraindicated, in the context of a clinical trial in 2009. However, updated ASTRO and/or GEC-ESTRO guidelines for APBI reconsider eligibility criteria and classify patients into three groups [46]. A systemic review of four prospective RCTs was done with median follow up of between 1 and 8 years along with 10 prospective single arm studies with follow-up of >4 years. Based on the inclusion criteria of patients well represented in studies reporting IBTR rates of <10%, a group "suitable" was defined "cautionary" group was defined to include females enrolled in studies but not well represented, and "unsuitable" group was defined as including characteristics of patients for whom there was less evidence from clinical trials. Patients who fall in unsuitable group for APBI are considered for whole breast irradiation and/or tumor breast boost [47].

Patient stratification criteria as per ASTRO/GEC-ESTRO Breast Cancer Working Group are the following:

A. Suitable (patient meets all criteria)
    1. Age >50 years
    2. Unifocal/unicentric invasive carcinoma
    3. Tumor size <2 cm, Tis or T1, pN0 axillary status
    4. Extensive intraductal component (EIC) or pure DCIS—If screen detected, low to intermediate grade, size <2.5 cm, resected with margins negative at >3 mm
    5. Margins negative
    6. Invasive ductal or favorable histology, associated lobular carcinoma in situ allowed
    7. No neoadjuvant treatment allowed
B. Cautionary (patient meets all criteria)
    1. Age 40–49 years
    2. Unicentric but multifocal carcinoma
    3. Tumor size 2.1–3 cm, T0-2
    4. Extensive intraductal component (EIC) or pure DCIS—< 3 cm and does not meet criteria for criteria
    5. Margins close (<2 mm)
    6. Invasive lobular histology
    7. No neoadjuvant treatment allowed
C. Unsuitable (patient meets all criteria)
    1. Age >50 years
    2. Multicentric or multifocal carcinoma
    3. Tumor size >3 cm, T3-4
    4. Extensive intraductal component (EIC) or pure DCIS—> 3 cm
    5. Margins positive
    6. Neoadjuvant treatment received

Management of Axilla The surgical approach to the axilla has taken a paradigm shift from axillary lymph node dissection to no surgery at all. The assessment of axilla incudes clinical examination and dedicated ultrasound of the axilla with or without FNAC of suspicious lymph nodes (Fig. 16.2) A marker may be placed in the suspicious lymph node for subsequent targeted axillary dissection. The present standard of care is sentinel lymph node biopsy with a dual-dye method in EBC patients with node-negative axilla. In patients with cN1 axilla, axillary lymph node dissection should be done in upfront surgery cases or if the patient remains node positive even after NACT. However, if the patient has received NACT and become clinically node negative, SLNB is recommended, provided that the dual-dye technique is used and a minimum of three lymph nodes are identified. The management is shown in the algorithm (Fig. 16.3).

Traditionally, in patients with clinically node-negative breast cancer who were SLN lymph node positive and clinical N2/N3 axillary lymph node positive, the standard of care had been axillary lymph node dissection followed by axillary radiation therapy. The benefit of complete axillary lymph node dissection (ALND) in patients with clinically node-negative patients was addressed by the American college of Surgeons Oncology Group (ACOSOG) Z0011 in patients with clinical T1/T2-N0 undergoing lumpectomy

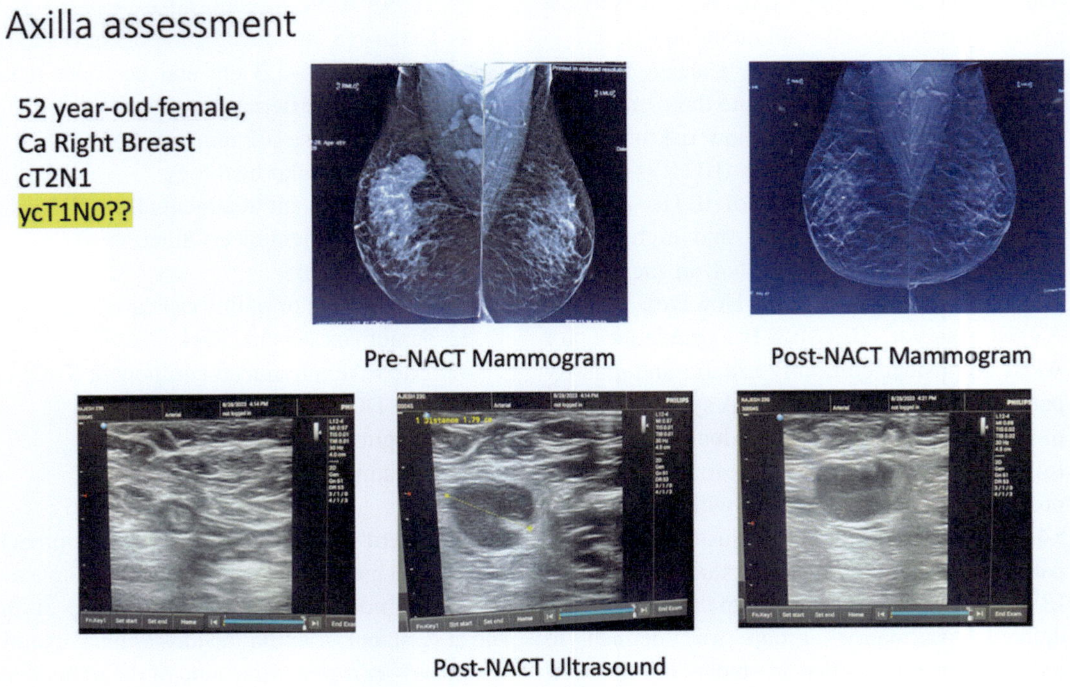

Fig. 16.2 Post NACT mammmogram: no axillary lymph nodes. Ultrasound of axilla: suspicious residual lymph nodes

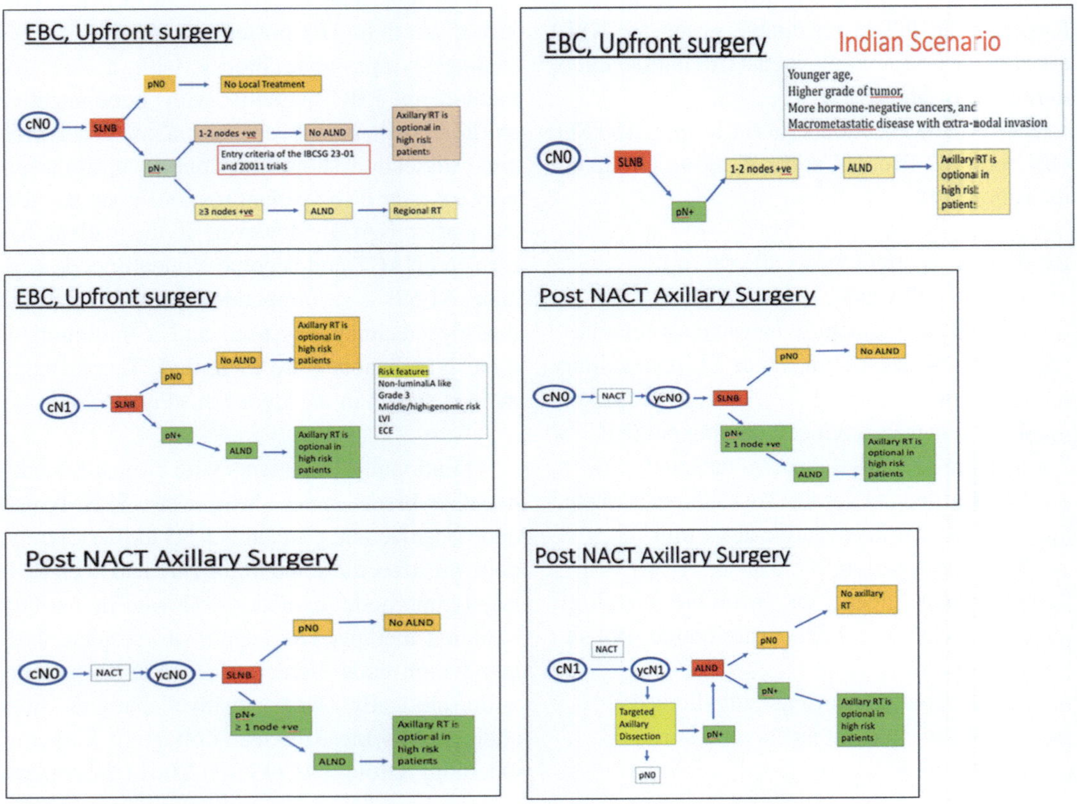

Fig. 16.3 Management algorithm for lymph nodes in the axilla

and SLNB with positive one or two lymph nodes. Similarly, the International Breast Cancer Study Group (IBCSG) 23-01 trial in patients with tumor size <5 cm and one or more SLNB lymph node positive addressed the issue of benefit of complete ALND. The results of both the trials after SLNB demonstrated no difference in recurrence after ALND after SLNB over the SLNB alone in patients with macroscopic and microscopic metastases [48–50].

The AMAROS trial compared ALND and axillary RT in patients with positive SLNB and negative clinical lymph node findings, which did not show any difference in recurrence rate. Overall survival and distant metastasis-free survival did not differ between the arms significantly. However, second primary breast carcinoma was more common in axillary RT arm in comparison to the ALND arm [51]. The results of these trials concluded that in selected patients with negative clinical findings in regional lymph nodes and positive SLNB without ALND, axillary RT can be given.

In patients with N0 disease and high risk with negative findings on axillary surgery, there is a trend to administer regional radiotherapy along with WBI, based on the results of MA20 trial. Regional lymph node irradiation includes supraclavicular lymph node, in case axillary lymph node dissection is not performed; axilla and internal mammary lymph nodes on an individual case basis. The risk factors T3 or T4 tumors and T2 with other risk factors like high grade, absence of estrogen receptor expression, or presence of lymphovascular invasion raise concern of adding regional lymph node to RT after WBI based on the results of MA 20 trial [52].

Patients presenting with clinical N2/3 and/or T4 disease, adjuvant RT with regional nodal irradiation (RNI), remains the standard of care irrespective of neoadjuvant treatment response, and for those with residual nodal involvement, complete axillary lymph node dissection and/or axillary RT remains the standard of care. Furthermore, in patients with pre-NACT clinical N1 disease, treatment paradigms have evolved. NSABP-51 recently completed accrual of patients randomly assigned to adjuvant RT and RNI group and adjuvant RT and no RNI group. The results of which are expected in the years to come [53].

In conclusion, the indications for axillary radiation are four or more lymph node positive, extracapsular extension, and SLNB-positive lymph node with inadequate or no lymph node dissection.

16.7 Management of Locally Advanced Breast Cancer

Locally advanced breast cancers (LABC) are tumors in the breast involving the skin or chest wall or spread to the regional lymph nodes and inflammatory breast cancers. This includes any cT, cN2/N3, cT3, cN+, and cT4, and any cN stage as shown in Fig. 16.4. LABC can be classified as an operable or inoperable disease. The criteria for resectable disease have changed over time with the introduction of effective neoadjuvant systemic therapies and extensive locoregional resections are abandoned. There is no unequivocal definition of unresectability, but a few defining properties have gained widespread acceptance such as fixation of the tumor to periosteum or intercostal muscles and inability to remove all gross disease, for example, because of invasion of the brachial plexus, axillary vessels, ribs, or skin nodules tracking toward or beyond inframammary fold or sternum or "cancer encuirasse." Inflammatory breast cancer is considered a locally advanced disease.

LABC accounts for a sizeable number (30–60%) of breast cancer cases and is a common clinical scenario in developing countries [54]. These patients are usually managed with multimodality therapy, that is, neoadjuvant systemic therapy and locoregional therapy. The rationale for systemic therapy, in the beginning, is to control the micrometastatic disease and to make the unresectable tumors eligible for surgery [55]. The surgery is a modified radical mastectomy for patients with cT4b and inflammatory breast cancer patients. Breast conservation surgery with oncoplasty may be an option in T1-T3, node-positive patients with good response to systemic therapy.

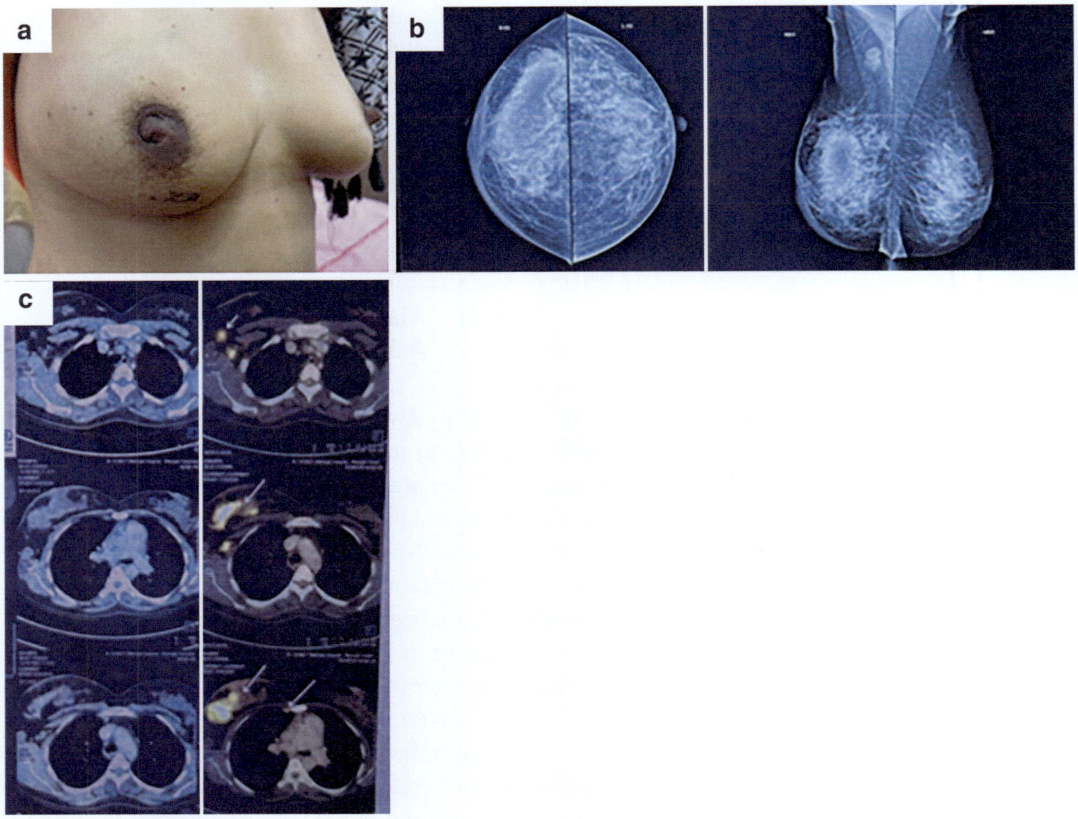

Fig. 16.4 (**a**) A 48-year-old female with right LABC (Peau d'orange) (**b**) Bilateral mammogram showing large mass involving upper outer and central quadrants with skin thickening and suspicious axillary lymph nodes. (**c**) FDG PET-CT scan showing FDG avid primary breast lesion and axillary lymph nodes and no evidence of distant metastasis

Modified radical mastectomy is the procedure after NACT in patients with locally advanced breast cancer. In high-risk patients who received NACT followed by MRM, it was observed that patients who received radiation had lower incidence of locoregional recurrence and distant metastases as compared to patients who did not receive radiation [56] (Fig. 16.5).

High-risk patients include patients with T3 and T4 disease, positive margins, gross extracapsular extension, four or more positive lymph nodes, or grade 3 and should receive PMRT and regional nodal irradiation to lower the risk of locoregional relapse by increasing the overall survival and breast-specific survival rates by 4–5% [15].

Intermediate-risk patients: The benefit of PMRT in this group, that is, T3N0 tumors is controversial. In a meta-analysis by NSABP trials, the role of PMRT was studied and in tumors >5 cm with no LN involvement, the incidence of locoregional failure was low as a first event; hence, it was concluded that PMRT should not be routinely used. However, from the SEER database, an analysis showed that PMRT was associated with significant improvement in overall survival and breast cancer-specific survival, which lead to conclusion that in patients with risk factors including age, lymphovascular invasion, and margin status, PMRT should be considered [57–59]. Another meta-analysis of chest wall and regional lymph nodal irradiation after MRM and axillary surgery or no radiation showed no additional benefit on locoregional recurrence in negative lymph node findings with axillary dissection was noted [60].

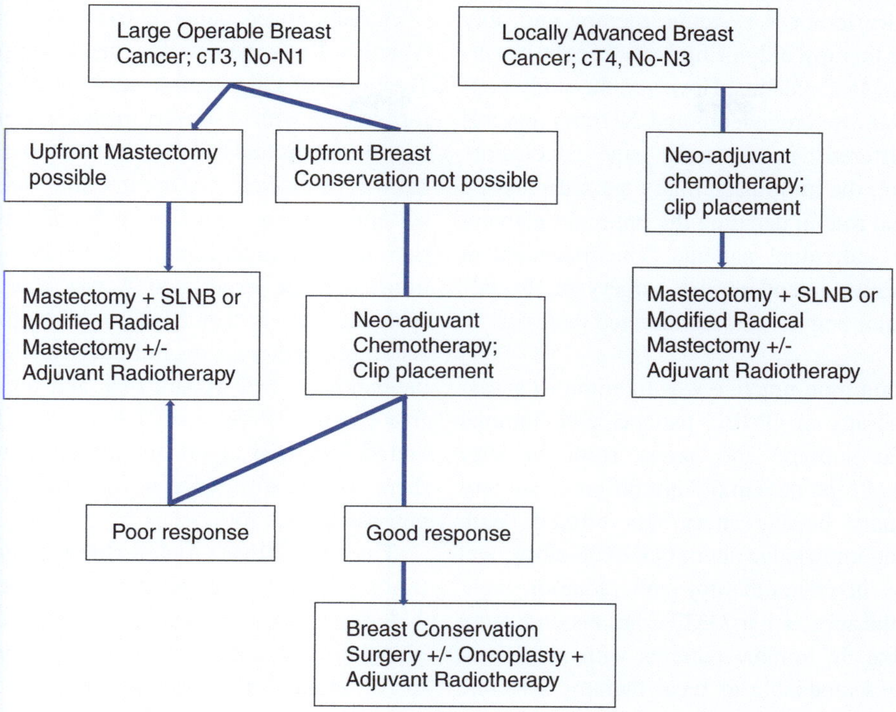

Fig. 16.5 Management algorithm for locally advanced breast cancers

Low-risk patients: In patients with T1/T2 N0 tumors, post-MRM, radiation therapy is not routinely recommended because of the low local recurrence risk. In these patients, the probability of locoregional failure is so low that the risk of toxicity associated with the treatment prevails. However, in selected patients with close/positive margins and patients aged <35 years, LVI positive, and/or grade 3 risk factors, who would otherwise be considered as low risk, PMRT may be indicated [61].

16.8 Role of Surgery in the Metastatic Breast Cancer

Metastatic breast cancer occurs in around 6% of patients presenting de novo and in 20–30% of patients as distant recurrence. In patients with metastases, systemic therapy remains the mainstay of treatment. However, surgery may be indicated for palliation of the primary tumor or metastatic site. The indications for palliative mastectomy are bleeding, tumor fungation, or intractable pain. Palliative surgery for bone metastases is indicated in fracture/imminent fracture, spinal cord compression, and unstable spine. Features of imminent fracture depend on the anatomical site, pain intensity, size of the deposit, and radiological characteristics. The new entity, oligometastatic breast cancer, is managed distinctly from the polymetastatic disease and is described in detail here.

Oligometastatic Breast Cancer (OMBC) It represents the spectrum of breast cancer lying between locoregional disease and overt metastases. As per the consensus statement by the European Society of Radiotherapy and Oncology (ESTRO) and the American Society of Radiation Oncology (ASTRO), OMBC is defined as 1–5 metastatic lesions safely treatable with local therapy; furthermore, the oligometastatic state must be assessed with high-resolution imaging [62]. The role of surgery in OMBC is controversial and no level I evidence is available at present. Randomized controlled trials comparing surgery of primary tumor + systemic therapy and only systemic therapy did not find any benefit of surgery in OMBC patients. However, the study population were heterogeneous and the trial protocols were different in reaching any conclusion. Therefore, the multidisciplinary team discussion has a vital role in deciding the optimal treatment plan for individual patients. The management with curative intent implies surgery of the primary tumor and metastases-directed therapy.

The common practice was to administer systemic therapy in OMBC patients with luminal molecular subtype and assess response after 3 months. If the patient did not progress, surgery for primary breast cancer was offered. With increasing knowledge about OMBC biology, and advances in chemotherapy and radiation techniques, the approach to OMBC has become more aggressive. In luminal patients with 3–5 metastatic sites amenable to local therapy, systemic therapy is started along with SBRT/surgery of the metastatic site followed by BCS/mastectomy [63]. A similar approach is also being tried in unfavorable subtypes like TNBC and Her2 neu [64]. Ongoing trials will guide in deciding the ideal management of OMBC.

Several phase III trials of stage IV breast cancer have shown no benefit in overall survival, but improvements in locoregional control have been reported with locoregional treatment. The ECOG-ACRIN Research group conducted a randomized phase III trial in 390 patients with stage IV breast cancer with systemic therapy plus early local therapy versus systemic therapy alone. If there was no progression post 4–8 months of systemic therapy, then patients were randomized to continued systemic therapy alone versus locoregional surgery and radiation therapy which showed no significant difference in 3-year overall survival, progression-free survival, or health-related quality of life. However, there was close association of lower locoregional recurrence/progression with locoregional treatment than with systemic therapy alone (10.2% vs. 25.6%, $p = 0.003$) [65].

A randomized phase II trial the Stereotactic Ablative Radiotherapy for the Comprehensive Treatment of Oligometastases (SABR-COMET) for patients with controlled primary tumor for at least 3 months and between one and five metastases was conducted. The control arm was standard systemic therapy alone or with palliative radiation of 8 Gy single fraction to 30 Gy to 10 fractions, and the experimental arm was standard systemic therapy with SBRT to all oligometastasis sites. An 8-year overall survival (OS) of all patients was 27% versus 14% and progression-free survival (PFS) was 21% and 0%. Both OS and PFS showed significant difference. However, there was no difference in the time to onset of new metastases [66].

The NRG BR002 trial, a phase II randomized trial exclusively for breast cancer patients with 1–4 extracranial metastases, controlled locoregional disease, and no clinical progression for up to 12 months on systemic therapy: included patients were randomized to standard systemic therapy versus standard systemic therapy plus metastasis-directed therapy. Among patients with oligometastasisss assigned to the ablative treatment arm 93% received SBRT, 2% underwent surgery, and 5%-78% received no treatment. Of these patients, 22% had metachronous metastases and 22% had synchronous metastases. With median follow-up of 19.5 months, 3-year PFS was 33% and 38% ($p = 0.36$), and the mean PFS was 23 months and 19.5 months. The 3-year OS was 72% and 69% ($p = 0.54$). There was lower progression rate within the oligometastases treated with SBRT, but there was no difference in time to appearance of new metastases [67].

Therefore, metastasis-directed radiation therapy to oligometastasis site is more effective for better local control along with standard systemic therapy and locoregional treatment. SBRT directed to metastatic sites could be used for improved durable long-term control. Clinical judgment is needed to determine when the local control benefit of SBRT provides survival benefit to metastasis-directed SBRT in stage IV breast cancer with 1–5 metastatic sites.

16.9 Management in Patients Referred from Outside

A significant proportion of breast cancer patients in India seek treatment at tertiary cancer centers after undergoing incomplete surgery for a breast lump [68]. These patients either have a prior diagnosis of cancer on fine needle aspiration biopsy or have directly undergone excision (Fig. 16.6). In the majority, the axilla is not addressed and staging workup is not adequate. All such patients are advised for breast imaging and pathology review. The need and extent of revision surgery depend on the margin status, residual disease, tumor-breast ratio, and lumpectomy scars. The breast conservation surgery is planned when negative margins can be achieved. This is done by rewide excision of tumor bed with or without oncoplasty. In patients presenting after mastectomy with positive margins or residual gross breast parenchyma/thick flaps, completion of mastectomy is advised (Fig. 16.7). If

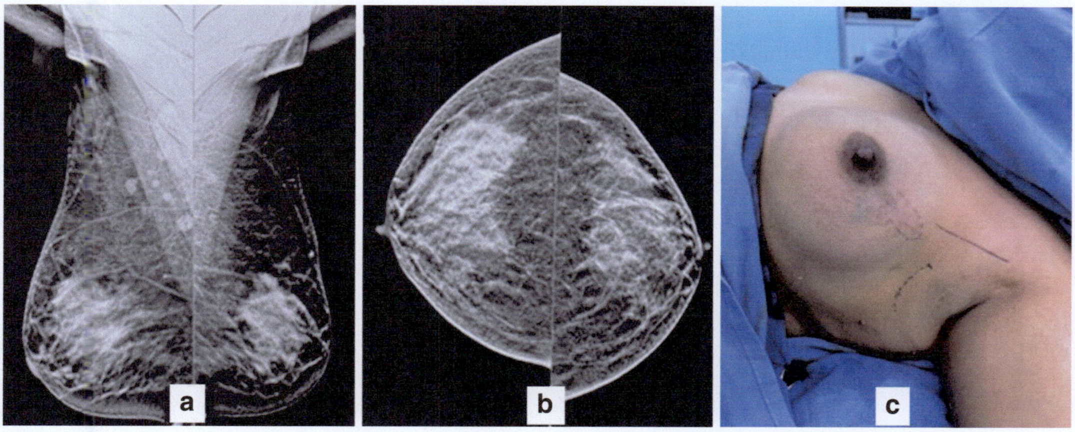

Fig. 16.6 A 31-year-old female presented with left breast carcinoma diagnosed after lumpectomy: Specimen size 3 × 4 cm. IDC, TPBC. Mammogram (**a**) MLO view and (**b**) CC view asymmetry in the right breast; no suspicious microcalcification. (**c**) No palpable lesion. Patient underwent rewide excision of the scar site along with SLNB

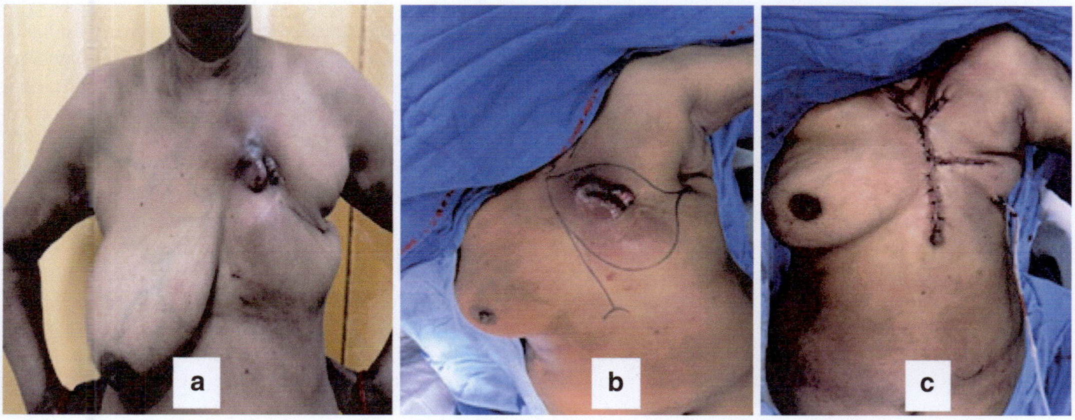

Fig. 16.7 A 59-year-old female with history of left mastectomy and no adjuvant treatment (**a**). PET-CT scan suggested of chest wall recurrence with left axillary lymph nodes (not shown)-Stage rcT4bN2M0, Luminal B. (**b**) Received systemic therapy but withheld after two cycles due to toxicity and had local progression. (**c**) Underwent completion MRM. Planned for adjuvant radiotherapy and hormonal therapy

revision surgery is not possible, radiotherapy is an option. Sentinel lymph node biopsy is recommended in axillary node-negative cases and axillary lymph node dissection in cN1 cases. In cN2 stage, axillary lymph node dissection is done after systemic therapy.

16.10 Conclusion

Adequate staging workup is a prerequisite for optimal management of breast cancer patients. The AJCC "TNM" staging along with hormone receptor and Her2neu status should be assigned to every patient before embarking on the multidisciplinary management. EBC patients should be offered BCS, unless contraindicated. Upfront surgery is preferred, except in the aggressive phenotypes like TNBC and Her2neu positive, wherein NACT is recommended after marker placement for tumor localization. LABC patients should be treated with systemic therapy first, followed by mastectomy. Selected patients with OMBC may be managed with a curative intent.

References

1. Amin MB, Greene FL, Edge SB, Compton CC, Gershenwald JE, Brookland RK, et al. The eighth edition AJCC cancer staging manual: continuing to build a bridge from a population-based to a more "personalized" approach to cancer staging. CA Cancer J Clin. 2017;67(2):93–9.
2. Giuliano AE, Connolly JL, Edge SB, Mittendorf EA, Rugo HS, Solin LJ, et al. Breast cancer-major changes in the American Joint Committee on Cancer eighth edition cancer staging manual. CA Cancer J Clin. 2017;67(4):290–303.
3. Veronesi U, Cascinelli N, Mariani L, Greco M, Saccozzi R, Luini A, et al. Twenty-year follow-up of a randomized study comparing breast-conserving surgery with radical mastectomy for early breast cancer. N Engl J Med. 2002;347(16):1227–32.
4. Blichert-Toft M, Nielsen M, Düring M, Møller S, Rank F, Overgaard M, et al. Long-term results of breast conserving surgery vs. mastectomy for early stage invasive breast cancer: 20-year follow-up of the Danish randomized DBCG-82TM protocol. Acta Oncol Stockh Swed. 2008;47(4):672–81.
5. Arthur DW, Winter KA, Kuerer HM, Haffty BG, Cuttino LW, Todor DA, et al. NRG Oncology-Radiation Therapy Oncology Group Study 1014: 1-year toxicity report from a phase 2 study of repeat breast-preserving surgery and 3-dimensional conformal partial-breast reirradiation for in-breast recurrence. Int J Radiat Oncol Biol Phys. 2017;98(5):1028–35.
6. Coopey S, Smith BL, Hanson S, Buckley J, Hughes KS, Gadd M, et al. The safety of multiple re-excisions after lumpectomy for breast cancer. Ann Surg Oncol. 2011;18(13):3797–801.
7. Chen AM, Obedian E, Haffty BG. Breast-conserving therapy in the setting of collagen vascular disease. Cancer J Sudbury Mass. 2001;7(6):480–91.
8. Wo J, Taghian A. Radiotherapy in setting of collagen vascular disease. Int J Radiat Oncol Biol Phys. 2007;69(5):1347–53.
9. Park CC, Mitsumori M, Nixon A, Recht A, Connolly J, Gelman R, et al. Outcome at 8 years after breast-conserving surgery and radiation therapy for invasive breast cancer: influence of margin status and systemic therapy on local recurrence. J Clin Oncol. 2000;18(8):1668–75.
10. Pierce LJ, Phillips KA, Griffith KA, Buys S, Gaffney DK, Moran MS, et al. Local therapy in BRCA1 and BRCA2 mutation carriers with operable breast cancer: comparison of breast conservation and mastectomy. Breast Cancer Res Treat. 2010;121(2):389–98.
11. Cowen D, Houvenaeghel G, Bardou V, Jacquemier J, Bautrant E, Conte M, et al. Local and distant failures after limited surgery with positive margins and radiotherapy for node-negative breast cancer. Int J Radiat Oncol Biol Phys. 2000;47(2):305–12.
12. Moran MS, Schnitt SJ, Giuliano AE, Harris JR, Khan SA, Horton J, et al. Society of Surgical Oncology-American Society for Radiation Oncology consensus guideline on margins for breast-conserving surgery with whole-breast irradiation in stages I and II invasive breast cancer. Ann Surg Oncol. 2014;21(3):704–16.
13. Morrow M, Van Zee KJ, Solin LJ, Houssami N, Chavez-MacGregor M, Harris JR, et al. Society of Surgical Oncology-American Society for Radiation Oncology-American Society of Clinical Oncology consensus guideline on margins for breast-conserving surgery with whole-breast irradiation in ductal carcinoma in situ. Pract Radiat Oncol. 2016;6(5):287–95.
14. Clough KB, Kaufman GJ, Nos C, Buccimazza I, Sarfati IM. Improving breast cancer surgery: a classification and quadrant per quadrant atlas for oncoplastic surgery. Ann Surg Oncol. 2010;17(5):1375–91.
15. Clarke M, Collins R, Darby S, Davies C, Elphinstone P, Evans V, Godwin J, Gray R, Hicks C, James S, et al. Early Breast Cancer Trialists' Collaborative Group (EBCTCG). Effects of radiotherapy and of differences in the extent of surgery for early breast cancer on local recurrence and 15-year survival: an overview of the randomized trials. Lancet. 2005;366 2087–106. [PubMed]
16. Fisher B, Anderson S, Bryant J, Margolese RG, Deutsch M, Fisher ER, Jeong JH, Wolmark N. Twenty-year follow-up of a randomized trial comparing total mastectomy, lumpectomy, and lumpectomy plus irra-

diation for the treatment of invasive breast cancer. N Engl J Med. 2002;347:1233–41. [CrossRef]

17. Early Breast Cancer Trialists' Collaborative Group (EBCTCG), Darby S, McGale P, Correa C, Taylor C, Arriagada R, Clarke M, Cutter D, Davies C, Ewertz M, et al. Effect of radiotherapy after breast-conserving surgery on 10-year recurrence and 15-year breast cancer death: meta-analysis of individual patient data for 10,801 women in 17 randomised trials. Lancet. 2011;378:1707–16.
18. Haviland JS, et al. The UK Standardisation of Breast Radiotherapy (START) trials of radiotherapy hypofractionation for treatment of early breast cancer: 10-year follow-up results of two randomised controlled trials. Lancet Oncol. 2013;14(11):1086–94., www.thelancet.com/journals/lanonc/article/PIIS1470-2045(13)70386-3/fulltext. https://doi.org/10.1016/s1470-2045(13)70386-3.
19. Brunt M, Adrian, et al. Hypofractionated breast radiotherapy for 1 week versus 3 weeks (FAST-forward): 5-year efficacy and late normal tissue effects results from a multicentre, non-inferiority, randomised, phase 3 trial. Lancet. 2020;395(10237):1613–26., www.thelancet.com/journals/lancet/article/PIIS0140-6736(20)30932-6/fulltext. https://doi.org/10.1016/s0140-6736(20)30932-6.
20. Swisher SK, Vila J, Tucker SL, Bedrosian I, Shaitelman SF, Litton JK, Smith BD, Caudle AS, Kuerer HM, Mittendorf EA. Locoregional control according to breast cancer subtype and response to Neoadjuvant chemotherapy in breast cancer patients undergoing breast-conserving therapy. Ann Surg Oncol. 2016;23:749–56. [CrossRef] [PubMed]
21. Nikyar N, Tegnelius E, Valachis A. Adjuvant locoregional radiation therapy in breast cancer patients with pathologic complete response after neoadjuvant chemotherapy: a systematic review and meta-analysis. Clin Transl Radiat Oncol. 2022;33:45–52. [CrossRef]
22. NCCN Clinical practice guidelines in oncology: breast cancer. Version 1. 2024. Available online: https://www.nccn.org/professionals/physician_gls/pdf/breast.pdf. Accessed on 6 February 2024.
23. Kaidar-Person O, Pfob A, Gentilini OD, Borisch B, Bosch A, Cardoso MJ, Curigliano G, De Boniface J, Denkert C, Hauser N, et al. The Lucerne toolbox 2 to optimise axillary management for early breast cancer: a multidisciplinary expert consensus. EClin Med. 2023;61:102085. [CrossRef]
24. Cardoso F, Kyriakides S, Ohno S, Penault-Llorca F, Poortmans P, Rubio IT, et al. Early breast cancer: ESMO clinical practice guidelines for diagnosis, treatment and follow-up†. Ann Oncol. 2019;30(8):1194–220.
25. van Paridon MW, Kamali P, Paul MA, Wu W, Ibrahim AMS, Kansal KJ, et al. Oncoplastic breast surgery: achieving oncological and aesthetic outcomes. J Surg Oncol. 2017;116(2):195–202.
26. Fisher B, Anderson S, Bryant J, Margolese RG, Deutsch M, Fisher ER, et al. Twenty-year follow-up of a randomized trial comparing total mastectomy, lumpectomy, and lumpectomy plus irradiation for the treatment of invasive breast cancer. N Engl J Med. 2002;347(16):1233–41.
27. Twenty-year follow-up of a randomized study comparing breast-conserving surgery with radical mastectomy for early breast cancer | NEJM [Internet]. [cited 2023 Nov 8]. Available from: https://www.nejm.org/doi/full/10.1056/nejmoa020989.
28. Chatterjee A, Gass J, Patel K, Holmes D, Kopkash K, Peiris L, et al. A consensus definition and classification system of oncoplastic surgery developed by the American Society of Breast Surgeons. Ann Surg Oncol. 2019;26(11):3436–44.
29. Macmillan RD, McCulley SJ. Oncoplastic breast surgery: what, when and for whom? Curr Breast Cancer Rep. 2016;8:112–7.
30. Nold RJ, Beamer RL, Helmer SD, McBoyle MF. Factors influencing a woman's choice to undergo breast-conserving surgery versus modified radical mastectomy. Am J Surg. 2000;180(6):413–8.
31. Albornoz CR, Matros E, Lee CN, Hudis CA, Pusic AL, Elkin E, et al. Bilateral mastectomy versus breast-conserving surgery for early stage breast cancer: the role of breast reconstruction. Plast Reconstr Surg. 2015;135(6):1518.
32. Somashekhar SP, Agarwal G, Deo SVS, Chintamani, Raghu Ram P, Sarkar D, et al. Indian solutions for Indian problems—Association of Breast Surgeons of India (ABSI) practical consensus statement, recommendations, and guidelines for the treatment of breast cancer in India. Indian J Surg. 2017;79(4):275–85.
33. Rubens RD, Sexton S, Tong D, Winter PJ, Knight RK, Hayward JL. Combined chemotherapy and radiotherapy for locally advanced breast cancer. Eur J Cancer. 1980;16(3):351–6.
34. Mougalian SS, Soulos PR, Killelea BK, Lannin DR, Abu-Khalaf MM, DiGiovanna MP, et al. Use of neoadjuvant chemotherapy for patients with stage I to III breast cancer in the United States. Cancer. 2015;121(15):2544–52.
35. Clough KB, Acosta-Marín V, Nos C, Alran S, Rouanet P, Garbay JR, et al. Rates of Neoadjuvant chemotherapy and oncoplastic surgery for breast cancer surgery: a French National Survey. Ann Surg Oncol. 2015;22(11):3504–11.
36. Vugts G, Maaskant-Braat AJG, Nieuwenhuijzen GAP, Roumen RMH, Luiten EJT, Voogd AC. Patterns of Care in the Administration of neo-adjuvant chemotherapy for breast cancer. A population-based study. Breast J. 2016;22(3):316–21.
37. Asselain B, Barlow W, Bartlett J, Bergh J, Bergsten-Nordström E, Bliss J, et al. Long-term outcomes for neoadjuvant versus adjuvant chemotherapy in early breast cancer: meta-analysis of individual patient data from ten randomised trials. Lancet Oncol. 2018;19(1):27–39.
38. Wolmark N, Wang J, Mamounas E, Bryant J, Fisher B. Preoperative chemotherapy in patients with operable breast cancer: nine-year results from National Surgical Adjuvant Breast and Bowel Project B-18. JNCI Monogr. 2001;2001(30):96–102.

39. Dhamija E, Singh R, Mishra S, Hari S. Image-guided breast interventions: biopsy and beyond. Indian J Radiol Imaging. 2021;31(02):391–9.
40. Denison CM, Lester SC. Essential components of a successful breast core needle biopsy program: imaging modalities, sampling techniques, specimen processing, radiologic/pathologic correlation, and appropriate follow-up. In: Shin SJ, Chen YY, Ginter PS, editors. A comprehensive guide to core needle biopsies of the breast [Internet]. Cham: Springer International Publishing; 2022. [cited 2024 Mar 27]. p. 1–46. https://doi.org/10.1007/978-3-031-05532-4_1.
41. Vicini FA, Cecchini RS, White JR, Arthur DW, Julian TB, Rabinovitch RA, et al. Long-term primary results of accelerated partial breast irradiation after breast-conserving surgery for early-stage breast cancer: a randomised, phase 3, equivalence trial. Lancet. 2019; https://doi.org/10.1016/s0140-6736(19)32514-0.
42. Shah C, et al. The American Brachytherapy Society consensus statement for accelerated partial-breast irradiation. Brachytherapy. 2018;17(1):154-170. 30.
43. Correa C, et al. Accelerated partial breast irradiation: executive summary for the update of an ASTRO evidence-based consensus statement. Pract Radiat Oncol. 2017;7(2):73–9.
44. Hughes KS, et al. Lumpectomy plus tamoxifen with or without irradiation in women age 70 years or older with early breast cancer: long-term follow-up of CALGB 9343. J Clin Oncol. 2013;31(19):2382–7. https://doi.org/10.1200/jco.2012.45.2615. Accessed 6 July 2021
45. Kunkler IH, Williams LJ, Jack WJL, et al. Breast-conserving surgery with or without irradiation in women aged 65 years or older with early breast cancer (PRIME II): a randomised controlled trial Lancet Oncol. 2013;16:266–73.
46. Kirby AM. Updated ASTRO guidelines on accelerated partial breast irradiation (APBI): to whom can we offer APBI outside a clinical trial? Br J Radiol. Published online March 23, 2018:20170565. https://doi.org/10.1259/bjr.20170565.
47. Smith BD, Arthur DW, Buchholz TA, Haffty BG, Hahn CA, Hardenbergh PH, et al. Accelerated partial breast irradiation consensus statement from the American society for radiation oncology (ASTRO). Int J Radiat Oncol Biol Phys. 2009;74:987–1001. https://doi.org/10.1016/j.ijrobp.2009.02.031. [PubMed] [CrossRef] [Google Scholar] [Ref list]
48. Jagsi R, Chadha M, Moni J, Ballman K, Laurie F, Buchholz TA, Giuliano A, Haffty BG. Radiation field design in the ACOSOG Z0011 (Alliance). Trial J Clin Oncol. 2014;32:3600–6. [CrossRef] [PubMed]
49. Giuliano AE, McCall L, Beitsch P, Whitworth PW, Blumencranz P, Leitch AM, Saha S, Hunt KK, Morrow M, Ballman K. Locoregional recurrence after sentinel lymph node dissection with or without axillary dissection in patients with sentinel lymph node metastases: the American College of Surgeons Oncology Group Z0011 randomized trial. Ann Surg. 2010;252:426–33. [CrossRef]
50. Galimberti V, Cole BF, Zurrida S, Viale G, Luini A, Veronesi P, Baratella P, Chifu C, Sargenti M, Intra M, et al. Axillary dissection versus no axillary dissection in patients with sentinel-node micrometastases (IBCSG 23-01): a phase 3 randomised controlled trial. Lancet Oncol. 2013;14:297–305. [CrossRef]
51. Bartels SAL, Donker M, Poncet C, Sauvé N, Straver ME, van de Velde CJH, Mansel RE, Blanken C, Orzalesi L, Klinkenbijl JHG, et al. Radiotherapy or surgery of the axilla after a positive sentinel node in breast cancer: 10-year results of the randomized controlled EORTC 10981-22023 AMAROS trial. J Clin Oncol. 2023;41:2159–65. [CrossRef]
52. Whelan TJ, Olivotto IA, Parulekar WR, Ackerman I, Chua BH, Nabid A, Vallis KA, White JR, Rousseau P, Fortin A, et al. MA.20 Study Investigators. Regional nodal irradiation in early-stage breast cancer. N Engl J Med. 2015;373:307–16. [CrossRef] [PubMed]
53. Standard or comprehensive radiation therapy in treating patients with early-stage breast cancer previously treated with chemotherapy and surgery. https://clinicaltrials.gov/ct2/show/NCT01872975
54. Dhanushkodi M, Sridevi V, Shanta V, Rama R, Swaminathan R, Selvaluxmy G, et al. Locally Advanced Breast Cancer (LABC): real-world outcome of patients from Cancer Institute, Chennai. JCO Glob Oncol. 2021;7:767–81.
55. Chia S, Swain SM, Byrd DR, Mankoff DA. Locally advanced and inflammatory breast cancer. J Clin Oncol. 2008;26(5):786–90.
56. Nielsen HM, Overgaard M, Grau C, Jensen AR, Overgaard J. Study of failure pattern among high-risk breast cancer patients with or without postmastectomy radiotherapy in addition to adjuvant systemic therapy: long-term results from the Danish Breast Cancer Cooperative Group DBCG 82 b and c randomized studies. J Clin Oncol. 2006;24:2268–75. [CrossRef] [PubMed]
57. Taghian AG, Jeong JH, Mamounas EP, Parda DS, Deutsch M, Costantino JP, Wolmark N. Low locoregional recurrence rate among node-negative breast cancer patients with tumors 5 cm or larger treated by mastectomy, with or without adjuvant systemic therapy and without radiotherapy: results from five national surgical adjuvant breast and bowel project randomized clinical trials. J Clin Oncol. 2006;24:3927–32.
58. Floyd SR, Buchholz TA, Haffty BG, Goldberg S, Niemierko A, Raad RA, Oswald MJ, Sullivan T, Strom EA, Powell SN, et al. Low local recurrence rate without postmastectomy radiation in node-negative breast cancer patients with tumors 5 cm and larger. Int J Radiat Oncol Biol Phys. 2006,66:358–64. [CrossRef]
59. Johnson ME, Handorf EA, Martin JM, Hayes SB. Postmastectomy radiation therapy for T3N0: a SEER analysis. Cancer. 2014;120:3569–74. [CrossRef]

60. EBCTCG (Early Breast Cancer Trialists' Collaborative Group), McGale P, Taylor C, Correa C, Cutter D, Duane F, Ewertz M, Gray R, Mannu G, Peto R, et al. Effect of radiotherapy after mastectomy and axillary surgery on 10-year recurrence and. Curr Oncol. 2024;31:1219.
61. 20-year breast cancer mortality: meta-analysis of individual patient data for 8135 women in 22 randomised trials. Lancet. 2014;383:2127–35.
62. Lievens Y, Guckenberger M, Gomez D, Hoyer M, Iyengar P, Kindts I, et al. Defining oligometastatic disease from a radiation oncology perspective: an ESTRO-ASTRO consensus document. Radiother Oncol J Eur Soc Ther Radiol Oncol. 2020;148:157–66.
63. Merloni F, Palleschi M, Casadei C, Romeo A, Curcio A, Casadei R, et al. Oligometastatic breast cancer and metastasis-directed treatment: an aggressive multimodal approach to reach the cure. Ther Adv Med Oncol. 2023;15:17588359231161412.
64. Selvarajan G, Dhanushkodi M, Radhakrishnan V, Kalaivarasi JP, Murali CS, Ananthi B, et al. The continuing conundrum in oligometastatic breast carcinoma: a real-world data. Breast. 2022;63:140–8.
65. Khan SA, Zhao F, Solin LJ, Goldstein LJ, Cella D, Basik M, Golshan M, Julian TB, Pockaj BA, Lee CA, et al. A randomized phase III trial of systemic therapy plus early local therapy versus systemic therapy alone in women with de novo stage IV breast cancer: a trial of the ECOG-ACRIN Research Group (E2108). J Clin Oncol. 2020;38(Suppl. S18):LBA2. [Google Scholar] [CrossRef]
66. Harrow S, Palma DA, Olson R, Gaede S, Louie AV, Haasbeek C, Mulroy L, Lock M, Rodrigues GB, Yaremko BP, et al. Stereotactic radiation for the comprehensive treatment of Oligometastases (SABR-COMET): extended long-term outcomes. Int J Radiat Oncol Biol Phys. 2022;114:611–6. [Google Scholar] [CrossRef]
67. Chmura SJ, Winter KA, Woodward WA, Borges VF, Salama JK, Al-Hallaq HA, Matuszak M, Milano MT, Jaskowiak NT, Bandos H, et al. A phase IIR/III trial of standard of care systemic therapy with or without stereotactic body radiotherapy (SBRT) and/or surgical resection (SR) for newly oligometastatic breast cancer (NCT02364557). J Clin Oncol. 2022;40:1007. [Google Scholar] [CrossRef]
68. Thorat MA, Rangole A, Nadkarni MS, Parmar V, Badwe RA. Revision surgery for breast cancer: single-institution experience. Cancer. 2008;113(8 Suppl):2347.
69. Hansen E, Roach M, III. Handbook of evidence-based radiation oncology. Berlin/Heidelberg: Springer International Publishing; 2018. ISBN 978-3-31-962642-0, 978-3-31-962641-3

Surgical Techniques of Axillary Lymph Node Dissection

17

Rashpal Singh and Sandeep Bhoriwal

Abstract

In breast cancer (BC), axillary staging of nodes has a pivotal role in deciding the management option and aids in prognostication. Before the institution of the concept of sentinel node biopsy, axillary node dissection was standard of care in all BC patients regardless of nodal status. Subsequently, the philosophy behind the treatment has shifted from a radical approach to a conservative and more pragmatic approach. The ACOSOGZ0011 trial that showed the omission of axillary nodal dissection in node negative axillae. Imaging of the axilla for characterisation of suspicious nodes plays an important role in staging axilla. Localisation of axillary nodes before giving neoadjuvant chemotherapy with different available options like clip, coil, radio-isotope seeds, etc. leading to the development of concept of targeted axillary nodal biopsy or dissection. All these nonradical/conservative options revolve around a common goal, that is, to avoid unnecessary and avoidable morbidity associated with axillary nodal dissection.

R. Singh
Department of Surgical Oncology, Indira Gandhi Medical College, Shimla, Himachal Pradesh, India

S. Bhoriwal (✉)
Department of Surgical Oncology, IRCH, AIIMS, New Delhi, India

Keywords

Breast cancer · Axillary lymph node dissection (ALND) · Sentinel node biopsy (SNB) · Targeted axillary node dissection

Abbreviations

ALND	axillary lymph node dissection
SLNB	sentinel lymph node biopsy
TAD	targeted axillary dissection

17.1 Introduction

As per GLOBOCAN 2022, breast cancer is one of the most common cancers globally as well as in India [1]. Axillary node involvement and number and location of nodes are all prognostic markers that further drive the treatment options [2]. Treatment of breast cancer depends on clinical stage of breast tumour, axillary node status and hormonal profile of the patients. Preoperative axillary assessment can be done with imaging modalities like mammogram, ultrasound, computed tomogram (CT) thorax, magnetic resonance imaging (MRI) breast and positron emission tomography (PET-CT).

Surgery for breast cancer has evolved from radical mastectomy to breast conservation. This

E. Dhamija, S. V. S. Deo (eds.), *Imaging in Management of Breast Diseases*,
https://doi.org/10.1007/978-981-96-4998-3_17

all has been possible due to an in-depth and better understanding of disease, tumour biology and advancement in molecular oncology. Surgery is generally divided into two parts, that is, surgery for tumour of breast and surgery for axillary nodes (ALND). The primary tumour may be addressed with breast conservative surgery (BCS) or complete removal of breast (mastectomy). Regarding axillary nodes, treatment is yet to be established due to the heterogeneity of treatment recommendation guidelines. It can be axillary dissection or sentinel node biopsy (SLNB) or radiotherapy depending upon the nodal status of axilla before and after chemotherapy.

Patients who have metastatic or clinically palpable axillary nodes before giving neoadjuvant chemotherapy achieve pathological complete response (pCR) after chemotherapy in 20–45% [3]. In such cases, axillary lymph node dissection (ALND) can be avoided; and other less invasive procedures like SLNB/targeted axillary dissection (TAD) can be considered. Broadly, to stage axilla, treatment options can range from sentinel node biopsy (SLNB) which can be done in patients planned for upfront surgery or after neoadjuvant chemotherapy [4, 5], axillary node dissection [6], or modified radical mastectomy (en bloc mastectomy + axillary node dissection) and targeted axillary node dissection (TAD).

In this chapter, we will discuss the indications, different techniques for staging of axilla and various treatment approaches to address axillary nodes in breast cancer.

17.2 Role of Imaging in Axillary Staging

Mammogram: It is the first investigation done in all breast cancer patients to help in establishing the diagnosis of malignancy. However, to assess axillary nodes, it is not a good imaging tool as it can assess only lateral group of nodes, that is, level 1 group. Level 2 nodes which are medial to pectoralis minor cannot be visualised on mammogram. It can detect microcalcification in axillary nodes which signifies suspicion of malignancy.

Ultrasound: In a newly diagnosed breast cancer, ultrasound axilla is one of the preferred modalities. It can differentiate between benign and suspicious nodes with a sensitivity and specificity of 60–75%. This can be enhanced up to 83–85% by using ultrasound-guided fine needle aspiration cytology (FNAC) of suspicious axillary node [7].

Radiomics: This is an emerging radiological tool that analyses certain radiological features like appearance, consistency, waveform of area of interest, or image in depth and a dataset is then created. As a result of this, status of suspicious axillary nodes can be estimated with an area under curve (AUC) > 0.9 [8].

CECT Thorax: This modality is generally used for locally advanced breast cancer (LABC) and stage III patients. Apart from providing comprehensive details of the local and regional extent of primary breast tumour, it also elucidates about axillary nodes, especially level 2, level 3 and also about internal mammary nodes and distant metastasis. However, its sensitivity and specificity in detecting metastatic axillary nodes are limited.

MRI Breast: This modality is not advised routinely in breast cancer patients. It is offered to young patients with dense breast where a mammogram is not recommended, and also when other imaging modality has equivocal findings. It is nonoperator dependent and provides a good objective overview of axillary nodes.

The treatment options for axillary nodes include the following:

1. Sentinel lymph node biopsy (SLNB)—Identification and removal of the sentinel lymph node, usually using radioactive tracer (Technetium-99) or blue dye
2. Targeted lymph node biopsy (TLNB)—Selective removal of metastatic lymph node(s) marked before neoadjuvant therapy
3. Axillary lymph node dissection (ALND)—Systematic removal of lymph nodes from the

axilla, usually levels I and II, sometimes including also level III
4. Targeted axillary dissection (TAD)—Combination of TLNB and SLNB

17.3 Sentinel Lymph Node Biopsy (SLNB)

Sentinel biopsy was first devised by Morton. The sentinel node is defined as the first node to receive lymphatic drainage from the affected organ. Specific afferent lymphatic channels are going from the primary tumour to these sentinel nodes. This sentinel node has the maximum chance of harbouring metastasis. This understanding of the sentinel node leads to the concept of sentinel node biopsy (SLNB) in different cancers.

The technique of SLNB has changed the historical perspective of treating breast cancer. It is a method to stage the axilla with less morbidity as compared to ALND. It has mitigated the negative aftereffects of ALND. NSABP-32 trial compared ALND vs SLNB and showed that SLNB identifies nodes in up to 95–97% cases with false-negative rate of only 9–10% [9].

Veronesi et al. also compared ALND and SLNB and showed similar results similar to NSABP-32 [10]. Currently, SLNB has dramatically changed the existing clinical practice.

Indications

- Clinically negative axilla (clinically N0)
- Patients who have received chemotherapy and have no nodes in the axilla, after chemotherapy
- DCIS (ductal carcinoma in situ) with high index of suspicion of invasive carcinoma

Contraindications

- Palpable axillary nodes.
- Matted or conglomerated nodal mass.
- All patients with clinical T4b stage.
- Inflammatory breast cancer (T4d).
- In pregnancy, blue dye is not recommended. Radio-labelled Sulfur colloid can be used safely.
- Previous axillary surgery, as the entire lymphatic system is disrupted which may lead to nonidentification of the sentinel node or removal of a non-sentinel node.

Landmark Trials Which Advocate SLNB in Breast Cancer

I. Effect of Axillary Dissection vs No Axillary Dissection on 10-Year Overall Survival Among Women With Invasive Breast Cancer and Sentinel Node Metastasis- The ACOSOG Z0011 (Alliance) Randomised Clinical Trial [11].

Study design: It was a phase 3 randomised controlled trial conducted in 115 centres in which patients were registered from May 1999 to December 2004.

Eligibility criteria: All patients with early breast cancer, that is, T1 and T2 with no clinically palpable axillary nodes and who had 1–2 sentinel nodes with micrometastasis after frozen section, were eligible for the study. After the sentinel node biopsy, patients were randomised into two arms, that is, to undergo axillary dissection and the other arm with no axillary dissection.

Outcome: Estimation of disease-free survival (DFS), overall survival (OS) and locoregional recurrence were the end points of this trial among both these arms.

Results: A total of 891 patients were enrolled; 446 patients were randomised to SNB alone and 445 to SNB plus ALND. Median follow-up was 6.2 years. The ten-year overall survival rate was 83.6% in the patient who underwent axillary dissection and 86.3% in the sentinel node biopsy-alone group. The ten-year disease-free survival (DFS) was 78.2% for the ALND group and 80.2% for the sentinel node dissection (SLND)-alone group.

Conclusions: Axillary dissection can be safely omitted in patients with a limited burden of nodal disease as there was no benefit in survival and without much risk of recurrence.

Limitation of the trial: The trial was closed early due to low accrual of patients and a lower event rate.

II. IBCSG 23-01 randomised controlled trial comparing axillary dissection vs no axillary dissection in patients with sentinel node micrometastases [10].

Study design: It was a two-arm, multicentre, phase 3 randomised controlled trial in which a total of 6681 breast cancer patients were registered from April 2001 to December 2010.

Inclusion criteria: Out of 6681 patients, only 934 patients were found to be eligible. Females of any age with biopsy-proven breast cancer having tumour size up to ≤5 cm and having only micrometastasis (≤2 mm) in sentinel nodes were included. Patients with palpable nodes in axilla, ductal carcinoma in situ (DCIS) and macrometastasis in the nodes were excluded from the study.

Outcome: This trial compared the overall survival (OS), disease-free survival (DFS), axillary recurrence and surgical complications after axillary dissection in patients who were randomised on a 1:1 basis to undergo axillary dissection vs no axillary dissection after the sentinel nodes were sent for frozen section.

Result: This trial showed that there was no difference in the DFS among patients who underwent axillary dissection and no axillary dissection group. Overall survival (OS) was also not different among the groups.

Axillary recurrence was less in the group that did'nt undergo axillary dissection as compared to the group that underwent axillary dissection. This was probably due to the effect of systemic chemotherapy and giving whole breast irradiation to affected breast which can completely remove the disease in less burdened axilla.

Limitation: Ninety percent of the patient had tumour size ≤3 cm and 90-95% patients received systemic chemotherapy, so these results cannot be extrapolated for larger breast tumour size or advanced stage breast cancer patients.

17.3.1 Technique of doing SLNB

SLNB can be performed in two ways—using blue-based dye (isosulfan blue or methylene blue) or dual dye technique involving blue dye with technetium-99 (Tc99) radioisotope. The surgical steps are being discussed in following sections-

(a) *Blue dye technique*: After the patient is intubated, the patient is placed in the supine position; SLNB begins with injection of dye into periareolar skin or peritumoral site (Fig. 17.1). The breast should be massaged for 5–7 minutes to dilate breast lymphatics, followed by small axillary incision to enter axillary fascia. All blue lymph nodes and any lymph nodes at the end of a blue lymphatic channel should be removed. Suspicious palpable nodes should also be removed as lymph nodes studded with tumour cells are likely not to take up the dye due to uptake due to occlusion of afferent lymphatics. At least 2–4 nodes should be removed because fewer the number of nodes harvested, the higher the chances of a false-negative rate.

(b) *Radioisotope-based SLNB*: It involves intradermal or subcutaneous periareolar injection of 0.5 mCi (millicurie) radioisotope technetium-99 (Tc^{99}) on the day of surgery or 2.5 mCi (millicurie) a day before surgery. Axilla is assessed using handheld gamma probe to detect the radioactivity value of axillary nodes which is displayed on the monitor as a numerical value (Fig. 17.2). There will be variable radioactivity values for individual axillary nodes.

As minimum nodes required in SLNB are 2–4 in number, hence in order to maintain the sensitivity of the SLNB procedure and minimise the false-negative rates (FNR) and morbidity

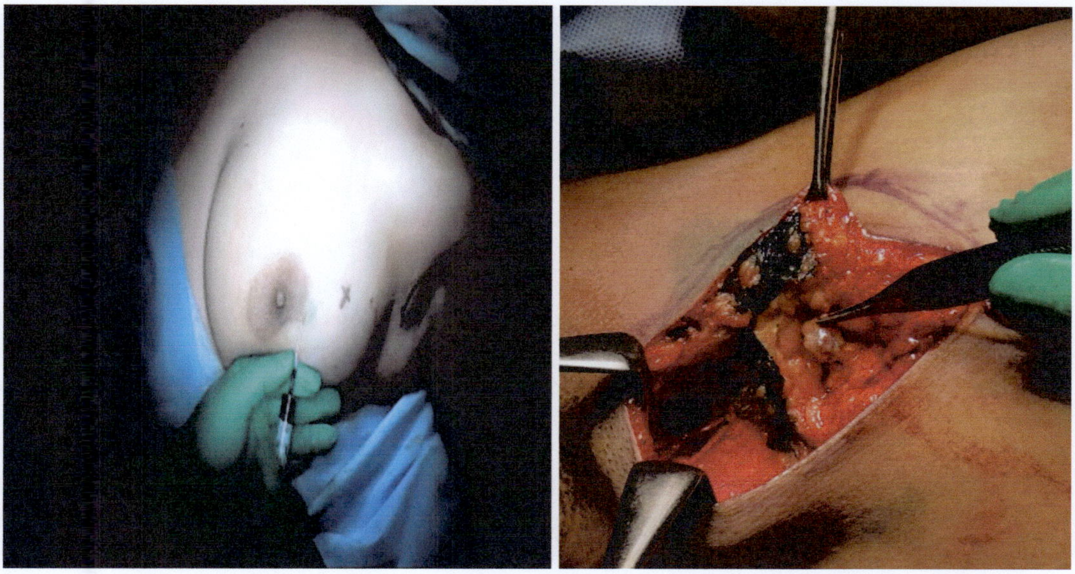

Fig. 17.1 SLNB with blue dye. The dye has been injected in periareolar location (left) and subsequent incision reveals uptake of the dye in axillary nodes (right)

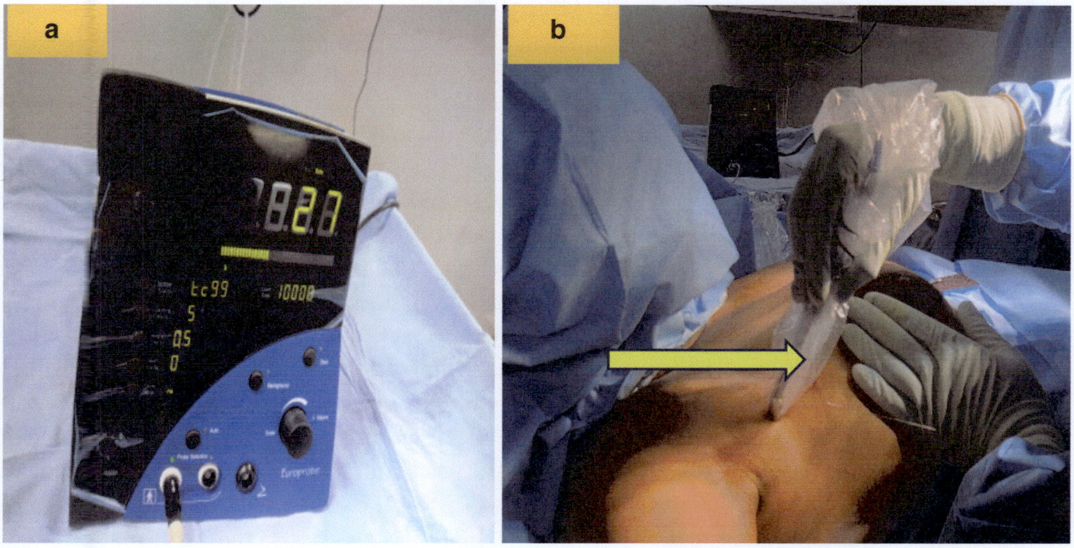

Fig. 17.2 (**a** and **b**) SLNB using radioisotope. The hand-held gamma probe is used to detect the radioactivity as shown in (**b**) with yellow arrow on the right side. The numerical reading on monitor showing "27" in (**a**) on left indicates radioactivity value of the axillary node

associated with the procedure at the same time. In order to circumvent this, we have to remove only the lymph node with maximum radioactivity which is called "hot node". This value is called "exvivo radioactivity count".

Based on this radioactivity count value, subsequent nodes will only be removed, if they carry the radioactivity value which should be at least more than or equal to 10% of the index node radioactivity value.

This is called "10 percent rule", that is, all nodes with radioactivity count >10% of ex-vivo count of the first "hot" radioactive node removed at the beginning of the procedure.

Generally, this technique is combined with the blue dye technique and called "10% + blue dye" technique in order to increase the diagnostic accuracy and sensitivity of the technique [5].

The diagnostic accuracy of up to 78.6% has been documented with the single dye technique using only blue dye and up to 90% with radioisotope dye, but the combination of both improves the accuracy to 93–94% with minimum false-negative rates (FNR) [3, 12].

All the nodes removed should be blue and hot (radioactive), and there should be no fatty tissue around the nodes, while sending them for pathological evaluation and these nodes should be sectioned into thin slices of 2–3 mm thickness for detailed assessment.

Recent advances in SLNB technique are the following:

(a) *Indocyanine green (ICG)-based SLNB*: This technique has shown promising result when combined with blue dye. The detection rate of sentinel nodes after combining with blue dye reaches to 92–93% which is comparable with radioisotope and blue dye for SLNB [13].

It can be used in settings where facilities or armamentarium of radioisotope provision or a nuclear medicine department are not available. It is cheaper and easily available and provides a real-time visualisation. It can be injected directly into the periareolar/peritumoural region and localised using a fluorescent imaging system. In this procedure, nodes which are blue and glowing on fluorescent imaging are removed and sent for frozen section. The number of nodes required is the same, that is, 2–4 as for other SLNB techniques.

17.4 Targeted Axillary Node Dissection (TAD)

As both ALND and SLNB are not completely devoid of complications due to their invasive nature and other associated side effects, SLNB is no doubt better than ALND in terms of less invasiveness and with less side effects. Even in highly experienced centres, SLNB carries a false-negative rate (FNR) of 7–10%. This was shown by meta-analysis in which 69 studies were included highlighting the FNR associated with SLNB [14].

Patients who had enlarged/metastatic nodes in the axilla at baseline may undergo neoadjuvant chemotherapy that sometimes results in complete clinical response in 40–75% of patients [3]. In such patients, there is no strong recommendation or guidelines issued by international societies regarding the accurate and best method of how to do axillary staging. The options being explored include surgery (ALND), focused or targeted axillary dissection (TAD), or SLNB and irradiation. In these cases, TAD definitely keeps a very good role in terms of less morbid, less invasive in nature and carrying the least false-negative rates (FNR) [15].

In India, too, there are no robust guidelines for such patients who receive neoadjuvant chemotherapy for clinically positive nodes in the axilla with subsequent complete response [16].

In TAD, we label the metastatic node under ultrasound guidance before chemotherapy or 1–5 days before surgery either by using radioactive material (iodine-125, technetium-99), magnetic seeds (Magseed), carbon tattooing, metallic clip, or coil, so that it will be easy to locate and facilitate the identification of targeted nodes during axillary dissection. After TAD, the false-negative rate (FNR) drops to 2–4.2% [15], as compared to FNR associated with other methods of SLNB methods in post-NACT axillary staging settings.

In the Netherlands, the same procedure is called the MARI (marking the axillary lymph node with radioactive seed) procedure where they place iodine seeds in suspicious nodes at the time of performing biopsy from these nodes [17].

For radioactive seed, gamma probe and for magseeds, the dedicated probe localises the nodes during surgery. For clip placement, wire-guided localisation is done before surgery and may require intraoperative ultrasound to identify the targeted node. This modality has maximum literature available and most widely used worldwide.

Limitations of TAD

- Requires close communication with the radiologist for wire localisation and seed placement.
- As TAD is a new method, it is not yet clear how many nodes are to be marked, which node is to be marked and how many nodes are to be removed during TAD.
- TAD is not cost-effective if magseeds are used for the localisation of nodes.

17.5 Axillary Lymph Node Dissection (ALND)

There are three levels of axillary nodes defined with respect to pectoralis minor muscle [18]:

Level 1: Lateral to pectoralis minor
Level 2: Posterior to pectoralis minor
Level 3: Medial to pectoralis minor

Definition of ALND: It is a surgical procedure in which en bloc removal of lymph nodes at levels 1 and 2 along with fibrofatty tissue lying inferior to the axillary vein, laterally up to latissimus dorsi muscle and medially up to the pectoralis minor muscle after safeguarding the axillary vein, nerve to serratus anterior and latissimus dorsi pedicle.

Pectoral nerves and intercostobrachial nerves can be spared or sacrificed depending upon the discretion of surgeon.

Currently, as per NCCN (National Comprehensive Cancer Network) guidelines, level 2 axillary nodal dissection is recommended for all breast cancer patients [19].

Level 3 axillary dissection are only recommended for higher T stage (T4), matted axillary nodes/extracapsular nodal spread, invasive lobular carcinoma type, or palpable nodes at level 3.

Removal of level 3 nodes does not improve overall survival (OS) and disease-free survival (DFS) as it is not an independent prognostic marker [20]. Moreover, it is associated with more morbidity in terms of seroma formation and increased paraesthesia compared to level 2 axillary dissection [21].

Hence it is imperative to consider the risk factors and predictive factors responsible for level 3 nodes involvement preoperatively to decide the axillary node level dissection during surgery.

Indications

1. More than two nodes were found positive after SLNB.
2. Suboptimally or inadequately treated axilla (less number of nodes harvested in previous surgery). Normally ten or more nodes are required for adequate staging of axilla after surgery for breast cancer patients; if less than this number is harvested, it is defined as suboptimally or inadequately treated axilla and patient will require further systemic chemotherapy/radiotherapy.
3. Axillary node metastasis without any detectable primary lesion in the breast.
4. Palpable nodes in axilla which are proven by fine needle aspiration (FNA) in patients who are planned for upfront surgery.
5. In all locally advanced breast cancer (LABC).

Technique

Position: Supine with arm flexed at 90 degrees and rotated outward to the body.

Anaesthesia—General anaesthesia.

Procedure: Axillary dissection in all breast cancer patients should follow the standard template boundaries which are mentioned as follows:

Superiorly: Till anterior and inferior surface of the axillary vein

Medially: Nerve to serratus anterior muscle

Laterally: Lateral border of latissimus dorsi muscle

Inferiorly: Angular vein

Posteriorly: Subscapularis muscle

Incision: Curvilinear/lazy "S" incision parallel to anterior axillary fold juxtaposition to axillary hairline for a length of 5–7 cm

Standard template of axillary dissection is followed, and removal of all nodes and fibrofatty tissue at level 2 is removed after safeguarding axillary vein, nerve to serratus anterior and thoracodorsal pedicle.

Pectoralis minor can be divided or split to gain access to the apex of the axilla.

Intercostobrachial sensory nerves, generally 2 in number, can be sacrificed to facilitate axillary dissection without many postoperative sequelae.

Complications of ALND

1. Seroma formation—it is one of the most common complications after ALND with an incidence rate of 20–30%. It happens as a result of the complex interplay between proinflammatory cytokines and antiinflammatory cytokines [22]. However its rate has been decreased after breast conservative surgery as compared to modified radical mastectomy. Rate of seroma formation also depends upon patient body habitus, axillary nodal burden of disease, type of energy source used during surgery and whether chemotherapy was received or not received before surgery [23].

   To mitigate the seroma formation, there are a few precautions which the surgeon should keep in mind while performing the surgery:
   (a) Obliteration of all dead spaces and ensuring complete haemostasis
   (b) Judicious use and appropriate selection of energy sources
   (c) Minimum usage or early removal of drains
   (d) Maintaining less negative suction pressure in drains kept in axilla
   (e) Gentle delayed shoulder exercises
   (f) Use of compression dressings to axilla
   (g) Use of subcutaneous/intravenous injection of octreotide during/after surgery
2. Wound infection: it can be decreased by maintaining the proper sterilisation during surgery, administration of intravenous antibiotics at the time of induction of anaesthesia and preventing the seroma formation and proper dressing after surgery.
3. Drain-associated discomfort.
4. Numbness and paraesthesia along the medial aspect of the operated arm.
5. Limited mobility of shoulder and arm.
6. Impaired quality of life and increased time duration to resume normal routine activities
7. Arm lymphedema: When the operated side arm is swollen and has a circumference difference of ≥2 cm as compared to contralateral arm after surgery [24].

   It is more common in patient who underwent ALND as compared to SLNB. The incidence of lymphedema is 20–25% in patient who underwent ALND and less than 10 % in SLNB patients [25].

   Other factors which are responsible are patients who are obese and having bulky nodes in axilla, who underwent extensive lymphadenectomy and who had received adjuvant radiotherapy.

Lymphedema preventive strategies during surgery:

(a) Avoiding overtreating of axilla by doing SLNB
(b) Preservation of lymphatic channel in axilla going to arm by doing axillary reverse mapping (ARM)
(c) Performing microsurgical venous-lymphatic anastomosis during surgery in high-risk patients
(d) Avoiding intravenous (i.v.) cannulation of the same arm

Treatment of Lymphedema

(a) Compression-layered bandage of the affected arm
(b) Manual decongestive therapy (MDT)
(c) Pneumatic compression stockings
(d) Arm exercises
(e) Surgical by either reducing or removing lymphedema tissue or by reconstructing lymphatics channel with a vein

17.6 Conclusion

Axillary nodal dissection (ALND) is a valid option for node-positive axilla. Sentinel node biopsy (SLNB) should be considered for all patients with negative axilla or having less nodal burden disease. Clipping of axillary nodes should be considered for patients who are planned for neoadjuvant chemotherapy in order to consider targeted axillary nodal dissection. Indocyanine green (ICG) and magseeds are emerging options with promising results in the management of axilla.

References

1. Bray F, Laversanne M, Sung H, Ferlay J, Siegel RL, Soerjomataram I, Jemal A. Global cancer statistics 2022: GLOBOCAN estimates of incidence and mortality worldwide for 36 cancers in 185 countries. CA Cancer J Clin. 2024; https://doi.org/10.3322/caac.21834.
2. Soerjomataram I, Louwman MW, Ribot JG, Roukema JA, Coebergh JW. An overview of prognostic factors for long-term survivors of breast cancer. Breast Cancer Res Treat. 2008;107(3):309–30.
3. Boughey JC, Suman VJ, Mittendorf EA, et al. Alliance for Clinical Trials in Oncology: Sentinel lymph node surgery after neoadjuvant chemotherapy in patients with node-positive breast cancer: the ACOSOG Z1071 (Alliance) clinical trial. JAMA. 2013;310:1455–61.
4. Maguire A, Brogi E. Sentinel lymph nodes for breast carcinoma: an update on current practice. Histopathology. 2016;68(1):152–67. https://doi.org/10.1111/his.12853.
5. Kuehn T, Bauerfeind I, Fehm T, Fleige B, Hausschild M, Helms G, Lebeau A, Liedtke C, von Minckwitz G, Nekljudova V, et al. Sentinel-lymph-node biopsy in patients with breast cancer before and after neoadjuvant chemotherapy (SENTINA): a prospective, multicentre cohort study. Lancet Oncol. 2013;14:609–18.
6. Beck AC, Morrow M. Axillary lymph node dissection: dead or still alive? https://doi.org/10.1016/j.breast.2023.01.009
7. Singh R, Deo SVS, Dhamija E, Mathur S, Thulkar S. To evaluate the accuracy of axillary staging using ultrasound and ultrasound-guided fine-needle aspiration cytology (USG-FNAC) in early breast cancer patients – a prospective study. Indian J Surg Oncol. 2020;11(4):726–34. https://doi.org/10.1007/s13193-020-01222-3.
8. Gong X, Guo Y, Zhu T, Peng X, Xing D, Zhang M. Diagnostic performance of radiomics in predicting axillary lymph node metastasis in breast cancer: A systematic review and meta-analysis. Front Oncol. 2022;28(12):1046005. https://doi.org/10.3389/fonc.2022.1046005.
9. Krag DN, Anderson SJ, Julian TB, Brown AM, Harlow SP, Costantino JP, Ashikaga T, Weaver DL, Mamounas EP, Jalovec LM, Frazier TG, Noyes RD, Robidoux A, Scarth HM, Wolmark N. Sentinel-lymph-node resection compared with conventional axillary-lymph-node dissection in clinically node-negative patients with breast cancer: overall survival findings from the NSABP B-32 randomised phase 3 trial. Lancet Oncol. 2010;11(10):927–33. https://doi.org/10.1016/S1470-2045(10)70207-2.
10. Veronesi U, Paganelli G, Viale G, Luini A, Zurrida S, Galimberti V, Intra M, Veronesi P, Robertson C, Maisonneuve P, Renne G, De Cicco C, De Lucia F, Gennari R. A randomized comparison of sentinel-node biopsy with routine axillary dissection in breast cancer. N Engl J Med. 2003;349(6):546–53. https://doi.org/10.1056/NEJMoa012782.
11. Giuliano AE, Ballman KV, McCall L, et al. Effect of axillary dissection vs no axillary dissection on 10-year overall survival among women with invasive breast cancer and sentinel node metastasis: the ACOSOG Z0011 (Alliance) randomized clinical trial. JAMA. 2017;318(10):918–26. https://doi.org/10.1001/jama.2017.11470.
12. Kim T, Giuliano AE, Lyman GH. Lymphatic mapping and sentinel lymph node biopsy in early-stage breast carcinoma: a meta-analysis. Cancer. 2006;106:4–16.
13. Mandal P, Mishra A, Deo SVS, et al. A pilot study evaluating sentinel lymph node biopsy using dual dye technique with ICG and methylene blue for early breast carcinoma (EBC). Indian J Surg. 2022;84(Suppl3):771–8. https://doi.org/10.1007/s12262-021-03124-2.
14. Chehade HEH, Headon H, El Tokhy O, Heeney J, Kasem A, Mokbel K. Is sentinel lymph node biopsy a viable alternative to complete axillary dissection following neoadjuvant chemotherapy in women with node-positive breast cancer at diagnosis? An updated meta-analysis, involving 3398 patients. Am J Surg. 2016;212:969–81.
15. Caudle AS, Yang WT, Krishnamurthy S, Mittendorf EA, Black DM, Gilcrease MZ, Bedrosian I, Hobbs BP, DeSnyder SM, Hwang RF, Adrada BE, Shaitelman SF, Chavez-MacGregor M, Smith BD, Candelaria RP, Babiera GV, Dogan BE, Santiago L, Hunt KK, Kuerer HM. Improved axillary evaluation following neoadjuvant therapy for patients with node-positive breast cancer using selective evaluation of clipped nodes: implementation of targeted axillary dissection. J Clin Oncol. 2016;34(10):1072–8. https://doi.org/10.1200/JCO.2015.64.0094.
16. Indian Council of Medical Research Consensus Document for Management of Breast Cancer; Department of Health Research MoHFW: New Delhi, India, 2016.
17. Donker M, Straver ME, Wesseling J, Loo CE, Schot M, Drukker CA, van Tinteren H, Sonke GS, Rutgers EJ, Vrancken Peeters MJ. Marking axillary lymph nodes with radioactive iodine seeds for axillary staging after neoadjuvant systemic treatment in breast cancer patients: the MARI procedure. Ann Surg. 2015;261(2):378–82. https://doi.org/10.1097/SLA.0000000000000558.
18. Cirocchi R, Amabile MI, De Luca A, et al. New classifications of axillary lymph nodes and their anatomical-clinical correlations in breast sur-

gery. World J Surg Onc. 2021;19:93. https://doi.org/10.1186/s12957-021-02209-2.
19. Gradishar WJ, Anderson BO, Balassanian R, et al. NCCN guidelines insights: breast cancer, version 1.2017. J Natl Compr Canc Netw. 2017;15(4):433–51. https://doi.org/10.6004/jnccn.2017.0044.
20. Hu J, Xia X, Yang H, Yu Y. Dissection of level III axillary lymph nodes in breast cancer. Cancer Manag Res. 2021;26(13):2041–6. https://doi.org/10.2147/CMAR.S290345.
21. Gonzalez EA, Saltzstein EC, Riedner CS, Nelson BK. Seroma formation following breast cancer surgery. Breast J. 2003;9(5):385–8.
22. Mettler L, Salmassi A, Heyer M, Schmutzier A, Schollmeyer T, Jonat W. Perioperative levels of interleukin-1beta and interleukin-6 in women with breast cancer. Clin Exp Obstet Gynecol. 2004;31(1):20–2.
23. Spiekerman van Weezelenburg MA, Bakens MJAM, Daemen JHT, et al. Prevention of seroma formation and its sequelae after axillary lymph node dissection: an up-to-date systematic review and guideline for surgeons. Ann Surg Oncol. 2024;31:1643–52. https://doi.org/10.1245/s10434-023-14631-9.
24. Ancukiewicz M, Miller CL, Skolny MN, et al. Comparison of relative versus absolute arm size change as criteria for quantifying breast cancer-related lymphedema: the flaws in current studies and need for universal methodology. Breast Cancer Res Treat. 2012;135:145–52.
25. Miller CL, Specht MC, Skolny MN, et al. Risk of lymphedema after mastectomy: potential benefit of applying ACOSOG Z0011 protocol to mastectomy patients. Breast Cancer Res Treat. 2014;144:71–7.

Data Science and Precision Medicine in Oncology

18

Himanshu Singh, S Senthil Kumaran, and Ekta Dhamija

Abstract

The collection of data during breast cancer screening holds significant potential for improving patient outcomes in the realm of data science. As the field of data science continues to evolve, the integration of technology with medicine offers a promising avenue for the development of personalized or precision medicine. By utilizing a multiomic approach, which incorporates multiple datasets, outcomes can be achieved that surpass those of single data analyses. Data mining and machine learning techniques are already being employed in the medical field and are being tested for integration into precision medicine. However, it is crucial to understand the associated challenges and risks in the long term. Protecting the privacy of patients is of utmost importance, as the data collected is closely tied to individual patients. Therefore, it is essential to maintain ethical boundaries in clinical and intellectual pursuits. Furthermore, the successful integration of technology into precision medicine requires standardization and interdisciplinary collaboration across all fields.

In this chapter, we will investigate the utilization of artificial intelligence (AI) in the field of oncology, focusing specifically on its role in cancer prognosis, prediction, and treatment selection. We will examine the ways in which AI and machine learning (ML) are employed to enhance healthcare outcomes and accuracy. Furthermore, the chapter will discuss the potential applications of AI and ML algorithms in cancer prediction, emphasizing their potential to revolutionize cancer research, diagnosis, and rehabilitation.

Keywords

Artificial intelligence · Machine learning · Precision medicine · Breast cancer

18.1 Introduction

Artificial intelligence (AI) refers to the computer science field that focuses on the development of intelligent agents and systems that can mimic human reasoning and memory capabilities autonomously. This includes the creation of algorithms for machine learning which involves learning from data and deep learning which involves learning from patterns. AI is an emerging discipline that often intersects with interdisciplinary fields such as data science. Data science (DS) utilizes scientific methods, processes, algorithms,

H. Singh · S. S. Kumaran (✉)
Department of Nuclear Magnetic Resonance (NMR), AIIMS, New Delhi, India

E. Dhamija
Department of Diagnostic and Interventional Onco-Radiology, IRCH, AIIMS, New Delhi, India

E. Dhamija, S. V. S. Deo (eds.), *Imaging in Management of Breast Diseases*,
https://doi.org/10.1007/978-981-96-4998-3_18

and systems to extract knowledge and insights from various forms of data. It involves a systematic examination of data to uncover patterns and relationships that can affect decision-making and problem-solving [1, 2].

AI and DS are distinct fields which are intricately connected. The integration of AI algorithms and tools within DS has led to the development of predictive and prescriptive insights. Additionally, the use of AI in analytics enhances the efficiency and effectiveness of data interpretation, which is crucial in the pharmaceutical and medical industries [1, 2]. Machine learning, a subset of AI, involves the use of algorithms and statistical models to perform tasks without explicit instructions based on informed decision presets. It is a form of data analysis that is automated and capable of adapting to new information and learning from experience [3]. Machine learning (ML) is an established concept that has practical applications in various fields, including finance, education, and network management. In the financial sector, machine learning is used to improve client experiences. In the field of education, machine learning supports both teaching and learning processes. Additionally, the integration of machine learning with software-defined networking is transforming the way network management is conducted [4, 5].

Deep learning is a subdivision of machine learning that employs algorithms that mimic the architecture of neuron clusters to extract features from data. This method can often be used for unsupervised learning and has the ability to learn directly from raw data, allowing it to uncover intricate patterns and representations. As a result, it has led to significant improvements in tasks such as image recognition. In contrast to traditional machine learning models, which require an understanding of the data and structure, deep learning models have a pattern learning-based approach that allows them to autonomously discover complex patterns within large datasets [6]. This distinction is particularly evident in the field of assistive technologies, where deep learning is outperforming conventional machine learning models in applications that involve human and medical connections [7]. The utilization of artificial intelligence and machine learning in cancer research has proven to be a valuable tool in recent years. These techniques have been applied in various areas of oncology, including imaging, drug discovery, predictive markers, and omics studies. AI and ML have demonstrated the potential to enhance existing methods for efficient detection and to predict patient outcomes and personalize treatment strategies. Various algorithms, such as convolutional neural networks (CNNs), support vector machines (SVMs), transfer learning, and deep learning methods, have shown promise in this field [8–11].

AI is a transformative force in oncology, offering advancements in personalized cancer care and drug discovery. While the potential is vast, the field must navigate challenges related to data management, computational resources, and the need for personalized biomarkers. AI's significance in breast cancer is extensive, encompassing various aspects such as early detection, diagnosis, prognosis, and personalized treatment. Breast cancer poses a significant threat to public health, as it is the most prevalent cancer among women and a leading cause of cancer-related fatalities [12]. Numerous research studies have pinpointed a range of risk factors, including hereditary tendencies, lifestyle choices, and reproductive history. Modifiable risk factors such as body mass index (BMI) and breast density have been demonstrated to significantly impact breast cancer incidence, suggesting potential areas for intervention and prevention [13, 14]. The field of precision medicine has witnessed substantial advancements in recent years, particularly in the context of cancer care. Accurately diagnosing breast abnormalities remains a significant challenge [15]. To address this issue, various tools such as mammography and ultrasound have been developed to screen for breast cancer. However, accurately categorizing patient into high risk presents a considerable challenge. Integrating advanced AI techniques, such as machine learning and deep learning, with traditional histopathology and biomarkers, can yield more precise and personalized insights (Fig. 18.1). Successfully integrating AI into clin-

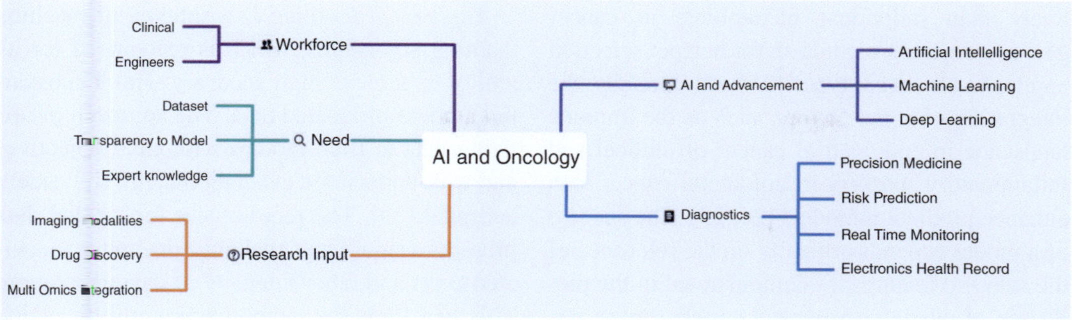

Fig. 18.1 Comprehensive view of AI and oncology

ical practice requires close collaboration between physicians, technologists, and engineers to optimize patient outcomes [12, 16].

ML tools can be utilized to develop predictive algorithms for treatment planning and risk of recurrence, ultimately fostering personalized therapy decisions. However, it is crucial to recognize that although AI offers powerful automation and analysis tools, it lacks the nuanced understanding, clinical context, and ethical considerations inherent to human pathologists in patient care. This chapter aims to illustrate these concerns too.

18.2 Machine Learning and Medicine

Machine learning (ML) is a subfield of artificial intelligence (AI) in which computers are designed to learn from data and enhance their performance iteratively. This learning process is achieved by exposing the system to training data and allowing it to adjust and improve its algorithms autonomously, without the need for explicit programming for each new task or piece of information [17, 18]. Notably, while ML is a subset of AI, it lays the foundation for more complex systems, specifically deep learning (DL), which utilizes neural network-based architecture for data processing in layers, thereby enabling the handling of highly complex tasks. Deep learning is capable of automatic feature extraction. DL models, such as convolutional neural networks (CNNs) and recurrent neural networks (RNNs), have been applied across various domains, including bioinformatics, optical communications, and medical image analysis [19–21]. It is noteworthy that DL models generally surpass traditional ML methods in tasks involving intricate data, but hybrid approaches that combine DL for feature extraction and traditional ML algorithms for classification have shown to be more effective in specific contexts. These hybrid models are referred to as hybrid DL-ML models. These findings imply that the integration of DL and ML can leverage the strengths of both approaches [22]. The development of hybrid DL-ML models presents an intriguing avenue for research, as they have demonstrated enhanced performance in certain applications, potentially offering a balance between the high capability of DL and the efficiency of traditional ML methods.

In the realm of oncology, the choice of model and anticipated outcome depends on the valuable information that can be obtained from the predictions. It is widely recognized that medicine is a multifaceted discipline. ML models are employed for predicting cancer-related outcomes, pathologic risk factors in cervical cancer, breast cancer recurrence, and survivability in gastric cancer [23, 24]. The selection of a model typically involves evaluating various algorithms based on their mathematical model and predictive accuracy, sensitivity, specificity, and other performance metrics such as the area under the receiver operating characteristic curve (AUC) [24]. However, it is crucial to consider contradictions and intriguing facts. For example, while machine learning models can predict hotspots more effectively than individual breakpoints in cancer genomes, no single criterion for hotspot selection applies to all cancer types [25]. Additionally, the integration of novel factors, such as the immune landscape in endometrial cancer or clinical and inflammatory markers in colorectal cancer, can enhance prediction models [26, 27]. The success of a model depends critically on the relevance of the selected features, as demonstrated in the prediction of ovarian cancer and gastric cancer survivability [24, 28]. Since it is a computer-derived model, it is essential to consider a range of performance metrics and tailor the model selection to the characteristics of the cancer being studied. The ultimate objective of any model-based outcome is to improve clinical decision-making and personalize treatment strategies, which may involve combining machine learning predictions with expert clinical judgment.

In the field of breast cancer research, data computation plays a crucial role, encompassing various methodologies and objectives. The application of systems biology approaches entails the utilization of computational models for predicting drug responses, underscoring the importance of extensive datasets. Furthermore, the identification of molecular and genetic markers, which are essential for the diagnosis and treatment of breast cancer, is facilitated through in silico analysis studies. However, it is vital to conduct comprehensive statistical evaluations to ensure the reliability of the findings.

18.2.1 Machine Learning Systems

Machine learning systems are classified according to their learning methodologies and the nature of the data they process. The main learning paradigms comprise supervised learning, where algorithms learn from data that has been labeled; unsupervised learning, which deals with data that is unlabeled; semisupervised learning, which utilizes both labeled and unlabeled data; and reinforcement learning, where algorithms learn to make decisions by receiving either rewards or penalties.

Supervised learning is a subtype of machine learning algorithms, which is recognized for its ability to achieve high accuracy with a substantial amount of labeled data. The approach of utilizing data to train models with clear objectives and well-understood evaluation metrics is widely accepted [29]. The requirement for labeled data presents a significant challenge due to the associated costs and labor intensity of data annotation. This can limit the generalization ability of the models and make them susceptible to biases [30–32]. Despite these limitations, various studies have proposed methods to mitigate them. For instance, *semisupervised learning* techniques that combine a small amount of labeled data with a larger pool of unlabeled data have been shown to improve classification accuracy and generalization ability [33]. Additionally, methods such as Random Erasing in data augmentation, similarity learning with Siamese networks, and self-supervised pretraining have been developed to enhance performance in scenarios with limited labeled data. Moreover, the incorporation of fairness constraints in semisupervised learning frameworks has been suggested to address the issue of bias, aiming for a better tradeoff between accuracy and fairness. While supervised learning is highly effective when ample labeled data is available, its limitations are acknowledged in the literature. The proposed solutions, such as semisupervised learning and innovative training strategies, demonstrate potential for improving model performance and fairness in the face of limited labeled data and potential biases [31–33].

The discussion of learning algorithms continues with the recognition of the potency of unsupervised learning models. These models are highly effective in identifying intricate patterns and connections within data that may be beyond human perception, especially when dealing with copious amounts of unlabeled data [34]. They are capable of autonomously discovering valuable patterns, which become increasingly significant given the prevalence of data that cannot practically be labeled for supervised learning. However, one of the primary challenges associated with unsupervised learning is the difficulty in evaluating the performance of these algorithms. Unlike supervised learning, where performance can be assessed against known outcomes, unsupervised learning lacks a clear benchmark for success due to the absence of labeled data. This issue is further exacerbated in applications such as anomaly detection, where the scarcity of anomalies renders it challenging to gauge the efficacy of the detection methods. This underscores the importance of developing robust evaluation metrics and methodologies to better understand and validate the outcomes of unsupervised learning [34, 35].

Reinforcement learning (RL) is a model that is designed to learn from experience and improve over time, particularly in dynamic environments where it can handle complex tasks [36–38]. However, it is also susceptible to unexpected or undesirable behaviors when faced with conditions that differ significantly from the training data or when the environment changes unpredictably [39]. Various approaches have been developed to enhance the adaptability of RL in such environments. For instance, incremental learning schemes have been proposed to adjust optimal policies automatically as the environment changes [40]. Time Adaptive Markov Decision Processes and associated algorithms have been introduced to adapt RL agents to different time restrictions. Moreover, robust proactive scheduling schemes have been developed to maintain stability in dynamic manufacturing environments [41]. These advancements suggest that while RL can be susceptible to unexpected behaviors, there are ongoing efforts to mitigate these issues.

18.2.2 Machine Learning and Imaging

Machine learning (ML) has established itself as a fundamental component of medical imaging, bolstering diagnostic capabilities and facilitating the development of precision medicine. The ongoing advancement of ML techniques is anticipated to bring about further enhancements in medical diagnostics. However, it is imperative to address the accompanying challenges to fully realize the potential of ML in this domain. ML algorithms, such as convolutional neural networks (CNNs), support vector machines (SVMs), and decision trees, are employed for tasks like image segmentation, classification, and detection across a variety of imaging modalities, including computed tomography (CT), magnetic resonance imaging (MRI), and positron emission tomography (PET) scans [42].

Convolutional neural networks (CNNs), a subtype of deep learning (DL) algorithms, have significantly impacted the field of medical image analysis. These algorithms excel in tasks such as classification, detection, segmentation, and registration of medical images. The adoption of CNNs in medical imaging is attributed to their ability to preserve local image relations and reduce dimensionality, which is crucial for accurate diagnosis and treatment planning [42]. Interestingly, while CNNs are acclaimed for their performance, they also face challenges, particularly in the availability of training datasets. Moreover, CNNs draw inspiration from the neural structure of living organisms, which contributes to their success in object recognition and classification tasks [6, 43].

The application of CNNs extends beyond medical imaging to areas such as language processing and recognition of moving objects, showcasing their versatility. These algorithms have become indispensable tools in medical image analysis, offering a viable alternative to traditional hand-crafted feature extraction methods [44]. Their ability to handle large volumes of data and learn complex patterns makes them highly effective for diagnosing conditions like pneumonia and analyzing brain MRI data [45]. As a result, the use of CNNs in medical imaging is expected to continue to grow in the coming years, with the potential to revolutionize the field of radiology and improve patient outcomes.

18.2.3 Machine Learning and Diagnostics

Medical diagnostics have been enhanced by the exploration of various machine learning techniques, such as convolutional neural networks

(CNNs), decision trees, and support vector machines (SVMs). These algorithms analyze medical data to identify patterns that may not be evident to human clinicians, thereby improving diagnostic processes [46, 47]. SVM. s are optimized for their high generalization ability in pattern recognition, while decision trees offer a more interpretable model structure, and random forests provide robustness against overfitting due to their ensemble nature [48, 49]. However, challenges are associated with these methods. For instance, conventional SVMs may struggle with multiclass problems, leading to unclassifiable regions in the feature space, necessitating the development of decision tree-based SVMs or other multiclass strategies [49]. Therefore, researchers often use a combination of these models to achieve the best of both worlds, with the high generalization ability of SVMs. and the interpretability and robustness of decision trees and random forests. Moreover, the integration of SVMs with decision trees in a stacked architecture, as seen in the SMKSVM-RF model, can further enhance predictive performance by leveraging the strengths of both algorithms [50]. SVMs, . decision trees, and random forests play a crucial role in advancing medical diagnostics [51]. However, the choice of algorithm and its configuration must be carefully considered to address the specific challenges of medical data and disease complexity.

18.2.4 Machine Learning in Drug Discovery

To effectively utilize machine learning in drug discovery, it is crucial to carefully select the appropriate algorithm and configure it to address the unique challenges posed by medical data and disease complexity. In the field of cancer drug discovery, machine learning (ML) plays a pivotal role in identifying potential drug candidates. Generative adversarial networks (GANs) and reinforcement learning are among the advanced ML techniques that contribute to this process. GANs which involve a system of two competing neural network models, have been utilized to generate synthetic molecular and patient data, aiding in the identification of novel biological targets and the generation of new molecular compounds with desired properties [52]. Reinforcement learning is applied to optimize various aspects of drug discovery, including the selection of promising compounds and the design of molecules with optimal pharmacological profiles [53]. The integration of GANs and reinforcement learning in ML-driven drug discovery processes is expected to enhance the efficiency, reduce the time and costs associated with drug development, and ultimately lead to the discovery of effective cancer therapies [54, 55]. These technologies are integral to the development of personalized, effective, and patient-centered treatments, marking a significant advancement in the pharmaceutical industry's efforts to combat cancer. One example of a technology that has made significant contributions to personalized cancer treatments is the use of next-generation sequencing (NGS) to analyze genomic data. This has enabled the identification of genetic mutations that drive cancer growth and has opened new avenues for targeted therapies [56].

18.2.5 Machine Learning in Personalized Medicine

Machine learning (ML) algorithms can analyze vast amount of data to identify patterns and make predictions, which can be utilized to develop personalized treatment plans for cancer patients. Natural language processing (NLP) can also be employed to analyze patient data and medical records to identify potential treatment options [57]. By employing these technologies, healthcare providers can make more informed decisions and develop more effective treatment plans, ultimately resulting in improved patient outcomes. NLP is of paramount importance in advancing personalized medicine, especially in the field of cancer care. By analyzing unstructured medical data, NLP facilitates the creation of tailored treatment plans. Predictive analytics, a subset of ML, utilizes patterns in existing data to forecast future outcomes, which is crucial for developing personalized treatment strategies. However, the application of NLP and ML in personalized medicine is not without challenges.

Issues such as privacy concerns, biases in models, and the need for interpretability highlight the complexity of integrating these technologies into clinical practice. Furthermore, the generalizability of NLP models remains a significant hurdle to overcome. Nevertheless, the full potential of these technologies can only be realized by addressing the associated challenges and ensuring the models are robust, interpretable, and generalizable across diverse patient populations. Therefore, it is imperative to invest in ongoing research and development of machine learning algorithms specifically designed for electronic health records, in order to maximize the benefits of these technologies while minimizing their limitations and potential risks [57–59].

18.2.6 Machine Learning in Electronics Health Records

The utilization of machine learning (ML) and natural language processing (NLP) techniques, including recurrent neural networks (RNNs), has demonstrated substantial enhancements in the management and analysis of patient records within electronic health records (EHRs). These technologies have the capacity to automate and optimize essential processes such as cohort dataset of patients and mapping pharmaceutical names to standardized codes, which are vital for clinical research and interoperability [60]. However, it should be acknowledged that the majority of EHR data remains unstructured and difficult to process automatically. Despite the potential benefits, the field has witnessed relatively slow progress, and there is a need for collaborative efforts to develop open-source software and infrastructure to accelerate the application of these technologies in healthcare. Although there are obstacles to overcome, further research and development in this field are necessary to fully realize the potential of ML and NLP in healthcare [61]. In addition to overcoming obstacles, there is a need for continued research and development to maximize the potential of machine learning and natural language processing in patient monitoring and other healthcare applications [59, 60, 62].

18.2.7 Machine Learning in Real-Time Monitoring

Over the past decade, significant advancements have been made in patient monitoring systems through the integration of machine learning and the Internet of Things (IoT), particularly with the use of wearable devices and sensor technology. These technologies enable real-time patient monitoring and the early detection of health issues by analyzing data collected from various sensors, such as SPO2, heart rate, and body temperature, to identify patterns and detect anomalies that may indicate a clinical issue [63–65]. This real-time analysis is essential for timely medical interventions and improving patient outcomes. However, these technologies also present various challenges, including data privacy concerns, device interoperability, and the need for standardized data collection and analysis methods [66]. Additionally, there are issues related to the acceptability of these technologies among the medical community and the potential for the misuse of private health-related information. The integration of ML, IoT, and wearable sensor technology in patient monitoring represents a transformative development, enabling continuous, noninvasive data collection and analysis for early detection and intervention. This convergence has the potential to revolutionize healthcare by providing more personalized and proactive care, allowing healthcare professionals to intervene before a patient's condition worsens.

18.2.8 Machine Learning and Precision Medicine

Precision medicine leverages machine learning to parse genetic information and implement customized treatment strategies. This approach relies on the analysis of existing databases to carry out patient-centric assessments. ML algorithms are vital in deciphering intricate genomic sequencing and gene expression profiling, which are fundamental pillars of bioinformatics. These technologies help in identifying genetic variants and expression patterns that can tailor therapeutic interventions [67]. Notably, while ML significantly enhances the analysis of genomic data, it also presents challenges, such as the need for scalable solutions to manage the increasing dimensionality of genomics datasets [68]. A hybrid model of ML and bioinformatics is crucial in advancing precision medicine by enabling personalized genetic analysis [69]. The confluence of these fields promotes the formulation of precise diagnoses and treatments, although it also necessitates careful consideration of the accompanying ethical and data management challenges. This confluence is particularly relevant in fields such as risk prediction, where the integration of data from multiple sources can culminate in more accurate forecasts and decision-making, but also raises questions about data privacy, consent, and the potential biases in algorithms. Therefore, it is crucial to strike a balance between the benefits of interdisciplinary collaboration and the need to mitigate these ethical concerns to ensure responsible and effective risk prediction [69]. AI has the potential to revolutionize oncology by providing significant advancements in personalized cancer care and drug discovery. However, there are several challenges that must be addressed, such as the management of large amounts of data, the need for adequate computational resources, and the development of personalized biomarkers. To fully realize the potential of AI in improving cancer diagnosis, treatment, and patient outcomes, continued research and development are necessary.

18.2.9 Machine Learning in Risk Prediction

The utilization of machine learning algorithms for predicting cancer-related patient outcomes is on the rise, particularly in identifying high-risk cases and supporting clinical decision-making (Fig. 18.2). Numerous studies have demonstrated

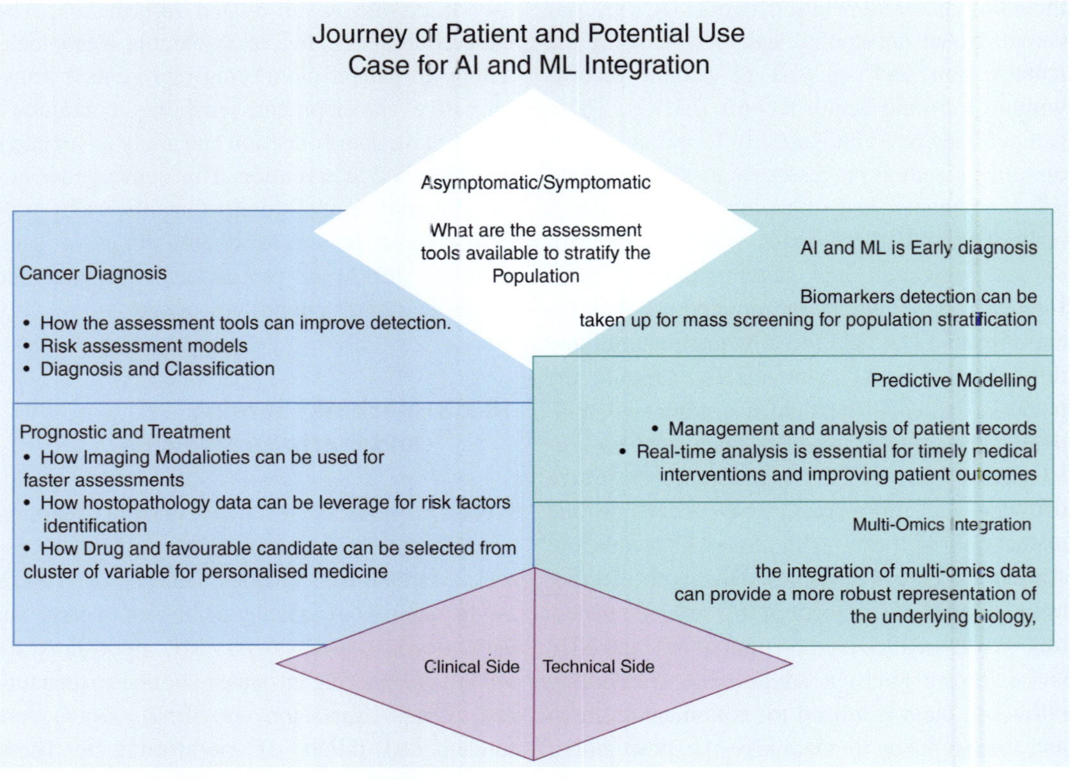

Fig. 18.2 Integration of AI and ML of patient data to clinical and technical aspects

the efficacy of various ML algorithms, including Bayesian networks, logistic regression, and gradient boosting, in predicting patient outcomes in cancer [70–73]. While logistic regression is a widely utilized method for developing predictive models, recent studies have shown that gradient boosting algorithms, particularly XGBoost, have outperformed other models in several applications. For instance, XGBoost has surpassed other ML models in predicting lymph node metastasis in prostate cancer, venous thromboembolism risk in hospitalized cancer patients, and 90-day mortality in ICU trauma patients [72–74]. Similarly, in the context of cervical cancer, XGBoost has exhibited superior prediction capabilities compared to other models [70, 75]. However, it is important to note that the random forest algorithm was found to be the most accurate for predicting kidney cancer in one study, indicating that the optimal ML algorithm may vary depending on the specific cancer type and the dataset utilized. Bayesian networks, logistic regression, and gradient boosting are valuable tools for risk prediction in cancer, and these predictive models can aid clinicians in identifying high-risk cancer patients and tailoring treatment strategies accordingly [70–73, 76].

18.3 Data Sciences in Oncology and Breast Cancer

Data science, which incorporates data mining and machine learning methods, holds significant importance in breast cancer research. By analyzing large datasets, these methodologies assist in improving the detection, diagnosis, and prognosis of breast cancer [77, 78]. However, the effectiveness of various techniques can vary. For instance, studies have shown that logistic regression models have achieved high classification accuracy in some cases, while other research has highlighted the superior performance of the C5.0 classifier in terms of accuracy and error reduction [79]. The choice of method is contingent upon the specific goals of the research, the nature of the data, and the desired outcomes. Hence, ongoing comparative analyses of these techniques are essential to optimize their application in breast cancer detection and treatment. Therefore, it is crucial to evaluate and compare different techniques to determine their effectiveness in breast cancer detection and treatment [80].

The utilization of data science in medical imaging, especially in radiology, has led to significant advancements in diagnostic accuracy and workflow efficiency. Artificial intelligence algorithms have been successfully applied to various imaging modalities, including MRI, X-ray, ultrasound, angiography, and echocardiography, enhancing the decision-making process and facilitating computer-aided diagnosis [81, 82]. AI has demonstrated notable improvements in tissue detection and characterization, outperforming experienced radiologists in certain cases [83]. These interdisciplinary approaches are revolutionizing radiology by enhancing diagnostic processes, personalizing medicine, and optimizing clinical workflows. The continuous collaboration between radiologists and AI developers is necessary to overcome the challenges and fully realize the potential benefits of AI in radiology [84]. This approach ensures that the tools are designed to address specific clinical needs and are thoroughly tested before being integrated into healthcare systems. By bringing together expertise from fields such as oncology, radiology, computer science, and bioinformatics, this collaborative effort can effectively address the multifaceted challenges of cancer diagnosis and treatment [9, 85].

Radiomics has gained significant attention in breast cancer detection and treatment monitoring. Radiomics involves extracting detailed features from medical images, which can be analyzed by AI algorithms to detect subtle patterns indicative of cancer [86]. There are interesting contrasts in the application of these technologies. The integration of clinical records with mammography images in DL models has demonstrated improved accuracy over using imaging data alone [87]. DL has been embedded in various imaging modalities, showing similar or superior performance to radiologists in some cases, but requiring further large-scale trials for validation [88]. On the other hand, radiomics offers a complementary approach by enabling the extraction of complex image features for early cancer detection [86].

18.4 Oncology Profile

A variety of data types are utilized, including genomic, transcriptomic, proteomic, and other omics data, as well as clinical, anatomopathological, and medical imaging data for research and outcome assessments [89–91]. These data types provide a comprehensive view of the biological processes involved in cancer and are essential for accurate prognosis and treatment planning. The integration of these diverse data modalities using advanced computational methods has the potential to contribute significantly to personalized medicine [91]. Some of these data types are summarized as follows.

18.4.1 Pathology Profiles

The evaluation of tissue samples for the identification of cancerous traits is a vital aspect of cancer diagnosis and treatment planning. Several diagnostic modalities and methodologies exist for analyzing tissue samples, each with its own benefits and potential applications in clinical practice. For example, fluorescence spectroscopy is used to differentiate between healthy and cancerous gastrointestinal tissues based on autofluorescence characteristics [92], proteomics, and high-performance liquid chromatography coupled with laser-induced fluorescence used to differentiate between normal, benign, and malignant breast tissue samples by detecting specific molecular or protein profiles indicative of cancerous changes within tissues [93]. Other techniques such as DNA methylation profiles provide a minimally invasive approach to identify tumors and their tissue of origin, which is crucial for treatment decisions [94]. Furthermore, ambient mass spectrometry is used to rapidly evaluate tumor cell percentage in glial tumor tissues, which is essential for molecular testing sensitivity [95]. Finally, the utility of CD147 expression is used in early hepatocellular carcinoma diagnosis through fine needle aspiration biopsy [96].

The significance of precise pathology profiles and the obstacles posed by intratumor variability, as well as the necessity for molecular analysis to complement morphological examination, represents a crucial area where machine learning and artificial intelligence are anticipated to serve as supportive technologies [97]. Additionally, other forms of data, such as the potential of microRNA analysis in fine needle aspiration biopsy samples to enhance diagnoses and optimize therapeutic options and a hybrid model for classifying upper aerodigestive tract cancer, contribute to a more refined understanding and diagnosis of cancer [98]. These methods hold the potential to improve clinical practice through the integration of AI algorithm methods, resulting in more accurate diagnoses, better treatment planning, and improved patient outcomes.

18.4.2 Imaging Data

Radiographic imaging is a vital tool in the detection and management of cancer. The accurate interpretation of imaging tests, such as mammograms, PET scans, and ultrasounds, is essential for diagnosing, staging, and monitoring treatment response in cancer patients [99]. Mammograms are critical for breast cancer screening, while PET scans, which utilize tracers like F-18 fluorodeoxyglucose (FDG), are highly sensitive in detecting metabolically active cancer cells across various cancer types [100]. Ultrasound offers a noninvasive, real-time imaging option, particularly useful for assessing lymph node metastases in conditions like melanoma [101]. These imaging modalities provide noninvasive means to visualize internal structures, aiding in the diagnosis, staging, and monitoring of cancerous growths [102, 103].

Besides computed tomography (CT) and magnetic resonance imaging (MRI), affordable imaging methods like ultrasound imaging technologies are available. These are crucial in breast cancer management, offering valuable tools for detection, diagnosis, and guiding biopsies [104, 105]. The interpretation of medical images is a complex task that requires consideration of the specific imaging modality's strengths and limitations. The choice of imaging technique should be tailored to the specific clinical context to ensure accurate detection and characterization of tumors or abnormalities associated with cancer.

18.4.3 Genetic and Molecular Data

Genetic alterations, including point mutations, recombinations, amplifications, and deletions affecting oncogenes, tumor-suppressor genes, and other genes that regulate cell proliferation and metastasis, play a critical role in the development of cancer [106]. The majority of these genetic alterations are somatically acquired, with a smaller fraction being inherited [107]. Traditional theories of carcinogenesis focus on the accumulation of somatic mutations, but they do not fully explain the role of nonmutagenic carcinogens or the observed cancer rates and latencies [108]. This has led to the exploration of genomic instability as a driving force in carcinogenesis, with preneoplastic cells displaying such instability that allows for the accumulation of genetic and epigenetic alterations [108]. Protein kinase "driver" mutations have also been instrumental in understanding tumorigenesis and developing personalized cancer therapeutics. Genetic variations, such as different alleles of the MICA gene, have been associated with varying risks of breast cancer development [109]. Additionally, genetic testing and molecular profiling are increasingly being used to refine breast cancer risk models, allowing for personalized screening and treatment decisions [110]. However, there are complexities and limitations to consider. While a genomic model has been developed to predict breast cancer in high-risk women with significant accuracy, it highlights the need for further identification of genetic components contributing to breast cancer. Moreover, environmental factors and lifestyle choices also play a substantial role in breast cancer occurrence and progression, which can be analyzed using ML algorithms to predict outcomes [3, 111].

The examination of molecular markers and gene expression patterns is a vital component of cancer research, aimed at improving the prediction and comprehension of cancer progression and treatment response. Several studies have shown the potential of gene expression data in identifying molecular signatures that can serve as prognostic or diagnostic biomarkers across various cancer types [112–115]. However, these studies also highlight challenges such as the cancer tissue's heterogeneity and the complexity of gene interactions. The use of multiplex gene expression assays has been effective in distinguishing between normal, adenomatous polyp, and carcinoma tissues in colon cancer [112]. The CAERUS approach has demonstrated high accuracy in predicting cancer outcomes by analyzing protein interaction networks [116]. The integration of development and cancer expression patterns has been proposed as a framework for identifying effective molecular signatures in lung cancer [117]. Despite these challenges, the integration of comprehensive gene expression data, advanced statistical methods, and machine learning algorithms can lead to the development of robust predictive models for cancer outcomes.

18.4.4 Clinical History, Patient Records, and Electronics Health Records

The collection of clinical history data, encompassing past treatments, family history, and lifestyle factors, is essential for accurately predicting cancer. Patient medical records serve as a repository for this information, which can be employed to identify patterns and risk factors associated with cancer development. However, the accuracy of such data can vary depending on the source, with discrepancies often noted between patient self-reports and medical records [118]. Moreover, behavioral risk factors derived from personal health records have been shown to be significant for monitoring and predicting cancer, emphasizing the importance of these data in public health and individual patient care. Notably, predictive modeling using electronic health records (EHRs) demonstrates promise for improving healthcare outcomes through early detection, although challenges persist due to data sparsity and the need for enhanced model interpretability [119]. Sociodemographic factors also influence the uptake and quality of family health history-based risk assessments, suggesting that patient engagement with health IT platforms may be affected by these variables [120]. To improve patient outcomes, early-warning methods that predict nonadherence to treatment regimens based on clinical and psychosocial risk factors in medical records have been developed, demonstrating the potential for targeted interventions [121]. Furthermore, multimodal modeling approaches that integrate various data sources, including clinical information, have shown encouraging performance in cancer prognosis prediction [122]. The quality of medical documentation, as evaluated against standards such as those set by the National Accreditation Board of Hospitals, is also critical for reducing medical errors and ensuring effective patient care [123]. Lastly, the improvement of paper-based medical records in low-resource settings has been identified as an area needed to support surgical and obstetric care [124].

18.4.5 Lifestyle, Environmental, and Community Data

Lifestyle and environmental factors are crucial in estimating cancer risk. Lifestyle decisions, such as diet, physical activity, alcohol consumption, and smoking, have been linked to the onset of breast cancer, with computational models evaluating the effects of these behaviors on estrogen levels and BRCA1 gene mutations [125]. Environmental factors, including exposure to carcinogens, are also recognized as contributors to cancer risk, although the specific role of environmental exposures in breast cancer is less well defined due to challenges in exposure assessment [126, 127]. The machine learning algorithms have been utilized to predict breast cancer risk using various data sources, including lifestyle and environmental data, demonstrating the potential for sophisticated analytical tools to enhance risk prediction.

18.4.6 Treatment Response Data, Clinical Investigation, and Outcomes

Oncology research plays a crucial role in the integration of treatment response data to predict cancer outcomes and tailor future therapies. For instance, neoadjuvant therapy (NAT) in HER2-positive early-stage breast cancer has demonstrated that a pathologic complete response can indicate a favorable prognosis. Similarly, in advanced colon and rectal cancer, the tumor response to neoadjuvant chemoradiation therapy has been directly linked to prognosis, although the best methods for monitoring this response are still under debate [128]. PET imaging, particularly with FDG, has also been recognized for its utility in monitoring response to treatment and predicting patient outcomes. The use of treatment response data, whether through pathologic assessments, imaging techniques like PET, or genomic profiling, is essential in predicting cancer outcomes and customizing future treatments [129]. Predictive modeling can also be used to track and forecast clinical outcomes, such as patient responses to treatments, disease progression, and survival rates. In advanced metastatic colorectal cancer (mCRC), a novel quantitative cancer-immunity cycle (QCIC) model has been developed to analyze treatment responses and predict tumor dynamics, introducing the treatment response index (TRI) and the death probability function (DPF) as evaluation tools [130]. However, the field must overcome challenges related to the interpretation and application of these data to maximize patient benefit and reduce unnecessary treatment burdens.

18.4.7 Multiomic Data Integration

The integration of various omics data types, such as genomics, proteomics, and metabolomics, is increasingly being recognized as a powerful approach for enhancing cancer prediction models. By combining multimodality data, researchers can obtain a more comprehensive analysis of the biological processes involved in cancer, potentially leading to improved prognostic capabilities [131, 132]. Interestingly, while the integration of multiomic data can provide a more robust representation of the underlying biology, it also presents analytical challenges due to high dimensionality and modest sample sizes. One can opt for knowledge-guided learning methods that incorporate biological knowledge and have shown to effectively address these challenges, improving prediction, feature selection, and other analytical tasks [130]. The use of advanced techniques like denoising autoencoders have demonstrated the potential to enhance the accuracy of cancer prognosis prediction by reducing the impact of data noise [133]. In future, application of knowledge-guided learning methods and advanced computational techniques can help overcome the inherent challenges of multiomic data integration, leading to more accurate and robust predictions.

18.5 Clinical and Ethical Consideration of AI in Medicine

The incorporation of artificial intelligence and machine learning into the healthcare sector has sparked concerns about ethical and clinical implications that must be addressed to establish a cohesive environment between medicine and data science. The literature consistently emphasizes the importance of navigating these ethical complexities to ensure responsible deployment of AI and ML in healthcare [134]. Critical issues such as privacy and data security, algorithmic bias, transparency, and professional responsibility are essential to safeguard patient welfare and upholding ethical principles [135]. Notably, while AI and ML offer transformative potential in healthcare, they also pose risks of perpetuating existing inequalities and unintentionally causing harm if ethical considerations are not adequately managed. The necessity for transparent, responsible, and socially accountable AI practices is highlighted across the literature, with a focus on preserving fundamental human rights and dignity [136]. Furthermore, the societal impact of AI and ML, including their influence on public opinion and political processes, adds another layer of ethical complexity that must be taken into account [137]. Providing healthcare professionals with education about AI tools is of utmost importance, particularly in the field of cancer prediction. The integration of AI into healthcare education is recognized as a vital step to ensure that the future health workforce is prepared to utilize these technologies effectively. Continuous education and training in AI tools will be necessary to keep pace with technological advancements and to maintain a high standard of patient care.

Compliance with regulations and openness are significant elements for successfully incorporating artificial intelligence into cancer imaging. Adherence to regulations ensures that AI systems adhere to established criteria for safety and efficacy, while transparency is crucial for fostering trust among healthcare professionals and patients and for addressing concerns about biases in algorithms and the comprehensibility of AI-driven decisions. Tackling these challenges is essential for the ethical and responsible use of AI in healthcare, and ongoing research and cooperation are vital for progressing AI applications in cancer imaging [135].

The ethical and legal implications of AI in radiology are complex and vital for the ethical integration of AI technologies in medical imaging. Data consent is a crucial aspect of utilizing patient information for the improvement of artificial intelligence (AI) applications in medicine. It ensures that patients are well informed and agree to the use of their data for research and development purposes, which is essential for maintaining trust and ethical standards in healthcare [138]. While the significance of data consent is widely acknowledged, there are complexities associated with obtaining it, especially in the context of AI where data is often used for continuous learning and improvement of algorithms. The dynamic nature of AI systems requires a framework that allows for ongoing consent, rather than a one-time approval process, to reflect the evolving use of data over time. This approach upholds ethical principles and fosters patient trust, which is vital for the feedback loop that informs software improvements.

Open access image repositories and data sharing platforms have been widely recognized as vital resources for advancing research in breast cancer. These repositories provide large, high-quality datasets that are essential for the application of machine learning techniques in medical research, particularly in the analysis of radiology and pathology image data [139]. The significance of such repositories is further emphasized by their role in promoting open science and reproducibility and accelerating scientific discovery through the sharing of research data. However, there are challenges associated with the development and use of these repositories that need to be addressed. For example, the effectiveness of search queries and the visibility of research results in search engines are crucial for the practical use of data, and these aspects can be hindered by poor development and lack of representation in global catalogues [140]. Additionally, while the number of open source medical imaging databases is growing, continuous statistical research is necessary to monitor their existence and ensure they meet the needs of the research community.

18.6 Importance of Transparency and Interpretability in AI Models

As AI continues to play an increasingly significant role in sectors such as healthcare, finance, and criminal justice, it is crucial to develop an understanding and trust in the decisions made by these systems. To achieve this, transparency and interpretability are essential. Transparency refers to an AI system's ability to make its decision-making processes and operations clear for observation, while interpretability involves the degree to which human experts can comprehend the mechanisms and outputs of the model [141]. Despite the general agreement on the importance of transparency and interpretability, there is a lack of consistency in how these concepts are defined across different domains. Some fields prioritize model-agnostic techniques, while others focus on the understandability of models. Additionally, the pursuit of interpretability sometimes comes at the cost of model performance, highlighting the need for careful management of this trade-off [142].

Transparency in AI models is a multifaceted concept that encompasses the visibility of the processes and decisions made by AI systems, which is crucial for scrutiny, accountability, and trust in healthcare applications [143]. The integration of explainable AI (XAI) is particularly significant, as it facilitates a better understanding of AI-generated predictions and decisions, thereby enhancing the trustworthiness of AI systems in clinical settings [142, 144]. Moreover, transparency is closely linked to the ethical implications of AI, such as ensuring fairness and mitigating biases, which are essential for maintaining the integrity of healthcare services. It is important to distinguish between trustworthiness and trust itself, as AI systems, lacking emotive states and moral agency, cannot be trusted in the human sense but can be deemed trustworthy based on their performance and reliability within the healthcare system [145]. The development of metrics for assessing the transparency of AI systems contributes to the confidence stakeholders can place in AI applications, ensuring that data sources and contributions are valid and up to date. The challenge lies in achieving a balance between interpretability and model performance, as well as establishing clear definitions and standards for explainability in AI. Addressing these aspects ensures that AI systems are not only technically proficient but also ethically sound and socially responsible, thereby securing their role as beneficial tools in the healthcare industry.

18.7 Practical Challenges in Using AI in Oncology and Breast Cancer

The practical challenges encountered in clinical settings when applying machine learning (ML) include integrating AI systems into regular clinical practice, requiring large amounts of training data, and ensuring the representativeness of retrospective datasets. In addition, achieving a balance between sensitivity and accuracy in ML algorithms is crucial to ensure their reliability and effectiveness for clinical decision-making. Sensitivity, or the true positive rate, is essential for correctly identifying patients with a condition, while accuracy ensures that predictions are correct overall. Notably, while ML algorithms have exhibited high accuracy in retrospective studies, their translation into practical medical settings has been limited, raising concerns about their usability and interaction with healthcare professionals. Furthermore, the requirement for large volumes of training data adds to the expenses and can be a barrier to the deployment of ML in healthcare. The representativeness of datasets is also a concern, as they may be subject to filtering and cleaning biases, which can affect the performance of ML algorithms. Achieving a balance between sensitivity and accuracy is a critical aspect of ML algorithm development and validation, as it directly impacts the clinical utility and trustworthiness of the AI systems [146].

18.8 Funding and Other Challenges for AI Implementation in Healthcare

The literature consistently concludes that education is crucial for equipping stakeholders to evaluate artificial intelligence (AI) technologies in medicine. According to various studies, medical education must adapt to incorporate AI-related topics to ensure that healthcare professionals are proficient in the clinical applications of AI. There is a growing need to prepare the healthcare workforce for the integration of machine learning (ML) , which suggests that AI and ML should be incorporated into curriculum and training programs [147]. The findings also indicate diverse stakeholder perspectives on AI understanding, suggesting the need for standardized AI comprehension in medical education to prevent misrepresentation and ensure coherent understanding across different levels [148]. Therefore, it is imperative to develop and implement comprehensive educational strategies that encompass AI-related topics to prepare stakeholders for the evolving landscape of AI in medicine.

As knowledge is gained by stakeholders, several other factors become crucial. Accuracy, privacy, and security have been identified as critical factors for optimizing healthcare with AI, implying that significant investment is required to meet these criteria. Another aspect of AI is the need for investment in governance structures to facilitate AI adoption, which includes addressing barriers such as trust and regulatory frameworks [149]. Additionally, the importance of organizational governance in healthcare AI adoption suggests that adequate funding is necessary to support informed decision-making and the development of governance structures. Interestingly, while funding is a recognized challenge, it is not the sole barrier. Trust is a significant catalyst for AI adoption, indicating that financial investment must also be accompanied by efforts to build trust among stakeholders. Furthermore, organizational governance suggests that funding should be directed not only toward technology acquisition but also toward building capabilities for the safe and responsible adoption of AI.

Data quality and availability are crucial elements for the successful implementation of machine learning (ML) algorithms in healthcare. High-quality data is necessary for the training of robust ML models that can accurately predict outcomes and assist in clinical decision-making [150]. The availability of comprehensive datasets allows for the development of algorithms that can generalize well to new, unseen cases, which is particularly important in healthcare applications where the stakes are high. Despite the potential of ML to revolutionize healthcare by improving diagnostics and patient care, the practical application of these algorithms in medical settings is often hindered by the quality and representativeness of the data used for training these models [151]. Retrospective datasets, commonly used for developing ML algorithms, may not always accurately reflect real-world clinical scenarios due to potential biases introduced during data collection and preprocessing.

Standardization and reproducibility of data and its results are essential elements for accurate and reliable diagnosis of breast cancer, as they ensure consistent findings across various studies and applications [85, 152, 153]. Proper feature selection is equally critical, as it directly impacts the accuracy of diagnostic models. Despite the general agreement on the importance of feature selection, there are differences in the methods used and the optimal number of features. For example, one study achieved a high classification accuracy of 99.03% using a feed-forward neural network with seven features selected through sequential forward selection, while another study reported 100% accuracy with a reduced feature set from 30 to 19 using a particle swarm optimization algorithm [154, 155]. These discrepancies demonstrate that different feature selection methods can lead to varying levels of diagnostic performance, and there is no universal solution [152]. Nevertheless, the studies suggest that the primary goal of feature selection remains consistent: to enhance the precision of diagnostic models and potentially improve patient survival rates through early detection.

18.9 Future Consideration of Using AI in Breast Cancer

The integration of artificial intelligence (AI) in oncology is expected to progress through the utilization of data intelligence, a deeper understanding of tumor biology, and the improvement of decision-making processes. AI applications in oncology are anticipated to benefit from the synergy between sophisticated data analytics and AI, which can lead to more personalized and effective cancer treatments [156]. The use of AI in clinical decision support systems (CDSS) is already being promoted worldwide, with systems like Watson for Oncology and CSCO AI, which are expected to evolve further in the coming years [157]. However, there are challenges to be addressed, such as the ethical considerations of AI applications in clinical decision-making, the need for transparency and interpretability in AI models, and the integration of AI into healthcare workflows. Additionally, the translation of molecular sequencing data into actionable insights remains a significant hurdle. The future consideration of using AI in cancer suggests that oncology will evolve into a more specialized field, with the potential for patients to receive more frequent and personalized treatment [158, 159]. AI's role in cancer management is multifaceted, encompassing screening, diagnosis, risk assessment, and treatment recommendations. Moreover, the ethical, legal, and social implications of AI in healthcare, including patient trust, data ownership, and professional responsibility, necessitate careful consideration and proactive governance. The realization of this potential depends on overcoming current challenges and ensuring that AI's integration into healthcare is ethically sound and clinically validated. Continued research and development, coupled with robust ethical frameworks and stakeholder engagement, are essential for harnessing AI's capabilities to improve patient outcomes in cancer care.

Summarizing, the prospects for future oncology AI applications are encouraging, as advancements in data intelligence and tumor biology knowledge contribute to improved decision-making processes. The successful implementation of these applications hinges on overcoming current challenges and ensuring that AI systems are ethically sound, interpretable, and well-integrated into clinical practice. A collaborative approach that combines AI automation with human expertise is ideal for optimizing patient care in oncology. By integrating AI's advanced analytical capabilities with the critical insights of healthcare professionals, personalized and effective cancer care can be achieved while upholding ethical considerations and patient privacy at the same time. This holistic approach fosters a more patient-centered healthcare system.

References

1. Raj P, Soundarabai PB, Augustine P. Data science: the artificial intelligence (AI) algorithms-inspired use cases. In: Demystifying graph data science: graph algorithms, analytics methods, platforms, databases, and use cases. Institution of Engineering and Technology; 2022. p. 15–37. https://doi.org/10.1049/pbpc048e_ch2.
2. Kosuru SK, et al. Data analytics and artificial intelligence. J Clin Pharm Res. 2023:15–7. https://doi.org/10.61427/jcpr.v3.i3.2023.112.
3. Ilyassov DK, Kitapova K, Kenc T. Overview and advantages of machine learning (ML) in statistics. Bull Karaganda Univ Econ Ser. 2023;109:59–66. https://doi.org/10.31489/2023ec1/59-66.
4. Le HD, Nguyen GH, Bui AT, Le TQ, Nguyen TH. Applications of machine learning (ML) – the real situation of the Vietnam Fintech market. J Soc Commer. 2022;2:60–70. https://doi.org/10.56209/jommerce.v2i2.28.
5. Perera Jayasuriya Kuranage M, Piamrat K, Hamma S. Network traffic classification using machine learning for software defined networks. In: Lecture notes in computer science. Springer International Publishing; 2020. p. 28–39. https://doi.org/10.1007/978-3-030-45778-5_3.
6. Sharif H, Rehman F, Rida A. Deep learning: convolutional neural networks for medical image analysis – a quick review. In: 2022 2nd international conference on digital futures and transformative technologies (ICoDT2). IEEE; 2022. https://doi.org/10.1109/icodt255437.2022.9787469.
7. Sahu A, Das PK, Meher S. Recent advancements in machine learning and deep learning-based breast cancer detection using mammograms. Physica Medica. 2023;114:103138. https://doi.org/10.1016/j.ejmp.2023.103138.
8. Chukwujindu E, Faiz H, AI-Douri S, Faiz K, De Sequeira A. Role of artificial intelligence in brain tumour imaging. Eur J Radiol. 2024;176:111509. https://doi.org/10.1016/j.ejrad.2024.111509.
9. Odeh M. Artificial intelligence (AI) and machine learning (ML) in diagnosing cancer: current trends; 2024. https://doi.org/10.20944/preprints202403.0433.v1.
10. Elemento O, Leslie C, Lundin J, Tourassi G. Artificial intelligence in cancer research, diagnosis and therapy. Nat Rev Cancer. 2021;21:747–52. https://doi.org/10.1038/s41568-021-00399-1.
11. Wei L, et al. Artificial intelligence (AI) and machine learning (ML) in precision oncology: a review on enhancing discoverability through multiomics integration. Br J Radiol. 2023;96:20230211. https://doi.org/10.1259/bjr.20230211.
12. Bhushan A, Gonsalves A, Menon JU. Current state of breast cancer diagnosis, treatment, and theranostics. Pharmaceutics. 2021;13:723. https://doi.org/10.3390/pharmaceutics13050723.
13. Ho PJ, et al. Incidence of breast cancer attributable to breast density, modifiable and non-modifiable breast cancer risk factors in Singapore. Sci Rep. 2020;10:503. https://doi.org/10.1038/s41598-019-57341-7.
14. Barnard ME, Boeke CE, Tamimi RM. Established breast cancer risk factors and risk of intrinsic tumor subtypes. Biochim Biophys Acta Rev Cancer. 2015;1856:73–85. https://doi.org/10.1016/j.bbcan.2015.06.002.
15. Wu P-Y, et al. Omic and electronic health record big data analytics for precision medicine. IEEE Trans Biomed Eng. 2017;64:263–73. https://doi.org/10.1109/TBME.2016.2573285.
16. Xie J. Computer aided diagnosis of early breast cancer by multimodal imaging. In: Cyber security intelligence and analytics. Springer International Publishing; 2020. p. 710–6. https://doi.org/10.1007/978-3-030-43306-2_100.
17. Marwaha S, Deb CK, Haque MA, Naha S, Maji AK. Application of artificial intelligence and machine learning in agriculture. In: Translating physiological tools to augment crop breeding. Springer Nature Singapore; 2023. p. 441–57. https://doi.org/10.1007/978-981-19-7498-4_21.
18. De Molina D, Rius A. Foundations of artificial intelligence and machine learning. In: Artificial intelligence in finance. Edward Elgar Publishing; 2023. p. 2–18. https://doi.org/10.4337/9781803926179.00009.
19. Liu W, Zhang J, Zhao Y. A comparison of deep learning and traditional machine learning approaches in detecting cognitive impairment using MRI scans. In: 2022 IEEE 46th annual computers, software, and applications conference (COMPSAC). IEEE; 2022. https://doi.org/10.1109/compsac54236.2022.00154.
20. Mavaie P, Holder L, Beck D, Skinner MK. Predicting environmentally responsive transgenerational differential DNA methylated regions (epimutations) in the genome using a hybrid deep-machine learning approach. BMC Bioinform. 2021;22:1–25. https://doi.org/10.1186/s12859-021-04491-z.
21. Wang D, Zhang M. Artificial intelligence in optical communications: from machine learning to deep learning. Front Commun Netw. 2021;2:656786. https://doi.org/10.3389/frcmn.2021.656786.
22. Chowdhury M, Li C, Poudel K. Combining deep learning with traditional machine learning to improve phonocardiography classification accuracy. In: 2021 IEEE signal processing in medicine and biology symposium (SPMB). IEEE; 2021. https://doi.org/10.1109/spmb52430.2021.9672296.

23. Ou Z, et al. Prediction of postoperative pathologic risk factors in cervical cancer patients treated with radical hysterectomy by machine learning. SSRN Electron J. 2020. https://doi.org/10.2139/ssrn.3722059.
24. Afrash MR, Mirbagheri E, Mashoufi M, Kazemi-Arpanahi H. Optimizing prognostic factors of five-year survival in gastric cancer patients using feature selection techniques with machine learning algorithms: a comparative study. BMC Med Inform Decis Mak. 2023;23:54. https://doi.org/10.1186/s12911-023-02154-y.
25. Cheloshkina K, Bzhikhatlov I, Poptsova M. Cancer breakpoint hotspots versus individual breakpoints prediction by machine learning models. In: Lecture notes in computer science. Springer International Publishing; 2020. p. 217–28. https://doi.org/10.1007/978-3-030-57821-3_19.
26. Bruno V, et al. Machine learning endometrial cancer risk prediction model: integrating guidelines of European Society for Medical Oncology with the tumor immune framework. Int J Gynecol Cancer. 2023;33:1708–14. https://doi.org/10.1136/ijgc-2023-004671.
27. Kang J. Skeletal muscle gauge prediction by a machine learning model in patients with colorectal cancer. Cancer Res. 2023;83:5428. https://doi.org/10.1158/1538-7445.AM2023-5428.
28. Ozhan O, Kucukakcali Z, Cicek I. Machine learning-based ovarian cancer prediction with XGboost and stochastic gradient boosting models. Med Sci. 2023;12:231. https://doi.org/10.5455/medscience.2022.09.207.
29. Suthaharan S. Supervised learning algorithms. In: Integrated series in information systems. Springer US; 2016. p. 183–206. https://doi.org/10.1007/978-1-4899-7641-3_8.
30. Chen Z, Xiao F, Guo F. Similarity learning-based fault detection and diagnosis in building HVAC systems with limited labeled data. Renew Sustain Energy Rev. 2023;185:113612. https://doi.org/10.1016/j.rser.2023.113612.
31. Felfeliyan B, et al. Self-supervised-RCNN for medical image segmentation with limited data annotation. Comput Med Imaging Graph. 2023;109:102297. https://doi.org/10.1016/j.compmedimag.2023.102297.
32. Okahana Y, Gotoh Y. A study for semi-supervised learning with random erasing. In: Lecture notes on data engineering and communications technologies. Springer International Publishing; 2020. p. 478–90. https://doi.org/10.1007/978-3-030-39746-3_49.
33. Mann GS, McCallum A. Simple, robust, scalable semi-supervised learning via expectation regularization. In: Proceedings of the 24th international conference on machine learning. ACM; 2007. https://doi.org/10.1145/1273496.1273571.
34. Pattanayak S. Unsupervised learning with restricted Boltzmann machines and autoencoders. In: Pro deep learning with TensorFlow 2.0. Apress; 2023. p. 407–510. https://doi.org/10.1007/978-1-4842-8931-0_5.
35. Unsupervised learning algorithms. Springer International Publishing; 2016. https://doi.org/10.1007/978-3-319-24211-8.
36. Pina R, Artaud C, Liu X, De Silva V. Staged reinforcement learning for complex tasks through decomposed environments. In: Intelligent systems and pattern recognition. Springer Nature Switzerland; 2023. p. 141–54. https://doi.org/10.1007/978-3-031-46338-9_11.
37. Goel R, Singla J. Enhancing robotic autonomy and deep reinforcement learning applications. In: Advances in logistics, operations, and management science. IGI Global; 2024. p. 295–312. https://doi.org/10.4018/979-8-3693-2849-1.ch020.
38. Nagayoshi M, Murao H, Tamaki H. Reinforcement learning for dynamic environment: a classification of dynamic environments and a detection method of environmental changes. Artif Life Robot. 2013;18:104–8. https://doi.org/10.1007/s10015-013-0106-0.
39. Liu H, Chen P, Zhao Z. Towards A robust meta-reinforcement learning-based scheduling framework for time critical tasks in Cloud environments. In: 2021 IEEE 14th international conference on CLOUD computing (CLOUD). IEEE; 2021. https://doi.org/10.1109/cloud53861.2021.00082.
40. Wang Z, Chen C, Li H-X, Dong D, Tarn T-J. A novel incremental learning scheme for reinforcement learning in dynamic environments. In: 2016 12th world congress on intelligent control and automation (WCICA). IEEE; 2016. https://doi.org/10.1109/wcica.2016.7578530.
41. Gan X, Zuo Y, Yang G, Zhang A, Tao F. Dynamic scheduling for dual-objective job shop with machine breakdown by reinforcement learning. Proc Inst Mech Eng B J Eng Manuf. 2023;238:3–17. https://doi.org/10.1177/09544054231167086.
42. Gogineni R, Chaturvedi A. Convolutional neural networks for medical image analysis. In: Convolutional neural networks for medical image processing applications. CRC Press; 2022. p. 75–90. https://doi.org/10.1201/9781003215141-4.
43. Kumar Sharma S. Use of AI in medical image processing. In: Advances in medical technologies and clinical practice. IGI Global; 2024. p. 1–18. https://doi.org/10.4018/979-8-3693-2359-5.ch001.
44. Bir P, Balas VE. A review on medical image analysis with convolutional neural networks. In: 2020 IEEE international conference on computing, power and communication technologies (GUCON). IEEE; 2020. https://doi.org/10.1109/gucon48875.2020.9231203.
45. Alqahtani S. A study on machine learning and deep learning in medical imaging emphasizes MRI: a systematic literature review. Int J Pharm Sci Res Allied Sci. 2023. https://doi.org/10.2196/preprints.47192.
46. Ibrahim I, Abdulazeez A. The role of machine learning algorithms for diagnosing diseases. J

Appl Sci Technol Trend. 2021;2:10–9. https://doi.org/10.38094/jastt20179.

47. Ramesh B, et al. Feasible prediction of multiple diseases using machine learning. E3S Web Conf. 2023;430:1051. https://doi.org/10.1051/e3sconf/202343001051.
48. Rodriguez-Galiano V, Sanchez-Castillo M, Chica-Olmo M, Chica-Rivas M. Machine learning predictive models for mineral prospectivity: an evaluation of neural networks, random forest, regression trees and support vector machines. Ore Geol Rev. 2015;71:804–18. https://doi.org/10.1016/j.oregeorev.2015.01.001.
49. Takahashi F, Abe S. Decision-tree-based support vector machines. Trans Inst Syst Control Inform Engrs. 2003;16:125–32. https://doi.org/10.1109/ICONIP.2002.1202854.
50. Saputra DCE, Ma'arif A, Sunat K. Optimizing predictive performance: hyperparameter tuning in stacked multi-kernel support vector machine random Forest models for diabetes identification. J Robot Control. 2024;4:896–904. https://doi.org/10.18196/jrc.v4i6.20898.
51. Choudhury A, Gupta D. A survey on medical diagnosis of diabetes using machine learning techniques. In: Recent developments in machine learning and data analytics. Springer Singapore; 2018. p. 67–78. https://doi.org/10.1007/978-981-13-1280-9_6.
52. Zhavoronkov A, et al. Artificial intelligence for aging and longevity research: recent advances and perspectives. Ageing Res Rev. 2019;49:49–66. https://doi.org/10.1016/j.arr.2018.11.003.
53. Quyen NH, Duy PT, Vy NC, Hien DTT, Pham V-H. Federated intrusion detection on non-IID data for IIoT networks using generative adversarial networks and reinforcement learning. In: Lecture notes in computer science. Springer International Publishing; 2022. p. 364–81. https://doi.org/10.1007/978-3-031-21280-2_20.
54. Ravindra Padalkar G, Dinkar Patil S, Mallikarjun Hegadi M, Kailash Jaybhaye N. Drug discovery using generative adversarial network with reinforcement learning. In: 2021 international conference on computer communication and informatics (ICCCI). IEEE; 2021. https://doi.org/10.1109/iccci50826.2021.9402449.
55. Paliwal A, Alam MA, Sharma P, Jain S, Dhoundiyal S. Revolutionizing cancer research and drug discovery: the role of artificial intelligence and machine learning. Curr Cancer Ther Rev. 2024;20:807–10. https://doi.org/10.2174/0115733947288355240305080236.
56. Kumari R, et al. Getting started with computational drug discovery: a comprehensive guide. In: Advances in healthcare information systems and administration. IGI Global; 2024. p. 235–58. https://doi.org/10.4018/979-8-3693-2897-2.ch012.
57. Lin H, Ni L, Phuong C, Hong J. Natural language processing for radiation oncology: personalizing treatment pathways. Pharmgenomics Pers Med. 2024;17:65–76. https://doi.org/10.2147/PGPM.S396971.
58. Liu Y. Natural language processing in data analytics. In: Data analytics and AI. Auerbach Publications; 2020. p. 117–32. https://doi.org/10.1201/9781003019855-7.
59. Houssein EH, Mohamed RE, Ali AA. Machine learning techniques for biomedical natural language processing: a comprehensive review. IEEE Access. 2021;9:140628–53. https://doi.org/10.1109/ACCESS.2021.3119621.
60. Manoharan A. Leveraging machine learning and NLP for enhanced cohorting and RxNorm mapping in electronic health records (EHRs). World J Adv Eng Techno. Sci. 2024;11:141–9. https://doi.org/10.30574/wjaets.2024.11.2.0083.
61. Ohno-Machado L. Realizing the full potential of electronic health records: the role of natural language processing. J Am Med Inform Assoc. 2011;18:539. https://doi.org/10.1136/amiajnl-2011-000501.
62. Li I, et al. Neural natural language processing for unstructured data in electronic health records: a review. Comput Sci Rev. 2022;46:100511. https://doi.org/10.48550/arXiv.2107.02975.
63. Yogesh V, Shanthakumara AH. Smart real-time health monitoring band using machine learning and IoT. In: 2021 2nd international conference on smart electronics and communication (ICOSEC). IEEE; 2021. https://doi.org/10.1109/icosec51865.2021.9591848.
64. Awotunde JB, Folorunso SO, Bhoi AK, Adebayo PO, Ijaz MF. Disease diagnosis system for IoT-based wearable body sensors with machine learning algorithm. In: Intelligent systems reference library. Springer Singapore; 2021. p. 201–22. https://doi.org/10.1007/978-981-16-2972-3_10.
65. Singh B, Kaunert C, Vig K, Gautam BK. Wearable sensors assimilated with internet of things (IoT) for advancing medical imaging and digital healthcare: real-time scenario. In: Inclusivity and accessibility in digital health. IGI Global; 2024. p. 275–97. https://doi.org/10.4018/979-8-3693-1463-0.ch018.
66. Sivaraman H. IoT-enabled healthcare monitoring: a systematic review of wearable devices. Inf Technol Ind. 2019;7:78–86. https://doi.org/10.17762/itii.v7i3.815.
67. Bioinformatics in precision medicine. In: Recent advances in molecular and translational medicine: updates in precision medicine. Bentham Science Publishers; 2021. p. 17–42. https://doi.org/10.2174/9789815036756121010005.
68. Moreno M, Vilaça R, Ferreira PG. Scalable transcriptomics analysis with Dask: applications in data science and machine learning. BMC Bioinform. 2022;23:514. https://doi.org/10.1186/s12859-022-05065-3.
69. Kausar A, Kausar A, Das S. AI in bioinformatics and computational biology. In: Advances in medical diagnosis, treatment, and care. IGI Global; 2024.

p. 278–90. https://doi.org/10.4018/979-8-3693-3629-8.ch014.
70. Edafetanure-Ibeh FT. Evaluating machine learning algorithms for cervical cancer prediction: a comparative analysis; 2024. https://doi.org/10.31219/osf.io/vyuf2.
71. Fatima N. Machine learning algorithms using logistic regression for predicting neurosurgical outcomes; 2020. https://doi.org/10.21203/rs.3.rs-37934/v1.
72. Meng L, et al. Development and validation of a machine learning model to predict venous thromboembolism among hospitalized cancer patients. Asia Pac J Oncol Nurs. 2022;9:100128. https://doi.org/10.1016/j.apjon.2022.100128.
73. Yang S, Cao L, Zhou Y, Hu C. A retrospective cohort study: predicting 90-day mortality for ICU trauma patients with a machine learning algorithm using XGBoost using MIMIC-III database. J Multidiscip Healthc. 2023;16:2625–40. https://doi.org/10.2147/jmdh.s416943.
74. Wang X, et al. Application of machine learning algorithm in prediction of lymph node metastasis in patients with intermediate and high-risk prostate cancer. J Cancer Res Clin Oncol. 2023;149:8759–68. https://doi.org/10.1007/s00432-023-04816-w.
75. Yu W, et al. A 5-year survival status prognosis of nonmetastatic cervical cancer patients through machine learning algorithms. Cancer Med. 2022;12:6867–76. https://doi.org/10.1002/cam4.5477.
76. Prathipati S. A comparative study on chronic kidney cancer prediction using supervised machine learning algorithms. Int J Sci Res Eng Manag. 2023;07. https://doi.org/10.55041/IJSREM18629.
77. Chellamuthu G, Kannimuthu S, Premalatha K. Data mining and machine learning approaches in breast cancer biomedical research. In: Research anthology on medical informatics in breast and cervical cancer. IGI Global; 2022. p. 792–822. https://doi.org/10.4018/978-1-6684-7136-4.ch042.
78. Laxmidas P, Faisal S, Indira B, Mekala S, Obaid S. Cancer tumor detection using machine learning. Int J Adv Res. 2023;11:71–5. https://doi.org/10.21474/IJAR01/16850.
79. Roseline R, Manikandan S. Determination of breast cancer using data mining techniques. Indian J Forensic Med Toxicol. 2018;12:259. https://doi.org/10.5958/0973-9130.2018.00169.X.
80. Patel H, Barot D, M. P. Big data analytics to predict breast cancer. Int J Res Appl Sci Eng Technol. 2022;10:2004–9. https://doi.org/10.22214/ijraset.2022.41045.
81. Niazi A. Applications of artificial intelligence in medical imaging: enhancing diagnostic accuracy and workflow efficiency; 2023. https://doi.org/10.31219/osf.io/t7uqe.
82. Stanciu S, et al. Artificial Intelligence in cardiovascular medical imaging. Rom J Mil Med. 2020;123:310–6. https://doi.org/10.55453/rjmm.2020.123.4.12.
83. Anam H, Ambad R, Singam A, Deshkar PA. Artificial intelligence: a new frontier in radiological imaging. E3S Web Conf. 2024;491:1004. https://doi.org/10.1051/e3sconf/202449101004.
84. Najjar R. Redefining radiology: a review of artificial intelligence integration in medical imaging. Diagnostics. 2023;13:2760. https://doi.org/10.3390/diagnostics13172760.
85. Koh D-M, et al. Artificial intelligence and machine learning in cancer imaging. Commun Med. 2022;2:133. https://doi.org/10.1038/s43856-022-00199-0.
86. Talwar R, Sharma M, Sonia. A comprehensive review on artificial intelligence-driven radiomics for early cancer detection and intelligent medical supply chain. In: AI and machine learning impacts in intelligent supply chain. IGI Global; 2024. p. 226–54. https://doi.org/10.4018/979-8-3693-1347-3.ch015.
87. Modi O, Subasi A. Breast tumor detection in ultrasound images using artificial intelligence. In: Applications of artificial intelligence in medical imaging. Elsevier; 2023. p. 137–81. https://doi.org/10.1016/b978-0-443-18450-5.00003-7.
88. Balkenende L, Teuwen J, Mann RM. Application of deep learning in breast cancer imaging. Semin Nucl Med. 2022;52:584–96. https://doi.org/10.1053/j.semnuclmed.2022.02.003.
89. Andrew Z, Charlie Z, Okyaz E. Advances in deep learning-based cancer outcome prediction using multi-omics data. Ann Proteom Bioinform. 2023;7:10–3. https://doi.org/10.29328/journal.apb.1001020.
90. Chai H, et al. Integrating multi-omics data through deep learning for accurate cancer prognosis prediction. Comput Biol Med. 2021;134:104481. https://doi.org/10.1016/j.compbiomed.2021.104481.
91. Lobato-Delgado B, Priego-Torres B, Sanchez-Morillo D. Combining molecular, imaging, and clinical data analysis for predicting cancer prognosis. Cancers (Basel). 2022;14:3215. https://doi.org/10.3390/cancers14133215.
92. Genova T, et al. Macro and micro spectroscopy parameters of cancerous and healthy gastrointestinal tissues. J Biomed Photonics Eng. 2017;3:40305. https://doi.org/10.18287/JBPE17.03.040305.
93. Menon S, et al. Protein profile study of breast cancer tissues using HPLC-LIF: a pilot study. In: Vo-Dinh T, Grundfest WS, Benaron DA, Cohn GE, Raghavachari R, editors. Advanced biomedical and clinical diagnostic systems V. SPIE; 2007. https://doi.org/10.1117/12.699935.
94. Pan Y, Liu G, Zhou F, Su B, Li Y. DNA methylation profiles in cancer diagnosis and therapeutics. Clin Exp Med. 2018;18(1):1–14. https://doi.org/10.1007/s10238-017-0467-0. Epub 2017 Jul 27. PMID: 28752221.

95. Pekov SI, et al. Rapid estimation of tumor cell percentage in brain tissue biopsy samples using inline cartridge extraction mass spectrometry. Anal Bioanal Chem. 2021;413:2913–22. https://doi.org/10.1007/s00216-021-03220-y.
96. Mamori S. Useful detection of CD147 (EMMPRIN) for pathological diagnosis of early hepatocellular carcinoma in needle biopsy samples. World J Gastroenterol. 2007;13:2913. https://doi.org/10.3748/wjg.v13.i21.2913.
97. Ryška A. Molecular pathology in real time. Cancer Metastasis Rev. 2016;35:129–40. https://doi.org/10.1007/s10555-016-9607-3.
98. Mathialagan P, Chidambaranathan M. Computer vision techniques for upper aero-digestive tract tumor grading classification – addressing pathological challenges. Pattern Recognit Lett. 2021;144:42–53. https://doi.org/10.1016/j.patrec.2021.01.002.
99. Ganesh PS, Kumar TS, Kumar M, Kumar M, S. R. Brain tumor detection and classification using image processing techniques. Int J Adv Res Sci Commun Technol. 2021;4:32–8. https://doi.org/10.48175/ijarsct-v4-i3-005.
100. Bornstein S, Young K, Tanyi J, Holland J. Heavy PETting: reducing radiation exposure from Intradepartment positron emission tomography scans. Int J Radiat Oncol Biol Phys. 2014;22:545. https://doi.org/10.1016/j.ijrobp.2013.11.015.
101. Blessing C. Positron emission tomography and ultrasonography. A comparative retrospective study assessing the diagnostic validity in lymph node metastases of malignant melanoma. Arch Dermatol. 1995;131:1394–8. https://doi.org/10.1001/archderm.131.12.1394.
102. Guo R, Lu G, Qin B, Fei B. Ultrasound imaging technologies for breast cancer detection and management: a review. Ultrasound Med Biol. 2018;44:37–70. https://doi.org/10.1016/j.ultrasmedbio.2017.09.012.
103. Mallidi S, Luke GP, Emelianov S. Photoacoustic imaging in cancer detection, diagnosis, and treatment guidance. Trends Biotechnol. 2011;29:213–21. https://doi.org/10.1016/j.tibtech.2011.01.006.
104. Kehagias D, Smyrniotis V, Gouliamos A, Vlahos L. Cystic pancreatic neoplasms: computed tomography and magnetic resonance imaging findings. Int J Gastrointest Cancer. 2000;28:223–30. https://doi.org/10.1385/IJGC:28:3:223.
105. Balandina AV, Kapishnikov AV, Kozlov SV. Magnetic resonance imaging and perfusion computed tomography capacities in brain glial tumors diagnosis. Kazan Med J. 2015;96:949–52. https://doi.org/10.17750/KMJ2015-949.
106. Sugimura T, Terada M, Yokota J, Hirohashi S, Wakabayashi K. Multiple genetic alterations in human carcinogenesis. Environ Health Perspect. 1992;98:5. https://doi.org/10.1289/ehp.92985.
107. Torkamani A, Verkhivker G, Schork NJ. Cancer driver mutations in protein kinase genes. Cancer Lett. 2009;281:117–27. https://doi.org/10.1016/j.canlet.2008.11.008.
108. Schneider BL. Destructive cycles: the role of genomic instability and adaptation in carcinogenesis. Carcinogenesis. 2004;25:2033–44. https://doi.org/10.1093/carcin/bgh204.
109. Vallian S, Rad MJ, Tavallaei M, Tavassoli M. Correlation of major histocompatibility complex class I related A (MICA) polymorphism with the risk of developing breast cancer. Med Oncol. 2011;29:5–9. https://doi.org/10.1007/s12032-010-9776-9.
110. Pesapane F, et al. Advances in breast cancer risk modeling: integrating clinics, imaging, pathology and artificial intelligence for personalized risk assessment. Future Oncol. 2023;19:2547–64. https://doi.org/10.2217/fon-2023-0365.
111. Bild A, et al. A genomic biomarker for breast cancer development in high-risk women. Cancer Res. 2009;69:4059. https://doi.org/10.1007/978-3-319-22909-6_1.
112. Drew JE, et al. Predictive gene signatures: molecular markers distinguishing colon adenomatous polyp and carcinoma. PLoS One. 2014;9:e113071. https://doi.org/10.1371/journal.pone.0113071.
113. Kaur H, Bhalla S, Kaur D, Raghava GPS. CancerLivER: a database of liver cancer gene expression resources and biomarkers. Database. 2020;2020:baaa012. https://doi.org/10.1093/database/baaa012.
114. Sharma S, Shah N, Singh R, Lokare R. Machine learning approach for predicting breast cancer using genomic data. SSRN Electron J. 2020. https://doi.org/10.2139/ssrn.3571724.
115. Yu X, et al. The pan-cancer analysis of gene expression patterns in the context of inflammation. Mol Biosyst. 2014;10:2270. https://doi.org/10.1039/c4mb00258j.
116. Zhang KX, Ouellette BFF. CAERUS: predicting CAncERoUtcomeS using relationship between protein structural information, protein networks, gene expression data, and mutation data. PLoS Comput Biol. 2011;7:e1001114. https://doi.org/10.1371/journal.pcbi.1001114.
117. Zhang C, et al. Integrative analysis of lung development–cancer expression associations reveals the roles of signatures with inverse expression patterns. Mol Biosyst. 2015;11:1271–84. https://doi.org/10.1039/C5MB00061K.
118. Ferrante JM, et al. Self-report versus medical records for assessing cancer-preventive services delivery. Cancer Epidemiol Biomarkers Prev. 2008;17:2987–94. https://doi.org/10.1158/1055-9965.epi-08-0177.
119. Li Z. A comparative study of clinical risk prediction using limited patient electronic health records. Appl Comput Eng. 2023;8:584–92. https://doi.org/10.54254/2755-2721/8/20230281.

120. Wu R, et al. Effect of sociodemographic factors on uptake of a patient-facing information technology family health history risk assessment platform. Appl Clin Inform. 2019;10:180–8. https://doi.org/10.1055/s-0039-1679926.
121. Kaskiris C, Sairamesh J, Rajagopal R. Risk prediction methods based on electronic medical records and social surveys for improving patient outcomes and enabling targeted care services. In: Advances in the human side of service engineering. AHFE International; 2019. https://doi.org/10.54941/ahfe100297.
122. Azher ZL, Vaickus LJ, Salas LA, Christensen BC, Levy JJ. Development of biologically interpretable multimodal deep learning model for cancer prognosis prediction; 2021. https://doi.org/10.1101/2021.10.30.466610.
123. Sinha RK, Shenoy N. Assessment of oncology medical records as per NABH standards. J Health Manag. 2013;15:329–43. https://doi.org/10.1177/0972063413492035.
124. Lodge W, et al. Assessing completeness of patient medical records of surgical and obstetric patients in Northern Tanzania. Glob Health Action. 2020;13:1765526. https://doi.org/10.1080/16549716.2020.1765526.
125. Das O, Pradhan I, Chatterjee R, Dash SR. A computational approach to assess breast cancer risk in relation with lifestyle factors. In: Smart innovation, systems and technologies. Springer Nature Singapore; 2022. p. 367–76. https://doi.org/10.1007/978-981-16-8739-6_34.
126. Wolff MS, Britton JA, Wilson VP. Environmental risk factors for breast cancer among African-American women. Cancer. 2002;97:289–310. https://doi.org/10.1002/cncr.11023.
127. Elespuru RK, Fischer C. Abstract 2612: personalized cancer risk and prevention: analysis of risk factors for specific cancers and integration into cancer risk assessment paradigms. Cancer Res. 2021;81:2612. https://doi.org/10.3390/jpm11060511.
128. Barot SV, Roesch E, Abraham J. Optimizing adjuvant and post-neoadjuvant therapy in HER2-positive early breast cancer. Expert Rev Anticancer Ther. 2022;22:1289–99. https://doi.org/10.1080/14737140.2022.2146580.
129. Naqa IE. The role of quantitative PET in predicting cancer treatment outcomes. Clin Transl Imaging. 2014;2:305–20. https://doi.org/10.1007/s40336-014-0063-1.
130. Li W, Ballard J, Zhao Y, Long Q. Knowledge-guided learning methods for integrative analysis of multi-omics data. Comput Struct Biotechnol. 2024;J23:1945–50. https://doi.org/10.1016/j.csbj.2024.04.053.
131. Eichner J, et al. Integrated enrichment analysis and pathway-centered visualization of metabolomics, proteomics, transcriptomics, and genomics data by using the InCroMAP software. J Chromatogr B. 2014;966:77–82. https://doi.org/10.1016/j.jchromb.2014.04.030.
132. Wu M, Jiang Y, Ma S. Integration of proteomics and other omics data. In: Proteomics data analysis. Springer US; 2021. p. 307–24. https://doi.org/10.1007/978-1-0716-1641-3_18.
133. Chen Z, et al. Artificial intelligence for assisting cancer diagnosis and treatment in the era of precision medicine. Cancer Commun. 2021;41:1100–15. https://doi.org/10.1002/cac2.12215.
134. Tiwari R. Ethical and societal implications of AI and machine learning. Int J Sci Res Eng Manag. 2023;07. https://doi.org/10.55041/IJSREM17505.
135. HarishbhaiTilala M, et al. Ethical considerations in the use of artificial intelligence and machine learning in health care: a comprehensive review. Cureus. 2024;16:e62443. https://doi.org/10.7759/cureus.62443.
136. Yadav KK, Gaurav A. Application and challenges of machine learning in healthcare. Int J Res Appl Sci Eng Technol. 2023;11:458–66. https://doi.org/10.22214/ijraset.2023.55678.
137. Kumar Jaiswal R, Sundar Sharma S, Kaushik R. Ethics in AI and machine learning. J Nonlinear Anal Optim. 2023;14:8–12. https://doi.org/10.36893/JNAO.2023.V14I1.0008-0012.
138. Aldhafeeri FM. Navigating the ethical landscape of artificial intelligence in radiography: a cross-sectional study of radiographers' perspectives. BMC Med Ethics. 2024;25:52. https://doi.org/10.1186/s12910-024-01052-w.
139. Prior F, et al. Open access image repositories: high-quality data to enable machine learning research. Clin Radiol. 2020;75:7–12. https://doi.org/10.1016/j.crad.2019.04.002.
140. Yumasheva SI. Open access medical repositories: status and development trends. Bibliosphere. 2023:83–95. https://doi.org/10.20913/1815-3186-2023-2-83-95.
141. Joyce DW, Kormilitzin A, Smith KA, Cipriani A. Explainable artificial intelligence for mental health through transparency and interpretability for understandability. NPJ Digit Med. 2023;6:1–7. https://doi.org/10.1038/s41746-023-00751-9.
142. Patidar N, Mishra S, Jain R, Prajapati D, Solanki A, Suthar R, Patel K, Patel H. Transparency in AI decision making: a survey of explainable AI methods and applications. Adv Robot Technol. 2024;2:1–10. https://doi.org/10.23880/art-16000110.
143. Barclay I, et al. A framework for fostering transparency in shared artificial intelligence models by increasing visibility of contributions. Concurr Comput. 2020;33:e6129. https://doi.org/10.1002/cpe.6129.
144. Shafik W, Lakshmi D. Explainable AI (EXAI) for smart healthcare automation. In: Advances in bioin-

formatics and biomedical engineering. IGI Global; 2024. p. 289–316. https://doi.org/10.4018/979-8-3693-4439-2.ch012.
145. Bilal Unver M, Asan O. Role of trust in AI-driven healthcare systems: discussion from the perspective of patient safety. In: Proceedings of the international symposium on human factors and ergonomics in health care, vol. 11; 2022. p. 129–34. https://doi.org/10.1177/2327857922111026.
146. Moldt J-A, et al. Assessing AI awareness and identifying essential competencies: insights from key stakeholders in integrating AI into medical education. JMIR Med Educ. 2024;10:e58355. https://doi.org/10.2196/58355.
147. Egon K, Karl L. Machine learning in healthcare education: preparing the future workforce; 2023. https://doi.org/10.31219/osf.io/yxg42.
148. Jackson P, Ponath Sukumaran G, Babu C, et al. Artificial intelligence in medical education - perception among medical students. BMC Med Educ. 2024;24:804. https://doi.org/10.1186/s12909-024-05760-0.
149. Kim JY, et al. Organizational governance of emerging technologies: AI adoption in healthcare. In: 2023 ACM conference on fairness, accountability, and transparency. ACM; 2023. https://doi.org/10.1145/3593013.3594089.
150. Judijanto L, Muda Priyangan D, Muthmainah HN, Jata IW. The influence of data quality and machine learning algorithms on AI prediction performance in business analysis in Indonesia. Eastasouth J Inform Syst Comput Sci. 2023;1:75–86. https://doi.org/10.58812/esiscs.v1i02.182.
151. Saeed A, Husnain A, Rasool S, Yousaf Gill A, Amelia A. Healthcare revolution: how AI and machine learning are changing medicine. J Res Soc Sci Econ Manag. 2023;3. https://doi.org/10.59141/jrssem.v3i3.558.
152. Bhardwaj H, Sakalle A, Tiwari A, Verma M, Bhardwaj A. Breast cancer diagnosis using simultaneous feature selection and classification: a genetic programming approach. In: 2018 IEEE symposium series on computational intelligence (SSCI). IEEE; 2018. https://doi.org/10.1109/ssci.2018.8628935.
153. Zheng D, Tang P, Lu D, Han L, Saberi S. A structured combination of ensemble classifier and filter-based feature selection to improve breast cancer diagnosis. J Cancer Res Clin Oncol. 2023;149:14519–34. https://doi.org/10.1007/s00432-023-05238-4.
154. Naveed N, Madhloom HT, Husain MS. Breast cancer diagnosis using wrapper-based feature selection and artificial neural network. Appl Comput Sci. 2021;17:19–30. https://doi.org/10.23743/acs-2021-18.
155. Kazerani R. Improving breast cancer diagnosis accuracy by particle swarm optimization feature selection. Int J Comput Intell Syst. 2024;17:44. https://doi.org/10.1007/s44196-024-00428-5.
156. Challa N, Kathiriya S, Munjala MB. Integrating advanced data analytics with artificial intelligence: unveiling synergies for enhanced decision-making. J Artif Intell Cloud Comput. 2022:1–6. https://doi.org/10.47363/jaicc/2022(1)185.
157. Somashekhar SP, et al. Watson for oncology and breast cancer treatment recommendations: agreement with an expert multidisciplinary tumor board. Ann Oncol. 2018;29:418–23. https://doi.org/10.1093/annonc/mdx781.
158. Ahn JS, et al. Artificial intelligence in breast cancer diagnosis and personalized medicine. J Breast Cancer. 2023;26:405. https://doi.org/10.4048/jbc.2023.26.e45.
159. Rentiya ZS, et al. Revolutionizing breast cancer detection with artificial intelligence (AI) in radiology and radiation oncology: a systematic review. Cureus. 2024;16:e57619. https://doi.org/10.7759/cureus.57619.

Journey of Breast Imaging

19

Pratyaksha Rana and Ekta Dhamija

Abstract

Breast cancer is the most common cancer and leading cause of mortality in females. The journey of breast imaging began in the first half of the twentieth century, with the aim to detect breast cancer in the early preclinical stage. Introduction of mammogram with subsequent technological advances over the years revolutionised breast cancer management, playing a pivotal role in screening, diagnosis, image-guided sampling, guiding treatment and surveillance. Subsequently, the other imaging modalities for breast-ultrasound and magnetic resonance imaging evolved and have undergone tremendous advancements over the years. The current scenario of all these modalities was a result of several path-breaking trials which have played a pivotal role in shaping breast imaging. This chapter highlights the several path-breaking trials which have played an indispensable role in evolution of breast imaging.

Keywords

Mammography · Ultrasound · Digital breast tomosynthesis · Synthesized mammogram · Stereotactic biopsy Contrast-enhanced mammogram Magnetic resonance imaging · Targeted axillary node dissection

19.1 Introduction

Breast cancer is the most common cancer and leading cause of mortality in females [1]. Early detection is crucial, as delayed diagnosis and advanced stage at presentation are associated with poor outcomes and decreased overall survival [1]. In the first half of the twentieth century, diagnosis was primarily based on clinical grounds, with most of the patients being diagnosed in the advanced stage of the disease, thus leading to poor prognosis and overall outcome [2]. In 1924, **Malvern Clopton** stated that "early breast cancer cannot be diagnosed by palpation or inspection", emphasising the need for surgical excision to make the diagnosis [3]. Attempts at obtaining surgical or in vivo breast radiographs in the 1920s and 1930s were unsuccessful due to extremely poor imaging quality. In the 1930s, **Stafford Warren and Lockwood**, in their individual works, successfully reported the usefulness of preoperative breast radiography to predict

P. Rana (✉)
Department of Radiology, UN Mehta Institute of Cardiology and Research Center, Ahmedabad, India

E. Dhamija
Department of Diagnostic and Interventional Onco-Radiology, IRCH, AIIMS, New Delhi, India

E. Dhamija, S. V. S. Deo (eds.), *Imaging in Management of Breast Diseases*,
https://doi.org/10.1007/978-981-96-4998-3_19

malignant and benign breast diseases but suffered the disadvantage of poor image quality [2, 4]. It was after the 1940s that a need for specialised breast imaging techniques was realised. In 1948, **Gershon-Cohen** demonstrated the feasibility of mammograms to depict occult breast cancer [5]. In 1960, **Egan** found mammograms to be useful for depicting unsuspected breast cancers [6].

Breast imaging since then has evolved overtime with tremendous advancements in technology, which have significantly affected mortality and made breast cancer a manageable disease. The routine use of mammographic screening has become much more widespread, expanding its coverage in lower-middle-income countries, primarily because of the positive results from randomised controlled trials and multi-institutional studies. Global usage of mammogram screening in asymptomatic women, along with an increasing level of general awareness of breast cancer as a public health problem, has prompted a series of governmental regulations, both at state and federal levels [7]. In developed nations like the United States, screening mammograms account for more than 75% of all mammography performed in the United States, thus detecting the smaller, nonpalpable lesions [8]. Notable evolution has taken place in the technique and technology of mammography, which has transitioned from the early days of direct-exposure film mammography to xeromammography to screen-film mammography to the current era of full-field digital mammogram (FFDM), digital breast tomosynthesis (DBT) and now contrast-enhanced mammograms (CEM). Not only mammogram, during the past several decades, substantial advancements in other breast imaging techniques, including ultrasonography (US), magnetic resonance imaging (MRI) and imaging-guided breast interventional procedures, have been witnessed. Alongside these, programmed screenings, federal regulations based on the Mammography Quality Standards Act and the development of the Breast Imaging Reporting and Data System (ACR BI-RADS) have helped to shape the specialty of breast imaging [9, 10]. Furthermore, we have entered the era of precision medicine, radiomics, radiogenomics and artificial intelligence for early detection, better characterisation and prognostication of breast cancer [11–13].

This chapter highlights the several path-breaking trials that have played an indispensable role in the evolution of breast imaging.

19.2 Mammogram

In the 1970s, most mammography was performed using the mammographic screen-film systems for mostly diagnostic indications in women with signs and symptoms of breast diseases [2]. Certain trials showed the pivotal role of mammogram in managing breast cancer and reducing the mortality associated with breast cancer [14–42]. There were takers on the other side as well, doubting and questioning its true role, highlighting the potential limitations such as radiation risk and unnecessary patient anxiety [43, 44]. Despite these hurdles, mammographic-based population screening gained widespread acceptance due to its unquestionable benefits and is currently implemented worldwide in most of the countries. The mortality benefit for the various age groups and the interval for screening continue to vary among the different nations, based on their local guidelines and population makeup.

The subsequent section discusses a few of the important studies that made mammogram a game changer for early detection of breast cancer. The first landmark study highlighting the importance of mammogram for early detection of breast cancer was carried out in the greater City of New York by a private insurance company (health insurance plan), in collaboration with **Sam Shapiro, Philip Strax and Louis Venet** and under the contract with the National Institutes of Health from 1963–1982. A total of 62,000 women aged 40–64 years were chosen at random from the members of the health insurance plan medical grounds, excluding women with a previous history of breast cancer or pregnant women. The mammogram was performed using the conventional Egan technique with no substantial breast compression, and mediolateral and craniocaudal views were obtained. The results demonstrated a higher proportion of breast cancer detection using mammography and clinical examination and subsequently a substantial reduction in mortality in the study group as compared to the control group (63 cancer-related deaths in the control group versus 40 in the study group) in women over the age of 50 years. The death rates for both groups were similar in women aged less than 50 years. The path-breaking results of the HIP **randomised controlled trial** encouraged several other multi-institutional screening studies for breast cancer detection [14, 15].

After the results of the HIP study in the 1970s, mammographic technique evolved with specialised mammographic tubes and adequate breast compression. In a 15-centre randomised screening trial, the reported sensitivity, specificity and positive predictive value of mammography were 0.75, 0.94 and 0.07, respectively [16].

The Swedish two-country trial estimated the long-term (29 years) effect of mammographic screening on breast cancer mortality. They found significant reduction in breast cancer mortality in women invited to screening according to both local end point committee data (relative risk [RR] = 0.69; 95% confidence interval: 0.56, 0.84; $P < 0.0001$) and consensus data (RR = 0.73; 95% confidence interval: 0.59, 0.89; $P = 0.002$). The updated results of the trial, in addition, also showed a better prognosis of the screen-detected cancers with smaller tumour sizes, node-negative tumours and lower grades at the time of detection [17–20].

The Malmo mammographic screening trial results also showed a 20% reduction in mortality from breast cancer in women aged 55 years and above with mammogram screening [21, 22].

The breast cancer demonstration projection in its initial round screened 8100 women aged 35 years and above and detected 67 women with breast cancer, predominantly in situ or minimal cancer. The highlights of the evidence of benefit for women aged 40–49 years from the 20-year follow-up of the BCDP showed that a high proportion of the cancers were detected by mammography alone and 28.6% of all the cancers were smaller than 1.0 cm. The adjusted survival rate for the entire group was 80.5%, and the observed survival rate was 61.7% [23–25].

The Edinburg randomised control trial recruited women aged 45–64 years from 1978 to 1981 (cohort 1) and those aged 45–49 years during 1982–1985 (cohorts 2 and 3). The result demonstrated difference in the study and control group in the mortality rates {rate ratio of 0.79 (95% CI 0.60–1.02)}, confirming the benefit of screening mammogram of lowering breast cancer mortality. However, at seven years follow-up, the mortality reduction achieved was 17% (relative risk = 0.83, 95% CI 0.58–1.18), which was not statistically significant, even when corrected for socioeconomic status [26, 27].

Tabar et al. investigated the efficacy of mass screening with single-view mammography in reducing mortality from breast cancer in Sweden. A 31% reduction in mortality and a 25% reduction in stage II or more advanced breast cancers were reported in the study group [28]. **Frisell et al**. undertook a randomised controlled trial in Stockholm for screening breast cancer in women between 40 and 64 years of age. The first round disclosed 128 breast cancers (113 invasive and 15 noninvasive) [29]. A study by **Addersson et al**. on 17,447 women demonstrated less advanced stages of breast cancer detected by screening in comparison to the control group [30].

The **Gothenburg breast cancer screening trial** evaluated 11,724 women aged 39–49 years with screening mammogram every 18 months. The results demonstrated a 44% reduction in mortality from breast cancer in the study group compared to the control group (relative risk [RR] = 0.56, $P = 0.042$, 95% confidence interval [CI]: 0.32–0.98). The updated results of the trial confirmed the mortality reduction benefit of mammogram, even in women younger than 50 years [31, 32].

The **UK Age Trial** evaluated the effect of mammographic screening from age 40 years on breast cancer mortality. They observed a significant reduction in breast cancer mortality at 10 years of follow-up, with 83 breast cancer deaths in the study group versus 219 in the control group (relative rate [RR] 0·75 [95% CI 0·58–0·97]; $p = 0·029$). They suggested reducing the lower age limit for screening from 50 to 40 years. The long-term follow-up of this trial also supported the initial results [33, 34].

The trial steering group also showed additional benefit in breast cancer mortality by reducing the age to 40–41 years [35]. **UKCCCR** trial showed two-view mammography to be medically more effective than one-view mammography. Two-view mammography detected 24% more women with breast cancer (95% confidence interval 16–31%) than one-view mammography [36]. **Warren et al.**, in their study on 33,734 women, also showed the advantage of adding the second view in screening mammogram [37].

On the other hand, the **Canadian National Breast Screening Studies 1 and 2** evaluated the efficacy of the combination of annual screening with mammography, physical examination of the breasts and the teaching of breast self-examination in reducing the rate of death from breast cancer among women aged 40–49 years and 50–59 years on entry, respectively. The results of both studies showed screen-detected breast cancer to be smaller and node-negative, however, with no impact on mortality from breast cancer. The 25-year follow-up of this trial also showed no reduction in mortality from breast cancer in women aged 40–59, with 22% overdiagnosis of screen-detected invasive breast cancer [38–42].

19.2.1 Switch to Digital Mammogram

With evolving techniques and digital technology, a digital system for mammography which used electronic image detectors instead of films was also introduced [2, 8]. During the initial period, several issues surfaced, like cost and doubtful diagnostic potential in comparison to screen-film mammography. However, with time, its advantages, including lower radiation dose, more accuracy in younger women and with dense breasts, no need for film development, etc., were realised, and currently, the vast majority of practices in various nations use full-field digital mammography (FFDM) systems [45, 46]. FFDM was approved by the US Food and Drug Administration in 2000 [47].

Few of the important clinical trials comparing FFDM with screen-film mammography:
The GE Senographe 2000 D trial led by Hendrick et al. compared the diagnostic accuracy of FFDM with screen-film mammogram in 641 women older than 40 years of age. This study showed a statistically significant, 2% reduction ($P < 0.001$) in the recall rate for FFDM versus that for screen-film mammograms, with no statistically significant difference in sensitivity and specificity between the two modalities [48].

The **Senoscan (Fischer imaging) FDA trial** also found no statistical difference between FFDM and screen-film mammogram in terms of sensitivity and specificity [49]. **Lewin et al.** compared the FFDM with screen-film mammography for cancer detection in 4954 examinations in women aged 40 years and older. Their results showed no significant difference in cancer detection rate; however, there were fewer recall rates and a higher positive biopsy rate with FFDM [50, 51].

Yamada et al., in their study on 480 women aged 50 years and above, showed no added benefit of screen-film mammograms over FFDM. The recall rate was not significantly different (2.9% with SFM vs. 4.2% with FFDM; $p = 0.253$). The positive predictive value was also not significantly different (14% with SFM vs. 10% with FFDM; $p = 0.69$) [52].

The Oslo 1 study (Norwegian senographe 2000D trial) also reported no statistically significant difference in cancer detection rate between FFDM and screen-film mammography [53]. However, the results of **Oslo II study** differed. They reported a significantly higher cancer detection rate with FFDM and comparable positive predictive value of both modalities [54].

The major landmark multi-institutional study, the **Digital Mammographic Imaging Screening Trial (DMIST)** of the American College of Radiology Imaging Network, comparing digital and analog mammography in a screening population, was the main game changer for the introduction of FFDM in screening settings. A total of 49,528 women were enrolled, who underwent both FFDM and screen-film mammography. The study demonstrated overall equivalence between the two techniques. However, for women younger than 50 years, pre- and perimenopausal women and women with heterogeneously dense or extremely dense breasts, digital mammography was more accurate than film mammography [55–57].

In a study by **Turco Del et al.,** a higher cancer detection rate for FFDM was noted over screen-film mammogram (0.72% vs. 0.58%, $p = 0.14$), particularly for cancers depicted as clustered microcalcifications (0.26% vs. 0.12%, $p = 0.007$), in younger (50–59 years) women (0.63% vs. 0.42%, $p = 0.09$) and in denser breasts (1.09% vs. 0.53%, $p = 0.24$) [58].

Vinnicombe et al., in a UK screening programme, reported no significant differences between FFDM and screen-film mammogram in terms of detection rates (0.68 [95% confidence interval {CI}: 0.47, 0.89] vs. 0.72 [95% CI: 0.58, 0.85], respectively, per 100 screening mammograms; $P = 0.74$), recall rates (3.2% [95% CI: 2.8, 3.6] vs. 3.4% [95% CI: 3.1, 3.6]; $P = 0.44$), positive predictive value (PPV) of an abnormal mammogram or characteristics of detected tumours. FFDM was found noninferior to screen-film mammogram in screen settings [59].

Hambly et al. reported a higher cancer detection rate for FFDM than screen-film mammography for initial screening and subsequent screening for invasive cancer and ductal carcinoma in situ and across all age groups. The cancer detection rate for cancers presenting as microcalcifications was also found to be significantly higher for FFDM than for screen-film mammography (1.9 vs. 1.3 per 1000, $p = 0.01$). The recall rate was significantly higher for FFDM than screen-film mammography (4.0% vs. 3.1%, $p < 0.001$). There was no significant difference in the PPVs of recall to assessment for FFDM and screen-film mammography (15.7% and 16.7%, $p = 0.383$) [60].

Fischman et al. compared the image quality and lesion detection for FFDM and screen-film mammography. They showed improved image quality with better depiction of microcalcification and nipple-areola region with FFDM, without the compromise on radiation dose [61]. **Karsseneujer et al.** also reported similar findings in their study on 56,518 digital mammogram [62].

Knox et al. studied the impact of FFDM on classification and mammographic characteristics of interval breast cancer. Although the rate of missed breast cancers did not differ between the FFDM and screen-film mammogram, there were significantly fewer cancers presenting as microcalcifications with the FFMD than with the screen-film mammogram (16% vs. 32%) [63].

19.2.2 The Evolution of Stereotactic-Guided Biopsy

With widespread implementation of the mammogram screening programmes, there was an increased detection rate of nonpalpable abnormalities such as microcalcifications, asymmetries and architectural distortion. Ultrasound correlate was available for a few of these screen-detected nonmass findings; however, the rest of the sonographically occult findings posed a diagnostic challenge. This paved the way for the introduction of stereotactic biopsy for determining the depth of the lesion; however, it had a significant error rate initially. Following this, an automated biopsy system was introduced, which led to much more precise lesion sampling. The famous Fischer prone table was modified to accommodate the stereotactic biopsy unit, which led to a more comfortable biopsy of the patients [64]. Currently, the stereotactic-guided biopsies and preoperative lesion localisation are state of the art for lesions not visualised on US and offer a good diagnostic yield. A study by **Fajardo et al.** determined the diagnostic accuracy of stereotactic and USG-guided core biopsy for diagnosing nonpalpable lesions. The sensitivity, specificity and accuracy by either imaging guidance method in this trial were 0.91, 1.00 and 0.98, respectively. The sensitivity, predictive value negative and accuracy for diagnosing masses (0.96, 0.99 and 0.99, respectively) were significantly greater ($P < 0.001$) than for calcifications (0.84, 0.94 and 0.96, respectively) [65].

19.2.3 Introduction to Digital Breast Tomosynthesis (DBT)

Screening mammogram for early detection and subsequent reduction of breast cancer mortality is now a widely accepted practice globally; however, recognised limitations of two-dimensional mammogram such as lower sensitivity in women with dense and texturally complex breasts and superimposed overlapping fibroglandular tissue with higher recall rates paved the way for the introduction of DBT [66]. In 1997, work by **Niklason et al**. demonstrated the feasibility of digital tomosynthesis using mastectomy specimens. Since then, many clinical studies have been undertaken investigating the role of DBT either alone or as an adjunct to FFDM [67]. The US Food and Drug Administration approved the first DBT commercial system for clinical use in 2011 [66].

Skaane et al. (Oslo Tomosynthesis Screening Trial) compared the FFDM alone and FFDM with DBT in a population-based screening programme. The cancer detection rate was found to be 6.1 per 1000 examinations for mammography alone and 8.0 per 1000 examinations for FFDM/DBT (27% increase, adjusted for reader; $P = 0.001$) [68]. Another prospective study by the same group (**OTST trial)** compared double readings when interpreting FFDM with DBT during a population-based screening programme and reported a significantly better cancer detection rate with double readings (7.1–9.4 per 1000). There was a reduction in false-positive rates from 10.3% to 8.5% [69].

Screening with tomosynthesis or standard mammography (STORM) trial included 7292 asymptomatic women aged 48 years and older for breast screening and compared conventional two-dimensional mammography with integrated two-dimensional and three-dimensional mammography/DBT. The results demonstrated higher cancer detection rates of two-dimensional/three-dimensional mammography in comparison to two-dimensional mammography. The incremental cancer detection rate attributable to integrated mammography was 2.7 cancers per 1000 screens, with a reduction in false-positive rates [70].

A malmo breast tomosynthesis screening trial was undertaken to assess the performance of one-view DBT as a stand-alone modality in breast cancer screening. Participants underwent one-view DBT and two-view FFDM, with independent double reading and scoring. The detection rate for one-view DBT was 8.9/1000 and 6.3/1000 for two-view FFDM ($p < 0.0001$). The recall rate was 3.8% for DBT and 2.6% for DM ($p < 0.0001$). The PPV was 24% for both DBT and FFDM [71].

The Proteus Donna study compared conventional FFDM with DBT in addition to FFDM over a period of approximately 3 years in population-based screening for women aged 46–68 years. The results demonstrated a lead time gain of DBT compared to DM, however, with an increase in false positives and moderate overdiagnosis [72].

The Reggio Emilia Tomosynthesis Randomised Trial compared FFDM plus DBT versus FFDM alone for breast cancer screening in women aged 45–70 years old. They reported a detection rate of 4.5 per 1000 and 8.6 per 1000, respectively. The greater detection rate for FFDM+DBT was stronger for ductal carcinoma in situ [73]. **Maxwell et al**. enrolled asymptomatic high-risk women aged 40–49 years to compare DBT + FFDM with FFDM alone and did not find any significant reduction in recall rate [74].

One of the potentially thought problems with the introduction of DBT for screening was the higher radiation dose per mammogram performed. However, several studies reported only a modest increase in radiation dose to the breast compared to FFDM.

Gennaro et al. compared the radiation dose delivered by FFDM and DBT for a single view and reported a modest increase in radiation dose to the breast by DBT compared to FFDM [75]. **Aase et al**., in their randomised controlled trial performed in Bergen (Breast Screen Norway), compared DBT with FFDM in a population-screen setting and reported significantly lower recall rates with DBT on the compromise of a higher readout time, with no significant increase in radiation dose [76]. *Another study by the similar group* assessed the distribution of findings of both the modalities and observed spiculated mass as the dominant feature for breast cancer among women screened with DBT, while calcifications were the most frequent feature for DM [77].

Recent results from the TOMMY **Trial** compared DBT with FFDM, which revealed improvement in AUC for the DBT group versus FFDM alone, with significantly improved specificity with DBT, higher sensitivity for invasive tumours of 11–20 mm in size and noninferior performance for depiction of microcalcifications [78].

The Tomosynthesis Mammography Imaging Screening Trial (TMIST) EA1151 is a randomised clinical trial (phase III) designed to assess the effectiveness for breast cancer screening with DBT compared to FFDM, which is currently under way [79].

Not only in the screen population, most of the studies report beneficial effects of DBT in the diagnostic settings as well. **MJ Michell et al**. reported improved sensitivity, specificity and overall diagnostic accuracy with DBT, with none of the malignant cases misinterpreted as benign or normal [80]. **Poplack et al**. also reported superior image quality for masses with lowered recall rates with DBT, however with inferior detection of microcalcifications [81]. Similar results were shown by **Waldherr et al**. with significantly improved sensitivity and negative predictive value [82].

Road to synthetic mammogram The growing use and benefits of DBT have now been well known; however, this increases the overall imaging time and the radiation doses, even if marginal [66]. Synthetic mammogram (SM) is a two-dimensional reconstruction of the tomosynthesis slice dataset that was designed to obviate the need for an additional FFDM. The US FDA approved SM for use in screening mammography in 2013 [83].

Earlier studies reported similar or even increased recall rates with SM/DBT (**Verona screening programme);** however, after the first large trial (**To-Be Trial, Norway**), the recall rates were found to be significantly improved with SM + DBT (3.1%) versus FFDM alone (4%) [84, 85].

A multicentre study by **Zuckerman et al**. also reported a significant reduction in recall rates of SM/DBT in comparison to FFDM/DBT with no significant difference in the positive predictive value [86]. The decreased recall rates with SM/DBT were further supported by meta-analysis and systematic review by **Alabousi et al**. They also reported the highest positive predictive value in patients screened with SM/DBT compared with those screened with FFDM alone, FFDM/DBT and DBT alone (16.0%, 10.0% and 7.0%, respectively) [87].

The **TOMSYMA trial** compared SM/DBT with FFDM alone in 99,689 women aged 50–69 years in Germany. They found 7.1 cancers per 1000 women in the SM/DBT group versus 4.8 cancers per 1000 women in the FFDM-alone group ($P < 0.0001$) [88–90]. **Hovda et al**., in their prospective study on women enrolled in the Breast Screen Norway programme, reported no significant difference in interval breast cancer rates and false-negative rates between the SM/DBT and FFDM groups [91]. In the **Trento trial**, the estimated interval cancer rate was not significantly different with SM versus FFDM (1.1 per 1000 vs. 1.36 per 1000) [92]. **Shin et al**., in their retrospective study on 189 patients, found DBT with synthetic mammogram to be superior to FFDM in terms of total diagnostic accuracy and lesion visibility for benign microcalcifications in dense breasts [93].

DBT-guided percutaneous procedures DBT has emerged as a powerful tool in screen and diagnostic settings, particularly for evaluation of architectural distortion, asymmetries and masses. The lesions detected on DBT should ideally be targeted on this modality, especially when the visibility on FFDM is poor and no correlate can be found on USG. DBT-guided biopsy or localisation would offer more accurate diagnostic yield in comparison to the traditional stereotactic-guided biopsy [94].

Bahl et al. compared the performance of upright DBT-guided vacuum-assisted breast biopsy (VABB) with that of prone stereotactic VABB and found a higher rate of technical success with DBT-guided biopsy, with lesser procedural time and radiation exposure. In addition, more architectural distortions and asymmetries were amenable to biopsy with DBT-guided biopsy [95]. **Ariaratnam et al**. also reported the beneficial role of DBT-guided biopsy for sonographically occult lesions [96].

19.3 Ultrasound and Magnetic Resonance Imaging

Mammogram is currently the gold standard screening tool for breast cancer and has shown to reduce the mortality rates due to breast cancer [97]. However, there are certain potential limitations of screening mammogram due to the intrinsic structural nature of the modality. There is significant underperformance in women with dense and texturally complex breasts, with reported sensitivity of 50–60% [98]. Moreover, women with extremely dense breasts have an increased risk of breast cancer. It lacks meaningful benefits for women aged 40–49 years. There is regional variation in occurrence of breast cancer, with 10–15 years earlier occurrence in Asian women compared to Western countries [99]. Additionally, Asian women, particularly of younger ages, tend to have denser breasts. There is also lower sensitivity of mammogram in carriers of BRCA mutation [100]. Another important potential challenge with mammogram is underdiagnosing the nonspiculated rapidly growing tumour subtypes (triple-negative, HER-2 Neu-positive group), which are especially more prone to develop in high-risk women. On the other hand, certain indolent cancers are often overdiagnosed with mammograms, which otherwise would have remained undetected throughout the woman's life [101, 102]. Despite the technical advancements in mammogram including DBT, the interval cancer rate remains substantially high (13–38%) [103]. These challenges are not only limited to the detection of lesions, but further lesion characterisation, treatment planning, response prediction and overall prognostication require additional imaging tools for optimal results. Another limitation is the availability of digital mammogram in underresource settings, which has contributed to unfavourable detection of breast cancer in low-income countries [104].

To overcome these potential challenges of mammogram, ultrasound (US) and dynamic contrast-enhanced breast MRI are now considered pivotal parts of breast imaging and treatment planning.

Ultrasound

USG is a low-cost, noninvasive, radiation-free modality which is easily available. With technological advancements like the introduction of high-frequency linear probes and automated breast US, its role in supplemental breast screening examination, characterisation of breast lesions, second-look tools in women with mammographically occult lesions and guided breast interventions has become indispensable. It is generally recommended as the primary modality in symptomatic women aged less than 35 years of age and an adjunct tool to mammogram for mammographically detected abnormalities. However, studies report conflicting results for the usage of US as a primary screening tool due to being an operator-dependent modality. Nevertheless, US shows a higher sensitivity and detection rate than mammogram, particularly in women with dense breasts or younger ages [105, 106].

A study by **Berg et al**. compared the diagnostic yield of screening US with mammogram versus mammogram alone in women at elevated risk of breast cancer. The study revealed the diagnostic yield for mammography of 7.6 per 1000 women (20 of 2637) as compared to 11.8 per 1000 for combined MG+ US. However, there was also a substantial increase in the false-positive rate. Another study by a similar group in women with high-risk of breast cancer reported 76% sensitivity, 84% specificity and 16% PPV with USG + MG in contrast to 52%, 91% and 38% for MG alone, respectively [107, 108].

A trial by **Corsetti et al**. evaluated the contribution of US in detecting breast cancer in women with dense breasts and negative mammogram. It showed early-stage detection of cancers in women with mammography-negative dense breasts, especially in women less than 50 years of age [109, 110]. A study by **Hooley et al**. also published similar results [111].

The J-START trial included 72,998 asymptomatic women aged 40–49 years from Japan to study the efficacy of US + FFDM in comparison to FFDM alone. They reported a significantly higher sensitivity with both modalities combined (91·1% vs. 77·0%, $p = 0.0004$) at the expense of lower specificity (87·7% vs. 91·4%, $p < 0.0001$) [112, 113].

Harada-Shoji et al. and Yamashita et al., in their respective studies, also demonstrated improved sensitivity of cancer detection in dense breasts with adjunctive US [114, 115]. **Benson et al**. also reported significantly better performance of US than mammography for detecting invasive breast cancer [116].

The added benefit of US for characterisation of breast lesions, especially detecting and characterisation of cystic lesions, dates back to the 1970s. Targeted US for breast complaints in younger women as the first-line technique and adjunctive US for lesions detected on mammogram is the standard of care applied at most of the places, with various studies showing the unmatched benefit of US for characterisation of breast lesions [117]. The recent **Breast US trial (BUST)** found US to be more accurate as a standalone breast imaging modality in the assessment of focal breast complaints in comparison to US plus DBT [118]. However, for further improved performance in characterising breast lesions, elastography was introduced. It was found useful in improving the specificity of US evaluation of BI-RADS 3 and 4A lesions. In a large study on 939 breast masses (**BE1 multinational study**), addition of elastography to B-mode US was found to significantly improve specificity (78.5% from 61.1%, $p < 0.001$) for characterisation of breast lesions [119]. In a randomised controlled trial by **Skerl et al**., anisotropy in a solid breast lesion was assessed to predict breast malignancy [120]. It found malignant lesions to be more anisotropic than benign lesions, especially the larger cancers. Shear wave elastography should be mentioned in the descriptors as per the fifth edition of the BIRADS lexicon.

Magnetic Resonance Imaging

The fundamentals of breast MRI revolve around its structural as well as the functional component of the imaging. The multiparametric MRI is based on the usage of contrast enhancement to depict neovascularity within the tumour in addition to its morphological features and has higher sensitivity in comparison to mammogram [103]. In a preliminary study on 20 patients, **Heywang et al**. showed promising results on using contrast-enhanced MRI to differentiate dysplastic scar tissue from carcinoma and in evaluation of dense breasts [121]. **Kaiser et al**. also reported similar observations in their study conducted around the same time [122]. These two studies paved the way for several multiinstitutional prospective studies to evaluate the role of breast MRI as a problem-solving diagnostic tool and an adjunct or independent breast screening modality. It remains a powerful modality as a screening tool in high-risk and intermediate-risk populations, a problem-solving tool for indeterminate lesions, presurgical staging in locally advanced breast cancer and an evaluation of response to chemotherapy [123].

Currently, it is recommended as a screening tool for women with high risk of breast cancer by multiple national and international guidelines. Women with a lifetime risk of more than 20% are considered a high-risk group, and the current recommendations in this subset included annual screening MRI and mammography. The coverage of screening MRI further expanded to include women with intermediate risk (15–20% lifetime risk), especially in women with personal histories of breast cancer and dense breasts. Currently, the American Cancer Society recommends against screening breast MRI in women at average risk; however, there is increasing evidence suggesting its positive performance even in women at average risk [124–129].

Few of the landmark studies highlighting the positive role of MRI in breast cancer detection: A screening study to evaluate the efficacy of MRI with that of mammogram for screening high-risk women was undertaken in 1909 women in the Netherlands. The reported sensitivity of clinical breast examination, mammography and MRI for detecting invasive breast cancer was 17.9%, 33.3% and 79.5%, respectively, and the specificity was 98.1%, 95.0% and 89.8%, respectively. The overall discriminating capacity of MRI was found to be significantly better than that of mammography ($P < 0.05$) [126].

The Dense Tissue and Early Neoplasm Screening (DENSE) trial was a randomised controlled trial conducted in the Netherlands to study the effect of supplemental magnetic resonance imaging (MRI) on the incidence of interval cancers in women with extremely dense breast tissue. A total of 40,373 women between the ages of 50 and 75 with extremely dense breast tissue and normal results on screening mammogram were enrolled in the study, and a subset of these women underwent supplemental MRI screening. The results concluded the substantial benefit of supplemental MRI screening in women with extremely dense breast tissue and normal results on mammography during a 2-year screening period [130]. The results of the second screening round of the **DENSE Trial** were even more promising, with a strong reduction in the number of false-positive results [131].

Berg et al., in their multiinstitutional study, determined the supplemental cancer detection yield of US and MRI in women at elevated risk of breast cancer. Their results suggested a higher yield of cancer detected on addition of MRI to mammogram in women with elevated risk of breast cancer (14.7 per 1000 (95% CI, 3.5–25.9; $P = 0.004$), although with a potential caveat of higher false-positive findings [108].

Kuhl et al., in their prospective observation study on 2120 women, showed additional detection of 60 breast cancers with breast MRI with an overall supplemental cancer detection rate of 15.5 per 1000 cases, a specificity of 97.1% and a PPV of 35.7% [132].

Despite these path-breaking studies clearly showing the added benefit of breast MRI in screen settings, wide spread coverage remains limited due to the cost, time and limited accessibility of the modality. Adherence to MRI screening even in the eligible high-risk women remains suboptimal [133].

To overcome these challenges of conventional breast MRI, the breakthrough concept of reducing the acquisition time of MRI was introduced in 2014, and the introduction of abbreviated MRI was proposed.

Kuhl et al. conducted a prospective observational reader study in 443 women with mild to moderate increased risk of breast cancer who underwent screening mammogram. The women included in the study had normal or benign findings on digital mammogram. An abbreviated MRI protocol was proposed, consisting of only one precontrast acquisition followed by post-contrast image acquisition, and first postcontrast subtracted (FAST) and maximum-intensity projection (MIP) images were studied. The abbreviated MRI protocol was compared with the conventional full diagnostic protocol. The reported specificity and positive predictive value of the abbreviated protocol were 94.3% and 24.4%, respectively, which was equivalent to the full diagnostic protocol. With an acquisition time of 3 min, an expert MIP image reading time of 2 s and a negative predictive value of 99.8%, abbreviated MRI was sort of a potential tool in breast cancer screening [134].

Several other studies also showed promising results for the usage of abbreviated MRI as a stand-alone or supplemental screening tool for breast cancer [135, 136]. The methods and protocol of abbreviated MRI continue to evolve.

Harvey et al. evaluated the ability of an abbreviated, high-risk screening breast MRI protocol for breast cancer detection. They demonstrated a significant reduction in scan acquisition time and interpretation times with no significant difference in cancer detection yield with abbreviated MRI in comparison to the conventional MRI [137]. Similar results were shown in a prospective study by **Panigrahi et al**. [138].

The EA1141 Trial is a prospective multicentre trial study for comparison of abbreviated breast MRI and DBT in breast cancer screening with dense breasts for asymptomatic average-risk category females aged 40–75 years. The trial was initiated in November 2016, intended to cover multiple international sites. Apart from its usage as a screening method, this study intended to address another important issue of overdiagnosis of low-grade indolent breast cancers by mammographic screening. The study results demonstrated 2.45-fold higher cancer detection using abbreviated MRI (15.2 per 1000 at prevalence screening) compared with DBT (6.2 per 1000), while the specificity was lower for abbreviated MRI in comparison to DBT (87% vs. 97%) [139].

A single-institutional prospective study on 246 participants compared the diagnostic performance of CEM, abbreviated MRI and standard full protocol MRI. The study results demonstrated significantly lower cancer detection rate (22.4 vs. 36.6) and sensitivity (61.1% vs. 100%) of CEM in comparison to standard MRI but lower recall rate (14.0% vs. 22.8%), lower false-positive biopsy recommendation rate per 1000 examinations (65.0 vs. 162.6) and higher specificity (87.8% vs. 80.2%). The performance differences between CEM and abbreviated MRI were similar to those observed between CEM and standard MRI. This study highlights the importance of further consideration of patient population characteristics before widespread screening with CEM [140].

Based on the concept of neoangiogenesis within the cancer with different enhancement kinetics of normal and/or benign tissue and that of malignant lesions, ultrafast MRI evolved, which may or may not be a part of abbreviated MRI. It captures early contrast material washin at high temporal resolution within the lesion using special sequences such as TWIST (time-resolved angiography with interleaved stochastic trajectories) and TRICKS (time-resolved imaging of contrast kinetics). Although ultrafast MRI is still highly investigational, early studies have shown that it has the potential to significantly improve the specificity while maintaining the sensitivity. It suffers the disadvantage of lower spatial resolution as a trade-off for higher temporal resolution, but the technique continues to evolve [141–144].

Diffusion-weighted imaging is currently part of the multiparametric MRI protocol for detection of breast cancer. A systematic review and meta-analysis by **Potsch et al**. found a pooled sensitivity and specificity of noncontrast DWI of 86.5% and 83.5%. The sensitivity of CE MRI was higher than noncontrast DWI (95.1% vs. 88.9%) while the specificity was comparable (82.2% vs. 82.0%). The sensitivity and specificity of noncontrast DWI and mammography were not found to be statistically different. Despite these promising results, further validation is needed with larger randomised controlled trials before clinical implementation [145].

MRI-guided biopsy Breast MRI is an established imaging modality for breast cancer, with higher detection of smaller and indeterminate lesions that need to be histologically proven to guide patient management. Most of the time, the lesions seen on MRI can be identified on second-look USG; however, in a subset of patients, a conclusive correlative finding cannot be obtained, which would require MRI-guided sampling. While the learning curve for this technique remains higher with technical challenges, the diagnostic yield has shown to be promising [146].

A study by **Lambert et al**. reported that MRI-guided VABB could obtain a larger yield of clinically relevant lesions with a false-negative biopsy rate of only 0.3% on a long-term follow-up of 7.6 years [147]. **Spick et al**. included 487 MR-guided VABB and showed it to be an accurate procedure for diagnosing MRI-only lesions with an agreement of 95.5% between the MRI-guided sample and the final diagnosis [148].

On the other hand, **Pinnamaneni et al**. conducted a study on the breast lesion outcome in patients after a cancelled MRI-guided biopsy due to nonvisualisation of the lesion and reported the majority of lesions got resolved on follow-up [149]. Therefore, due to its limited availability, smaller lesions are often followed up rather than referring for a guided biopsy, which is costly and time consuming.

19.4 Contrast-Enhanced Mammogram

FFDM and DBT rely on the detection of structural changes in the breast, and they play a pivotal role in breast cancer screening and assessment of patients. However, the accuracy is limited in women with dense breasts, and although supplemental imaging with US and especially MRI was found to be superior in such scenarios, these modalities had their own limitations. The cost, limited availability of equipment and expertise for MRI are major concerns in low- to middle-income countries. Contrast-enhanced mammogram (CEM) emerged as a functional imaging tool that uses iodinated contrast for the visualisation of breast neovascularity using the same mammography equipment with certain upgrades. It offers the advantage of easier accessibility, lower cost and scan time in comparison to MRI. In addition, the learning curve has been less steep as compared to MRI. The studies have evaluated its role for assessment of abnormalities detected in the screening population and reported higher sensitivity as well as specificity of CEM compared with FFDM. Recent studies have shown promising results where CEM has been found to outperform FFDM for diagnostic evaluation of women with palpable masses, assessment of extent of local disease and monitoring response to chemotherapy [150–152].

Currently, contrast-enhanced breast MRI is recommended for women at high risk for developing breast cancer and in certain subsets of women with intermediate risk. Despite attempts to reduce the scan time and protocol of MRI, it is still difficult to accommodate a large number of patients requiring breast MRI with additional cost issues, especially in a country like ours. Since CEM has shown to have additional benefits over structural imaging modalities, it can be a promising tool in comparison to MRI [153]. A prospective pilot study by **Jochelson et al.** reported the specificity of CEDM and MRI were 94.7% and 94.1%, respectively, in detected new cancers [154].

The CONTRRAST trial compared CEM with MRI in asymptomatic females and reported the mean AUC for DM, CEM, abbreviated MRI and full-protocol MRI as 0.79, 0.91, 0.89 and 0.91, respectively. CEM was found superior to digital mammography ($P < 0.001$) [155]. **Geel et al.** also showed superior diagnostic performance of CEM in comparison to FFDM, with quicker identification of abnormalities on recombined images in comparison to low-energy images [156].

An ongoing prospective **Tomosynthesis or Contrast-Enhanced Mammography, or TOCEM, trial** includes three annual screenings with both DBT and CEM in women with a personal history of breast cancer. The interim analysis has shown increased early breast cancer detection each year, with an increase of 5.0–6.6% recall rate on addition of CEM to DBT [157].

Contrast-enhanced mammography imaging screening trial (CMIST) is currently underway with the aim to determine whether CEM improves breast cancer detection for women with dense breasts [158]. With all these advances and additional lesions being picked up on CEM, **CEM-guided breast biopsy** is also being explored as an alternative method to MRI-guided biopsy, and the initial results of sampling under CEM guidance have been promising. **Alcantara et al.** evaluated the feasibility of CEM-guided biopsy for suspicious enhancing lesions and reported a success rate of 95.4% with a median total time per procedure of 15 min [159]. Similar results were shown by a large single-centre prospective study by **Kornecki et al.** [160].

19.5 Contrast-Enhanced Ultrasound

Contrast-enhanced ultrasound (CEUS) has created a significant opportunity for visualising microcirculation compared with traditional US techniques. Based on the concept of depicting neoangiogenesis in breast cancer, it has been extensively applied for various applications in breast imaging, including lesion characterisation, depicting the molecular subtype and response to chemotherapy. In a recent meta-analysis by **Wang et al.**, the reported pooled sensitivity and specificity for CEUS diagnosing malignant breast lesions were 0.87 [95% confidence intervals (CI), 0.81–0.90] and 0.79 (95% CI, 0.73–0.84), respectively, in the breast [161]. **Yan et al.** established a nomogram model, incorporating clinical data and imaging features of US and CEUS, for improving the diagnostic efficiency of solid breast lesions. As compared to the BI-RADS model, the nomogram model demonstrated satisfactory discriminative function with area under the receiver operating characteristic [ROC] curves [AUC] as 0.940 (95% confidence interval [CI] 0.909–0.971), sensitivity of 90.5% and specificity of 90.2% in the training cohort, and AUC, 0.968 (95% CI 0.941 to 0.995), sensitivity 97.1% and specificity 86.7% in the validation cohort [162].

Although the modality has not been able to find its place in the current imaging protocol, larger prospective studies are needed to assess its utility before clinical application.

19.6 Beyond the Breast: Imaging the Axilla

Management of axilla in breast cancer has significantly undergone changes in the past several decades. Before the mid-1990s, axillary lymph node dissection (ALND) was the main staging modality for locoregional lymph node disease, even in early breast cancer. It was in the late 1990s, the concept of sentinel lymph node (SLN) sampling gained importance and revolutionised staging.

Imaging currently plays a crucial role for pre-operative evaluation of axilla in clinically node negative patients. Image-guided sampling and localisation of positive lymph nodes prior to chemotherapy play a crucial role in targeted axillary dissection. The features of malignant lymph nodes are well described in the literature, and US remains the most commonly used and the technique of choice for imaging the axilla [163, 164].

The national surgical adjuvant breast and bowel project (NSABP) B-32 trial is one of the largest studies which evaluated the safety and efficacy of sentinel lymph node biopsy (SLNB). The results of the study showed no statistically significant difference in overall survival, disease-free survival and regional control for SLNB alone versus SLNB and ALND, with lesser rates of postoperative complications in the SLNB group [165].

The ACOSOG ZOO11 trial also reported a 10-year overall survival in women with T1 or T2 invasive primary breast cancer with no palpable axillary adenopathy and 1 or 2 sentinel lymph nodes containing metastases, treated with SLND alone, to be noninferior to overall survival for those treated with ALND [166].

A recent multicentre study by **Boniface et al. (SENOMAC trial)** also found omission of completion ALND to be noninferior to the more extensive surgery in patients with clinically node-negative breast cancer who had sentinel-node macrometastases, most of whom received nodal radiation therapy [167].

The SLNB gained widespread acceptance over time; however, the utility of SLN surgery after neoadjuvant chemotherapy was questioned due to high reported false-negative rates. An ACOSOG **Z1071** clinical trial was undertaken to determine the false-negative rates for SLN surgery following chemotherapy in patients initially presenting with biopsy-proven node-positive breast cancer. The false-negative rate (FNR) of SLND postchemotherapy was 13% in patients with stage T0–T4, N1–N2 and M0 breast cancer [168]. The SENTINA **study** also reported a higher FNR, precluding the use of standard SLND in patients converted to node-negative status after completion of chemotherapy [169]. *These reports suggested a change in approach and patient selection for greater sensitivity required for SLN surgery over ALND.*

This paved the way for the concept of targeted axillary dissection (TAD). A marker is inserted in a suspicious node prior to neoadjuvant chemo-

therapy, which allows for a targeted axillary dissection along with SLND. A study by **Kuemmel et al. reported** excellent clinical outcomes with TAD without ALND in a select group of patients [170]. A recent multi-institutional study highlighted that the 3-year cumulative incidence of axillary recurrence did not differ between TAD and SLNB (0.5% vs. 0.8%; $P = 0.55$), thus favouring the omission of ALND in node-negative patients after neoadjuvant chemotherapy [171]. Although TAD does seem like a promising alternative, further larger trials are needed for its validation and widespread application.

19.7 Conclusion

Breast cancer imaging continues to evolve. It is the large prospective multi-institutional trials which have shaped the current subspeciality of breast imaging. Further studies and validation are needed for broadening the horizon and overcoming the current challenges.

References

1. Wilkinson L, Gathani T. Understanding breast cancer as a global health concern. Br J Radiol. 2022;95(1130):20211033.
2. Joe BN, Sickles EA. The evolution of breast imaging: past to present. Radiology. 2014;273(2 Suppl):S23–44.
3. Clopton MB. The difficulty of diagnosis of carcinoma of the breast. Radiology. 1925;4(5):390–4.
4. Lockwood H. The value of breast radiography. Radiology. 1934;23(2):202–7.
5. Ingleby H, Gershon-Cohen J. Comparative anatomy, pathology and roentgenology of the breast. Philadelphia: University of Pennsylvania Press; 1960.
6. Egan RL. Experience with mammography in a tumor institution: evaluation of 1,000 studies. Radiology. 1960;75(6):894–900.
7. Ren W, Chen M, Qiao Y, Zhao F. Global guidelines for breast cancer screening: a systematic review. Breast. 2022;64:85–99.
8. Sickles EA. Breast imaging: from 1965 to the present. Radiology. 2000;215(1):1–16.
9. Houn F, Elliott ML, McCrohan JL. The mammography quality standards act of 1992. History and philosophy. Radiol Clin North Am. 1995;33(6):1059–65.
10. Sickles EA, D'Orsi CJ, Bassett LW, et al. ACR BI-RADS mammography. In: ACR BI-RADS atlas breast imaging re- porting and data system 2013. 5th ed. Reston: American College of Radiology; 2013. p. 1–175.
11. Grimm LJ, Mazurowski MA. Breast cancer radiogenomics: current status and future directions. Acad Radiol. 2020;27(1):39–46.
12. Yala A, Lehman C, Schuster T, Portnoi T, Barzilay R. A deep learning mammography-based model for improved breast cancer risk prediction. Radiology. 2019;292(1):60–6.
13. Dembrower K, Liu Y, Azizpour H, Eklund M, Smith K, Lindholm P, et al. Comparison of a deep learning risk score and standard mammographic density score for breast cancer risk prediction. Radiology. 2020;294(2):265–72.
14. Strax P, Venet L, Shapiro S. Value of mammography in reduction of mortality from breast cancer in mass screening. Am J Roentgenol Radium Ther Nucl Med. 1973;117(3):686–9.
15. Shapiro S. Periodic screening for breast cancer: the HIP randomized controlled trial. Health insurance plan. J Natl Cancer Inst Monogr. 1997;22:27–30.
16. Baines CJ, McFarlane DV, Miller AB. Sensitivity and specificity of first screen mammography in 15 NBSS centres. Can Assoc Radiol J. 1988;39(4):273–6.
17. Tabár L, Fagerberg G, Day NE, Duffy SW. The Swedish two-county trial of mammographic screening for breast cancer: recent results on mortality and tumor characteristics. Pathol Biol. 1992;39(9):846.
18. Tabar L, Duffy SW, Burhenne LW. New Swedish breast cancer detection results for women aged 40–49. Cancer. 1993;72(4 Suppl):1437–48.
19. Tabár L, Vitak B, Chen TH, Yen AM, Cohen A, Tot T, et al. Swedish two-county trial: impact of mammographic screening on breast cancer mortality during 3 decades. Radiology. 2011;260(3):658–63.
20. Yen AM, Duffy SW, Chen TH, Chen LS, Chiu SY, Fann JC, et al. Long-term incidence of breast cancer by trial arm in one county of the Swedish two-county trial of mammographic screening. Cancer. 2012;118(23):5728–32.
21. Andersson I, Aspegren K, Janzon L, Landberg T, Lindholm K, Linell F, et al. Mammographic screening and mortality from breast cancer: the Malmö mammographic screening trial. BMJ. 1988;297(6654):943–8.
22. Zackrisson S, Andersson I, Janzon L, Manjer J, Garne JP. Rate of over-diagnosis of breast cancer 15 years after end of Malmö mammographic screening trial: follow-up study. BMJ. 2006;332(7543):689–92.
23. Moskowitz M, Pemmaraju S, Fidler JA, Sutorius DJ, Russell P, Scheinok P, et al. On the diagnosis of minimal breast cancer in a screenee population. Cancer. 1976;37(5):2543–52.
24. Seidman H, Gelb SK, Silverberg E, LaVerda N, Lubera JA. Survival experience in the breast cancer detection demonstration project. CA Cancer J Clin. 1987;37(5):258–90.

25. Smart CR. Highlights of the evidence of benefit for women aged 40–49 years from the 14-year follow-up of the breast cancer detection demonstration project. Cancer. 1994;74(1 Suppl):296–300.
26. Roberts MM, Alexander FE, Anderson TJ, Chetty U, Donnan PT, Forrest P, et al. Edinburgh trial of screening for breast cancer: mortality at seven years. Lancet. 1990;335(8684):241–6.
27. Alexander FE, Anderson TJ, Brown HK, Forrest AP, Hepburn W, Kirkpatrick AE, et al. 14 years of follow-up from the Edinburgh randomised trial of breast-cancer screening. Lancet. 1999;353(9168):1903–8.
28. Tabár L, Fagerberg CJ, Gad A, Baldetorp L, Holmberg LH, Gröntoft O, et al. Reduction in mortality from breast cancer after mass screening with mammography. Randomised trial from the Breast Cancer Screening Working Group of the Swedish National Board of Health and Welfare. Lancet. 1985;1(8433):829–32.
29. Frisell J, Glas U, Hellström L, Somell A. Randomized mammographic screening for breast cancer in Stockholm. Design, first round results and comparisons. Breast Cancer Res Treat. 1986;8(1):45–54.
30. Andersson I, Andrén L, Hildell J, Linell F, Ljungqvist U, Pettersson H. Breast cancer screening with mammography: a population-based, randomized trial with mammography as the only screening mode. Radiology. 1979;132(2):273–6.
31. Bjurstam N, Björneld L, Duffy SW, Smith TC, Cahlin E, Erikson O, et al. The Gothenburg breast cancer screening trial: preliminary results on breast cancer mortality for women aged 39–49. J Natl Cancer Inst Monogr. 1997;22:53–5.
32. Bjurstam NG, Björneld LM, Duffy SW. Updated results of the Gothenburg trial of mammographic screening. Cancer. 2016;122(12):1832–5.
33. Duffy SW, Vulkan D, Cuckle H, Parmar D, Sheikh S, Smith RA, et al. Effect of mammographic screening from age 40 years on breast cancer mortality (UK age trial): final results of a randomised, controlled trial. Lancet Oncol. 2020;21(9):1165–72.
34. Duffy S, Vulkan D, Cuckle H, Parmar D, Sheikh S, Smith R, et al. Annual mammographic screening to reduce breast cancer mortality in women from age 40 years: long-term follow-up of the UK age RCT. Health Technol Assess. 2020;24(55):1–24.
35. Moss S. A trial to study the effect on breast cancer mortality of annual mammographic screening in women starting at age 40. J Med Screen. 1999;6(3):144–8.
36. Wald NJ, Murphy P, Major P, Parkes C, Townsend J, Frost C. UKCCCR multicentre randomised controlled trial of one and two view mammography in breast cancer screening. BMJ. 1995;311(7014):1189–93.
37. Warren RM, Duffy SW, Bashir S. The value of the second view in screening mammography. Br J Radiol. 1996;69(818):105–8.
38. Miller AB, Baines CJ, To T, Wall C. Canadian National Breast Screening Study: 1. Breast cancer detection and death rates among women aged 40 to 49 years. CMAJ. 1992;147(10):1459–76. Erratum in: Can Med Assoc J 1993 Mar 1;148(5):718.
39. Miller AB, Baines CJ, To T, Wall C. Canadian National Breast Screening Study: 2. Breast cancer detection and death rates among women aged 50 to 59 years. CMAJ. 1992;147(10):1477–88. Erratum in: Can Med Assoc J 1993 Mar 1;148(5):718.
40. Miller AB, To T, Baines CJ, Wall C. The Canadian National Breast Screening Study: update on breast cancer mortality. J Natl Cancer Inst Monogr. 1997;22:37–41.
41. Miller AB, To T, Baines CJ, Wall C. The Canadian National Breast Screening Study-1: breast cancer mortality after 11 to 16 years of follow-up. A randomized screening trial of mammography in women age 40 to 49 years. Ann Intern Med. 2002;137(5 Part 1):305–12.
42. Miller AB, Wall C, Baines CJ, Sun P, To T, Narod SA. Twenty five year follow-up for breast cancer incidence and mortality of the Canadian National Breast Screening Study: randomised screening trial. BMJ. 2014;348:g366.
43. Yaffe MJ, Mainprize JG. Risk of radiation-induced breast cancer from mammographic screening. Radiology. 2011;258(1):98–105.
44. Sutton S, Saidi G, Bickler G, Hunter J. Does routine screening for breast cancer raise anxiety? Results from a three wave prospective study in England. J Epidemiol Community Health. 1995;49(4):413–8.
45. Gater L. Digital mammography: state of the art. Radiol Technol. 2002;73(5):445–57. quiz 458-60.
46. Pisano ED, Yaffe MJ. Digital mammography. Radiology. 2005;234(2):353–62.
47. Gold LS, Klein G, Carr L, Kessler L, Sullivan SD. The emergence of diagnostic imaging technologies in breast cancer: discovery, regulatory approval, reimbursement, and adoption in clinical guidelines. Cancer Imaging. 2012;12(1):13–24.
48. Hendrick RE, Lewin JM, D'Orsi CJ, et al. Non-inferiority study of FFDM in an enriched diagnostic cohort: comparison with screen-film mammography in 625 women. In: Yaffe MJ, editor. IWDM 2000: 5th international workshop on digital mammography. Madison: Medical Physics; 2001. p. 475–81.
49. Cole E, Pisano ED, Brown M, Kuzmiak C, Braeuning MP, Kim HH, et al. Diagnostic accuracy of Fischer Senoscan Digital Mammography versus screen-film mammography in a diagnostic mammography population. Acad Radiol. 2004;11(8):879–86.
50. Lewin JM, Hendrick RE, D'Orsi CJ, Isaacs PK, Moss LJ, Karellas A, et al. Comparison of full-field digital mammography with screen-film mammography for cancer detection: results of 4,945 paired examinations. Radiology. 2001;218(3):873–80.
51. Lewin JM, D'Orsi CJ, Hendrick RE, Moss LJ, Isaacs PK, Karellas A, et al. Clinical comparison of full-field digital mammography and screen-film mammography for detection of breast cancer. AJR Am J Roentgenol. 2002;179(3):671–7.

52. Yamada T, Ishibashi T, Sato A, Saito M, Saito H, Matsuhashi T, et al. Comparison of screen-film and full-field digital mammography: image contrast and lesion characterization. Radiat Med. 2003;21(4):166–71.
53. Skaane P, Young K, Skjennald A. Population-based mammography screening: comparison of screen-film and full-field digital mammography with soft-copy reading–Oslo I study. Radiology. 2003;229(3):877–84.
54. Skaane P, Hofvind S, Skjennald A. Randomized trial of screen-film versus full-field digital mammography with soft-copy reading in population-based screening program: follow-up and final results of Oslo II study. Radiology. 2007;244(3):708–17.
55. Pisano ED, Gatsonis CA, Yaffe MJ, Hendrick RE, Tosteson AN, Fryback DG, et al. American College of Radiology Imaging Network digital mammographic imaging screening trial: objectives and methodology. Radiology. 2005;236(2):404–12.
56. Pisano ED, Gatsonis C, Hendrick E, Yaffe M, Baum JK, Acharyya S, et al. Digital mammographic imaging screening trial (DMIST) investigators group. Diagnostic performance of digital versus film mammography for breast-cancer screening. N Engl J Med. 2005;353(17):1773–83.
57. Galen B, Staab E, Sullivan DC, Pisano ED. Congressional update: report from the Biomedical Imaging Program of the National Cancer Institute. American College of Radiology Imaging Network: the digital mammographic imaging screening trial–an update. Acad Radiol. 2002;9(3):374–5.
58. Del Turco MR, Mantellini P, Ciatto S, Bonardi R, Martinelli F, Lazzari B, et al. Full-field digital versus screen-film mammography: comparative accuracy in concurrent screening cohorts. AJR Am J Roentgenol. 2007;189(4):860–6.
59. Vinnicombe S, Pinto Pereira SM, McCormack VA, Shiel S, Perry N, Dos Santos Silva IM. Full-field digital versus screen-film mammography: comparison within the UK breast screening program and systematic review of published data. Radiology. 2009;251(2):347–58.
60. Hambly NM, McNicholas MM, Phelan N, Hargaden GC, O'Doherty A, Flanagan FL. Comparison of digital mammography and screen-film mammography in breast cancer screening: a review in the Irish breast screening program. AJR Am J Roentgenol. 2009;193(4):1010–8.
61. Fischmann A, Siegmann KC, Wersebe A, Claussen CD, Müller-Schimpfle M. Comparison of full-field digital mammography and film-screen mammography: image quality and lesion detection. Br J Radiol. 2005;78(928):312–5.
62. Karssemeijer N, Bluekens AM, Beijerinck D, Deurenberg JJ, Beekman M, Visser R, et al. Breast cancer screening results 5 years after introduction of digital mammography in a population-based screening program. Radiology. 2009;253(2):353–8.
63. Knox M, O'Brien A, Szabó E, Smith CS, Fenlon HM, McNicholas MM, et al. Impact of full field digital mammography on the classification and mammographic characteristics of interval breast cancers. Eur J Radiol. 2015;84(6):1056–61.
64. Chakrabarthi S. Stereotactic breast biopsy: a review & applicability in the Indian context. Indian J Med Res. 2021;154(2):237–47.
65. Fajardo LL, Pisano ED, Caudry DJ, Gatsonis CA, Berg WA, Connolly J, et al. Radiologist investigators of the radiologic diagnostic oncology group V. Stereotactic and sonographic large-core biopsy of nonpalpable breast lesions: results of the radiologic diagnostic oncology group V study. Acad Radiol. 2004;11(3):293–308.
66. Vedantham S, Karellas A, Vijayaraghavan GR, Kopans DB. Digital breast tomosynthesis: state of the art. Radiology. 2015;277(3):663–84.
67. Niklason LT, Niklason LE, Kopans DB, Inventors; the General Hospital Corp, original assignee. Tomosynthesis system for breast imaging. USPTO 5872828 A. February 16, 1999.
68. Skaane P, Bandos AI, Gullien R, Eben EB, Ekseth U, Haakenaasen U, et al. Comparison of digital mammography alone and digital mammography plus tomosynthesis in a population-based screening program. Radiology. 2013;267(1):47–56.
69. Skaane P, Bandos AI, Gullien R, Eben EB, Ekseth U, Haakenaasen U, et al. Prospective trial comparing full-field digital mammography (FFDM) versus combined FFDM and tomosynthesis in a population-based screening programme using independent double reading with arbitration. Eur Radiol. 2013;23:2061–71.
70. Ciatto S, Houssami N, Bernardi D, Caumo F, Pellegrini M, Brunelli S, et al. Integration of 3D digital mammography with tomosynthesis for population breast-cancer screening (STORM): a prospective comparison study. Lancet Oncol. 2013;14(7):583–9.
71. Lång K, Andersson I, Rosso A, Tingberg A, Timberg P, Zackrisson S. Performance of one-view breast tomosynthesis as a stand-alone breast cancer screening modality: results from the Malmö breast tomosynthesis screening trial, a population-based study. Eur Radiol. 2016;26(1):184–90.
72. Armaroli P, Frigerio A, Correale L, Ponti A, Artuso F, Casella D, et al. A randomised controlled trial of digital breast tomosynthesis vs digital mammography as primary screening tests: screening results over subsequent episodes of the Proteus Donna study. Int J Cancer. 2022;151(10):1778–90.
73. Pattacini P, Nitrosi A, Giorgi Rossi P, Iotti V, Ginocchi V, Ravaioli S, et al. Digital mammography versus digital mammography plus Tomosynthesis for breast cancer screening: the Reggio Emilia Tomosynthesis randomized trial. Radiology. 2018;288(2):375–85.
74. Maxwell AJ, Michell M, Lim YY, Astley SM, Wilson M, Hurley E, et al. A randomised trial of screening with digital breast tomosynthesis plus conventional digital 2D mammography versus 2D mammography

alone in younger higher risk women. Eur J Radiol. 2017;94:133–9.
75. Gennaro G, Bernardi D, Houssami N. Radiation dose with digital breast tomosynthesis compared to digital mammography: per-view analysis. Eur Radiol. 2018;28(2):573–81.
76. Aase HS, Holen ÅS, Pedersen K, Houssami N, Haldorsen IS, Sebuødegård S, et al. A randomized controlled trial of digital breast tomosynthesis versus digital mammography in population-based screening in Bergen: interim analysis of performance indicators from the To-Be trial. Eur Radiol. 2019;29(3):1175–86.
77. Aase HS, Danielsen AS, Hoff SR, Holen ÅS, Haldorsen IS, Hovda T, et al. Mammographic features and screening outcome in a randomized controlled trial comparing digital breast tomosynthesis and digital mammography. Eur J Radiol. 2021;141:109753.
78. Gilbert FJ, Tucker L, Gillan MG, Willsher P, Cooke J, Duncan KA, et al. The TOMMY trial: a comparison of TOMosynthesis with digital MammographY in the UK NHS Breast Screening Programme–a multicentre retrospective reading study comparing the diagnostic performance of digital breast tomosynthesis and digital mammography with digital mammography alone. Health Technol Assess. 2015;19(4):i–xxv.
79. Maki AK, Mawdsley GE, Mainprize JG, Pisano E, Shen SZ, Alonzo-Proulx O, et al. Audit of data from examination image headers collected for quality assurance in the ECOG-ACRIN EA1151 tomosynthesis mammographic imaging screening trial (TMIST). Med Phys. 2023;50(12):7427–40.
80. Michell MJ, Iqbal A, Wasan RK, Evans DR, Peacock C, Lawinski CP, et al. A comparison of the accuracy of film-screen mammography, full-field digital mammography, and digital breast tomosynthesis. Clin Radiol. 2012;67(10):976–81.
81. Poplack SP, Tosteson TD, Kogel CA, Nagy HM. Digital breast tomosynthesis: initial experience in 98 women with abnormal digital screening mammography. AJR Am J Roentgenol. 2007;189(3):616–23.
82. Waldherr C, Cerny P, Altermatt HJ, Berclaz G, Ciriolo M, Buser K, et al. Value of one-view breast tomosynthesis versus two-view mammography in diagnostic workup of women with clinical signs and symptoms and in women recalled from screening. AJR Am J Roentgenol. 2013;200(1):226–31.
83. Chikarmane SA, Offit LR, Giess CS. Synthetic mammography: benefits, drawbacks, and pitfalls. Radiographics. 2023;43(10):e230018.
84. Caumo F, Romanucci G, Hunter K, Zorzi M, Brunelli S, Macaskill P, et al. Comparison of breast cancers detected in the Verona screening program following transition to digital breast tomosynthesis screening with cancers detected at digital mammography screening. Breast Cancer Res Treat. 2018;170(2):391–7.
85. Moshina N, Aase HS, Danielsen AS, Haldorsen IS, Lee CI, Zackrisson S, et al. Comparing screening outcomes for digital breast tomosynthesis and digital mammography by automated breast density in a randomized controlled trial: results from the to-be trial. Radiology. 2022;303(1):E23.
86. Zuckerman SP, Conant EF, Keller BM, Maidment AD, Barufaldi B, Weinstein SP, et al. Implementation of synthesized two-dimensional mammography in a population-based digital breast tomosynthesis screening program. Radiology. 2016;281(3):730–6.
87. Alabousi M, Wadera A, Kashif Al-Ghita M, Kashef Al-Ghetaa R, Salameh JP, Pozdnyakov A, et al. Performance of digital breast tomosynthesis, synthetic mammography, and digital mammography in breast cancer screening: a systematic review and meta-analysis. J Natl Cancer Inst. 2021;113(6):680–90.
88. Heindel W, Weigel S, Gerß J, Hense HW, Sommer A, Krischke M, et al. TOSYMA screening trial study group. Digital breast tomosynthesis plus synthesised mammography versus digital screening mammography for the detection of invasive breast cancer (TOSYMA): a multicentre, open-label, randomised, controlled, superiority trial. Lancet Oncol. 2022;23(5):601–11.
89. Weigel S, Heindel W, Hense HW, Decker T, Gerß J, Kerschke L. TOSYMA screening trial study group. Breast density and breast cancer screening with digital breast tomosynthesis: a TOSYMA trial subanalysis. Radiology. 2023;306(2):e221006.
90. Weigel S, Heindel W, Decker T, Weyer-Elberich V, Kerschke L, Gerß J, et al. TOSYMA screening trial study group. Digital breast tomosynthesis versus digital mammography for detection of early-stage cancers stratified by grade: a TOSYMA subanalysis. Radiology. 2023;309(3):e231533.
91. Hovda T, Holen ÅS, Lång K, Albertsen JL, Bjørndal H, Brandal SHB, et al. Interval and consecutive round breast cancer after digital breast tomosynthesis and synthetic 2D mammography versus standard 2D digital mammography in BreastScreen Norway. Radiology. 2020;294(2):256–64.
92. Bernardi D, Gentilini MA, De Nisi M, Pellegrini M, Fantò C, Valentini M, et al. Effect of implementing digital breast tomosynthesis (DBT) instead of mammography on population screening outcomes including interval cancer rates: results of the Trento DBT pilot evaluation. Breast. 2020;50:135–40.
93. Shin J, Woo OH, Shin HS, Song SE, Cho KR, Seo BK. Diagnostic performance of digital breast tomosynthesis with the two-dimensional synthesized mammogram for suspicious breast microcalcifications compared to full-field digital mammography in stereotactic breast biopsy. J Korean Soc Radiol. 2022;83(5):1090–103.
94. Tucunduva TCM, Bueno ATP, Chala LF, Lee MV, Torres US, Sato LT, et al. Prone tomosynthesis-guided breast biopsy: a primer. Radiographics. 2024;44(6):e230192.

95. Bahl M, Maunglay M, D'Alessandro HA, Lehman CD. Comparison of upright digital breast tomosynthesis-guided versus prone stereotactic vacuum-assisted breast biopsy. Radiology. 2019;290(2):298–304.
96. Ariaratnam NS, Little ST, Whitley MA, Ferguson K. Digital breast tomosynthesis vacuum assisted biopsy for tomosynthesis-detected sonographically occult lesions. Clin Imaging. 2018;47:4–8.
97. Nyström L, Andersson I, Bjurstam N, Frisell J, Nordenskjöld B, Rutqvist LE. Long-term effects of mammography screening: updated overview of the Swedish randomised trials. Lancet. 2002;359(9310):909–19.
98. von Euler-Chelpin M, Lillholm M, Vejborg I, Nielsen M, Lynge E. Sensitivity of screening mammography by density and texture: a cohort study from a population-based screening program in Denmark. Breast Cancer Res. 2019;21(1):111.
99. Leong SP, Shen ZZ, Liu TJ, Agarwal G, Tajima T, Paik NS, Sandelin K, et al. Is breast cancer the same disease in Asian and Western countries? World J Surg. 2010;34(10):2308–24.
100. Brekelmans CT, Seynaeve C, Bartels CC, Tilanus-Linthorst MM, Meijers-Heijboer EJ, Crepin CM, et al. Rotterdam Committee for Medical and Genetic Counseling. Effectiveness of breast cancer surveillance in BRCA1/2 gene mutation carriers and women with high familial risk. J Clin Oncol. 2001;19(4):924–30.
101. Kriege M, Brekelmans CT, Boetes C, Besnard PE, Zonderland HM, Obdeijn IM, et al. Magnetic Resonance Imaging Screening Study Group. Efficacy of MRI and mammography for breast-cancer screening in women with a familial or genetic predisposition. N Engl J Med. 2004;351(5):427–37.
102. Welch HG, Prorok PC, O'Malley AJ, Kramer BS. Breast-cancer tumor size, overdiagnosis, and mammography screening effectiveness. N Engl J Med. 2016;375(15):1438–47.
103. Burnside ES, Vulkan D, Blanks RG, Duffy SW. Association between screening mammography recall rate and interval cancers in the UK breast cancer service screening program: a cohort study. Radiology. 2018;288(1):47–54.
104. Sood R, Rositch AF, Shakoor D, Ambinder E, Pool KL, Pollack E, et al. Ultrasound for breast cancer detection globally: a systematic review and meta-analysis. J Glob Oncol. 2019;5:1–17.
105. Hooley RJ, Scoutt LM, Philpotts LE. Breast ultrasonography: state of the art. Radiology. 2013;268(3):642–5.
106. Devolli-Disha E, Manxhuka-Kërliu S, Ymeri H, Kutllovci A. Comparative accuracy of mammography and ultrasound in women with breast symptoms according to age and breast density. Bosn J Basic Med Sci. 2009;9(2):131–6.
107. Berg WA, Blume JD, Cormack JB, Mendelson EB, Lehrer D, Böhm-Vélez M, et al. CRIN 6666 investigators. Combined screening with ultrasound and mammography vs mammography alone in women at elevated risk of breast cancer. JAMA. 2008;299(18):2151–63.
108. Berg WA, Zhang Z, Lehrer D, Jong RA, Pisano ED, Barr RG, et al. ACRIN 6666 investigators. Detection of breast cancer with addition of annual screening ultrasound or a single screening MRI to mammography in women with elevated breast cancer risk. JAMA. 2012;307(13):1394–404.
109. Corsetti V, Ferrari A, Ghirardi M, Bergonzini R, Bellarosa S, Angelini O, et al. Role of ultrasonography in detecting mammographically occult breast carcinoma in women with dense breasts. Radiol Med. 2006;111(3):440–8. English, Italian
110. Corsetti V, Houssami N, Ferrari A, Ghirardi M, Bellarosa S, Angelini O, et al. Breast screening with ultrasound in women with mammography-negative dense breasts: evidence on incremental cancer detection and false positives, and associated cost. Eur J Cancer. 2008;44(4):539–44.
111. Hooley RJ, Greenberg KL, Stackhouse RM, Geisel JL, Butler RS, Philpotts LE. Screening US in patients with mammographically dense breasts: initial experience with Connecticut Public Act 09–41. Radiology. 2012;265(1):59–69.
112. Ishida T, Suzuki A, Kawai M, Narikawa Y, Saito H, Yamamoto S, et al. A randomized controlled trial to verify the efficacy of the use of ultrasonography in breast cancer screening aged 40-49 (J-START): 76 196 women registered. Jpn J Clin Oncol. 2014;44(2):134–40.
113. Ohuchi N, Suzuki A, Sobue T, Kawai M, Yamamoto S, Zheng YF, et al. J-START investigator groups. Sensitivity and specificity of mammography and adjunctive ultrasonography to screen for breast cancer in the Japan Strategic Anti-cancer Randomized Trial (J-START): a randomised controlled trial. Lancet. 2016;387(10016):341–8.
114. Harada-Shoji N, Suzuki A, Ishida T, Zheng YF, Narikawa-Shiono Y, Sato-Tadano A, Ohta R, et al. Evaluation of adjunctive ultrasonography for breast cancer detection among women aged 40–49 years with varying breast density undergoing screening mammography: a secondary analysis of a randomized clinical trial. JAMA Netw Open. 2021;4(8):e2121505.
115. Yamashita MW, Larsen LH, Perez J, Edwards AV, Papaioannou J, Jiang Y. Comparison of mammography and mammography with supplemental whole-breast US tomography for cancer detection in patients with dense breasts. Radiology. 2024;311(3):e231680.
116. Benson SR, Blue J, Judd K, Harman JE. Ultrasound is now better than mammography for the detection of invasive breast cancer. Am J Surg. 2004;188(4):381–5.
117. Ying X, Lin Y, Xia X, Hu B, Zhu Z, He P. A comparison of mammography and ultrasound in women

with breast disease: a receiver operating characteristic analysis. Breast J. 2012;18(2):130–8.
118. Appelman L, Siebers CCN, Appelman PTM, Go HLS, Broeders MJM, van Oirsouw MCJ, et al. US and digital breast tomosynthesis in women with focal breast complaints: results of the breast US trial (BUST). Radiology. 2023;307(4):e220361.
119. Berg WA, Cosgrove DO, Doré CJ, Schäfer FK, Svensson WE, Hooley RJ, et al. Shear-wave elastography improves the specificity of breast US: the BE1 multinational study of 939 masses. Radiology. 2012;262(2):435–49.
120. Skerl K, Vinnicombe S, Thomson K, McLean D, Giannotti E, Evans A. Anisotropy of solid breast lesions in 2D shear wave elastography is an indicator of malignancy. Acad Radiol. 2016;23(1):53–61.
121. Heywang SH, Hahn D, Schmidt H, Krischke I, Eiermann W, Bassermann R, et al. MR imaging of the breast using gadolinium-DTPA. J Comput Assist Tomogr. 1986;10(2):199–204.
122. Kaiser WA, Zeitler E. MR imaging of the breast: fast imaging sequences with and without Gd-DTPA. Preliminary observations. Radiology. 1989;170(3 Pt 1):681–6.
123. Saslow D, Boetes C, Burke W, Harms S, Leach MO, Lehman CD, et al. American Cancer Society guidelines for breast screening with MRI as an adjunct to mammography. CA Cancer J Clin. 2007;57(2):75–89.
124. Monticciolo DL, Newell MS, Moy L, Lee CS, Destounis SV. Breast cancer screening for women at higher-than-average risk: updated recommendations from the ACR. J Am Coll Radiol. 2023;20(9):902–14.
125. Mann RM, Balleyguier C, Baltzer PA, Bick U, Colin C, Cornford E, et al. Breast MRI: EUSOBI recommendations for women's information. Eur Radiol. 2015;25(12):3669–78.
126. Kriege M, Brekelmans CT, Boetes C, Besnard PE, Zonderland HM, Obdeijn IM, et al. Efficacy of MRI and mammography for breast-cancer screening in women with a familial or genetic predisposition. N Engl J Med. 2004;351(5):427–37.
127. Lo G, Scaranelo AM, Aboras H, Ghai S, Kulkarni S, Fleming R, et al. Evaluation of the utility of screening mammography for high-risk women undergoing screening breast MR imaging. Radiology. 2017;285(1):36–43.
128. Gweon HM, Cho N, Han W, Yi A, Moon HG, Noh DY, et al. Breast MR imaging screening in women with a history of breast conservation therapy. Radiology. 2014;272(2):366–73.
129. Lee JM, Ichikawa L, Valencia E, Miglioretti DL, Wernli K, Buist DSM, et al. Performance benchmarks for screening breast MR imaging in community practice. Radiology. 2017;285(1):44–52.
130. Bakker MF, de Lange SV, Pijnappel RM, Mann RM, Peeters PHM, Monninkhof EM, et al. DENSE trial study group. Supplemental MRI screening for women with extremely dense breast tissue. N Engl J Med. 2019;381(22):2091–102.
131. Veenhuizen SGA, de Lange SV, Bakker MF, Pijnappel RM, Mann RM, Monninkhof EM, et al. DENSE trial study group. Supplemental breast MRI for women with extremely dense breasts: results of the second screening round of the DENSE trial. Radiology. 2021;299(2):278–86.
132. Kuhl CK, Strobel K, Bieling H, Leutner C, Schild HH, Schrading S. Supplemental breast MR imaging screening of women with average risk of breast cancer. Radiology. 2017;283(2):361–70.
133. Do WS, Weiss JB, McGregor HF, Forte DM, Sheldon RR, Sohn VY. Poor compliance despite equal access: military experience with screening breast MRI in high risk women. Am J Surg. 2019;217(5):843–7.
134. Kuhl CK, Schrading S, Strobel K, Schild HH, Hilgers RD, Bieling HB. Abbreviated breast magnetic resonance imaging (MRI): first postcontrast subtracted images and maximum-intensity projection-a novel approach to breast cancer screening with MRI. J Clin Oncol. 2014;32(22):2304–10.
135. Leithner D, Moy L, Morris EA, Marino MA, Helbich TH, Pinker K. Abbreviated MRI of the breast: does it provide value? J Magn Reson Imaging. 2019;49(7):e85–e100.
136. Fonseca MM, Alhassan T, Nisha Y, Koszycki D, Schwarz BA, Segal R, et al. Randomized trial of surveillance with abbreviated MRI in women with a personal history of breast cancer- impact on patient anxiety and cancer detection. BMC Cancer. 2022;22(1):774.
137. Harvey SC, Di Carlo PA, Lee B, Obadina E, Sippo D, Mullen L. An abbreviated protocol for high-risk screening breast MRI saves time and resources. J Am Coll Radiol. 2016;13(4):374–80.
138. Panigrahi B, Mullen L, Falomo E, Panigrahi B, Harvey S. An abbreviated protocol for high-risk screening breast magnetic resonance imaging: impact on performance metrics and BI-RADS assessment. Acad Radiol. 2017;24(9):1132–8.
139. Kuhl CK. Abbreviated breast MRI for screening women with dense breast: the EA1141 trial. Br J Radiol. 2018;91(1090):20170441.
140. Lawson MB, Partridge SC, Hippe DS, Rahbar H, Lam DL, Lee CI, et al. Comparative performance of contrast-enhanced mammography, abbreviated breast MRI, and standard breast MRI for breast cancer screening. Radiology. 2023;308(2):e230576.
141. Gao Y, Heller SL. Abbreviated and ultrafast breast MRI in clinical practice. Radiographics. 2020;40(6):1507–27.
142. Honda M, Kataoka M. Quantitative evaluation of breast lesions using ultrafast MRI has come so far. Eur Radiol. 2024;34(10):6283–4.

143. Juliano M, Samreen N, Chacko C, Heller SL. Clinical role of abbreviated and ultrafast mri in breast imaging. Br J Radiol. 2024;27:tqae079.
144. Amitai Y, Freitas VAR, Golan O, Kessner R, Shalmon T, Neeman R, et al. The diagnostic performance of ultrafast MRI to differentiate benign from malignant breast lesions: a systematic review and meta-analysis. Eur Radiol. 2024;34:6285.
145. Pötsch N, Sodano C, Baltzer PAT. Performance of diffusion-weighted imaging-based noncontrast MRI protocols for diagnosis of breast cancer: a systematic review and meta-analysis. Radiology. 2024;311(2):e232508.
146. Papalouka V, Kilburn-Toppin F, Gaskarth M, Gilbert F. MRI-guided breast biopsy: a review of technique, indications, and radiological-pathological correlations. Clin Radiol. 2018;73(10):908.e17–25.
147. Lambert J, Steelandt T, Heywang-Köbrunner SH, Gieraerts K, Van Den Berghe I, Van Ongeval C, et al. Long-term MRI-guided vacuum-assisted breast biopsy results of 600 single-center procedures. Eur Radiol. 2021;31(7):4886–97.
148. Spick C, Schernthaner M, Pinker K, Kapetas P, Bernathova M, Polanec SH, et al. MR-guided vacuum-assisted breast biopsy of MRI-only lesions: a single center experience. Eur Radiol. 2016;26(11):3908–16.
149. Pinnamaneni N, Moy L, Gao Y, Melsaether AN, Babb JS, Toth HK, et al. Canceled MRI-guided breast biopsies due to nonvisualization: follow-up and outcomes. Acad Radiol. 2018;25(9):1101–10.
150. Ghaderi KF, Phillips J, Perry H, Lotfi P, Mehta TS. Contrast-enhanced mammography: current applications and future directions. Radiographics. 2019;39(7):1907–20.
151. Sensakovic WF, Carnahan MB, Czaplicki CD, Fahrenholtz S, Panda A, Zhou Y, et al. Contrast-enhanced mammography: how does it work? Radiographics. 2021;41(3):829–39.
152. Lorente-Ramos RM, Azpeitia-Armán J, Oliva-Fonte C, Pérez-Bartolomé A, Azpeitia HJ. Contrast-enhanced mammography artifacts and pitfalls: tips and tricks to avoid misinterpretation. Radiographics. 2023;43(10):e230021.
153. Pötsch N, Vatteroni G, Clauser P, Helbich TH, Baltzer PAT. Contrast-enhanced mammography versus contrast-enhanced breast MRI: a systematic review and meta-analysis. Radiology. 2022;305(1):94–103.
154. Jochelson MS, Pinker K, Dershaw DD, Hughes M, Gibbons GF, Rahbar K, et al. Comparison of screening CEDM and MRI for women at increased risk for breast cancer: a pilot study. Eur J Radiol. 2017;97:37–43.
155. Phillips J, Mehta TS, Portnow LH, Fishman MDC, Zhang Z, Pisano ED. Comparison of contrast-enhanced mammography with MRI utilizing an enriched reader study: a breast cancer study (CONTRRAST trial). Radiology. 2023;309(2):e230530.
156. van Geel K, Kok EM, Krol JP, Houben IPL, Thibault FE, Pijnappel RM, et al. Reversal of the hanging protocol of contrast enhanced mammography leads to similar diagnostic performance yet decreased reading times. Eur J Radiol. 2019;117:62–8.
157. Berg WA, Berg JM, Bandos AI, Vargo A, Chough DM, Lu AH, et al. Addition of contrast-enhanced mammography to tomosynthesis for breast cancer detection in women with a personal history of breast cancer: prospective TOCEM trial interim analysis. Radiology. 2024;311(1):e231991.
158. Contrast Enhanced Mammography Imaging Screening Trial (CMIST). American College of Radiology website. https://www.acr.org/Research/Clinical-Research/CMIST. Accessed 1 Nov 2021.
159. Alcantara R, Posso M, Pitarch M, Arenas N, Ejarque B, Iotti V, et al. Contrast-enhanced mammography-guided biopsy: technical feasibility and first outcomes. Eur Radiol. 2023;33(1):417–28.
160. Kornecki A, Bhaduri M, Khan N, Nachum IB, Muscedere G, Shmuilovich O, et al. Contrast-enhanced mammography-guided breast biopsy: single-center experience. AJR Am J Roentgenol. 2023;220(6):826–7.
161. Wang J, Zhao R, Cheng J. Diagnostic accuracy of contrast-enhanced ultrasound to differentiate benign and malignant breast lesions: a systematic review and meta-analysis. Eur J Radiol. 2022;149:110219.
162. Yan M, Peng C, He D, Xu D, Yang C. A nomogram for enhancing the diagnostic effectiveness of solid breast BI-RADS 3-5 masses to determine malignancy based on imaging aspects of conventional ultrasonography and contrast-enhanced ultrasound. Clin Breast Cancer. 2023;23(7):693–703.
163. Chang JM, Leung JWT, Moy L, Ha SM, Moon WK. Axillary nodal evaluation in breast cancer: state of the art. Radiology. 2020;295(3):500–15.
164. Chung HL, Le-Petross HT, Leung JWT. Imaging updates to breast cancer lymph node management. Radiographics. 2021;41(5):1283–99.
165. Harlow SP, Krag DN, Julian TB, Ashikaga T, Weaver DL, Feldman SA, et al. Prerandomization surgical training for the National Surgical Adjuvant Breast and Bowel Project (NSABP) B-32 trial: a randomized phase III clinical trial to compare sentinel node resection to conventional axillary dissection in clinically node-negative breast cancer. Ann Surg. 2005;241(1):48–54.
166. Giuliano AE, Ballman KV, McCall L, Beitsch PD, Brennan MB, Kelemen PR, et al. Effect of axillary dissection vs no axillary dissection on 10-year overall survival among women with invasive breast cancer and sentinel node metastasis: the ACOSOG Z0011 (Alliance) randomized clinical trial. JAMA. 2017;318(10):918–26.

167. de Boniface J, FiltenborgTvedskov T, Rydén L, Szulkin R, Reimer T, Kühn T, Kontos M, Gentilini OD, et al. Omitting axillary dissection in breast cancer with sentinel-node metastases. N Engl J Med. 2024;390(13):1163–75.
168. Boughey JC, Suman VJ, Mittendorf EA, Ahrendt GM, Wilke LG, Taback B, et al. Sentinel lymph node surgery after neoadjuvant chemotherapy in patients with node-positive breast cancer: the ACOSOG Z1071 (Alliance) clinical trial. JAMA. 2013;310(14):1455–61.
169. Kuehn T, Bauerfeind I, Fehm T, Fleige B, Hausschild M, Helms G, et al. Sentinel-lymph-node biopsy in patients with breast cancer before and after neoadjuvant chemotherapy (SENTINA): a prospective, multicentre cohort study. Lancet Oncol. 2013;14(7):609–18.
170. Kuemmel S, Heil J, Bruzas S, Breit E, Schindowski D, Harrach H, et al. Safety of targeted axillary dissection after Neoadjuvant therapy in patients with node-positive breast cancer. JAMA Surg. 2023;158(8):807–15.
171. Montagna G, Mrdutt MM, Sun SX, Hlavin C, Diego EJ, Wong SM, et al. Omission of axillary dissection following nodal downstaging with neoadjuvant chemotherapy. JAMA Oncol. 2024;10(6):793–8.

Index

E. Dhamija, S. V. S. Deo (eds.), *Imaging in Management of Breast Diseases*,
https://doi.org/10.1007/978-981-96-4998-3

O

P

R

S

T

U

V

Y

Z

MIX
Papier aus verantwortungsvollen Quellen
Paper from responsible sources
FSC® C105338

If you have any concerns about our products,
you can contact us on
ProductSafety@springernature.com

In case Publisher is established outside the EU,
the EU authorized representative is:
Springer Nature Customer Service Center GmbH
Europaplatz 3, 69115 Heidelberg, Germany

Printed by Libri Plureos GmbH
in Hamburg, Germany